COMPLETE GUIDE TO

SPORTS INJURIES

HOW TO TREAT—
Fractures, Bruises, Sprains, Strains, Dislocations, Head Injuries.

H. Winter Griffith, M.D.

Illustrations by Mark Pederson

THE BODY PRESS/PERIGEE

The Body Press/Perigee Books
are published by
The Berkley Publishing Group
200 Madison Avenue
New York, NY 10016
ISBN 0-399-51712-X Library of Congress Catalog Number 86-70726
© 1986 The Putnam Berkley Group, Inc.   Printed in U.S.A.

9   10

Notice: The information in this book is true and complete to the best of our knowledge. The book is intended only as a supplementary guide to medical treatment. It is not intended as a replacement for sound medical advice from a doctor. Only a doctor can include the variables of an individual's age, sex and past medical history needed for proper medical care. This book does not contain every possible factor relating to sports injuries, illness or rehabilitation. Important decisions about treating an injured or ill person must be made by the individual and their doctor. All recommendations herein are made without guarantees on the part of the author, the illustrator, the technical consultants or the publisher. The author and publisher disclaim all liability in connection with the use of this information.

Contents

About the Authors

H. Winter Griffith, M.D., a Fellow of the American Academy of Family Physicians, has had a lifelong participation and interest in athletics and exercise. A high school and college athlete, Dr. Griffith was team physician for several years for Florida State University athletic teams. Dr. Griffith has authored several medical books, including the best-selling *Complete Guide to Prescription & Non-Prescription Drugs* and *Complete Guide to Symptoms, Illness & Surgery*. Dr. Griffith received his medical degree from Emory University in 1953, and spent more than 20 years in private practice. He established a basic medical-science program at Florida State University and was director of the family practice residency program at Tallahassee Memorial Hospital. Dr. Griffith then became associate professor of Family & Community Medicine at the University of Arizona College of Medicine.

Mark Pederson's medical illustrations have been published in more than 100 journal articles and books. Since 1974 he has been head of the Medical Illustration Section, Division of Biomedical Communications, at the University Medical Center in Tucson, Arizona. Mr. Pederson taught in the Department of Anatomy at the University of Michigan while earning a M.S. degree in Medical & Biological Illustration. He received a B.S. degree in Art from Mankato State College in Minnesota. He is a member of the Association of Medical Illustrators.

Technical Consultants

Fred L. Allman, Jr., M.D.

Director, Sports Medicine Clinic, Atlanta, Georgia.
Orthopedic consultant, Georgia Institute of Technology and Atlanta Public Schools athletic teams.
Past President, American Orthopedic Society for Sports Medicine.
Past President, American College of Sports Medicine.

Susan Hillman, A.T.C., R.P.T.

Head Athletic Trainer, University of Arizona.

Fred J. Hirsch, M.D.

Team Physician, University of Arizona Intercollegiate Athletics.
Fellow, American Academy of Sports Medicine.

Daniel Levinson, M.D.

Associate Professor of Family and Community Medicine, University of Arizona College of Medicine.
Fellow, American Board of Family Practice.

James G. Mason, Ph.D.

Professor Emeritus, Department of Teacher Education, University of Texas at El Paso.
Former Chairman, Department of Physical Education, University of Texas at El Paso.

Preface

The recent increase in organized and recreational sports participation for all ages and both sexes has been accompanied by a significant increase in the number of injuries sustained by these athletes. Most of these injuries are minor sprains, strains and bruises, and many are due to overuse rather than to external force. Other injuries are more serious and usually require the attention of a physician or other members of the medical team. Some of these injuries require hospitalization and surgery. Rarely, athletic participation may result in a catastrophic injury with prolonged disability, paralysis or even death.

This book will be extremely beneficial in the recognition and care of minor injuries, helping the reader to know not only what is wrong, but also how to administer first aid and determine when to be seen by a physician. Even in the case of more serious injuries, the injured person and his or her family will be able to better understand the condition and what might be expected before full recovery is reached.

Dr. Griffith has many years of experience as an athlete, a team physician, a professor of the medical sciences, and a scholar.

This book is recommended reading for all coaches, parents and athletes—regardless of age or sex.

Fred L. Allman, Jr., M.D.

SPORTS, EXERCISE & YOUR HEALTH

We are living in a time when interest in sports and fitness has never been higher. Correspondingly, our knowledge about injury and illness as a result of physical activity has also increased. The purpose of this book is to share this knowledge with you, giving you some guidelines about prudent physical activity and athletic participation. But first, we must examine the relationship between physical activity and good health.

THE BENEFITS OF EXERCISE

Regular exercise or athletic activity plays a key role in staying healthy. Not only is exercise an important part of treating medical problems such as hypertension, depression and high blood-fat levels (especially high levels of low-density cholesterol)—it can also be important in *preventing* many of these same medical problems.

Regular exercise also improves your body image and increases your energy level. It helps control weight and reduces stress.

If you are an athlete engaged in a competitive sport, or if you are a fitness enthusiast participating in a regular exercise program, you are familiar with the many benefits of regular physical activity. If you do not participate in a sport or fitness program, the following suggestions will help you choose and begin the right program for you. Exercise comes in many forms—everyone should be able to find some activity enjoyable.

7 STEPS TO CHOOSING A SPORT OR EXERCISE PROGRAM

(1) Obtain a physical examination from your doctor so you will know if you have any limitations that affect your choice of activity.

(2) Choose an activity you enjoy. Some people prefer an exercise they can do alone so they don't have to coordinate plans with others. Other people enjoy the company and extra incentive provided by workout partners. The best sport or exercise for you is one you *do*. So look around, join a club, find others to join you or set out on your own—but begin!

(3) Set aside time to work out. It's best to start at three sessions per week, then increase gradually to four, five or more. Some people schedule a session every day. When interruptions occur, they still get the recommended minimum of three exercise sessions a week.

Most people find that setting aside a consistent time each day helps them get into the habit of working out. The time of day is not important, as long as you don't try to exercise or play on a full stomach. On the other hand, exercising on an empty stomach first thing in the morning is not a good idea either. A light meal 30 minutes before your workout should not interfere with your performance. Common-sense measures, such as avoiding the heat of the day and not exercising when sick, are important.

(4) Be prudent in the amount of time you exercise each day. The ideal duration is 30 minutes of continuous activity. Some people find it necessary to begin with 10 to 15 minutes and build up. Except for those who train for athletic competition, it is not necessary to spend many hours a day exercising.

(5) Choose the proper intensity of exercise. Appropriate intensity varies

greatly depending on your age, sex and medical condition. Many doctors recommend aerobic exercise as beneficial for most persons. It can be geared to an individual's fitness level and increased as his ability allows.

Exercise is aerobic if it accelerates the heart rate to a prescribed level, sustains the physical activity for at least 20 minutes, uses major muscle groups of the body, and is regulated in intensity and duration. Aerobic exercise should be done at least three times a week to achieve cardio-pulmonary-vascular fitness—a strong and healthy heart, lungs and blood vessels.

The best forms of aerobic exercise include brisk walking, swimming, bike riding, jogging, rope jumping, rowing or aerobic dance. Sports such as tennis and golf have good recreational effects, but they do not require enough sustained effort to reach and maintain aerobic levels for a sufficient period of time.

Although we have defined aerobic exercise here, we strongly recommend that you read one of the many books on this subject to get a broader view of the benefits and techniques of this important category of exercise. Two recommended ones are:

The New Aerobics by Dr. Kenneth Cooper, a recognized international authority on fitness and exercise.

MuscleAerobics: The Ultimate Workout for Body Shaping by Patricia Patano and Linette Savage, published by The Body Press. This is a new approach that combines aerobics with the use of body-shaping hand weights.
(6) Incorporate additional exercise into your day whenever you can. Park your car far enough from your destination to allow a good walk. Use the stairs instead of taking the elevator. Use manual rather than power tools.
(7) Vary your activity, alternating sports and forms of exercise to avoid boredom. It takes about a month of good, regular exercise before you will begin to see and feel the benefits. Meanwhile, use whatever tricks you can think of to keep yourself going.

THE RISKS OF EXERCISE

Despite the many healthy benefits obtained through sports and exercise, injuries and illnesses can occur as a result of physical activity. Anyone participating in a contact sport such as football can expect some of the contact to be hard on the body. Bruises, sprains, broken bones, concussions —even deaths—have been known to occur. We are now aware of many factors that can help prevent injuries, and prevention is the best cure. For example, protective equipment kept in good repair, a well-conditioned body, and adequate warm-up go a long way in preventing serious injuries in athletics. But accidents do happen.

In addition, certain pre-existing conditions can increase the danger or difficulty of participation in physical activity. For example, if a person has an infection, his performance will not be up to par—he may make himself sicker or be more prone to injury. Some pre-existing conditions are permanent, such as diabetes mellitus, and these have a bearing on how a person can participate. The whole body is involved in any kind of exercise program, and its state must be taken into account.

THE GOALS OF THIS BOOK

This book is designed to help you maintain or achieve a satisfactory level of good health. Good physical and mental health is essential to winning in competitive sports and achieving an optimal level of fitness in all areas. This book is *your* resource—it has been written for you with the following objectives:
● To present a concise, comprehensive, clear guide to sports injuries and illnesses.
● To address the benefits and risks of competitive athletics, and to minimize

the frequency of the only major risk: injury.

- To provide parents with information about the physical requirements for competing and the various aspects of injuries to athletes of all ages, including youngsters and adolescents. This will help parents make informed decisions regarding sports activities for their children.
- To equip young people with enough information to make wise decisions about their participation in sports.
- To encourage safe participation in sports among all age groups by outlining nutritional requirements and conditioning and rehabilitation procedures to prevent or treat illness and injury.
- To provide coaches and trainers with a guide for technical concepts they need to master to wisely instruct and supervise the athletes they direct. Trainers and coaches can be effective teachers—they have great influence over impressionable young people and they attract great devotion.
- To make it possible for athletes or parents to render self-care when it is appropriate.
- To call attention to situations when parents or athletes need to obtain professional help.
- To provide a second opinion when surgery or other drastic measures have been recommended.
- To provide an unbiased third opinion when two professional opinions differ. The information in this book comes from experienced, authoritative experts in the field of sports injuries and sports medicine, and it represents a consensus among professionals.

To organize and present information as clearly as possible, this book has been divided into two major sections, Sports Injuries and Sports Medicine. Each of these sections is made up of easy-to-use charts. A chart format was chosen to make it easy to find the information you need quickly. Other smaller sections—Rehabilitation, Appendix, Glossary, Index and Emergency First Aid—follow the first two sections. The smaller sections do not include charts.

Each sports-injury chart addresses one specific injury, including text and an illustration to compare normal and injured anatomy. It includes information about how to identify the injury, how to prevent the injury, and what first aid to administer if you find someone injured. It can serve as an informal second opinion for the treatment of each injury. It also covers what to expect as you are treated and during recovery, what activity level you can expect to be allowed, what rehabilitation you might need, and what sort of diet will help you heal quicker.

Each sports-medicine chart addresses a common, non-injury medical problem that might occur among athletes and others engaged in vigorous physical activity. Some problems are caused by conditions such as crowded locker rooms or the use of athletic equipment. Others are not unique to athletes but can affect athletic performance, either temporarily or permanently. Still others can be caused or made worse by athletic activity. Information on how to recognize the medical problem, how to prevent it, how it is usually treated, and how you can expect it to affect your performance is included.

The Guide to Sports-Injury Charts, page 14, and Guide to Sports-Medicine Charts, page 21, explain in detail what is included on each chart.

Following is a brief explanation of the other book sections.

The Rehabilitation section is an important adjunct to the sports-injury charts. This section provides a program of exercise and conditioning that can be followed after injury in 13 major body areas. Each injury chart contains a reference to this section. The exercises are simple and generally don't require special equipment. However, consult your doctor before attempting the exercises.

The Appendix section deals with sports-medicine topics of a more general nature that apply to most charts, such as Aging & Exercise, Safe Use of Crutches, or Nutrition for Athletes.

The Glossary gives brief definitions of medical terms and concepts associated with sports medicine, especially if they are referred to in the book.

The Index is your key to finding the information you need. Every topic is cross-referenced by its most-common names. Refer to the index to find your topic before trying to find it by leafing through the charts.

An Emergency First Aid section completes the major areas covered in this book. Most emergencies are covered under the individual injury entries, but life-threatening emergencies are dealt with separately in this section. *In case of emergency,* *refer to the last four pages of this book.* Emergencies are listed alphabetically in this section.

YOUR DOCTOR'S ROLE

Condensing the available mass of information about sports medicine and injuries into one volume has required some shortening and simplification. We have made every effort to include all major facts and concepts.

However, this book does not promise that you will always be able to diagnose and treat your own injuries or illnesses. Printed words cannot replace the knowledge and expertise that your doctor provides.

It is impossible to include in a book all the factors and circumstances that affect each *individual's* health. Your team physician or personal physician may take into account other factors not included here when he or she makes a precise diagnosis and recommends treatment for you. Most athletes are basically healthy people to begin with. More important, the athlete has great motivation to get well quickly so he or she can resume competition. All these factors make diagnosis, treatment and rehabilitation different—and usually quicker—for athletes than for the general population.

Your active participation in your medical program is a key element in winning, not only in athletic pursuits and sports competition, but also in life. We hope this book will be an important reference and guide to help you take care of your body so you can achieve your maximum athletic potential.

NORMAL ANATOMY

These illustrations are for general orientation of anatomy and provide brief explanations of function. They are frequently repeated throughout the book without further explanation. This section is by no means a complete explanation of anatomy or body parts. However, it concerns those body parts that are usually most affected by sports and exercise. These include the musculo-skeletal system, the brain and central nervous system, the cardiovascular system and the respiratory tract. Most sports injuries affect these areas—especially the musculo-skeletal system.

SKELETON

See Figure 1, front view of the female skeleton, and Figure 2, rear view of the male skeleton.

Both males and females have 206 bones: 29 in the skull, 26 in the spine, 25 in the chest, 64 in the arms, and 62 in the legs.

Female bones are slightly smaller and lighter than corresponding male bones. Limbs are shorter in proportion to total body length. Females have an increased shoulder slope and an increased angle at the elbow.

The hip joint is smaller and more delicate. The female pelvic cavity, surrounded by the hip bones and sacrum, is wider than the male pelvis to allow for childbirth.

BRAIN, SPINAL CORD & NERVES

See Figure 3.

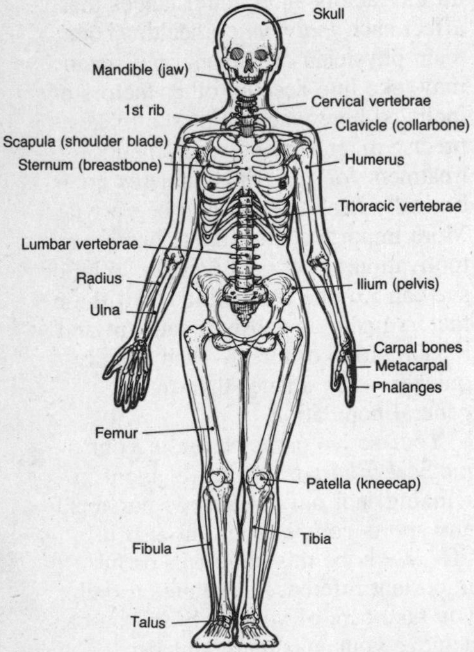

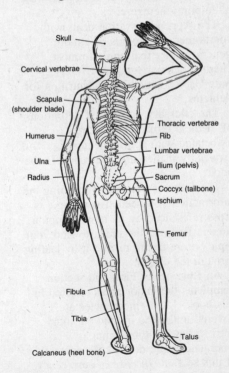

Figure 1:
- Skull
- Mandible (jaw)
- 1st rib
- Scapula (shoulder blade)
- Sternum (breastbone)
- Cervical vertebrae
- Clavicle (collarbone)
- Humerus
- Thoracic vertebrae
- Lumbar vertebrae
- Radius
- Ulna
- Ilium (pelvis)
- Carpal bones
- Metacarpal
- Phalanges
- Femur
- Patella (kneecap)
- Fibula
- Tibia
- Talus

FIGURE 1

Figure 2:
- Skull
- Cervical vertebrae
- Scapula (shoulder blade)
- Humerus
- Ulna
- Radius
- Thoracic vertebrae
- Rib
- Lumbar vertebrae
- Ilium (pelvis)
- Sacrum
- Coccyx (tailbone)
- Ischium
- Femur
- Fibula
- Tibia
- Talus
- Calcaneus (heel bone)

FIGURE 2

Billions of nerve cells in the brain control body movement and other functions associated with speech, learning, emotions and memory. The spinal cord and nerves branching from it are an extension of the same complicated nerve cells that form the brain. They provide the path by which messages are transmitted from the brain to all parts of the body.

The brain is protected by the rigid bones of the skull; the spinal cord is protected by the bones of the spine (vertebral column). The nerves outside the brain and spine are less well protected and more subject to injury during competitive sports and other vigorous activity.

HEART & MAJOR BLOOD VESSELS

See Figure 4.

The heart is a thick, strong muscle about the size of a clenched fist. The blood vessels are of two types: arteries and veins. To avoid confusion, the illustration shows only arteries. Veins and arteries usually run parallel. Arteries carry blood from the heart through narrower and narrower branches to capillaries that provide oxygen and nourishment to every body cell. In the capillaries, the blood absorbs waste materials from cells. Beyond the capillaries, veins begin. Veins carry the blood back to the heart to be pumped to the lungs. There carbon dioxide is eliminated and oxygen from the inhaled air is

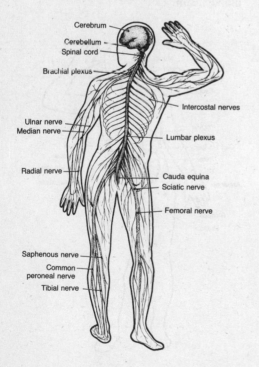

Cerebrum
Cerebellum
Spinal cord
Brachial plexus
Intercostal nerves
Ulnar nerve
Median nerve
Lumbar plexus
Radial nerve
Cauda equina
Sciatic nerve
Femoral nerve
Saphenous nerve
Common peroneal nerve
Tibial nerve

FIGURE 3

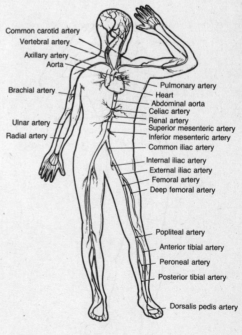

Common carotid artery
Vertebral artery
Axillary artery
Aorta
Brachial artery
Pulmonary artery
Heart
Abdominal aorta
Celiac artery
Renal artery
Ulnar artery
Superior mesenteric artery
Radial artery
Inferior mesenteric artery
Common iliac artery
Internal iliac artery
External iliac artery
Femoral artery
Deep femoral artery
Popliteal artery
Anterior tibial artery
Peroneal artery
Posterior tibial artery
Dorsalis pedis artery

FIGURE 4

absorbed. The oxygenated blood then returns to the heart to be pumped once again through arteries to the body cells. Nourishment enters the blood stream by absorption through capillaries of the intestinal tract. Waste materials (other than carbon dioxide) pass through the kidneys to be eliminated. Gases pass into the lung capillaries to be eliminated along with carbon dioxide.

RESPIRATORY SYSTEM

See Figure 5.

The major parts of the respiratory system include the nose and mouth, trachea, bronchial tubes and lungs. The lungs contain about 300 million tiny air sacs where absorption of oxygen from inhaled air takes place.

Carbon dioxide and other waste gases are eliminated by exhaling.

The respiratory rate is closely related to the intensity of exercise Exercise immediately increases the respiratory rate to provide more oxygen to sustain increased body needs.

GASTROINTESTINAL SYSTEM & URINARY TRACT

See Figure 6.

During the process of digestion, food passes through the esophagus to the stomach, then into the small and large intestines. The liver and pancreas (among other functions) manufacture enzymes that pass into the intestinal tract to aid in the digestion and absorption of the nutrients into the bloodstream.

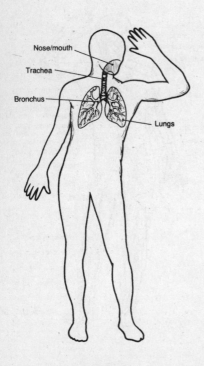

FIGURE 5

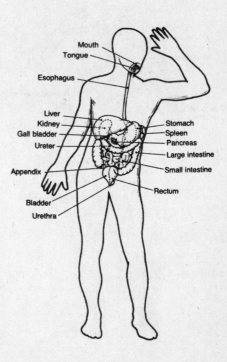

FIGURE 6

The urinary tract is composed of the kidneys, ureters, bladder and urethra. Blood brought to the functioning part of the kidney is filtered, and waste materials are extracted and become urine. Urine passes through the ureters to the bladder, where it is stored until it is eliminated through the urethra.

MAJOR MUSCLE GROUPS

See Figure 7, front view, and Figure 8, rear view, of major muscle groups.

There are over 600 named muscles in the body that attach to bone to allow our bodies to move. Females and males have the same muscles. The muscles shown here are all under voluntary control (skeletal muscles). That is, we can command the movement of these muscles. Chemical and electrical activity generated in our brains is transmitted through nerves to the muscles we wish to contract or relax.

Another set of muscles in the body, mainly those in the heart, blood vessels, intestines and other body organs, functions automatically— completely out of conscious control.

Muscles receive nutrition through the bloodstream via the circulatory system. Extra nutrition and oxygen are needed by muscles during exercise. These needs are met in three ways: (1) increased respiratory rate; (2) increased cardiac output (the amount of blood pumped per minute by the heart); and (3) redistribution of blood flow from inactive organs, such as the gastrointestinal tract, to active skeletal muscles.

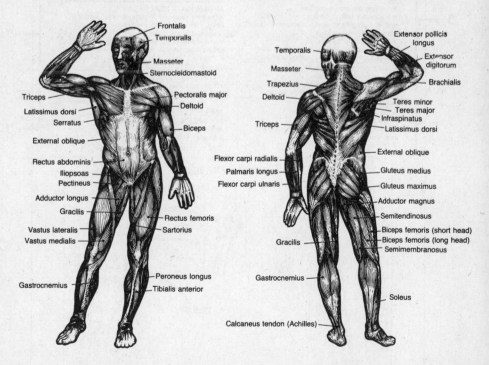

FIGURE 7

FIGURE 8

GUIDE TO SPORTS-INJURY CHARTS

In this guide, the information about injuries associated with sports and vigorous physical exercise is organized in easy-to-read, illustrated charts.

The injuries described in this section are the most-common ones that occur during vigorous physical activity or in competitive sports. Some injuries, such as those of the ankle, are quite common. Others are relatively rare,

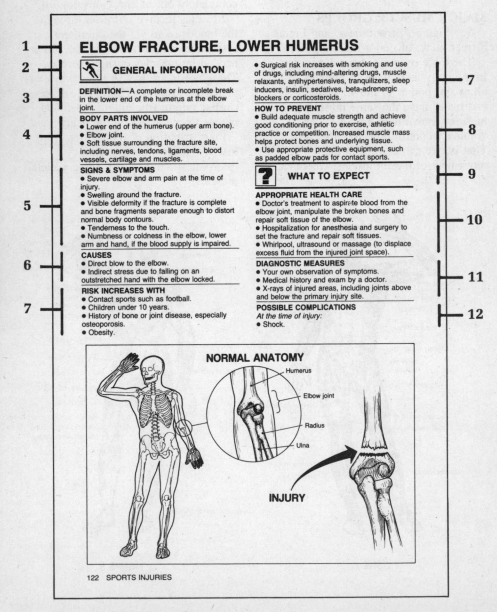

ELBOW FRACTURE, LOWER HUMERUS

GENERAL INFORMATION

DEFINITION—A complete or incomplete break in the lower end of the humerus at the elbow joint.

BODY PARTS INVOLVED
- Lower end of the humerus (upper arm bone).
- Elbow joint.
- Soft tissue surrounding the fracture site, including nerves, tendons, ligaments, blood vessels, cartilage and muscles.

SIGNS & SYMPTOMS
- Severe elbow and arm pain at the time of injury.
- Swelling around the fracture.
- Visible deformity if the fracture is complete and bone fragments separate enough to distort normal body contours.
- Tenderness to the touch.
- Numbness or coldness in the elbow, lower arm and hand, if the blood supply is impaired.

CAUSES
- Direct blow to the elbow.
- Indirect stress due to falling on an outstretched hand with the elbow locked.

RISK INCREASES WITH
- Contact sports such as football.
- Children under 10 years.
- History of bone or joint disease, especially osteoporosis.
- Obesity.

- Surgical risk increases with smoking and use of drugs, including mind-altering drugs, muscle relaxants, antihypertensives, tranquilizers, sleep inducers, insulin, sedatives, beta-adrenergic blockers or corticosteroids.

HOW TO PREVENT
- Build adequate muscle strength and achieve good conditioning prior to exercise, athletic practice or competition. Increased muscle mass helps protect bones and underlying tissue.
- Use appropriate protective equipment, such as padded elbow pads for contact sports.

WHAT TO EXPECT

APPROPRIATE HEALTH CARE
- Doctor's treatment to aspirate blood from the elbow joint, manipulate the broken bones and repair soft tissue of the elbow.
- Hospitalization for anesthesia and surgery to set the fracture and repair soft tissues.
- Whirlpool, ultrasound or massage (to displace excess fluid from the injured joint space).

DIAGNOSTIC MEASURES
- Your own observation of symptoms.
- Medical history and exam by a doctor.
- X-rays of injured areas, including joints above and below the primary injury site.

POSSIBLE COMPLICATIONS
At the time of injury:
- Shock.

NORMAL ANATOMY

Humerus

Elbow joint

Radius

Ulna

INJURY

122   SPORTS INJURIES

but still possible.

Each injury is presented in a two-page format, including text and detailed illustrations. A sample chart, *ELBOW FRACTURE, LOWER*

HUMERUS, is used here as an example. The major sections of this chart are explained on the following pages to help you become familiar with the chart format.

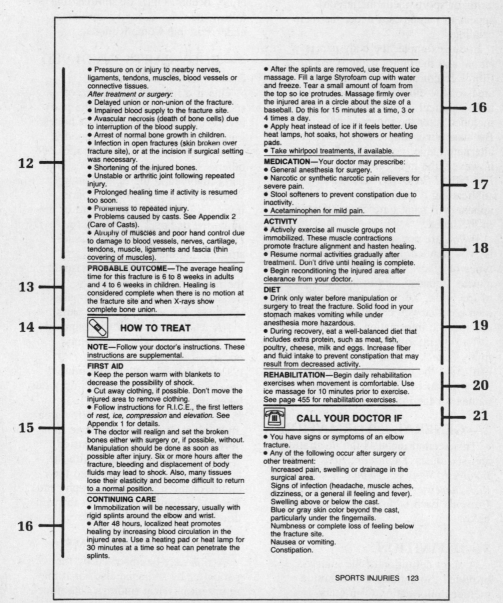

12

• Pressure on or injury to nearby nerves, ligaments, tendons, muscles, blood vessels or connective tissues.
After treatment or surgery:
• Delayed union or non-union of the fracture.
• Impaired blood supply to the fracture site.
• Avascular necrosis (death of bone cells) due to interruption of the blood supply.
• Arrest of normal bone growth in children.
• Infection in open fractures (skin broken over fracture site), or at the incision if surgical setting was necessary.
• Shortening of the injured bones.
• Unstable or arthritic joint following repeated injury.
• Prolonged healing time if activity is resumed too soon.
• Proneness to repeated injury.
• Problems caused by casts. See Appendix 2 (Care of Casts).
• Atrophy of muscles and poor hand control due to damage to blood vessels, nerves, cartilage, tendons, muscle, ligaments and fascia (thin covering of muscles).

13

PROBABLE OUTCOME—The average healing time for this fracture is 6 to 8 weeks in adults and 4 to 6 weeks in children. Healing is considered complete when there is no motion at the fracture site and when X-rays show complete bone union.

14

🖊 **HOW TO TREAT**

NOTE—Follow your doctor's instructions. These instructions are supplemental.

FIRST AID
• Keep the person warm with blankets to decrease the possibility of shock.
• Cut away clothing, if possible. Don't move the injured area to remove clothing.
• Follow instructions for R.I.C.E., the first letters of *rest, ice, compression* and *elevation*. See Appendix 1 for details.

15

• The doctor will realign and set the broken bones either with surgery or, if possible, without. Manipulation should be done as soon as possible after injury. Six or more hours after the fracture, bleeding and displacement of body fluids may lead to shock. Also, many tissues lose their elasticity and become difficult to return to a normal position.

CONTINUING CARE
• Immobilization will be necessary, usually with rigid splints around the elbow and wrist.

16

• After 48 hours, localized heat promotes healing by increasing blood circulation in the injured area. Use a heating pad or heat lamp for 30 minutes at a time so heat can penetrate the splints.

16

• After the splints are removed, use frequent ice massage. Fill a large Styrofoam cup with water and freeze. Tear a small amount of foam from the top so ice protrudes. Massage firmly over the injured area in a circle about the size of a baseball. Do this for 15 minutes at a time, 3 or 4 times a day.
• Apply heat instead of ice if it feels better. Use heat lamps, hot soaks, hot showers or heating pads.
• Take whirlpool treatments, if available.

17

MEDICATION—Your doctor may prescribe:
• General anesthesia for surgery.
• Narcotic or synthetic narcotic pain relievers for severe pain.
• Stool softeners to prevent constipation due to inactivity.
• Acetaminophen for mild pain.

18

ACTIVITY
• Actively exercise all muscle groups not immobilized. These muscle contractions promote fracture alignment and hasten healing.
• Resume normal activities gradually after treatment. Don't drive until healing is complete.
• Begin reconditioning the injured area after clearance from your doctor.

19

DIET
• Drink only water before manipulation or surgery to treat the fracture. Solid food in your stomach makes vomiting while under anesthesia more hazardous.
• During recovery, eat a well-balanced diet that includes extra protein, such as meat, fish, poultry, cheese, milk and eggs. Increase fiber and fluid intake to prevent constipation that may result from decreased activity.

20

REHABILITATION—Begin daily rehabilitation exercises when movement is comfortable. Use ice massage for 10 minutes prior to exercise. See page 455 for rehabilitation exercises.

21

☎ **CALL YOUR DOCTOR IF**

• You have signs or symptoms of an elbow fracture.
• Any of the following occur after surgery or other treatment:
  Increased pain, swelling or drainage in the surgical area.
  Signs of infection (headache, muscle aches, dizziness, or a general ill feeling and fever).
  Swelling above or below the cast.
  Blue or gray skin color beyond the cast, particularly under the fingernails.
  Numbness or complete loss of feeling below the fracture site.
  Nausea or vomiting.
  Constipation.

SPORTS INJURIES 123

1—CHART NAME

The charts are arranged alphabetically by body part, followed by the most common name for the injury. Other names (usually medical terms or sports-medicine jargon) appear in parentheses under the main heading.

In our example, the body part is *elbow* and the injury name is *fracture*. Elbow fractures can affect different areas of the elbow, so the specific bone segment, *lower humerus,* is included after the injury name. Because our example does not have an alternate name, none is listed. If, however, the injury in question were *ELBOW, EPICONDYLITIS,* a subheading *(Tennis Elbow)* would also appear. All names are cross-referenced in the index.

If you are not sure what your injury is, you may compare the different types of elbow injuries because they appear alphabetically in the same part of the book. Yet each injury has its own chart so you can quickly obtain the specific information you need.

To find information about a sports injury, check first in the index. If you can't find the injury chart you need, ask your doctor or trainer for alternate names for the injury.

2—GENERAL INFORMATION

This section includes the illustration and six topics: *Definition; Body Parts Involved; Signs & Symptoms; Causes; Risk Increases With;* and *How to Prevent.* Each is discussed separately below.

3—DEFINITION

A short definition of the injury is provided. Sometimes the definition includes information from other categories, such as causes, risks or general treatment. It also includes the primary body parts (bones, muscles, ligaments, nerves and other tissues) involved in the injury at the time the injury occurs. Other disabilities that follow the original injury are listed under Possible Complications.

4—BODY PARTS INVOLVED & ILLUSTRATION

This is a list and illustration of specific anatomical parts of the body involved in the injury, such as bones, joints, muscles, ligaments, blood vessels, nerves, lining membranes and others. The list usually includes body parts involved at the time of injury.

In our example, the body parts involved include the lower end of the humerus, or upper arm bone, the elbow joint, and many soft tissues surrounding the injury area.

The illustration helps you visualize the nature of the injury and the detailed anatomy of the body parts involved. It consists of three parts:
(1) A whole-body view to designate the general area where the injury occurs.
(2) An enlarged view of the injured area as it appears before the injury has taken place (normal anatomy).
(3) A close-up illustration of the area after injury showing the change in normal anatomy that has occurred.

By using the illustration with the text, the reader can understand the nature of the injury. Photographs and X-rays are harder to interpret than line drawings and are not used here.

5—SIGNS & SYMPTOMS

A *sign* may be observed by the patient or by someone else, or it may represent physical findings determined by X-ray examinations and other diagnostic measures. A *symptom* can only be felt or experienced by the patient.

In our example, the first item under this heading is: "Severe elbow and arm pain at the time of injury." This is a symptom that can be experienced only by the patient. The next two items, "swelling" and "deformity," are signs. They can be observed by others around the patient.

6—CAUSES

The cause of most athletic injuries is usually obvious because the symptoms begin immediately after the injury. However, some injuries produce delayed symptoms, and their cause is not readily apparent. Other injuries may occur simultaneously as a complication of a primary injury. For example, indirect elbow injuries frequently accompany direct trauma to the wrist. Both types of causes are mentioned in our sample injury.

7—RISK INCREASES WITH

Risk factors are usually pre-existing medical disorders. For example, an athlete with arthritis may be at increased risk for joint and bone injuries because these body parts are already weakened or misshapen.

The type of sport in which a person participates can also be a risk factor. For example, boxing is a sport particularly likely to lead to fractures of bones in the hand.

Our example includes risk factors in both categories. A person with osteoporosis has a greater risk of suffering an elbow fracture, and elbow fractures of the lower humerus are most likely in contact sports.

8—HOW TO PREVENT

Prevention may be of two kinds, prevention of the initial injury or prevention of a reinjury after healing. Prevention of any injury is the best of all possible treatments.

In general, the most important way to prevent injury is to follow a strenuous, carefully supervised conditioning program before beginning competition. Protective equipment designed for individual sports, such as elbow pads in our example, can also prevent or lessen the severity of injuries.

9—WHAT TO EXPECT

This section includes four topics: *Appropriate Health Care; Diagnostic Measures; Possible Complications;* and *Probable Outcome.* Each is discussed separately below.

10—APPROPRIATE HEALTH CARE

A doctor's diagnosis and prescription of treatment are usually the most appropriate forms of health care for all moderate or serious injuries. In a few cases, total self-care is sufficient, especially if the patient has had previous experience in treating a specific sports injury. Then he can use this book to verify his approach and as a source of additional information concerning treatment and rehabilitation. In no case should this book replace a doctor's instructions.

Even the simplest injuries sometimes result in the development of complications. These usually require professional care. To cover such cases, a doctor's treatment is listed on some charts as appropriate even though it may apply to only a small fraction of cases.

One of the most important aspects of appropriate health care—but one that is not listed on the charts—is a positive mental attitude about getting well. Having a positive outlook, being determined to heal quickly, and maintaining a sense of humor can be powerful assets in helping you regain strength, flexibility and skill so you can return quickly to your athletic activities.

If you have a particularly serious athletic injury, you may benefit by seeking care from a sports-medicine specialist. But beware! Sports medicine is a new medical specialty. As of this writing, this specialty has no certifying board. Therefore, some people who designate themselves as sports-medicine specialists may not have any relevant special training and may use the term "sports medicine" merely as a marketing tool.

Check out the credentials of any physician you choose. Your family doctor or a nearby medical school can usually provide referrals to qualified sports-medicine specialists. Be certain that the doctor you select communicates well with you. The best doctor-patient relationship is one of mutual respect.

11—DIAGNOSTIC MEASURES

Your own observation of signs and symptoms is usually the first—and often, the most important—diagnostic measure. It is the first step toward appropriate medical treatment. For this reason, it is listed under this heading on almost all injury charts. Exceptions are made for a few injuries, such as those involving unconsciousness, when self-observation is impossible.

A medical history and physical examination by a doctor, trainer or physical therapist are almost universal requirements before treatment of any serious injury. Additional studies include X-rays, laboratory studies or other specialized tests. See the Glossary for an explanation of any diagnostic tests you don't understand.

You may not require all the diagnostic tests listed on the chart, or conversely, you may undergo tests not listed. Some tests are performed only if previous tests have not provided enough information. Others are performed only when complications develop.

12—POSSIBLE COMPLICATIONS

Complications are additional medical problems triggered by or resulting from the original injury. Complications can sometimes occur despite accurate diagnosis and competent treatment. In our example, possible complications of an elbow fracture range from shock at the time of injury to long-term problems, such as arrested bone growth in children. As a rule, serious complications occur in only a small percentage of cases.

13—PROBABLE OUTCOME

The outcome of an injury or illness is generally the area of greatest concern to the patient. Athletes are keenly concerned with how the injury will affect future performance. Unfortunately, doctors can't always provide definite answers. No one can predict how long an injury will require to heal—or even how completely it will heal—with absolute accuracy.

The predictions in this section are educated guesses based on the average expected outcome. For instance, an elbow fracture of the lower humerus requires an *average* healing time of 6 to 8 weeks in adults and 4 to 6 weeks in children. Responses to treatment vary greatly from person to person. They are affected by such variables as age, sex, general state of health before the injury, specific pre-existing medical conditions, and fitness level.

14—HOW TO TREAT

This section provides a summary and reminder of instructions given you by your trainer or doctor. It is not intended to replace your doctor's instructions. If the instructions don't seem to fit your problem, ask your doctor or trainer for answers that apply uniquely to you.

The six major headings include: *First Aid; Continuing Care; Medication; Activity; Diet;* and *Rehabilitation.*

15—FIRST AID

The instructions here are intended for people who have not had previous training in first aid.

Our example gives simple instructions for treating someone with a fracture at the elbow. The victim should be covered to prevent shock, the arm should not be moved, and the steps for R.I.C.E. (rest, ice, compression and elevation) should be followed.

16—CONTINUING CARE

The instructions under this heading apply to home treatment, including treatment following surgery when that has been necessary. They cover common matters, such as applications of heat or cold, post-operative care of surgical wounds, appropriate clothing, bandages, and bathing.

The continuing care instructions cannot be complete or apply to everybody, but they provide a good review of general measures helpful for most injured athletes.

17—MEDICATION

Information listed under this heading is generally of two types: drugs your doctor may prescribe or administer, and non-prescription medicines you can safely administer yourself.

Prescription drugs are named by generic name or drug class. A brief description of a drug's purpose and effect is given.

You may obtain complete information regarding drugs and medications by referring to my book, *Complete Guide To Prescription & Non-Prescription Drugs,* published by HPBooks. It is available in most bookstores, or you can order direct from the publisher at P.O. Box 5367, Tucson, Arizona 85703.

18—ACTIVITY

This section is of vital interest to an injured person accustomed to vigorous exercise. It tells you whether to stay in bed, when to rest the injured part, and when you may resume activity.

As a rule, you should keep the uninjured parts of the body active while the injured part rests. Rest is essential for recovery. For example, someone with an elbow fracture of the lower humerus should begin exercising the uninjured arm, legs, shoulders and other muscle groups—as well as cardiovascular (aerobic) training—as soon as possible. See your doctor for specific instructions.

19—DIET

Diet information for an injured

person can vary from "no special diet" to references to diets that include extra protein for most efficient healing. Nutrition plays an important part in healing. The body requires certain nutritional building blocks to repair tissue. Opinions vary about diet for competitive athletes, but the general rules of good nutrition are the same for athletes as for others. See Appendix 5, page 482, for a complete discussion of nutrition.

20—REHABILITATION

Rehabilitation is a crucial part of treating any injury, particularly injuries to competitive athletes. Its importance cannot be overemphasized. Details of rehabilitation for specific regions of the body may be found in the Rehabilitation section in this book. Each chart refers you to the appropriate page for your injury.

21—CALL YOUR DOCTOR IF

The person with no previous medical experience should be able to determine from the chart whether he or she needs to see a doctor. For example, our sample chart leaves no doubt that a doctor should be seen immediately following a possible elbow fracture.

In addition, instructions are given for signs of complications that may arise after the initial injury. These instructions are especially important for injuries that are more serious than they first appear.

After your doctor has made a diagnosis, the course of recovery may differ from what is expected. Your doctor wants to be the first to know. Many developing complications can be averted with prompt medical treatment. Specific symptoms are listed that indicate the most common complications.

For example, a person with an elbow fracture would almost certainly have a cast. Our example lists telltale signs of problems due to a cast, including swelling and color changes in the hand.

Of course, if you have any symptoms other than those listed in this section that you believe are related to the injury or the medicines you take, call your doctor about them, too.

GUIDE TO SPORTS-MEDICINE CHARTS

Sports-medicine charts cover topics that affect or result from your participation in sports, physical exercise or athletic competition.

Any illness or disorder that affects health has some effect on physical activity. This book deals only with those most applicable to sports and exercise.

Each of the medical problems is described on a one-page format as shown in the sample chart, *DEHYDRATION,* on page 23. The format is similar but slightly different from the one used for the Sports Injuries section.

Major sections of the chart format are numbered and explained in the next few pages.

1—CHART NAME

Charts are arranged alphabetically by the most common name for the illness, disorder or medical problem. Other names for these appear in parentheses below the main heading. *DEHYDRATION* does not have another name, so it appears alone. However, a disease such as *ATHLETE'S FOOT* is also known as "Ringworm of the Foot", so this second name appears as a subheading. All names in this book, including alternate names, are cross-referenced in the index.

To find information about a medical problem, check the index. If you can't find the illness chart that you need, ask your team physician, trainer or personal doctor for alternate names for the disorder.

2—GENERAL INFORMATION

This section includes four topics: *Definition; Signs & Symptoms; Causes & Risk Factors;* and *How to Prevent.* Each is discussed separately below.

3—DEFINITION

Here you will find a short definition of the problem or disease. In the *DEHYDRATION* chart, the definition is short and simple. Charts for other ailments may be more detailed. Sometimes an illness or disorder cannot be defined without including information about causes, risks or general treatment—even if this information is covered in greater detail elsewhere on the chart.

4—SIGNS & SYMPTOMS

The distinction between signs and symptoms is important. A *sign* is observed. A *symptom* is felt or experienced.

In our sample chart, the first item mentioned under this heading is "dry mouth." This is a symptom that only the patient can experience. The next three items ("decreased or absent urination, sunken eyes, wrinkled skin") are signs. They can be observed by the patient or by others.

Signs and symptoms are listed together in this book. No attempt has been made to separate the two. A wide range of possible signs and symptoms is listed on most charts. *It is unlikely that any patient will have all, or even most, of the possible signs and symptoms.*

The presence or absence of signs and symptoms may vary according to:
● The age and sex of the patient.
● His general state of health at the onset of the disorder.
● The extent and stage of the illness.

The charts in this book are written from the perspective of the effect of disease on an athlete. For more general information, including a separate section devoted to symptoms, please refer to my book *Complete*

Guide to Symptoms, Illness & Surgery, published by The Body Press.

5—CAUSES & RISK FACTORS

Many times the cause of a disorder is unknown. At the same time, many disorders have factors that are known to increase the risk of succumbing to a disease. These include factors that may trigger the problem, make it more likely to occur or cause it to increase in duration or intensity. Because it is sometimes hard to know when risks end and causes begin, these two factors are listed together on the illness charts.

Common causes of illness in athletes include:
● Inherited (congenital) defects.
● Infections from bacteria, viruses, parasites, yeast or fungi. All of these are sometimes referred to as "germs," but most people associate "germs" with bacteria only.
● Allergies.
● Physical injury, including that caused by cold or heat.
● Toxins (poisons) from a wide range of sources, including environmental pollution.

Risk factors affecting how a person reacts to the causes above include:
● Age.
● Stress, either physical or emotional.
● Fatigue or overwork.
● Poor nutrition due to improper diet, disease, or the special demands of strenuous physical activity.
● Obesity.
● Recent or chronic illness that can lower resistance to other disorders.
● Recent surgery or injury.
● Use of drugs, such as alcohol, tobacco, caffeine, narcotics, psychedelics, hallucinogens, marijuana, sedatives, hypnotics or cocaine.
● Use of prescription or non-prescription medications. Even necessary drugs may cause adverse reactions and side effects that can complicate the treatment and outcome of medical problems and affect athletic performance.
● Crowded or unsanitary conditions, including locker rooms.
● Poor personal hygiene.
● Mental or emotional disorders, such as anxiety and depression.
● Defects in the body's immune system.

6—HOW TO PREVENT

Prevention can be of two types—prevention of the initial disease or prevention of a relapse or recurrence after recovery.

Prevention of any medical problem is the best treatment. Many diseases cannot be prevented because we cannot control all of their causes. However, we *can* control many risk factors. In our example, an athlete can decrease the risk of becoming severely dehydrated by remembering to drink adequate water, especially during hot weather and when sweating heavily.

7—WHAT TO EXPECT

This section includes four topics: *Diagnostic Measures; Surgery; Normal Course of Illness;* and *Possible Complications.* Each is discussed separately below.

8—DIAGNOSTIC MEASURES

As with injuries, your own observation of symptoms is usually the first diagnostic measure of an illness. The next logical step is often a medical history and physical exam by

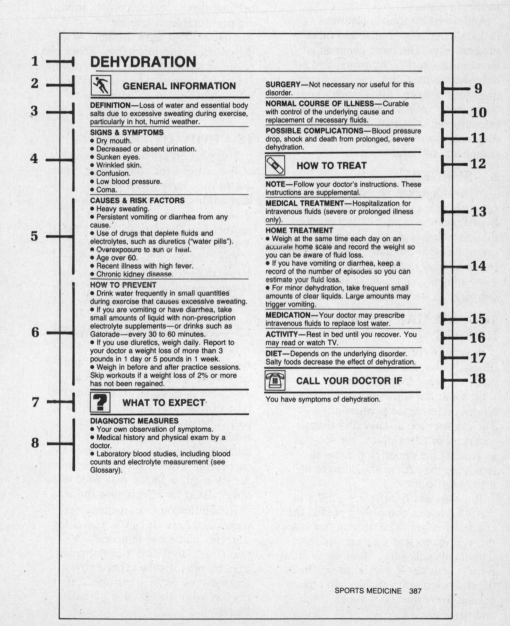

1 **DEHYDRATION**

2 📋 **GENERAL INFORMATION**

3 **DEFINITION**—Loss of water and essential body salts due to excessive sweating during exercise, particularly in hot, humid weather.

SIGNS & SYMPTOMS
4
- Dry mouth.
- Decreased or absent urination.
- Sunken eyes.
- Wrinkled skin.
- Confusion.
- Low blood pressure.
- Coma.

CAUSES & RISK FACTORS
- Heavy sweating.
- Persistent vomiting or diarrhea from any cause.
5
- Use of drugs that deplete fluids and electrolytes, such as diuretics ("water pills").
- Overexposure to sun or heat.
- Age over 60.
- Recent illness with high fever.
- Chronic kidney disease.

HOW TO PREVENT
- Drink water frequently in small quantities during exercise that causes excessive sweating.
- If you are vomiting or have diarrhea, take small amounts of liquid with non-prescription electrolyte supplements—or drinks such as Gatorade—every 30 to 60 minutes.
6
- If you use diuretics, weigh daily. Report to your doctor a weight loss of more than 3 pounds in 1 day or 5 pounds in 1 week.
- Weigh in before and after practice sessions. Skip workouts if a weight loss of 2% or more has not been regained.

7 ❓ **WHAT TO EXPECT**

DIAGNOSTIC MEASURES
- Your own observation of symptoms.
- Medical history and physical exam by a doctor.
8
- Laboratory blood studies, including blood counts and electrolyte measurement (see Glossary).

SURGERY—Not necessary nor useful for this disorder. **9**

NORMAL COURSE OF ILLNESS—Curable with control of the underlying cause and replacement of necessary fluids. **10**

POSSIBLE COMPLICATIONS—Blood pressure drop, shock and death from prolonged, severe dehydration. **11**

🩹 **HOW TO TREAT** **12**

NOTE—Follow your doctor's instructions. These instructions are supplemental.

MEDICAL TREATMENT—Hospitalization for intravenous fluids (severe or prolonged illness only). **13**

HOME TREATMENT
- Weigh at the same time each day on an accurate home scale and record the weight so you can be aware of fluid loss.
- If you have vomiting or diarrhea, keep a record of the number of episodes so you can estimate your fluid loss.
14
- For minor dehydration, take frequent small amounts of clear liquids. Large amounts may trigger vomiting.

MEDICATION—Your doctor may prescribe intravenous fluids to replace lost water. **15**

ACTIVITY—Rest in bed until you recover. You may read or watch TV. **16**

DIET—Depends on the underlying disorder. Salty foods decrease the effect of dehydration. **17**

☎ **CALL YOUR DOCTOR IF** **18**

You have symptoms of dehydration.

a doctor. Even if a problem can be treated at home, a doctor's history and exam will be necessary if complications develop that require medical treatment.

Additional diagnostic measures include laboratory studies and other medical tests. The most common are listed in this section by name, and are described in the Glossary. The list of diagnostic tests is only a guide. Your doctor may not need every one listed, or additional ones may be required if diagnosis is difficult or if complications develop.

9—SURGERY

When surgery is necessary or useful for cure, it is indicated here. Sometimes the name or description of the procedure is given. If you are uncertain what the name means, refer to the Glossary. As is the case with most ailments, our sample shows that dehydration does not require surgery.

10—NORMAL COURSE OF ILLNESS

A very important concern in any illness is how the illness will affect the patient's life. Most illnesses last a short time, but some may continue to hinder performance permanently. These issues are discussed in this section. For dehydration, we see that as soon as the underlying cause is removed, the patient should have no lasting difficulties.

Illnesses and injuries are similar in that no one can completely predict the course of either. This section describes the average patient's experience, but individuals will vary. Medicine is an inexact science. Response to treatment depends on many variables, and there remain many questions about health and disease.

11—POSSIBLE COMPLICATIONS

Complications are additional medical problems triggered by the original illness. Some complications are preventable, a few are inevitable—but most are rare. With dehydration, life-threatening shock can occur as a complication. However, this is a rare occurrence resulting only when dehydration is ignored and untreated in its earlier stages.

12—HOW TO TREAT

This section provides a general list of instructions for your illness. Your doctor may have given you instructions, and this information should not replace your doctor's instructions. Treatments vary a great deal from individual to individual.

The five major headings include: *Medical Treatment; Home Treatment; Medication; Activity;* and *Diet.* They are explained in detail below.

13—MEDICAL TREATMENT

Some ailments can be treated successfully at home. This section covers those cases when medical treatment is essential. It explains the type of treatment usually used for a particular disorder. Many times, medical treatment is necessary only if home treatment has not proven successful. For instance, in the case of dehydration, a person may need to be hospitalized for intravenous fluids.

Rehabilitation is sometimes mentioned here. It can be useful for illnesses that cause temporary or permanent disability. Rehabilitation may be provided by trained physical therapists or physiatrists (medical doctors who specialize in physical therapy).

14—HOME TREATMENT

This section covers the various things a patient can do at home to help himself get better. Some of the instructions elaborate on what your doctor may have told you to do. Others give you suggestions for treating yourself. The measures mentioned here are not complete and may not apply to everyone, but they provide a good review of home treatment helpful for many patients. For example, our sample chart for dehydration explains the importance of weighing daily and recording rapid fluid loss.

15—MEDICATION

Medication is often an important part of treatment. This chart section tells you which non-prescription drugs you can take safely, and it lists the prescription drugs your doctor is most likely to recommend. Drugs are named by generic name or drug class.

16—ACTIVITY

Patients are often confused about whether they must stay in bed during an illness. They are often concerned about returning to their favorite sport or physical activity, and want to know if activity will be restricted after recovery. These questions are answered under this heading.

Exercise references are often included, and when not specified otherwise, references to regular physical exercise mean aerobic exercise.

In the case of dehydration, it is only necessary to rest in bed until you recover. No permanent reduction in activity is necessary, nor is it useful.

17—DIET

Diet information can vary from "no special diet" to references to the diets which hasten healing or recovery time. Nutrition plays a big part in health and disease.

In the case of dehydration, the diet prescribed depends on the underlying cause of the disorder. For additional specialized diet instructions, consult your doctor or a dietitian.

18—CALL YOUR DOCTOR IF

For most medical problems, a phone call or visit to your doctor is recommended to establish a diagnosis.

After diagnosis, when the course of an illness differs from what is expected, your doctor wants to know. Many developing complications can be averted with prompt medical treatment. The symptoms listed usually indicate complications.

Of course, if any other symptoms begin that you believe are related to your illness or the drugs you take, call your doctor about them, too.

ABDOMINAL-WALL STRAIN

GENERAL INFORMATION

DEFINITION—Injury to the muscles or tendons of the abdominal wall, or injury to the places where muscles or tendons attach to pelvic bones. Tendons, muscles and bones comprise units. These units stabilize the pelvis and rib cage and allow their motion. A strain occurs at the weakest part of a unit. Strains are of 3 types:
- Mild (Grade I)—Slightly pulled muscle without tearing of muscle or tendon fibers. There is no loss of strength.
- Moderate (Grade II)—Tearing of fibers in a muscle, tendon or at the attachment to bone. Strength is diminished.
- Severe (Grade III)—Rupture of the muscle-tendon-bone attachment with separation of fibers. Severe strain requires surgical repair. Chronic strains are caused by overuse. Acute strains are caused by direct injury or overstress.

BODY PARTS INVOLVED
- Abdominal muscles and tendons.
- Bones in the abdominal area (ribs, pubic bone and iliac-crest bone).
- Soft tissue surrounding the strain, including nerves, periosteum (covering to bone), blood vessels and lymph vessels.

SIGNS & SYMPTOMS
- Pain when moving or stretching abdominal muscles.
- Muscle spasm, especially with hard breathing or twisting.
- Swelling in the abdominal area.
- Loss of strength (moderate or severe strain).
- Crepitation ("crackling") feeling and sound when the injured area is pressed with fingers.
- Calcification of the muscle or its tendon (visible with X-ray).
- Inflammation of the tendon sheath.

CAUSES
- Prolonged overuse of muscle-tendon units in the abdominal wall.
- Single violent injury or force applied to the muscle-tendon units in the abdominal wall.

RISK INCREASES WITH
- Stretching exercises.
- Pole vaulting, high jumping and hurdling.
- Contact sports.
- Any cardiovascular medical problem that results in decreased circulation.
- Medical history of any bleeding disorder.
- Obesity.
- Poor nutrition.
- Previous abdominal-wall strain.
- Poor muscle conditioning.

HOW TO PREVENT
- Participate in a strengthening and conditioning program appropriate for your sport.
- Warm up before practice or competition.

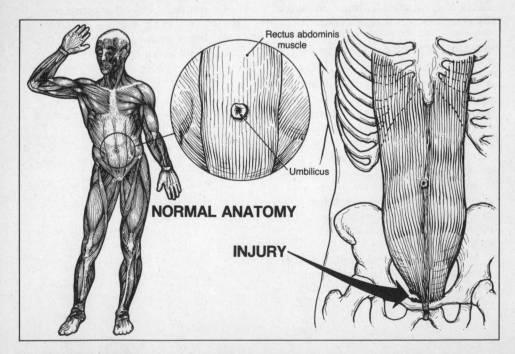

Rectus abdominis muscle

Umbilicus

NORMAL ANATOMY

INJURY

WHAT TO EXPECT

APPROPRIATE HEALTH CARE
- Doctor's diagnosis.
- Self-care during rehabilitation.
- Physical therapy (moderate or severe strain).
- Surgery (severe strain).

DIAGNOSTIC MEASURES
- Your own observation of symptoms.
- Medical history and exam by a doctor.
- X-rays of injured areas to rule out fractures.

POSSIBLE COMPLICATIONS
- Prolonged healing time, if activity is resumed too soon.
- Proneness to repeated injury.
- Inflammation at attachment to bone (periostitis).
- Prolonged disability (sometimes).

PROBABLE OUTCOME—If this is a first-time injury, proper care and sufficient healing time before resuming activity should prevent permanent disability. Torn ligaments and tendons require as long to heal as fractured bones. Average healing times are:
- Mild strain—2 to 10 days.
- Moderate strain—10 days to 6 weeks.
- Severe strain—6 to 10 weeks.

If this is a repeat injury, complications listed above are more likely to occur.

HOW TO TREAT

NOTE—Follow your doctor's instructions. These instructions are supplemental.

FIRST AID—Follow instructions for R.I.C.E., the first letters of *rest, ice, compression* and *elevation* (if possible). See Appendix 1 for details.

CONTINUING CARE
- Use ice massage 3 or 4 times a day for 15 minutes at a time. Fill a large Styrofoam cup with water and freeze. Tear a small amount of foam from the top so ice protrudes. Massage firmly over the injured area in a circle about the size of a softball.
- After the first 24 hours, apply heat instead of ice, if it feels better. Use heat lamps, hot soaks, hot showers, heating pads, or heat liniments and ointments.
- Take whirlpool treatments, if available.
- Wrap the injured abdominal-wall muscles loosely with an elasticized bandage or wear a corset between treatments.
- Massage gently and often to provide comfort and decrease swelling.

MEDICATION
- For minor discomfort, you may use:
  Aspirin, acetaminophen or ibuprofen.
  Topical liniments and ointments.
- Your doctor may prescribe:
  Stronger pain relievers.
  Injection of a long-acting local anesthetic to reduce pain.
  Injection of a corticosteroid, such as triamcinolone, to reduce inflammation.

ACTIVITY—Resume your normal activities gradually after pain subsides.

DIET—Eat a well-balanced diet that includes extra protein, such as meat, fish, poultry, cheese, milk and eggs. Increase fiber and fluid intake to prevent constipation that may result from decreased activity.

REHABILITATION—Begin a supervised weight-lifting program when supportive wrapping is no longer needed. Use ice massage for 10 minutes prior to exercise.

CALL YOUR DOCTOR IF

- You have symptoms of a moderate or severe abdominal-wall strain, or a mild strain persists longer than 10 days.
- Pain or swelling worsens despite treatment.

ACHILLES' TENDINITIS

 GENERAL INFORMATION

DEFINITION—Inflammation of the Achilles' tendon.

BODY PARTS INVOLVED
- Achilles' tendon, which attaches the lower leg muscles to the heel.
- Soft tissue in the surrounding area, including blood vessels, nerves, ligaments, periosteum (covering to bone) and connective tissue.

SIGNS & SYMPTOMS
- Constant pain or pain with motion.
- Limited motion of the ankle.
- Crepitation (a "crackling" sound when the tendon moves or is touched).
- Heat and redness over the inflamed Achilles' tendon.

CAUSES
- Strain from unusual use or overuse of the lower leg muscles and Achilles' tendon.
- Direct blow or injury to the lower leg, foot or ankle. Tendinitis becomes more likely with repeated injury.
- Infection introduced through broken skin at the time of injury.

RISK INCREASES WITH—Contact sports, especially those involving kicking, jumping and quick starts.

HOW TO PREVENT
- Engage in a vigorous program of physical conditioning before beginning regular sports participation.
- Warm up adequately before practice or competition.
- Learn proper moves and techniques for your sport.

 WHAT TO EXPECT

APPROPRIATE HEALTH CARE
- Doctor's examination and diagnosis.
- Self-care during recovery.

DIAGNOSTIC MEASURES
- Your own observation of symptoms and signs.
- Medical history and physical examination by your doctor.
- X-rays of the area to rule out other abnormalities.

POSSIBLE COMPLICATIONS
- Prolonged healing time if activity is resumed too soon.
- Proneness to repeated injury.

PROBABLE OUTCOME—Achilles' tendinitis is usually curable in about 6 weeks with heat treatments and rest of the inflamed area. Recovery is usually quicker if the inflammation is caused by a direct blow rather than by a strain or sprain.

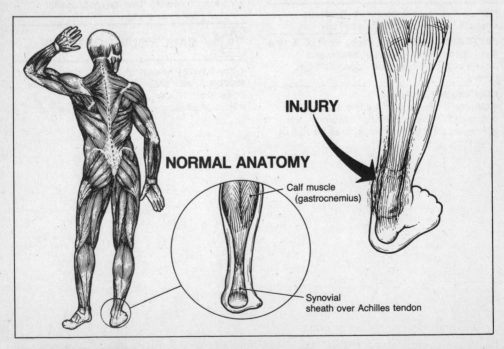

INJURY

NORMAL ANATOMY

Calf muscle (gastrocnemius)

Synovial sheath over Achilles tendon

HOW TO TREAT

NOTE—Follow your doctor's instructions. These instructions are supplemental.

FIRST AID—None. This problem develops slowly.

CONTINUING CARE
• You may need a walking-boot cast for 10 to 14 days. See Appendix 2 (Care of Casts). Then wrap the ankle area with an elasticized bandage until healing is complete.
• Apply heat frequently. Use heat lamps, hot soaks, hot showers, heating pads, or heat liniments and ointments.
• Take whirlpool treatments, if available.
• To prevent a recurrence, wear protective strapping or an adhesive bandage for several weeks after healing is complete.

MEDICATION
• You may use non-prescription drugs such as acetaminophen for minor pain.
• Your doctor may prescribe stronger pain relievers. Don't take prescription pain medication longer than 4 to 7 days. Use only as much as you need.

ACTIVITY—Resume normal activities gradually.

DIET—During recovery, eat a well-balanced diet that includes extra protein, such as meat, fish, poultry, cheese, milk and eggs. Increase fiber and fluid intake to prevent constipation that may result from decreased activity. Your doctor may suggest vitamin and mineral supplements to promote healing.

REHABILITATION
• Begin daily rehabilitation exercises when supportive wrapping is no longer needed and you can walk without pain.
• Use ice massage for 10 minutes before and after exercise. Fill a large Styrofoam cup with water and freeze. Tear a small amount of foam from the top so ice protrudes. Massage firmly over the injured area in a circle about the size of a softball.
• See pages 446 and 462 for rehabilitation exercises.

 ## CALL YOUR DOCTOR IF

• You have symptoms of Achilles' tendinitis.
• New, unexplained symptoms develop. Drugs used in treatment may produce side effects.

ACHILLES'-TENDON STRAIN

GENERAL INFORMATION

DEFINITION—Injury to the Achilles' tendon or its adjoining muscle or bone. These 3 parts comprise a unit. The strain occurs at the weakest part of the unit. Strains are of 3 types:
● Mild (Grade I)—Slightly pulled muscle without tearing of muscle or tendon fibers. There is no loss of strength.
● Moderate (Grade II)—Tearing of fibers in a muscle, tendon or at the attachment to bone. Strength is diminished.
● Severe (Grade III)—Rupture of the muscle-tendon-bone attachment with separation of fibers. Severe strain requires surgical repair. Chronic strains are caused by overuse. Acute strains are caused by direct injury or overstress.

BODY PARTS INVOLVED
● Achilles' tendon.
● Muscle attached to the Achilles' tendon.
● Heel bone.
● Soft tissue surrounding the strain, including nerves, periosteum (bone covering), blood vessels and lymph vessels.

SIGNS & SYMPTOMS
● Pain when flexing or extending the foot.
● Muscle spasm at the rear of the calf.
● Swelling around the Achilles' tendon.
● Loss of strength (moderate or severe strain).
● Crepitation ("crackling") feeling and sound

when the injured area is pressed with fingers.
● Calcification of the muscle or its tendon (visible with X-ray).
● Inflammation of the sheath covering the Achilles' tendon.

CAUSES
● Prolonged overuse of muscle-tendon units in the ankle.
● Single episode of stressful overactivity, as in hurdling, long-jumping, high-jumping or starting a sprint.

RISK INCREASES WITH
● Contact sports.
● Running.
● Sports that require quick starts, such as long-jumping, hurdling or running races.
● Any cardiovascular medical problem that results in decreased circulation.
● Medical history of any bleeding disorder.
● Obesity.
● Poor nutrition.
● Previous Achilles'-tendon injury.
● Poor muscle conditioning.

HOW TO PREVENT
● Participate in a strengthening and conditioning program appropriate for your sport.
● Warm up before practice or competition.
● Tape the Achilles' area before practice or competition.
● Wear proper protective shoes.

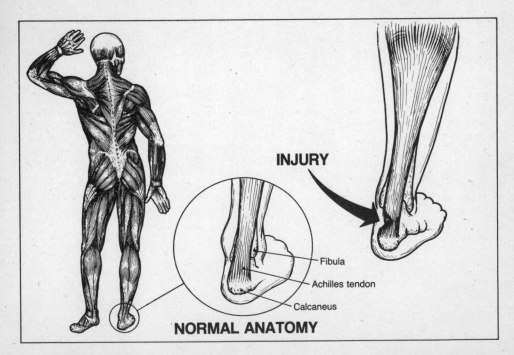

INJURY

Fibula

Achilles tendon

Calcaneus

NORMAL ANATOMY

WHAT TO EXPECT

APPROPRIATE HEALTH CARE
- Doctor's diagnosis.
- Application of tape, plaster splints or casts (sometimes).
- Self-care during rehabilitation.
- Physical therapy (moderate or severe strain).
- Surgery (severe strain).

DIAGNOSTIC MEASURES
- Your own observation of symptoms.
- Medical history and exam by a doctor.
- X-rays of injured areas to rule out fractures.

POSSIBLE COMPLICATIONS
- Prolonged healing time if activity is resumed too soon.
- Proneness to repeated injury.
- Unstable or arthritic ankle following repeated injury.
- Inflammation at the attachment to bone (periostitis).
- Prolonged disability (sometimes).

PROBABLE OUTCOME—If this is a first-time injury, proper care and sufficient healing time before resuming activity should prevent permanent disability. Torn ligaments and tendons require as long to heal as bone fractures. Average healing times are:
- Mild strain—2 to 10 days.
- Moderate strain—10 days to 6 weeks.
- Severe strain—6 to 10 weeks.

If this is a repeat injury, complications listed above are more likely to occur.

 HOW TO TREAT

NOTE—Follow your doctor's instructions. These instructions are supplemental.

FIRST AID—Follow instructions for R.I.C.E., the first letters of *rest, ice, compression* and *elevation*. See Appendix 1 for details.

CONTINUING CARE—If a cast or splints are used, leave toes free and exercise them occasionally. If a cast or splints are not used:
- Use ice massage 3 or 4 times a day for 15 minutes at a time. Fill a large Styrofoam cup with water and freeze. Tear a small amount of foam from the top so ice protrudes. Massage firmly over the injured area in a circle about the size of a softball.
- After the first 24 hours, apply heat instead of ice, if it feels better. Use heat lamps, hot soaks, hot showers, heating pads, or heat liniments and ointments.
- Take whirlpool treatments, if available.
- Wrap the injured ankle with an elasticized bandage between treatments. Insert a heel lift in your shoe.
- Massage gently and often to provide comfort and decrease swelling.

MEDICATION
- For minor discomfort, you may use:
  Aspirin, acetaminophen, or ibuprofen.
  Topical liniments and ointments.
- Your doctor may prescribe:
  Stronger pain relievers.
  Injection of a long-acting local anesthetic to reduce pain (rare).
  Injection of a corticosteroid, such as triamcinolone, to reduce inflammation (rare).

ACTIVITY
- For a moderate or severe strain, walk with crutches for at least 72 hours—longer with a cast or splints. See Appendix 3 (Safe Use of Crutches).
- Resume normal activities gradually after pain has subsided.

DIET—Eat a well balanced diet that includes extra protein, such as meat, fish, poultry, cheese, milk and eggs. Increase fiber and fluid intake to prevent constipation that may result from decreased activity.

REHABILITATION—Begin daily rehabilitation exercises when supportive wrapping is no longer needed. See pages 446 and 455 for rehabilitation exercises.

 CALL YOUR DOCTOR IF

- You have symptoms of a moderate or severe Achilles'-tendon strain, or a mild strain persists longer than 10 days.
- Pain or swelling worsens despite treatment.
- The following occurs with a cast or splints:
  Pain, numbness or coldness below the injury.
  Dusky, blue or gray toenails.

ANKLE-BONE FRACTURE

GENERAL INFORMATION

DEFINITION—A fracture, usually in either side of the ankle, often including a total tear of one or more ankle ligaments. A temporary dislocation of the ankle joint may also occur. Ankle sprains are among the most common injuries in sports.

BODY PARTS INVOLVED
● Lowest part of the lower leg bones (tibia and fibula).
● Ligaments on either side of the ankle that support the ankle joint.
● Three main bones of the ankle joint (talus, tibia, and fibula) may be involved with the dislocation or sprain.
● Blood vessels, nerves, periosteum (covering of bone), and other soft tissue close to the injury site.

SIGNS & SYMPTOMS
● Severe ankle pain immediately after injury.
● Popping or feeling of tearing in the outer or inner part of the ankle. Sometimes there will be a sensation that the ankle joint is dislocated or has popped back into joint.
● Severe tenderness at the injury site.
● The injured person usually falls at the time of injury and has difficulty walking.

● Forcing the ankle in the direction of pain may reveal some looseness in the joint.
● General swelling throughout the ankle and foot.
● Bruising immediately or soon after injury.

CAUSES—Stress imposed from either side of the ankle joint that temporarily forces or pries the ankle or heel bone (talus) out of its normal socket. The ligament or ligaments that normally hold the joint in place are stretched and torn.

RISK INCREASES WITH
● Previous ankle injury.
● Contact sports.
● Runners, walkers and those who jump in such sports as basketball, soccer, volleyball, skiing or distance and high-jumping. These persons often accidentally land on the side of the foot.
● Shoes with inadequate support to prevent lateral displacement when stress occurs.
● Poor nutrition, especially calcium deficiency.
● Poor muscle strength or conditioning.
● Inadequate strapping prior to participation in contact sports.
● Walking or running on rough surfaces, such as roads with potholes.

HOW TO PREVENT
● Engage in vigorous presport strengthening and conditioning.

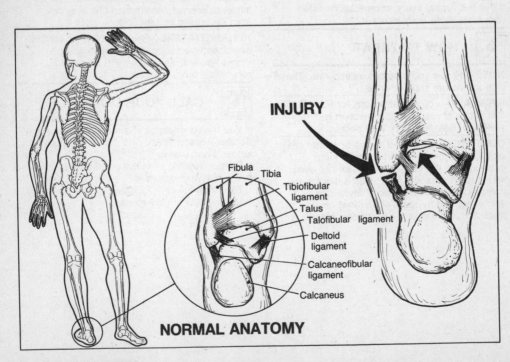

INJURY

Fibula Tibia
Tibiofibular ligament
Talus
Talofibular ligament
Deltoid ligament
Calcaneofibular ligament
Calcaneus

NORMAL ANATOMY

- Wear high-top athletic shoes for contact sports.
- Have adequate taping (midfoot to midcalf) before participation in activities at risk.
- Wear supportive elastic ankle wraps (not as good as tape, but better than nothing).
- Support the ankle well during sports activities for 12 months after any significant ankle injury.

 ## WHAT TO EXPECT

APPROPRIATE HEALTH CARE
- Hospitalization for surgery to pin broken bones together and to repair ruptured tendons.
- Doctor's care.
- Physical therapy after the cast is removed.

DIAGNOSTIC MEASURES
- Your own observation of symptoms.
- Medical history and exam by a doctor.
- X-rays of injured areas to assess total injury.

POSSIBLE COMPLICATIONS
- Full extent of the injury may not be recognized immediately, delaying treatment.
- Excessive postoperative bleeding or infection.
- Prolonged healing time if usual activities are resumed too soon.
- Proneness to repeated ankle injury.
- Unstable or permanently arthritic ankle joint, if many repeat injuries occur.

PROBABLE OUTCOME
- After surgery, ankle fracture-sprains require an average of 18 to 20 weeks to heal completely. The pins or screws inserted surgically to hold bones together are usually removed in 8 to 12 weeks. If this is a first-time injury, proper care, surgery and sufficient healing time before resuming activity should prevent permanent disability. Torn ligaments require as much healing time as fractured bones.
- If non-surgical treatment is chosen, healing time while completely avoiding putting weight on the ankle may require 12 months.

 ## HOW TO TREAT

NOTE—Follow your doctor's instructions. These instructions are supplemental.

FIRST AID—Use instructions for R.I.C.E., the first letters of *rest, ice, compression* and *elevation*. See Appendix 1 for details.

CONTINUING CARE
- Following surgery, the doctor may apply a stirrup boot splint from below the knee to the toes. Stirrup boots are less likely to cause problems with swelling than an immediate cast may cause. This will support the ankle effectively enough to walk on crutches, but you should not bear weight on the injured ankle.

- When the swelling subsides several days later, sutures may be removed. The splint is replaced by a walking-boot cast for 10 to 21 days. See Appendix 2 (Care of Casts). Start walking on the walking cast immediately.
- After the cast has been removed, strapping or a brace will be necessary for at least 6 weeks.
- Bathe and shower as usual after the cast is removed, even if sutures are still in place.
- After cast removal, use frequent ice massage. Fill a large Styrofoam cup with water and freeze. Tear a small amount of foam from the top so ice protrudes. Massage firmly over the injured area in a circle about the size of a baseball. Do this for 15 minutes at a time, 3 or 4 times a day.
- Apply heat instead of ice, if it feels better. Use heat lamps, hot soaks, hot showers or heating pads.
- Take whirlpool treatments, if available.
- Gentle massage will frequently provide comfort and decrease swelling.

MEDICATION
- For minor discomfort, you may use aspirin, acetaminophen, or topical liniments and ointments.
- Your doctor may prescribe stronger medicine for pain, if needed.

ACTIVITY—Walk with crutches until you have a walking cast. See Appendix 3 (Safe Use of Crutches). Resume your normal activities gradually. Don't drive until healing is complete.

DIET
- Drink only water before manipulation or surgery to treat the fracture. Solid food in your stomach makes vomiting while under anesthesia more hazardous.
- During recovery, eat a well-balanced diet that includes extra protein, such as meat, fish, poultry, cheese, milk and eggs. Increase fiber and fluid intake to prevent constipation that may result from decreased activity.

REHABILITATION—Begin daily rehabilitation exercises when supportive wrapping is no longer needed. Use ice massage for 10 minutes prior to exercise. See pages 446 and 455 for rehabilitation exercises.

 ## CALL YOUR DOCTOR IF

- You have signs or symptoms of any severe ankle injury.
- Pain, swelling or bruising increase during treatment or rehabilitation.
- You notice numbness or discoloration of the toes when the walking cast is in place.
- Signs of postoperative infection occur, such as fever, drainage from the surgical wound or increasing pain at the surgical site.

ANKLE CONTUSION

GENERAL INFORMATION

DEFINITION—Bruising of skin and underlying tissues of the ankle due to a direct blow. Contusions cause bleeding from ruptured small capillaries that allow blood to infiltrate muscles, tendons or other soft tissue. Ankle contusions are common, but they are not serious injuries.

BODY PARTS INVOLVED—Ankle tissues, including blood vessels, muscles, tendons, nerves, covering to bone (periosteum) and connective tissue.

SIGNS & SYMPTOMS
- Local swelling—either superficial or deep.
- Pain and tenderness over the bruise.
- Feeling of firmness when pressure is exerted at the injury site.
- Discoloration under the skin, beginning with redness and progressing to the characteristic "black and blue" bruise.

CAUSES—Direct blow to the ankle, usually from a blunt object.

RISK INCREASES WITH
- Violent contact sports such as field hockey, ice hockey and soccer, especially when ankles are not adequately protected.
- Medical history of any bleeding disorder such as hemophilia.

- Poor nutrition, including vitamin deficiency.
- Use of anticoagulants or aspirin.

HOW TO PREVENT—Wear appropriate protective gear and equipment, such as high-ankle shoes, during competition or other athletic activity if there is risk of an ankle contusion.

WHAT TO EXPECT

APPROPRIATE HEALTH CARE
- Doctor's care unless the contusion is quite small.
- Self-care for minor contusions, and for serious contusions during rehabilitation.
- Physical therapy for serious contusions.

DIAGNOSTIC MEASURES
- Your own observation of symptoms.
- Medical history and physical exam by a doctor for all except minor injuries.
- X-rays of the injured area to assess total injury to soft tissue and to rule out the possibility of underlying fracture. The total extent of injury may not be apparent for 48 to 72 hours.

POSSIBLE COMPLICATIONS
- Excessive bleeding leading to disability. Infiltrative-type bleeding can sometimes lead to calcification and impaired function of the injured muscle.

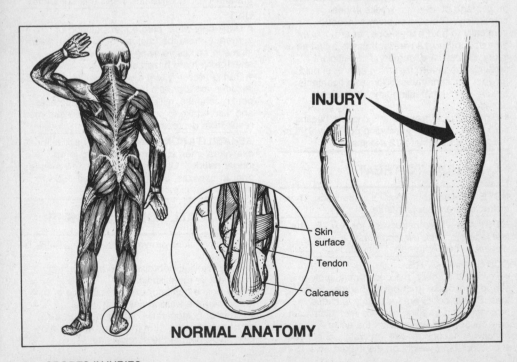

INJURY

Skin surface

Tendon

Calcaneus

NORMAL ANATOMY

• Infection if skin over the contusion is broken.

PROBABLE OUTCOME—Healing time varies with the extent of injury, but uncomplicated ankle contusions usually heal within 2 to 4 days.

 ## HOW TO TREAT

NOTE—Follow your doctor's instructions. These instructions are supplemental.

FIRST AID—Use instructions for R.I.C.E., the first letters of *rest, ice, compression* and *elevation*. See Appendix 1 for details.

CONTINUING CARE
• Wrap an elasticized bandage over a piece of sponge rubber on the injured area. Keep the area compressed for about 72 hours.
• Continue ice massage. Fill a large Styrofoam cup with water and freeze. Tear a small amount of foam from the top so ice protrudes. Massage gently over the injured area in a circle about the size of a softball. Do this for 15 minutes at a time, 3 or 4 times a day, and before workouts or competition.
• After 72 hours, apply heat instead of ice if it feels better. Use heat lamps, hot soaks, hot showers, heating pads, heat liniments or ointments, or whirlpool treatments.
• Massage gently and often to provide comfort and decrease swelling. Stroke toward the heart from the toes.

MEDICATION
• For minor discomfort, you may use:
  Acetaminophen or ibuprofen.
  Topical liniments and ointments.
• Your doctor may prescribe stronger medicine for pain.

ACTIVITY—As soon as underlying damage can be ruled out, normal activity can begin within a day or two.

DIET—For serious injuries, eat a well-balanced diet that includes extra protein, such as meat, fish, poultry, cheese, milk and eggs. Your doctor may prescribe vitamin and mineral supplements to promote healing.

REHABILITATION
• For serious contusions, begin daily rehabilitation exercises when supportive wrapping is no longer needed.
• See pages 446 and 462 for rehabilitation exercises.

 ## CALL YOUR DOCTOR IF

• You have a contusion that doesn't improve in 1 or 2 days.
• Skin is broken and signs of infection (drainage, increasing pain, fever, headache, muscle aches, dizziness or a general ill feeling) occur.

ANKLE DISLOCATION

GENERAL INFORMATION

DEFINITION—An injury to the ankle so that the adjoining bones are displaced and no longer touch each other. Ankle dislocations are almost always associated with sprains (damage to ligaments) and fractures.

BODY PARTS INVOLVED
- Bones of the ankle, including the tibia, fibula and talus.
- Ligaments that hold the bones of the ankle together.
- Soft tissue surrounding the dislocated bones, including nerves, tendons, muscles and blood vessels.

SIGNS & SYMPTOMS
- Excruciating pain at the time of injury.
- Loss of ankle function and severe pain when attempting to move the ankle.
- Locking of the dislocated bones in the abnormal position or spontaneous reposition, leaving no apparent deformity.
- Tenderness over the site of the dislocation, fracture and sprain.
- Ankle swelling and bruising.
- Numbness or paralysis in the foot from pressure, pinching or cutting of blood vessels or nerves.

CAUSES
- Serious injury with stress on the side of the ankle, forcing the ankle through a motion for which it is not designed.
- End result of a severe ankle sprain (injury to ligaments, fibers or attachment due to overstress).
- Recurrent sprains and strains that leave weakened ligaments.
- Powerful muscle contractions.

RISK INCREASES WITH
- Running or fast walking, especially on uneven terrain.
- Participation in contact sports.
- Repeated ankle injury of any sort, especially dislocations or sprains.
- Arthritis of any type (rheumatoid, gout).
- Poor muscle conditioning.

HOW TO PREVENT
- Protect ankle joints with protective devices, such as wrapped elastic bandages or tape wraps.
- Develop a high level of lower leg and ankle strength and conditioning.
- Warm up adequately before physical activity.
- Avoid irregular surfaces for running or track events.

? WHAT TO EXPECT

APPROPRIATE HEALTH CARE
- Doctor's care.
- Surgery (sometimes) to insert metal pins or screws to hold broken bits of bone together and to repair ruptured tendons.

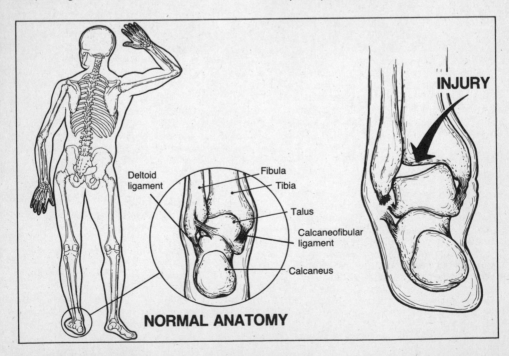

Deltoid ligament
Fibula
Tibia
Talus
Calcaneofibular ligament
Calcaneus

NORMAL ANATOMY

INJURY

- Physical therapy after the cast is removed.
- Self-care during rehabilitation.

DIAGNOSTIC MEASURES
- Your own observation of symptoms.
- Medical history and exam by a doctor.
- X-rays of injured areas to assess total injury. Dislocations of the ankle bones are frequently associated with fractures and sprains (torn ligaments) of the ankle.

POSSIBLE COMPLICATIONS
- Excessive bleeding or postoperative infection.
- Prolonged healing time if usual activities are resumed too soon.
- Proneness to repeated ankle injury.
- Unstable or permanently arthritic ankle joint, if many repeat injuries occur.

PROBABLE OUTCOME
- A dislocated ankle with a fracture-sprain requires an average of 18 to 20 weeks to heal completely. Surgical pins or screws are usually removed in 8 to 12 weeks. If this is a first-time injury, proper care, surgery and sufficient healing time before resuming activity should prevent permanent disability.
- If non-surgical treatment is chosen, healing time with total lack of weight-bearing may require 12 months.

 ## HOW TO TREAT

NOTE—Follow your doctor's instructions. These instructions are supplemental.

FIRST AID—Use instructions for R.I.C.E., the first letters of *rest, ice, compression* and *elevation.* See Appendix 1 for details.

CONTINUING CARE
- The doctor will reduce (realign) the dislocated bones with surgery or, if possible, without. The setting lines up the dislocated bones as close to their normal position as possible. Manipulation should be done as soon as possible after injury. Six or more hours after the dislocation, bleeding and displacement of body fluids may lead to shock. Also, many tissues lose their elasticity and become difficult to return to a normal position.
- Following surgery, the physician may apply a stirrup boot splint from below the knee to the toes. Stirrup boots are less likely to cause problems with swelling at this time than a cast may cause. This will support the ankle enough to allow you to walk with crutches, but you should not put weight on the injured ankle.
- When the swelling subsides several days later, sutures may be removed and the splint replaced by a walking-boot cast. This cast may need to stay in place for 10 to 21 days. Start walking on the walking cast immediately.
- After the cast has been removed, strapping will be necessary for a minimum of 6 weeks.
- Bathe and shower as usual after the cast is removed, even if sutures are still in place.
- Use ice massage. Fill a large Styrofoam cup with water and freeze. Tear a small amount of foam from the top so ice protrudes. Massage firmly over the injured area in a circle about the size of a baseball. Do this for 15 minutes at a time, 3 or 4 times a day, and before workouts or competition.
- Apply heat instead of ice, if it feels better. Use heat lamps, hot soaks, hot showers, heating pads, or heat liniments or ointments.
- Take whirlpool treatments, if available.
- Gentle massage will frequently provide comfort and decrease swelling.

MEDICATIONS
- For minor discomfort, you may use:
  Non-prescription medicines such as aspirin, acetaminophen or ibuprofen.
  Topical liniments and ointments.
- Your doctor may prescribe stronger medicine for pain, if needed.

ACTIVITY
- Walk with crutches until your doctor applies the walking cast. See Appendix 3 (Safe Use of Crutches).
- Resume your normal activities gradually.
- Don't drive until healing is complete. Use a vehicle with an automatic transmission, if possible.

DIET—During recovery, eat a well-balanced diet that includes extra protein, such as meat, fish, poultry, cheese, milk and eggs. Increase fiber and fluid intake to prevent constipation that may result from decreased activity. Your doctor may suggest vitamin and mineral supplements to promote healing.

REHABILITATION
- Begin daily rehabilitation exercises when supportive wrapping is no longer needed. Use ice massage for 10 minutes prior to exercise.
- See pages 446 and 462 for rehabilitation exercises.

 ## CALL YOUR DOCTOR IF

- You have symptoms of any severe ankle injury.
- Pain, swelling or bruising increases despite treatment.
- You notice numbness or discoloration of the toes when the walking cast is in place.
- Signs of postoperative infection occur, such as fever, drainage from the surgical wound or increasing pain at the operative site.

ANKLE EXOSTOSIS

GENERAL INFORMATION

DEFINITION—A piling up of bone at the site of a new or repeat injury, usually caused by direct trauma.

BODY PARTS INVOLVED
- Lower part of the tibia (lower-leg bone).
- Heel and other foot bones.
- Other areas of the foot (sometimes).
- Blood vessels, nerves, periosteum (covering of bone), and other soft tissue close to the exostosis.

SIGNS & SYMPTOMS
- Loss of "push" or "drive" (the ability to push off rapidly and forcefully in running).
- Inability to run, cut or jump at full speed.
- Low level of ankle pain with activity. Sometimes no pain exists.
- No tenderness or pressure with a physical examination. Sometimes pain and tenderness in the ankle and top of the heel bone can be detected only by special examination from a trained medical professional.
- Change in ankle-bone contours. This begins as a small irregular bump that progresses to a large calcified spur (1cm or more in length). In the worst cases, the exostosis may break away and appear on the X-ray as a calcified foreign body.

- "Locking" if the tendon catches on the exostosis during exercise.

CAUSES
- Repeated ankle or foot injury, even mild injury.
- Participation in sports that require "pushing off" or "springing" from a position with the foot bent upward.

RISK INCREASES WITH
- Medical history of repeated ankle injury.
- Vitamin and mineral deficiency, which makes complications following injury more likely.
- Poor muscle strength or conditioning, which fosters improper movement and allows undue stress on the ankle and foot bones.
- Improper or inadequate strapping prior to participation in contact sports.
- If surgery is necessary, surgical risk increases with smoking and use of drugs, including mind-altering drugs, muscle relaxants, tranquilizers, sleep inducers, insulin, sedatives, beta-adrenergic blockers or corticosteroids.

HOW TO PREVENT
- Engage in vigorous muscle strengthening and conditioning prior to regular participation in sports.
- Allow full healing time after an ankle or foot injury before resuming any sport that requires you to push off and run.

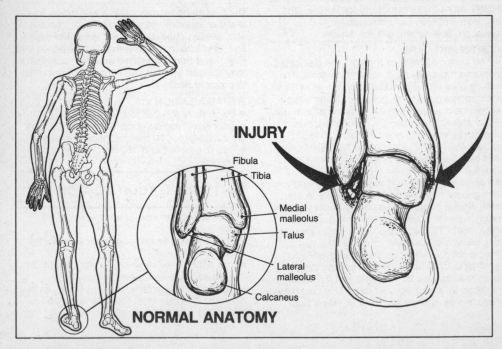

INJURY

Fibula
Tibia
Medial malleolus
Talus
Lateral malleolus
Calcaneus

NORMAL ANATOMY

- Warm up adequately before competition or workouts.

WHAT TO EXPECT

APPROPRIATE HEALTH CARE
- Doctor's diagnosis and care.
- Surgery to remove the exostosis (sometimes).
- Self-care during recovery.

DIAGNOSTIC MEASURES
- Your own observation of symptoms.
- Medical history and physical exam by a doctor.
- X-rays of the foot, ankle and knee.

POSSIBLE COMPLICATIONS
- Disability severe enough to diminish an athlete's competitive ability if the exostosis is untreated. Because mild exostosis is not readily apparent, coaches and other athletes often attribute the decline in performance to emotional causes or a loss of competitive drive in the athlete, rather than understanding that it is caused by a physical disability (exostosis).
- Proneness to repeated injury.
- Degenerative arthritic changes in the ankle joint and cartilage in later life.
- Pressure on or injury to nearby nerves, ligaments, tendons, blood vessels or connective tissue.

PROBABLE OUTCOME—Exostosis usually causes no disability with proper treatment, including rest of the injured ankle, heat treatments, corticosteroid injections, and protection against additional injury. In a few cases, surgery is necessary. No surgical treatment is required for mild conditions that do not interfere with performance.

HOW TO TREAT

NOTE—Follow your doctor's instructions. These instructions are supplemental.

FIRST AID—None. The problem develops gradually.

CONTINUING CARE
- Apply heat frequently. Use heat lamps, hot soaks, hot showers, heating pads, or heat liniments and ointments.
- Take whirlpool treatments, if available.
- Gentle massage will frequently provide comfort and decrease swelling.

MEDICATION—Medicine usually is not necessary for this disorder. For minor discomfort, you may use non-prescription drugs such as aspirin or ibuprofen.

ACTIVITY—Rest the injured ankle for 2 to 4 weeks. Use splints or crutches, if necessary, to prevent weight-bearing. Elevate the foot when sitting or lying down. Resume your normal activities gradually.

DIET—During recovery, eat a well-balanced diet that includes extra protein, such as meat, fish, poultry, cheese, milk and eggs. Increase fiber and fluid intake to prevent constipation that may result from decreased activity. Your doctor may suggest vitamin and mineral supplements to promote healing.

REHABILITATION
- Begin daily rehabilitation exercises when pain subsides and you have clearance from your doctor.
- Use ice massage for 10 minutes before and 10 minutes after exercise. Fill a large Styrofoam cup with water and freeze. Tear a small amount of foam from the top so ice protrudes. Massage firmly over the injured area in a circle about the size of a baseball.
- See pages 446 and 462 for rehabilitation exercises.

CALL YOUR DOCTOR IF

- Your ability to push off with the foot and ankle diminishes for no apparent reason.
- Any of the following occurs after surgery: Numbness or discoloration of the toes when the walking cast is in place.
  Signs of infection (headache, muscle aches, dizziness, or a general ill feeling and fever).
  Increased pain, swelling, redness, drainage, or bleeding in the surgical area.
  New, unexplained symptoms. Drugs used in treatment may cause side effects.

ANKLE FRACTURE, BIMALLEOLAR

GENERAL INFORMATION

DEFINITION—A break in the bones of both sides of the ankle. A temporary dislocation and rupture of ligaments of the ankle joint may also accompany this injury. The fracture sites include both of the mallet-shaped sides of the lower end of the tibia (leg bone) and the corresponding side of the fibula (leg bone). The full extent of injury may not be recognized immediately.

BODY PARTS INVOLVED
● Three main bones of the ankle joint—the talus, tibia and fibula.
● Ligaments that support the ankle joint.
● Blood vessels, nerves, periosteum (covering of bone), and other soft tissue close to the injury site.

SIGNS & SYMPTOMS
● Severe, immediate ankle pain.
● A feeling of popping or tearing in the outer or inner part of the ankle. Sometimes it will feel as if the ankle joint was temporarily dislocated and popped back into joint. A sound may be heard at the time of fracture.
● Severe tenderness at the injury site.
● The injured person usually falls at the time of injury and has great difficulty walking.
● General swelling and bruising immediately throughout the ankle and foot.

CAUSES—Direct blow or stress imposed from either side of the ankle joint. The ligament or ligaments that normally hold the joint in place are stretched and sometimes torn.

RISK INCREASES WITH
● Sports that demand quick changes in direction, such as football and skiing.
● Activities involving jumping, such as basketball, soccer, volleyball, distance-jumping and high-jumping. Participants often accidentally land on the side of the foot or someone else lands on their foot.
● Walking or running on rough surfaces, such as roads with potholes.
● Shoes with inadequate support to prevent the foot from rolling over when stress occurs.
● Poor nutrition.
● Poor muscle strength or conditioning.
● Inadequate strapping prior to contact or collision sports.
● Previous ankle injury.

HOW TO PREVENT
● Build your strength with a conditioning program appropriate for your sport.
● Warm up before practice or competition.
● Tape the ankle from midfoot to midcalf before practice or competition. If you cannot use tape, wrap the ankle with elastic bandages.
● Wear proper protective shoes.
● Provide the ankle with substantial support

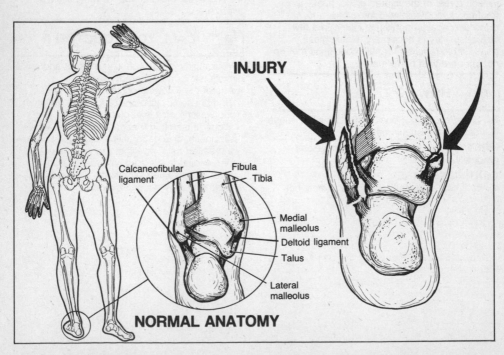

INJURY

Calcaneofibular ligament
Fibula
Tibia
Medial malleolus
Deltoid ligament
Talus
Lateral malleolus

NORMAL ANATOMY

during sports activities for 12 months following any significant ankle injury.

 ## WHAT TO EXPECT

APPROPRIATE HEALTH CARE
- Surgery to pin broken bones.
- Doctor's care.
- Physical therapy after the cast is removed.
- Self-care during rehabilitation.

DIAGNOSTIC MEASURES
- Your own observation of symptoms.
- Medical history and exam by a doctor.
- X-rays of injured areas to assess total injury. Fractures of the ankle bones are often associated with torn ligaments (sprains).

POSSIBLE COMPLICATIONS
- Excessive postoperative bleeding or infection.
- Prolonged healing time if usual activities are resumed too soon.
- Proneness to repeated ankle injury.
- Unstable or permanently arthritic ankle joint, if many repeat injuries occur. Arthritic changes may also occur in the knee joint because the ankle fracture sometimes causes added stress on the knee due to changes in weight-bearing.

PROBABLE OUTCOME—Ankle fractures require an average of 18 to 20 weeks to heal completely. Surgical pins or screws are usually removed in 8 to 12 weeks. If this is a first-time injury, proper care, surgery and sufficient healing time before resuming activity should prevent permanent disability. If non-surgical treatment is chosen, healing time and inability to bear weight may require 12 months.

 ## HOW TO TREAT

NOTE—Follow your doctor's instructions. These instructions are supplemental.

FIRST AID—Use instructions for R.I.C.E., the first letters of *rest, ice, compression* and *elevation*. See Appendix 1 for details.

CONTINUING CARE
- Following surgery, the physician may apply a stirrup boot splint from below the knee to the toes. Stirrup boots are less likely to cause problems with swelling than a cast may cause. This will support the joint effectively enough to walk on crutches, but you should not bear weight on the injured ankle.
- When the swelling subsides in several days, sutures are usually removed and the splint is replaced by a walking-boot cast. This cast may need to stay in place for 10 to 21 days. You may walk on the walking cast immediately.
- After the cast is removed, strapping will be necessary for a minimum of 6 weeks.
- Bathe and shower as usual after the cast is removed, even if sutures are still in place.
- Use an ice pack 3 or 4 times a day. Wrap ice chips or cubes in a plastic bag. Wrap the bag in a moist towel, and place it over the injured ankle. Use for 20 minutes at a time.
- Apply heat instead of ice, if it feels better. Use heat lamps, hot soaks, hot showers, heating pads, or heat liniments and ointments.
- Take whirlpool treatments, if available.
- Massage the ankle gently and often to provide comfort and decrease swelling.

MEDICATIONS
- For minor discomfort, you may use:
  Non-prescription medicines such as aspirin, acetaminophen or ibuprofen.
  Topical liniments and ointments.
- Your doctor may prescribe stronger medicine for pain, if needed.

ACTIVITY—Walk with crutches until your surgeon applies the walking cast. See Appendix 3 (Safe Use of Crutches). Resume your normal activities gradually, but don't drive until healing is complete.

DIET—During recovery, eat a well-balanced diet that includes extra protein, such as meat, fish, poultry, cheese, milk and eggs. Increase fiber and fluid intake to prevent constipation that may result from decreased activity.

REHABILITATION
- Begin daily rehabilitation exercises when movement is comfortable.
- Use ice massage for 10 minutes before and 10 minutes after exercise. Fill a large Styrofoam cup with water and freeze. Tear a small amount of foam from the top so ice protrudes. Massage firmly over the injured area in a circle.
- See pages 446 and 462 for rehabilitation exercises.

 ## CALL YOUR DOCTOR IF

- You have symptoms of any severe ankle injury.
- Pain, swelling or bruising increase during treatment or rehabilitation.
- You notice numbness or discoloration of the toes when the walking cast is in place.
- You develop signs of postoperative infection (fever or increasing pain or drainage from the surgical wound).

ANKLE FRACTURE, CHONDRAL

GENERAL INFORMATION

DEFINITION—A fracture of the ankle involving both bone and cartilage, accompanied by a total tear (or sprain) of one or more ligaments. A temporary dislocation of the ankle joint may also occur. Two-ligament sprains with a chondral fracture of the ankle will cause more disability than a single-ligament sprain.

BODY PARTS INVOLVED
- Bones and cartilage of the foot and heel.
- Ligaments that support the ankle joint.
- Weight-bearing surfaces of the ankle.

SIGNS & SYMPTOMS
- Severe pain in the ankle appearing at the time of the injury.
- Popping or a feeling of tearing in the outer or inner part of the ankle. Sometimes there will be a sensation that the ankle joint is dislocated or was temporarily dislocated and popped back into joint.
- Severe tenderness at the injury site.
- Loss of function. The injured person usually falls at the time of injury and has great difficulty when attempting to walk. The ankle loses its stability.
- Looseness in the joint if the foot is forced in the direction of pain.
- Generalized swelling immediately throughout the ankle and foot.
- Bruising immediately or soon after injury.

- Continuing signs and symptoms with little improvement, indicating an injury more severe than a simple sprain.

CAUSES—Stress imposed from either side of the ankle joint that temporarily forces or pries the ankle or heel bone (talus) out of its normal socket. The ligaments that normally hold the joint in place are stretched and torn.

RISK INCREASES WITH
- Previous ankle injury.
- Activities in which the foot may land sideways, such as running, walking, and jumping in such sports as basketball, soccer, volleyball, skiing, distance and high jumping.
- Shoes with inadequate support to prevent sideways displacement when stress occurs.
- Poor nutrition, especially calcium deficiency.
- Poor muscle strength or conditioning.
- Inadequate ankle strapping prior to participation in contact sports.
- Walking or running on rough surfaces, such as roads with potholes.

HOW TO PREVENT
- Engage in vigorous presport strengthening and conditioning.
- Tape ankle adequately (midfoot to midcalf) before participation in contact sports. Otherwise, wear supportive elastic ankle wraps (not as good as tape, but better than nothing).
- Provide the ankle with substantial support during sports activities for 12 months following any significant ankle injury.

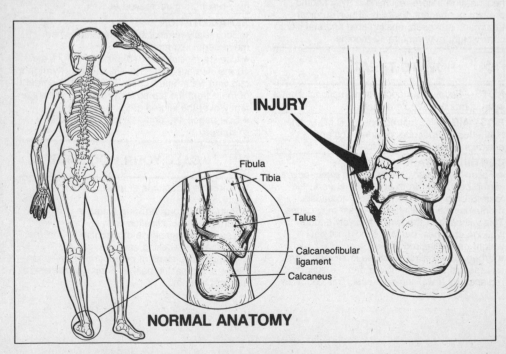

INJURY

Fibula
Tibia
Talus
Calcaneofibular ligament
Calcaneus

NORMAL ANATOMY

WHAT TO EXPECT

APPROPRIATE HEALTH CARE
• Hospitalization for surgery to insert metal pins or screws to hold broken bits of bone together and to repair the ruptured ligaments.
• Doctor's care for application of a walking cast after surgery and ankle taping when the cast is no longer needed.
• Physical therapy after the cast is removed.

DIAGNOSTIC MEASURES
• Your own observation of symptoms.
• Medical history and exam by a doctor.
• X-rays of injured areas to assess total injury. Chondral fractures of ankle bones are often associated with torn ligaments (sprains).

POSSIBLE COMPLICATIONS
• Full extent of the injury is sometimes not recognized immediately, delaying treatment.
• Prolonged healing time if activity is resumed too soon.
• Proneness to repeated ankle injury.
• Unstable or arthritic ankle joint following repeated injury.

PROBABLE OUTCOME—Healing time after
surgery averages 18 to 20 weeks. The pins or screws inserted surgically to hold bones together are usually removed in 8 to 12 weeks. If this is a first-time injury, proper care (including surgery) and sufficient time for healing before resuming activity should prevent permanent disability. Torn ligaments require as much time to heal as fractured bones. If non-surgical treatment is chosen and no weight is put on the ankle, healing time may take up to 12 months.

 HOW TO TREAT

NOTE—Follow your doctor's instructions. These instructions are supplemental.

FIRST AID
• Use instructions for R.I.C.E., the first letters of *rest, ice, compression* and *elevation.* See Appendix 1 for details.
• To prevent further injury to the ankle, avoid any weight-bearing. Go to your doctor's office or hospital emergency room as soon as possible.

CONTINUING CARE
• Following surgery, the doctor may apply a stirrup boot splint from below the knee to the toes. Stirrup boots are less likely to cause problems with swelling than a cast may cause. This will support the joint effectively enough to walk on crutches, but you should not bear weight on the injured ankle.
• When the swelling subsides several days later, sutures may be removed and the splint

will be replaced by a walking-boot cast. See Appendix 2 (Care of Casts). This cast may need to stay in place for 10 to 21 days. Start walking on the walking cast immediately.
• After the cast has been removed, strapping will be necessary for a minimum of 6 weeks.
• After cast removal, use frequent ice massage. Fill a large Styrofoam cup with water and freeze. Tear a small amount of foam from the top so ice protrudes. Massage firmly over the injured area in a circle about the size of a baseball. Do this for 15 minutes at a time, 3 or 4 times a day.
• Apply heat instead of ice if it feels better. Use heat lamps, hot soaks, hot showers, heating pads, or heat liniments or ointments.
• Take whirlpool treatments, if available.
• Gentle, frequent massage will provide comfort and decrease swelling.

MEDICATION
• For minor discomfort, you may use:
  Non-prescription medicines such as aspirin, acetaminophen or ibuprofen.
  Topical liniments and ointments.
• Your doctor may prescribe stronger medicine for pain, if needed.

ACTIVITY—Walk with crutches until your doctor
applies the walking cast. See Appendix 3 (Safe Use of Crutches.) Resume your normal activities gradually. Don't drive until healing is complete.

DIET
• Drink only water before manipulation or surgery to treat the fracture. Solid food in your stomach makes vomiting while under anesthesia more hazardous.
• During recovery, eat a well-balanced diet that includes extra protein, such as meat, fish, poultry, cheese, milk and eggs. Increase fiber and fluid intake to prevent constipation that may result from decreased activity.

REHABILITATION—Begin daily rehabilitation
exercises when supportive wrapping is no longer needed. Use ice massage for 10 minutes prior to exercise. See pages 446 and 462 for rehabilitation exercises.

 CALL YOUR DOCTOR IF

• You have signs or symptoms of any severe ankle injury.
• Pain, swelling or bruising increase during treatment or rehabilitation.
• You notice numbness or discoloration of toes when the walking cast is in place.
• Signs of postoperative infection occur, including fever, drainage from the surgical wound or increasing pain at the surgical site.

ANKLE SPRAIN, GRADE 1
(Mild or 1st Degree Ankle Sprain)

 GENERAL INFORMATION

DEFINITION—Stretching and slight or partial tearing of one or more ligaments in the ankle. A two-ligament sprain causes more disability than a single-ligament sprain.

BODY PARTS INVOLVED
● Ligaments that support the ankle joint.
● Three main bones of the ankle joint—the talus (heel bone), and the tibia and fibula (lower leg bones).
● Blood vessels, nerves, periosteum (covering of bone), and other soft tissue close to the injury.

SIGNS & SYMPTOMS
● Ankle pain at the time of injury.
● A feeling of popping or tearing in the outer part of the ankle.
● Mild tenderness at the injury site.
● Little loss of function. The injured person can bear weight and walk without help for 30 minutes or so following injury. Then, depending on the extent of injury, the joint may seem to lose some of its stability.
● Swelling in the ankle.
● Little or no visible bruising for several hours after injury. Then some bruising may appear.

CAUSES—Stress imposed from either side of the ankle joint, temporarily forcing or prying the ankle or heel bone out of its normal socket. The ligaments that normally hold the joint in place are stretched and sometimes torn.

RISK INCREASES WITH
● Previous ankle injury.
● Any sport in which sideways displacement of the ankle is likely. Runners, walkers, and participants in such sports as basketball, soccer, volleyball, skiing, distance jumping and high jumping are prone to ankle sprains. When jumping, they often accidentally land on the side of the foot.
● Use of shoes with insufficient support to prevent sideways displacement when stress occurs.
● Poor muscle strength or conditioning.
● Inadequate strapping prior to participation in contact sports.
● Walking or running on rough surfaces, such as roads with potholes.

HOW TO PREVENT
● Build your strength with a conditioning program appropriate for your sport.
● Warm up before practice or competition.
● Tape the ankle from midfoot to midcalf before practice or competition. If you cannot use tape,

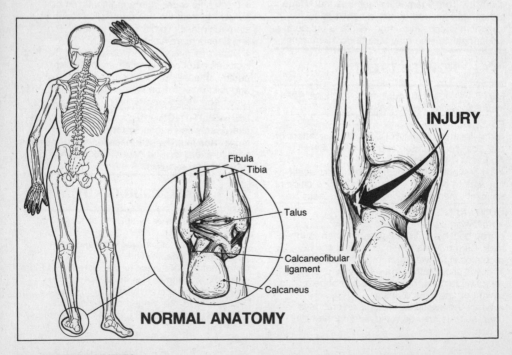

Fibula
Tibia
Talus
Calcaneofibular ligament
Calcaneus

NORMAL ANATOMY

INJURY

wrap the ankle with elastic bandages or use an elastic brace.
- Wear proper protective shoes.
- Provide the ankle with substantial support during sports activities for 12 months following any significant ankle injury.

 ## WHAT TO EXPECT

APPROPRIATE HEALTH CARE
- Doctor's care only if discomfort is great or doesn't improve in 24 hours.
- Self-care after diagnosis.
- Whirlpool, ultrasound or massage (to displace fluid from the injured joint space).

DIAGNOSTIC MEASURES
- Your own observation of symptoms.
- Medical history and exam by a doctor.
- X-rays of the ankle, foot and knee to rule out fractures.

POSSIBLE COMPLICATIONS
- Prolonged healing time if activity is resumed too soon.
- Proneness to repeated injury.
- Unstable or arthritic ankle joint following repeated injury.

PROBABLE OUTCOME—The full extent of the injury cannot be determined for 12 to 24 hours. A first-degree ankle sprain usually heals enough in 5 to 7 days to allow modified activity. Complete healing requires an average of 6 weeks.

 ## HOW TO TREAT

NOTE—Follow your doctor's instructions. These instructions are supplemental.

FIRST AID—The goal is to prevent further injury to the torn ligaments. Follow instructions for R.I.C.E., the first letters of *rest, ice, compression* and *elevation*. See Appendix 1 for details.

CONTINUING CARE
- Continue using an ice pack 3 or 4 times a day. Wrap ice chips or cubes in a plastic bag. Wrap the bag in a moist towel, and place it over the injured area. Use for 20 minutes at a time.

- After 72 hours, apply heat instead of ice if it feels better. Use heat lamps, hot soaks, hot showers, heating pads, or heat liniments or ointments.
- Take whirlpool treatments, if available.
- Keep the foot elevated whenever possible to decrease swelling.
- Massage the ankle gently and often to provide comfort and decrease swelling.

MEDICATION
- For minor discomfort, you may use:
  Non-prescription medicines such as aspirin, acetaminophen or ibuprofen.
  Topical liniments or ointments.
- Your doctor may prescribe:
  Injection of procaine and hyaluronidase to decrease pain soon after injury.
  Stronger medicine for pain, if needed.

ACTIVITY—Except for very minor injuries, walk with crutches for about 72 hours. See Appendix 3 (Safe Use of Crutches). Resume your normal activities gradually.

DIET—During recovery, eat a well-balanced diet that includes extra protein, such as meat, fish, poultry, cheese, milk and eggs. Increase fiber and fluid intake to prevent constipation that may result from decreased activity. Your doctor may suggest vitamin and mineral supplements to promote healing.

REHABILITATION
- Begin daily rehabilitation exercises when supportive wrapping is no longer needed.
- Use ice massage for 10 minutes before and 10 minutes after exercise. Fill a large Styrofoam cup with water and freeze. Tear a small amount of foam from the top so ice protrudes. Massage firmly over the injured area in a circle about the size of a baseball.
- See pages 446 and 462 for rehabilitation exercises.

 ## CALL YOUR DOCTOR IF

- You have symptoms of an ankle sprain that does not improve within 1 week.
- Ankle pain, swelling or bruising increase despite treatment.

ANKLE SPRAIN, GRADE 2
(Moderate or 2nd Degree Ankle Sprain)

 GENERAL INFORMATION

DEFINITION—Stretching and partial tearing of one or more ligaments of the ankle, resulting in weakening and some loss of ankle function. A two-ligament sprain causes more disability than a single-ligament sprain.

BODY PARTS INVOLVED
- Ligaments that support the ankle joint.
- Three main bones of the ankle joint—the talus (heel bone), and the tibia and fibula (lower leg bones).
- Blood vessels, nerves, periosteum (covering of bone), and other soft tissue close to the injury.

SIGNS & SYMPTOMS
- Severe ankle pain at the time of injury.
- A feeling of popping or tearing in the outer part of the ankle.
- Extreme tenderness at the injury site.
- Loss of function. The injured person usually falls, but can walk a little since direct weight-bearing does not place stress on the injured ankle. Then, depending on the extent of injury, the joint may seem to lose some stability.
- Looseness in the joint if the foot is forced in the direction of pain.
- Generalized swelling immediately throughout the ankle and foot.
- Bruising that appears soon after injury.

CAUSES—Stress imposed from either side of the ankle joint, temporarily forcing or prying the ankle or heel bone out of its normal socket. The ligaments that normally hold the joint in place are stretched and torn.

RISK INCREASES WITH
- Previous ankle injury.
- Any sport in which sideways displacement of the ankle is likely. Runners, walkers, and participants in sports such as basketball, soccer, volleyball, skiing, distance jumping and high jumping are prone to ankle sprains. They often accidentally land on the side of the foot.
- Use of shoes with inadequate support to prevent sideways displacement when stress occurs.
- Poor muscle strength or conditioning.
- Inadequate strapping prior to participation in contact sports.
- Walking or running on rough surfaces, such as roads with potholes.

HOW TO PREVENT
- Build your strength with a conditioning program appropriate for your sport.
- Warm up before practice or competition.
- Tape the ankle from midfoot to midcalf before practice or competition. If you cannot use tape, wrap the ankle with elastic bandages or use an elastic brace.

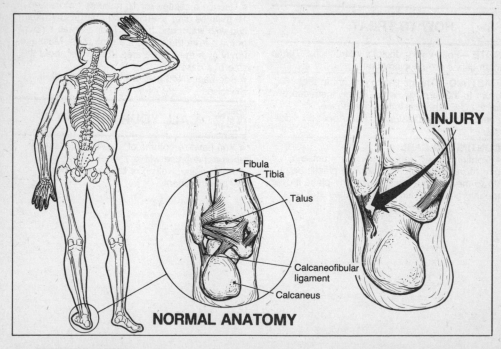

Fibula
Tibia
Talus
Calcaneofibular ligament
Calcaneus

NORMAL ANATOMY

INJURY

- Wear proper protective shoes.
- Provide the ankle with substantial support during sports activities for 12 months following any significant ankle injury.

 ## WHAT TO EXPECT

APPROPRIATE HEALTH CARE
- Doctor's care to apply a walking cast, and to apply tape after cast removal.
- Whirlpool, ultrasound and massage (to displace accumulated fluid in injured joint spaces).

DIAGNOSTIC MEASURES
- Your own observation of symptoms.
- Medical history and exam by a doctor.
- X-rays of the injured areas to rule out fractures.

POSSIBLE COMPLICATIONS
- Prolonged healing time if activity is resumed too soon.
- Proneness to repeated injury.
- Unstable or arthritic ankle joint following repeated injury.

PROBABLE OUTCOME—The full extent of injury cannot be determined for 12 to 24 hours. A second-degree ankle sprain requires an average of 6 to 10 weeks to heal completely. If this is a first-time injury, proper treatment and sufficient healing time before resuming activity should prevent permanent disability. Ligaments have a poor blood supply, and torn ligaments require as much healing time as fractures.

 ## HOW TO TREAT

NOTE—Follow your doctor's instructions. These instructions are supplemental.

FIRST AID—The goal is to prevent further injury to the torn ligaments. Follow instructions for R.I.C.E., the first letters of *rest, ice, compression* and *elevation*. See Appendix 1 for details.

CONTINUING CARE
- Keep ice packs on the injured area almost continuously for 24 hours.
- Wrap an elastic bandage over a sponge-rubber donut over the sprained area to compress the area for about 72 hours.
- After the first 24 hours, your doctor may apply a stirrup boot splint from below the knee to the toes. This will support the ankle enough to walk on crutches, but you should not bear weight on the injured ankle yet.
- When the swelling subsides in several days,

the splint is replaced by a walking-boot cast for 10 to 21 days. You may walk on the walking cast immediately.
- After the cast has been removed, strapping will be necessary for a minimum of 6 weeks.
- After cast removal (or if a cast was not used), continue using an ice pack 3 or 4 times a day. Wrap ice chips or cubes in a plastic bag. Wrap the bag in a moist towel, and place it over the injured area. Use for 20 minutes at a time.
- Apply heat Instead of ice, if it feels better. Use heat lamps, hot soaks, hot showers, heating pads, or heat liniments or ointments.
- Take whirlpool treatments, if available.
- Keep the foot elevated whenever possible to decrease swelling.
- Gentle massage will frequently provide comfort and decrease swelling.

MEDICATION
- For minor discomfort, you may use:
  Non-prescription medicines such as aspirin, acetaminophen or ibuprofen.
  Topical liniments and ointments.
- Your doctor may prescribe:
  Injection of procaine and hyaluronidase to decrease pain soon after injury.
  Stronger medicine for pain, if needed.

ACTIVITY—Use a splint and crutches or a walking-boot cast as prescribed by your doctor. After the cast is removed, resume your normal activities gradually. Don't drive until the ankle is completely healed.

DIET—During recovery, eat a well-balanced diet that includes extra protein, such as meat, fish, poultry, cheese, milk and eggs. Increase fiber and fluid intake to prevent constipation that may result from decreased activity.

REHABILITATION
- Begin daily rehabilitation exercises when supportive wrapping is no longer needed.
- Use ice massage for 10 minutes before and 10 minutes after exercise. Fill a large Styrofoam cup with water and freeze. Tear a small amount of foam from the top so ice protrudes. Massage firmly in a circle over the injured area.
- See pages 446 and 462 for rehabilitation exercises.

 ## CALL YOUR DOCTOR IF

- You have symptoms of a second-degree ankle sprain.
- Ankle pain, swelling or bruising increases despite treatment.
- You experience numbness or discoloration of toes when the walking cast is in place.

ANKLE SPRAIN, GRADE 3
(Severe or 3rd Degree Ankle Sprain)

 GENERAL INFORMATION

DEFINITION—A severe injury to the ankle in which one or more ligaments are stretched and totally torn. A severe sprain may include a temporary or lasting dislocation. A two-ligament sprain causes more disability than a single-ligament sprain.

BODY PARTS INVOLVED
● Ligaments that support the ankle joint.
● Three main bones of the ankle joint—the talus (heel bone), and the tibia and fibula (lower leg bones).
● Blood vessels, nerves, periosteum (covering of bone) and other soft tissue close to the injury.

SIGNS & SYMPTOMS
● Severe ankle pain at the time of injury.
● A feeling of popping or tearing in the outer or inner part of the ankle. Sometimes there will be a sensation that the ankle joint is dislocated or was temporarily dislocated and popped back into joint.
● Severe tenderness at the injury site.
● Loss of function. The injured person usually falls and has great difficulty walking. The joint loses its stability.
● Looseness in the joint if the foot is forced in the direction of pain.

● Immediate, generalized swelling throughout the ankle and foot.
● Bruising that appears immediately or soon after injury.

CAUSES—Stress imposed from either side of the ankle joint, temporarily forcing or prying the ankle or heel bone out of its normal socket. The ligament or ligaments that normally hold the joint in place are stretched and torn.

RISK INCREASES WITH
● Previous ankle injury.
● Any sport in which sideways displacement of the ankle is likely. Runners, walkers and participants in such sports as basketball, soccer, volleyball, skiing, distance jumping and high jumping are prone to ankle sprains. They often accidentally land on the side of the foot.
● Use of shoes with inadequate support to prevent sideways displacement when stress occurs.
● Poor muscle strength or conditioning.
● Inadequate strapping prior to participation in contact sports.
● Walking or running on rough surfaces, such as roads with potholes.

HOW TO PREVENT
● Build your strength with a conditioning program appropriate for your sport.
● Warm up before practice or competition.

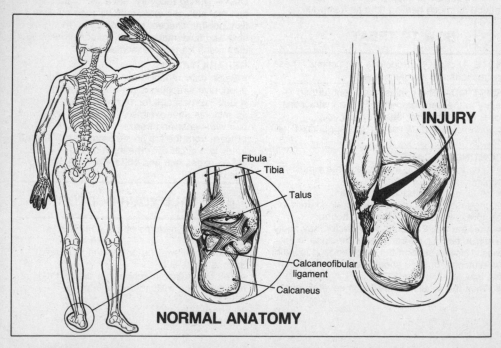

Fibula
Tibia
Talus
Calcaneofibular ligament
Calcaneus
NORMAL ANATOMY

INJURY

- Tape the ankle from midfoot to midcalf before practice or competition. If you cannot use tape, wrap the ankle with elastic bandages or use an elastic brace.
- Wear proper protective shoes.
- Provide the ankle with substantial support during sports activities for 12 months following any significant ankle injury.

WHAT TO EXPECT

APPROPRIATE HEALTH CARE
- Doctor's care.
- Application of a walking cast, and taping of the ankle when the cast is no longer needed.
- Physical therapy after the cast is removed.
- Hospitalization for surgery (sometimes) to repair the torn ligaments.

DIAGNOSTIC MEASURES
- Your own observation of symptoms.
- Medical history and exam by a doctor.
- X-rays of injured areas to assess total injury. Grade 3 sprains are often accompanied by fractures of the ankle bones.

POSSIBLE COMPLICATIONS
- Prolonged healing time if activity is resumed too soon.
- Proneness to repeated injury.
- Unstable or arthritic ankle joint following repeated injury.

PROBABLE OUTCOME—The full extent of injury cannot be determined for 12 to 24 hours. Third-degree ankle sprains require an average of 12 to 16 weeks to heal completely. If this is a first-time injury, proper care, surgery and sufficient healing time before resuming activity should prevent permanent disability. Ligaments have a poor blood supply, and torn ligaments require as much healing time as fractures.

HOW TO TREAT

NOTE—Follow your doctor's instructions. These instructions are supplemental.

FIRST AID—The goal is to prevent further injury to the torn ligaments. See a doctor immediately for proper diagnosis and care. Follow instructions for R.I.C.E., the first letters of *rest, ice, compression* and *elevation*. See Appendix 1 for details.

CONTINUING CARE
- The doctor may apply a stirrup-boot splint from below the knee to the toes. Stirrup boots are less likely to cause problems with swelling than an immediate cast may cause. This will support the joint effectively enough to walk on crutches, but you should not bear weight on the injured ankle.
- When the swelling subsides in several days, any sutures will probably be removed and the splint replaced by a walking-boot cast for 10 to 21 days. You may walk on the walking cast immediately.
- After the cast has been removed, ankle taping will be necessary for a minimum of 6 weeks.
- After cast removal, use an ice pack 3 or 4 times a day. Wrap ice chips or cubes in a plastic bag. Wrap the bag in a moist towel, and place it over the injured area. Use for 20 minutes at a time.
- Apply heat instead of ice if it feels better. Use heat lamps, hot soaks, hot showers, heating pads, or heat liniments or ointments.
- Take whirlpool treatments, if available.
- Keep the foot elevated whenever possible to decrease swelling.
- Massage the ankle gently and often to provide comfort and decrease swelling.

MEDICATION
- For minor discomfort, you may use:
  Non-prescription medicines such as aspirin, acetaminophen or ibuprofen.
  Topical liniments and ointments.
- Your doctor may prescribe:
  Injection of procaine and hyaluronidase to decrease pain soon after injury.
  Stronger medicine for pain, if needed.

ACTIVITY—Walk with crutches until your surgeon applies the walking cast. See Appendix 3 (Safe Use of Crutches). Resume your normal activities gradually. Don't drive until healing is complete.

DIET—During recovery, eat a well-balanced diet that includes extra protein, such as meat, fish, poultry, cheese, milk and eggs. Increase fiber and fluid intake to prevent constipation that may result from decreased activity.

REHABILITATION
- Begin daily rehabilitation exercises when supportive wrapping is no longer needed.
- Use ice massage for 10 minutes before and 10 minutes after exercise. Fill a large Styrofoam cup with water and freeze. Tear a small amount of foam from the top so ice protrudes. Massage firmly in a circle over the injured area.
- See pages 446 and 462 for rehabilitation exercises.

CALL YOUR DOCTOR IF

- You have symptoms of a third-degree ankle sprain.
- Ankle pain, swelling or bruising increases despite treatment.
- You notice numbness or discoloration of the toes when the walking cast is in place.
- You develop signs of postoperative infection (increased pain or drainage from the surgical wound, or fever).

ANKLE STRAIN

GENERAL INFORMATION

DEFINITION—Strain to any muscles or tendons that surround the ankle. Muscles, tendons and bones comprise units. These units stabilize the ankle and allow its motion. A strain occurs at the weakest part of a unit. Strains are of 3 types:
- Mild (Grade I)—Slightly pulled muscle without tearing of muscle or tendon fibers. There is no loss of strength.
- Moderate (Grade II)—Tearing of fibers in a muscle, tendon or at the attachment to bone. Strength is diminished.
- Severe (Grade III)—Rupture of the muscle-tendon-bone attachment with separation of fibers. Severe strain requires surgical repair. Chronic strains are caused by overuse. Acute strains are caused by direct injury or overstress.

BODY PARTS INVOLVED
- Tendons and muscles surrounding the ankle.
- Lower-leg bones (tibia and fibula) and foot bones.
- Soft tissue surrounding the strained muscle and attached tendon, including nerves, periosteum (covering to bone), blood vessels and lymph vessels.

SIGNS & SYMPTOMS
- Pain when moving or stretching the ankle.
- Muscle spasm in the calf.
- Tenderness to the touch.
- Swelling in the ankle.
- Loss of strength (moderate or severe strain).
- Crepitation ("crackling") feeling and sound when the ankle is pressed with fingers.
- Calcification of the muscle or its tendon (visible with X-ray).
- Inflammation of the sheath covering the tendon.

CAUSES
- Prolonged overuse of muscle-tendon units in the ankle.
- Single violent injury or force applied to the muscle-tendon unit in the ankle.

RISK INCREASES WITH
- Sports that require quick starts, such as starting a race.
- Contact sports.
- Any cardiovascular medical problem that results in decreased circulation.
- Medical history of any bleeding disorder.
- Obesity.
- Poor nutrition.
- Previous ankle injury.
- Poor muscle conditioning.

HOW TO PREVENT
- Participate in a strengthening and conditioning program appropriate for your sport.
- Warm up before practice or competition.
- Tape the ankle area before practice or competition.
- Wear proper shoes and protective equipment.

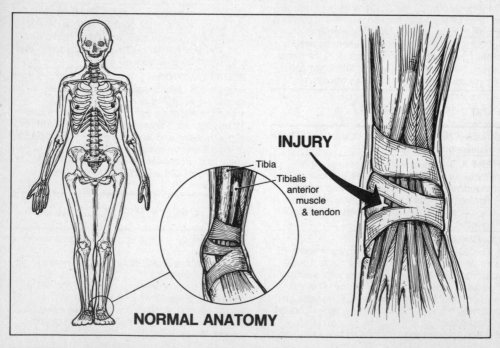

INJURY

Tibia

Tibialis anterior muscle & tendon

NORMAL ANATOMY

WHAT TO EXPECT

APPROPRIATE HEALTH CARE
- Doctor's diagnosis.
- Application of tape, splints or walking casts (sometimes).
- Self-care during rehabilitation.
- Physical therapy (moderate or severe strain).
- Surgery (severe strain).

DIAGNOSTIC MEASURES
- Your own observation of symptoms.
- Medical history and exam by a doctor.
- X-rays of the leg, foot and ankle to rule out fractures.

POSSIBLE COMPLICATIONS
- Prolonged healing time if activity is resumed too soon.
- Proneness to repeated injury.
- Unstable or arthritic ankle following repeated injury.
- Inflammation at the attachment to bone (periostitis).
- Prolonged disability (sometimes).

PROBABLE OUTCOME—If this is a first-time injury, proper care and sufficient healing time before resuming activity should prevent permanent disability. Torn ligaments and tendons require as long to heal as fractured bones. Average healing times are:
- Mild strain—2 to 10 days.
- Moderate strain—10 days to 6 weeks.
- Severe strain—6 to 10 weeks.

If this is a repeat injury, complications listed above are more likely to occur.

 HOW TO TREAT

NOTE—Follow your doctor's instructions. These instructions are supplemental.

FIRST AID—Use instructions for R.I.C.E., the first letters of *rest, ice, compression* and *elevation*. See Appendix 1 for details.

CONTINUING CARE
- Use ice massage 3 or 4 times a day for 15 minutes at a time. Fill a large Styrofoam cup with water and freeze. Tear a small amount of foam from the top so ice protrudes. Massage firmly over the injured area in a circle about the size of a softball.
- After the first 24 hours, apply heat instead of ice, if it feels better. Use heat lamps, hot soaks, hot showers, heating pads, or heat liniments or ointments.
- Take whirlpool treatments, if available.
- If a cast was used, wrap the injured ankle with an elasticized bandage between treatments after the cast is removed.
- Massage gently and often to provide comfort and decrease swelling.

MEDICATION
- For minor discomfort, you may use:
  Aspirin, acetaminophen or ibuprofen.
  Topical liniments and ointments.
- Your doctor may prescribe:
  Stronger pain relievers.
  Injection of a long-acting local anesthetic to reduce pain (rare).
  Injection of a corticosteroid, such as triamcinolone, to reduce inflammation (rare).

ACTIVITY
- For a moderate or severe strain, walk with crutches for at least 72 hours—longer with a cast or splints. See Appendix 3 (Safe Use of Crutches).
- Resume your normal activities gradually.

DIET—Eat a well-balanced diet that includes extra protein, such as meat, fish, poultry, cheese, milk and eggs. Increase fiber and fluid intake to prevent constipation that may result from decreased activity.

REHABILITATION—Begin daily rehabilitation exercises when supportive wrapping is no longer needed. Use ice massage for 10 minutes prior to exercise. See pages 446 and 462 for rehabilitation exercises.

 CALL YOUR DOCTOR IF

- You have symptoms of a moderate or severe ankle strain, or a mild strain persists longer than 10 days.
- Pain or swelling worsens despite treatment.
- The following occurs with a cast or splints:
  Pain, numbness or coldness below the injury.
  Dusky, blue or gray toenails.

ANKLE SYNOVITIS

GENERAL INFORMATION

DEFINITION—Inflammation of the synovium, the smooth, lubricated lining of the ankle joint. The synovium's lubricating fluid helps the ankle move freely and prevents bone surfaces from rubbing against each other. Synovitis is often a complication of an injury, such as a fracture, or of collagen diseases, such as gout or rheumatoid arthritis.

BODY PARTS INVOLVED
- Ankle joint.
- Synovial membrane surrounding the entire joint.
- Space between the joint and the synovial membrane.

SIGNS & SYMPTOMS
- Pain and heat in the ankle.
- No visible ankle swelling. Swelling and fluid accumulation is deep within the joint.

CAUSES
- Any injury to the ankle and ankle joint.
- Bacterial infection (frequently gonorrhea).
- Metabolic disturbance, such as an acute attack of gout or rheumatoid arthritis.

RISK INCREASES WITH
- Repeated ankle injury.
- Poor muscle strength or conditioning, which makes ankle injury more likely.
- Inadequate ankle strapping prior to participation in contact sports.
- Medical history of gout, rheumatoid arthritis, or other inflammatory joint diseases.
- Infection in another joint.
- Vitamin or mineral deficiency, which makes complications following injury more likely.

HOW TO PREVENT
- Tape the ankle securely from midfoot to midcalf before participation in contact sports. If taping is not possible, wear supportive elastic ankle wraps.
- Protect the ankle with substantial support during sports activities for 12 months after a significant ankle injury.

WHAT TO EXPECT

APPROPRIATE HEALTH CARE
- Doctor's diagnosis and application of a walking cast and tape.
- Self-care during rehabilitation.
- Whirlpool, ultrasound or massage to displace excess fluid from the injured joint space.

DIAGNOSTIC MEASURES
- Your own observation of symptoms.
- Medical history and exam by a doctor.
- X-rays of the ankle, foot and knee to rule out fractures.

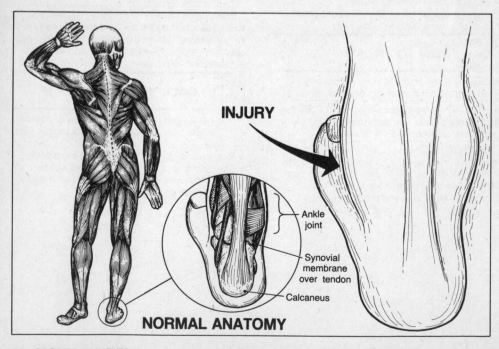

INJURY

Ankle joint

Synovial membrane over tendon

Calcaneus

NORMAL ANATOMY

POSSIBLE COMPLICATIONS
- Prolonged healing time if activity is resumed too soon.
- Proneness to repeated ankle injury.
- Unstable or arthritic ankle joint following repeated bouts of synovitis.
- Chronic synovitis that may prevent athletic participation.

PROBABLE OUTCOME—Healing is possible in 3 to 5 weeks with heat treatments, corticosteroid injections and rest (of the ankle). In many cases, ankle synovitis does not heal completely and becomes chronic. This is because the ankle joint is subjected to continual stress.

HOW TO TREAT

NOTE—Follow your doctor's instructions. These instructions are supplemental.

FIRST AID—No first aid. This condition develops gradually.

CONTINUING CARE
- Obtain treatment for any underlying medical condition, such as gout or infection.
- For greater comfort, keep the foot elevated whenever possible.
- You may need a walking plaster boot cast for 10 to 14 days. See Appendix 2, Care of Casts.
- After the cast is removed, apply heat frequently. Use heat lamps, hot soaks, hot showers, heating pads, or heat liniments and ointments.
- Take whirlpool treatments, if available.
- Massage gently and often to provide comfort and decrease swelling.
- Chronic synovitis may require ankle strapping before any workout or competition.

MEDICATION
- Your doctor may prescribe:
  Antibiotics if infection is present.
  Non-steroidal anti-inflammatory drugs or antigout medicine.
  Injection of a long-acting local anesthetic mixed with a corticosteroid to help reduce pain and inflammation.
- You may take aspirin or ibuprofen for minor discomfort.

ACTIVITY—Resume normal activities slowly as swelling, pain, redness and disability diminish.

DIET—During recovery, eat a well-balanced diet that includes extra protein, such as meat, fish, poultry, cheese, milk and eggs. Increase fiber and fluid intake to prevent constipation that may result from decreased activity. Your doctor may suggest vitamin and mineral supplements to promote healing.

REHABILITATION
- Rest the ankle for 3 to 5 weeks. Elevate it whenever possible.
- Begin daily rehabilitation exercises when a walking cast is no longer needed.
- Use ice massage for 10 minutes before and 10 minutes after exercise. Fill a large Styrofoam cup with water and freeze. Tear a small amount of foam from the top so ice protrudes. Massage firmly over the injured area in a circle about the size of a baseball.
- See pages 446 and 462 for rehabilitation exercises.

CALL YOUR DOCTOR IF

- You have symptoms of ankle synovitis.
- Symptoms worsen or persist longer than 5 weeks despite treatment outlined above.

ANKLE TENOSYNOVITIS

 GENERAL INFORMATION

DEFINITION—Inflammation of a tendon or the lining of a tendon sheath in the ankle. This lining secretes a fluid that lubricates the tendon. When the lining becomes inflamed, the tendon cannot glide smoothly in its covering.

BODY PARTS INVOLVED
- Any ankle tendon and its lining.
- Soft tissue in the surrounding area, including blood vessels, nerves, ligaments, periosteum (covering to bone) and connective tissue.

SIGNS & SYMPTOMS
- Constant pain or pain with motion.
- Limited motion of the ankle.
- Crepitation (a "crackling" sound when the tendon moves or is touched).
- Heat and redness over the inflamed tendon.

CAUSES
- Strain from unusual use or overuse of muscles and tendons in the ankle.
- Direct blow or injury to the ankle. Tenosynovitis becomes more likely with repeated ankle injury.
- Infection introduced through broken skin at the time of injury or through a surgical incision after injury.

RISK INCREASES WITH
- Contact sports, especially kicking sports such as football or soccer.

- Skiing.
- If surgery is needed, surgical risk increases with smoking, poor nutrition, alcoholism or drug abuse, and recent or chronic illness.

HOW TO PREVENT
- Engage in a vigorous program of physical conditioning before beginning regular sports participation.
- Warm up adequately before practice or competition.
- Wear protective footgear appropriate for your sport.
- Learn proper moves and techniques for your sport.

 WHAT TO EXPECT

APPROPRIATE HEALTH CARE
- Doctor's examination and diagnosis.
- Surgery (sometimes) to enlarge the tendon's covering and restore a smooth gliding motion. The surgical procedure under general anesthesia is performed in an outpatient surgical facility or hospital operating room.

DIAGNOSTIC MEASURES
- Your own observations of symptoms and signs.
- Medical history and physical examination by your doctor.
- X-rays of the area to rule out other abnormalities.

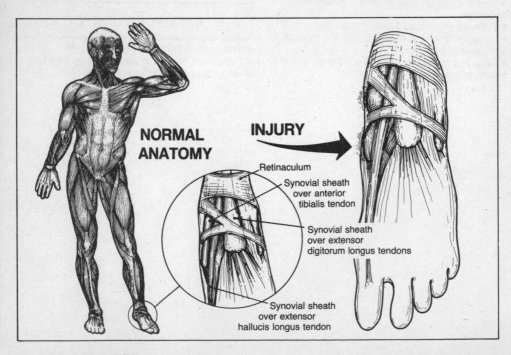

NORMAL ANATOMY

INJURY

Retinaculum

Synovial sheath over anterior tibialis tendon

Synovial sheath over extensor digitorum longus tendons

Synovial sheath over extensor hallucis longus tendon

- Laboratory studies:
  Blood and urine studies before surgery.
  Tissue examination after surgery.

POSSIBLE COMPLICATIONS
- Prolonged healing time if activity is resumed too soon.
- Proneness to repeated injury.
- Adhesive tenosynovitis: The tendon and its covering become bound together. Restriction of motion may be complete or partial. Surgery is necessary to remove the covering or transfer the tendon to a less constrictive area.
- Constrictive tenosynovitis: The walls of the covering thicken and narrow, preventing the tendon from sliding through. Surgery is necessary to cut away part of the covering.

PROBABLE OUTCOME—Tenosynovitis of the ankle is usually curable in about 6 weeks with heat treatments, corticosteroid injections and rest of the inflamed area. Recovery is usually quicker if the inflammation is caused from a direct blow rather than from a sprain or strain.

 ## HOW TO TREAT

NOTE—Follow your doctor's instructions. These instructions are supplemental.

FIRST AID—None. This problem develops slowly.

CONTINUING CARE
- If surgery is not necessary, you may need a walking-boot cast for 10 to 14 days. See Appendix 2 (Care of Casts). Then wrap the ankle with an elasticized bandage until healing is complete.
- Apply heat frequently. Use heat lamps, hot soaks, hot showers, heating pads, or heat liniments and ointments.
- Take whirlpool treatments, if available.

MEDICATION—You may use non-prescription drugs such as acetaminophen for minor pain. Your doctor may prescribe:
- Stronger pain relievers. Don't take prescription pain medication longer than 4 to 7 days. Use only as much as you need.
- Injection of the tendon covering with a long-acting local anesthetic and a non-absorbable corticosteroid to relieve pain and inflammation.

ACTIVITY—Resume normal activity slowly.

DIET—During recovery, eat a well-balanced diet that includes extra protein, such as meat, fish, poultry, cheese, milk and eggs. Increase fiber and fluid intake to prevent constipation that may result from decreased activity. Your doctor may suggest vitamin and mineral supplements to promote healing.

REHABILITATION
- Begin daily rehabilitation exercises when supportive wrapping is no longer needed.
- Use ice massage for 10 minutes before and after exercise. Fill a large Styrofoam cup with water and freeze. Tear a small amount of foam from the top so ice protrudes. Massage firmly over the injured area in a circle about the size of a softball.
- See pages 446 and 462 for rehabilitation exercises.

 ## CALL YOUR DOCTOR IF

- You have symptoms of ankle tenosynovitis.
- Any of the following occur after surgery:
  Increased pain, swelling, redness, drainage or bleeding in the surgical area.
  Signs of infection (headache, muscle aches, dizziness, or a general ill feeling and fever).
  New, unexplained symptoms. Drugs used in treatment may produce side effects.

ARM CONTUSION, FOREARM

GENERAL INFORMATION

DEFINITION—Bruising of skin and underlying tissues of the forearm caused by a direct blow. Contusions cause bleeding from ruptured small capillaries, allowing blood to infiltrate muscles, tendons or other soft tissue.

BODY PARTS INVOLVED—Tissues of the forearm, including blood vessels, muscles, tendons, nerves, covering to bone (periosteum) and connective tissue.

SIGNS & SYMPTOMS
- Forearm swelling—either superficial or deep.
- Pain and tenderness in the forearm.
- Feeling of firmness when pressure is exerted on the injured area.
- Discoloration under the skin, beginning with redness and progressing to the characteristic "black and blue" bruise.
- Restricted forearm activity proportional to the extent of injury.

CAUSES—Direct blow to the forearm, usually from a blunt object.

RISK INCREASES WITH
- Violent contact sports, especially when the forearm is not adequately protected.
- Medical history of any bleeding disorder such as hemophilia.
- Poor nutrition, including vitamin deficiency.
- Use of anticoagulants or aspirin.

HOW TO PREVENT—Wear appropriate protective gear and equipment during competition or other athletic activity if you have had a recent contusion or the activity makes a contusion likely.

WHAT TO EXPECT

APPROPRIATE HEALTH CARE
- Doctor's care, unless the contusion is quite small.
- Self-care for minor contusions and for serious contusions during rehabilitation.
- Physical therapy for serious contusions.

DIAGNOSTIC MEASURES
- Your own observation of symptoms.
- Medical history and physical exam by a doctor for all except minor injuries.
- X-rays of the injured area to assess total injury to soft tissue and to rule out the possibility of underlying fracture. Total extent of injury may not be apparent for 48 to 72 hours.

POSSIBLE COMPLICATIONS
- Excessive bleeding, leading to disability. Infiltrative-type bleeding can sometimes lead to calcification and impaired function of injured muscles and tendons.

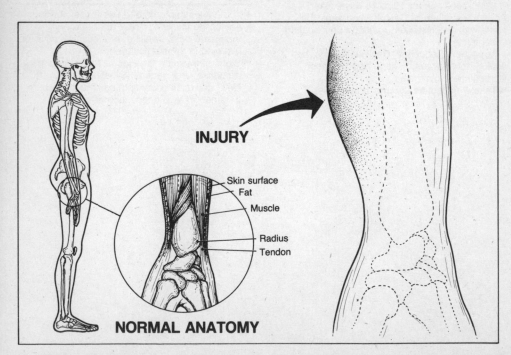

INJURY

Skin surface
Fat
Muscle
Radius
Tendon

NORMAL ANATOMY

- Decreased blood supply to forearm muscles, causing tissue death, loss of function and contraction of affected muscles.
- Prolonged healing time if usual activities are resumed too soon.
- Possible infection if skin is broken over the contusion.

PROBABLE OUTCOME—Healing time varies with the extent of injury, but average healing time for forearm contusions is 2 to 3 weeks.

 ## HOW TO TREAT

NOTE—Follow your doctor's instructions. These instructions are supplemental.

FIRST AID—Use instructions for R.I.C.E., the first letters of *rest, ice, compression* and *elevation*. See Appendix 1 for details.

CONTINUING CARE
- Use a sling to immobilize the arm.
- Wrap an elasticized bandage over a felt pad on the injured area. Keep the area compressed for about 72 hours.
- Continue ice massage. Fill a large Styrofoam cup with water and freeze. Tear a small amount of foam from the top so ice protrudes. Massage gently over the injured area in a circle about the size of a softball. Do this for 15 minutes at a time, 3 or 4 times a day, and before workouts or competition.
- After 72 hours, apply heat instead of ice if it feels better. Use heat lamps, hot soaks, hot showers, heating pads, heat liniments or ointments, or whirlpool treatments.
- Massage gently and often to provide comfort and decrease swelling.

MEDICATION
- For minor discomfort, you may use:
  Acetaminophen or ibuprofen.
  Topical liniments and ointments.
- Your doctor may prescribe stronger medicine for pain.

ACTIVITY—Begin activities slowly and stop exercise as soon as pain begins. Increase activity as healing progresses.

DIET—During recovery, eat a well-balanced diet that includes extra protein, such as meat, fish, poultry, cheese, milk and eggs. Your doctor may prescribe vitamin and mineral supplements to promote healing.

REHABILITATION
- Begin daily rehabilitation exercises when supportive wrapping is no longer needed.
- See page 474 for rehabilitation exercises.

 ## CALL YOUR DOCTOR IF

- You have symptoms of a forearm contusion that doesn't improve within a day or two.
- Skin is broken and signs of infection (drainage, increasing pain, fever, headache, muscle aches, dizziness or a general ill feeling) occur.

ARM CONTUSION, RADIAL NERVE

GENERAL INFORMATION

DEFINITION—Injury from a direct blow to the area over the radial nerve in the upper arm, close to the elbow. Contusions cause bleeding from ruptured small capillaries that allow blood to infiltrate nerves, muscles, tendons or other soft tissue.

BODY PARTS INVOLVED
● Radial nerve.
● Blood vessels, muscles, tendons, covering to bone (periosteum) and connective tissue.

SIGNS & SYMPTOMS
● Swelling at the contusion site—either superficial or deep.
● Pain and tenderness at the elbow.
● Shocking, tingling sensation with numbness in the wrist and hand.
● Dropped wrist and loss of some movement in the fingers and thumb.
● Feeling of firmness when pressure is exerted at the injury site.
● Discoloration under the skin, beginning with redness and progressing to the characteristic "black and blue" bruise.
● Restricted elbow activity proportional to the extent of injury.

CAUSES
● Direct blow to the elbow and radial nerve from a blunt object.
● Falling on an elbow.

RISK INCREASES WITH
● Contact sports such as football, hockey or baseball, especially when elbows and arms are not adequately protected.
● Medical history of any bleeding disorder such as hemophilia.
● Poor nutrition, including vitamin deficiency.

HOW TO PREVENT—Wear appropriate protective gear and equipment, such as elbow pads, during competition or other athletic activity if there is risk of an elbow or radial-nerve contusion.

WHAT TO EXPECT

APPROPRIATE HEALTH CARE
● Doctor's care unless the contusion is quite small.
● Surgery (sometimes) to treat the contused nerve. This usually involves transferring and transplanting the nerve into muscle, where it is sutured in place.
● Self-care for minor contusions or for serious nerve contusions during rehabilitation after surgery.

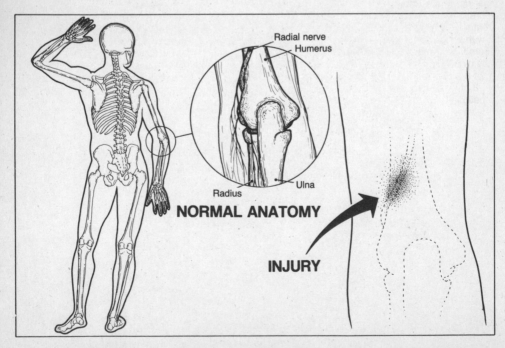

Radial nerve
Humerus
Radius
Ulna
NORMAL ANATOMY

INJURY

- Physical therapy following surgery.

DIAGNOSTIC MEASURES
- Your own observation of symptoms.
- Medical history and physical exam by a doctor for all except minor injuries.
- X-rays of the elbow to assess total injury to soft tissue and to rule out the possibility of underlying fracture. The total extent of injury may not be apparent for 48 to 72 hours.

POSSIBLE COMPLICATIONS
- Permanent damage to the radial nerve, leading to disability in the forearm and hand.
- Prolonged healing time if usual activities are resumed too soon.
- Infection if skin over the contusion is broken.

PROBABLE OUTCOME—Healing time varies greatly with the extent of injury and whether surgery is required or not. Healing is usually complete within 2 months, but in a few cases, symptoms never disappear.

 # HOW TO TREAT

NOTE—Follow your doctor's instructions. These instructions are supplemental.

FIRST AID—Use instructions for R.I.C.E., the first letters of *rest, ice, compression* and *elevation*. See Appendix 1 for details.

CONTINUING CARE
- Support the arm in a sling.
- Wrap an elasticized bandage over a sponge-rubber donut on the injured area. Keep the area compressed for about 72 hours.
- Continue ice massage. Fill a large Styrofoam cup with water and freeze. Tear a small amount of foam from the top so ice protrudes. Massage gently over the injured area in a circle about the size of a softball. Do this for 15 minutes at a time, 3 or 4 times a day, and before workouts or competition.

- Apply heat instead of ice when skin warmth over the injury becomes the same as for the non-injured areas. Use heat lamps, hot soaks, hot showers, heating pads, heat liniments or ointments, or whirlpool treatments.
- Massage gently and often to provide comfort and decrease swelling.

MEDICATION
- For minor discomfort, you may use:
  Acetaminophen or ibuprofen.
  Topical liniments and ointments.
- Your doctor may prescribe stronger medicine for pain.

ACTIVITY—Begin activities slowly and stop exercise as soon as pain begins. Increase activity as healing progresses.

DIET—Eat a well-balanced diet that includes extra protein, such as meat, fish, poultry, cheese, milk and eggs. Your doctor may prescribe vitamin and mineral supplements to promote healing.

REHABILITATION
- Begin daily rehabilitation exercises when supportive wrapping is no longer needed.
- See page 455 for rehabilitation exercises.

 # CALL YOUR DOCTOR IF

- You have symptoms of a radial-nerve contusion.
- Any of the following occur after surgery:
  Increased pain, swelling, redness, drainage or bleeding in the surgical area.
  Signs of infection: headache, muscle aches, dizziness, fever, or a general ill feeling.
  Nausea or vomiting.
  Constipation.
- New, unexplained symptoms develop. Drugs used in treatment may produce side effects.

ARM CONTUSION, UPPER ARM

GENERAL INFORMATION

DEFINITION—Bruising of the skin, muscle and underlying tissues of the upper arm due to a direct blow. Contusions cause bleeding from ruptured small capillaries, allowing blood to infiltrate muscles, tendons or other soft tissue. Muscle tissue is damaged most by a contusion in this area.

BODY PARTS INVOLVED
● Upper arm, particularly the biceps and triceps muscles.
● Other soft tissues, including blood vessels, tendons, nerves, covering to bone (periosteum) and connective tissue.

SIGNS & SYMPTOMS
● Local swelling—either superficial or deep.
● Pain and tenderness over the bruised area.
● Feeling of firmness when pressure is exerted on the injured area.
● Discoloration under the skin, beginning with redness and progressing to the characteristic "black and blue" bruise.
● Restricted arm activity proportional to the extent of injury.

CAUSES—Direct blow to the upper arm, usually from a blunt object.

RISK INCREASES WITH
● Violent contact sports such as football or hockey, especially when the upper arm is not protected adequately.
● Medical history of any bleeding disorder such as hemophilia.
● Poor nutrition, including vitamin deficiency.
● Use of anticoagulants or aspirin.

HOW TO PREVENT—Wear appropriate protective gear and equipment, such as foam-rubber or felt pads, during competition or other athletic activity if there is risk of an upper-arm contusion.

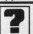

WHAT TO EXPECT

APPROPRIATE HEALTH CARE
● Doctor's care unless the injury is quite small.
● Self-care for minor contusions, or for serious contusions during rehabilitation.
● Physical therapy for serious contusions.

DIAGNOSTIC MEASURES
● Your own observation of symptoms.
● Medical history and physical exam by a doctor for all except minor injuries.
● X-rays of the arm, shoulder and elbow to assess total injury to soft tissue and to rule out the possibility of underlying fracture. The total

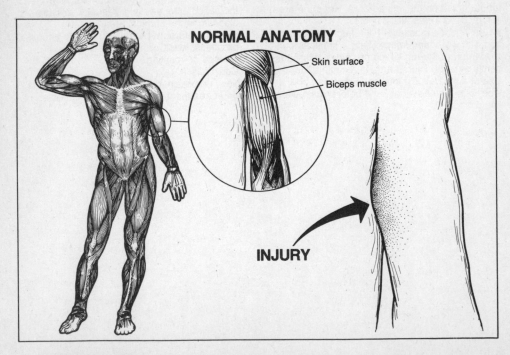

NORMAL ANATOMY

— Skin surface

— Biceps muscle

INJURY

extent of injury may not be apparent for 48 to 72 hours.

POSSIBLE COMPLICATIONS
• Excessive bleeding leading to disability. Infiltrative-type bleeding can occasionally lead to calcification and impaired function of injured muscle.
• Prolonged healing time if usual activity is resumed too soon.
• Infection if skin over the contusion is broken.

PROBABLE OUTCOME—Healing time varies with the extent of injury, but all but the most serious upper-arm contusions should heal in 1 to 2 weeks.

 # HOW TO TREAT

NOTE—Follow your doctor's instructions. These instructions are supplemental.

FIRST AID—Use instructions for R.I.C.E., the first letters of *rest, ice, compression* and *elevation*. See Appendix 1 for details.

CONTINUING CARE
• Wrap felt or sheet wadding over the injured area. Then wrap the arm with an elasticized bandage from armpit to fingertips. Keep the area compressed for about 72 hours.
• Continue ice massage. Fill a large Styrofoam cup with water and freeze. Tear a small amount of foam from the top so ice protrudes. Massage gently over the injured area in a circle about the size of a softball. Do this for 15 minutes at a time, 3 or 4 times a day, and before workouts or competition.

• After 72 hours, apply heat instead of ice if it feels better. Use heat lamps, hot soaks, hot showers, heating pads, heat liniments or ointments, or whirlpool treatments.
• Massage gently and often to provide comfort and decrease swelling.

MEDICATION
• For minor discomfort, you may use:
  Acetaminophen or ibuprofen.
  Topical liniments and ointments.
• Your doctor may prescribe stronger medicine for pain.

ACTIVITY—Begin activities slowly and stop exercise as soon as pain begins. Increase activity as healing progresses.

DIET—During recovery, eat a well-balanced diet that includes extra protein, such as meat, fish, poultry, cheese, milk and eggs. Your doctor may prescribe vitamin and mineral supplements to promote healing.

REHABILITATION
• Begin daily rehabilitation exercises when supportive wrapping is no longer needed.
• See pages 455 and 465 for rehabilitation exercises.

 # CALL YOUR DOCTOR IF

• You have an upper-arm contusion that doesn't improve in 1 or 2 days.
• Skin is broken and signs of infection (drainage, increasing pain, fever, headache, muscle aches, dizziness or a general ill feeling) occur.

ARM EXOSTOSIS
(Blocker's Exostosis)

GENERAL INFORMATION

DEFINITION—An overgrowth of bone in the upper arm. An exostosis occurs at the site of repeated injury, usually from direct blows. This benign overgrowth of bone can be mistaken for a bone tumor.

BODY PARTS INVOLVED
- Middle third (usually) of the humerus, the upper arm bone.
- Soft tissue surrounding the exostosis, including muscles, nerves, lymph vessels, blood vessels and periosteum (covering to bone).

SIGNS & SYMPTOMS
- No symptoms for mild cases.
- Pain and tenderness in the upper arm at the site of the exostosis.
- Extreme sensitivity in the upper arm to pressure or minor injury.
- Change in the contour of the bone, ranging from a slight lump to a large calcified spur (1cm or more in length) on the humerus. In the worst cases, the exostosis may break away and feel like a distinct foreign body in the arm. An X-ray will show it to be loose in the tissues of the upper arm.

CAUSES
- Repeated injury (contusions, sprains or strains) that involve the upper arm bone.
- Chronic irritation to an already damaged bone area.

RISK INCREASES WITH
- Contact sports, particularly football or other sports that require blocking with the arms.
- Other direct blows to the arms.
- History of bone or joint disease, such as osteomyelitis, osteomalacia or osteoporosis.
- Vitamin or mineral deficiency.
- Poor muscle strength or conditioning, making injury more likely.
- If surgery or anesthesia are needed, surgical risk increases with smoking, use of mind-altering drugs, muscle relaxants, tranquilizers, sleep inducers, insulin, sedatives, beta-adrenergic blockers or corticosteroids.

HOW TO PREVENT
- Allow adequate time for recovery from any arm injury.
- During participation in contact sports, wear a fiberboard pad over the upper arms and shoulder pads to prevent injuries.
- Learn proper moves and techniques for the sports activities you pursue to decrease the risk of injury.

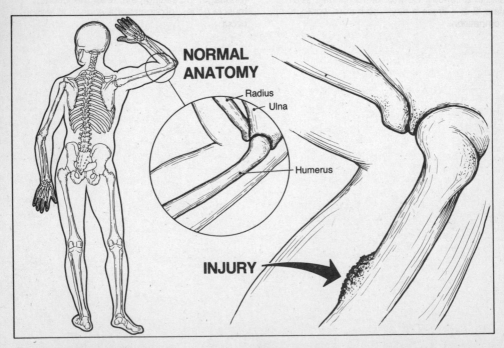

NORMAL ANATOMY

Radius

Ulna

Humerus

INJURY

WHAT TO EXPECT

APPROPRIATE HEALTH CARE
- Doctor's care.
- Surgery (sometimes) to remove the exostosis.
- Self-care during rehabilitation.
- Physical therapy.

DIAGNOSTIC MEASURES
- Your own observation of signs and symptoms.
- Medical history and physical exam by a doctor.
- X-rays of the elbow, arm and shoulder.

POSSIBLE COMPLICATIONS
- Overlooking a mild exostosis that produces no symptoms, despite signs of diminished performance. Athletes and coaches frequently assume that decreased performance results from loss of competitive drive or emotional causes rather than from the physical disability that actually exists.
- Prolonged healing time if activity is resumed too soon.
- Proneness to repeated arm injury.
- Unstable or arthritic shoulder or elbow following repeated injury.
- Pressure on or injury to nearby muscles, nerves, ligaments, tendons, blood vessels or connective tissue.
- Impaired blood supply to the injured area.

PROBABLE OUTCOME—Upper-arm exostosis usually causes no disability if it is treated properly. Treatment usually involves resting the injured arm for 2 to 4 weeks, heat treatments, corticosteroid injections and protection against additional injury. In a few cases, surgery is necessary to remove the exostosis.

 HOW TO TREAT

NOTE—Follow your doctor's instructions. These instructions are supplemental.

FIRST AID—None. This condition develops gradually.

CONTINUING CARE
- Rest the injured arm. Use a sling if needed to prevent weight-bearing. Don't subject yourself to reinjury until completely healed.
- Apply heat frequently. Use heat lamps, hot soaks, hot showers, heating pads, or heat liniments and ointments.
- Take whirlpool treatments, if available.
- Follow instructions under How to Prevent to avoid a recurrence of the injury. Use proper protection during competition and workouts.

MEDICATION
- Medicine usually is not necessary for this disorder. For minor pain, you may use non-prescription drugs such as aspirin.
- If surgery is necessary, your doctor may prescribe:
    Non-steroidal anti-inflammatory drugs to help control swelling.
    Stronger pain relievers.
    Antibiotics to fight infection.

ACTIVITY—Decrease activity for 2 to 4 weeks. If surgery is necessary, resume normal activity gradually.

DIET—During recovery, eat a well-balanced diet that includes extra protein, such as meat, fish, poultry, cheese, milk and eggs. Increase fiber and fluid intake to prevent constipation that may result from decreased activity. Your doctor may suggest vitamin and mineral supplements to promote healing.

REHABILITATION
- Begin daily rehabilitation exercises when movement is comfortable. Weight-lifting under supervision can provide a quick return of strength and flexibility.
- Use ice massage for 10 minutes prior to exercise. Fill a large Styrofoam cup with water and freeze. Tear a small amount of foam from the top so ice protrudes. Massage firmly over the injured area in a circle about the size of a softball.
- See pages 455 and 465 for rehabilitation exercises.

 CALL YOUR DOCTOR IF

- You have symptoms of upper-arm exostosis.
- You notice no improvement despite treatment.
- Any of the following occur after surgery:
    Increased pain, swelling, redness, drainage, or bleeding in the surgical area.
    Signs of infection (headache, muscle aches, dizziness, or a general ill feeling and fever).
    New, unexplained symptoms. Drugs used in treatment may cause side effects.

ARM FRACTURE, FOREARM

GENERAL INFORMATION

DEFINITION—A complete or incomplete break in one or both bones of the forearm (the radius and the ulna).

BODY PARTS INVOLVED
- Ulna and radius bones.
- Elbow and wrist joints.
- Soft tissue around the fracture site, including nerves, tendons, ligaments and blood vessels.

SIGNS & SYMPTOMS
- Severe arm pain at the time of injury.
- Swelling of soft tissue around the fracture.
- Visible deformity if the fracture is complete and the bone fragments separate enough to distort normal arm contours.
- Tenderness to the touch.
- Numbness and coldness in the lower arm and hand if the blood supply is impaired.

CAUSES—Direct blow or indirect stress to the bone. Indirect stress may be caused by twisting or violent muscle contraction.

RISK INCREASES WITH
- Contact sports, especially football, soccer or hockey.
- History of bone or joint disease, especially osteoporosis.
- Poor nutrition, especially calcium deficiency.
- If surgery or anesthesia is needed, surgical risk increases with smoking and use of drugs, including mind-altering drugs, muscle relaxants, antihypertensives, tranquilizers, sleep inducers, insulin, sedatives, beta-adrenergic blockers or cortisone.

HOW TO PREVENT
- Build your strength with a good conditioning program before beginning regular athletic practice or competition. Increased muscle mass helps protect bones and underlying tissue.
- If you have had a previous arm injury, use padded arm splints when competing in contact sports.

WHAT TO EXPECT

APPROPRIATE HEALTH CARE
- Doctor's treatment.
- Hospitalization (sometimes) for anesthesia and surgery to set the fracture or to insert a metal plate that immobilizes broken bones until they heal.
- Whirlpool, ultrasound or massage (to displace excess fluid from the elbow and wrist).

DIAGNOSTIC MEASURES
- Your own observation of symptoms.
- Medical history and exam by a doctor.
- X-rays of injured areas, including the elbow above and the wrist below the primary injury site. In young people, X-rays of the normal side should be made for comparison.

POSSIBLE COMPLICATIONS
At the time of injury:
- Shock.

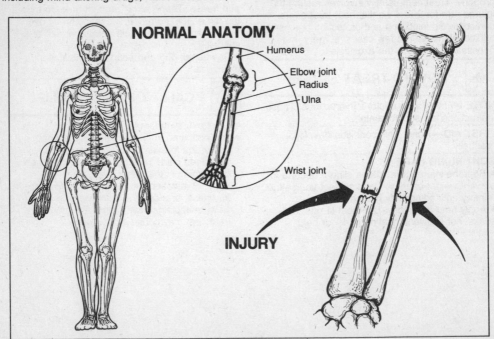

NORMAL ANATOMY

Humerus
Elbow joint
Radius
Ulna
Wrist joint

INJURY

● Pressure on or injury to nearby nerves, ligaments, tendons, muscles, blood vessels, or connective tissues.

After treatment or surgery:
● Delayed union or non-union of the fracture.
● Impaired blood supply to the fracture site.
● Avascular necrosis (death of bone cells) due to interruption of the blood supply.
● Death of muscle cells if the arm swells inside the cast.
● Arrest of normal bone growth in children.
● Infection in open fractures (skin broken over fracture site), or at the incision if surgical setting was necessary.
● Shortening of the injured bones.
● Proneness to repeated injury.
● Unstable or arthritic wrist or elbow following repeated injury.
● Prolonged healing time if activity is resumed too soon.
● Problems caused by casts. See Appendix 2 (Care of Casts).

PROBABLE OUTCOME—The average healing time for this fracture is 6 to 8 weeks in adults and 5 to 6 weeks in children. Healing is complete when there is no motion at the fracture site and when X-rays show complete bone union.

 HOW TO TREAT

NOTE—Follow your doctor's instructions. These instructions are supplemental.

FIRST AID
● Keep the person warm with blankets to decrease the possibility of shock.
● Cut away clothing, if possible, but don't move the injured arm to do so.
● Follow instructions for R.I.C.E., the first letters of *rest, ice, compression* and *elevation.* See Appendix 1 for details.
● The doctor will manipulate and set the broken bones with surgery or, if possible, without. Manipulation should be done as soon as possible after injury. Six or more hours after the fracture, bleeding and displacement of body fluids may lead to shock. Also, many tissues lose their elasticity and become difficult to return to a normal position.

CONTINUING CARE
● Immobilization will be necessary. A rigid cast or plaster splints will be placed around the injured arm to immobilize the elbow and wrist.
● After 48 hours, localized heat promotes healing by increasing blood circulation in the injured area. Use a heat lamp or heating pads so heat can penetrate the cast.
● After the cast is removed, use frequent ice massage. Fill a large Styrofoam cup with water and freeze. Tear a small amount of foam from the top so ice protrudes. Massage firmly over the injured area in a circle about the size of a baseball. Do this for 15 minutes at a time, 3 or 4 times a day.
● Apply heat instead of ice if it feels better. Use heat lamps, hot soaks, hot showers, heating pads, or heat liniments or ointments.
● Take whirlpool treatments, if available.

MEDICATION—Your doctor may prescribe:
● General anesthesia, local anesthesia, or muscle relaxants to make bone manipulation and fixation of bone fragments possible.
● Narcotic or synthetic narcotic pain relievers for severe pain.
● Stool softeners to prevent constipation due to inactivity.
● Acetaminophen (available without prescription) for mild pain after initial treatment.

ACTIVITY
● Actively exercise all muscle groups not immobilized. These muscle contractions promote fracture alignment and hasten healing.
● Begin reconditioning the injured arm after clearance from your doctor.
● Resume normal activities gradually after treatment. Don't drive until healing is complete.

DIET
● Drink only water before manipulation or surgery to treat the fracture. Solid food in your stomach makes vomiting while under anesthesia more hazardous.
● During recovery, eat a well-balanced diet that includes extra protein, such as meat, fish, poultry, cheese, milk and eggs. Increase fiber and fluid intake to prevent constipation that may result from decreased activity.

REHABILITATION—Begin daily rehabilitation exercises when movement is comfortable. Use ice massage for 10 minutes prior to exercise. See pages 455 and 474 for rehabilitation exercises.

 CALL YOUR DOCTOR IF

● You have signs or symptoms of a forearm fracture.
● Any of the following occur after surgery or other treatment:
    Increased pain, swelling or drainage in the surgical area.
    Signs of infection (headache, muscle aches, dizziness, or a general ill feeling and fever).
    Swelling above or below the cast.
    Blue or gray skin color beyond the cast, particularly under the fingernails.
    Numbness or complete loss of feeling below the fracture site.
    Nausea or vomiting.
    Constipation.

ARM FRACTURE, HUMERUS

GENERAL INFORMATION

DEFINITION—A complete or incomplete break in the humerus, the large bone in the upper arm extending from the elbow to the shoulder. The most common fractures of the humerus occur in the tubercle (top part of the humerus that fits into the shoulder joint) or in the neck or shaft of the humerus.

BODY PARTS INVOLVED
● Humerus.
● Elbow and shoulder joints.
● Soft tissue around the fracture site, including nerves, tendons, ligaments and blood vessels.

SIGNS & SYMPTOMS
● Severe arm pain at the time of injury.
● Swelling of soft tissue around the fracture.
● Visible deformity if the fracture is complete and the bone fragments separate enough to distort normal arm contours.
● Tenderness to the touch.
● Numbness and coldness in the arm and hand if the blood supply is impaired.

CAUSES—Direct blow or indirect stress to the bone. Indirect stress may be caused by twisting or violent muscle contraction.

RISK INCREASES WITH
● Contact sports such as football or hockey.
● History of bone or joint disease, especially osteoporosis.
● Children under 12 or adults over 60.
● Obesity.
● If surgery or anesthesia is needed, surgical risk increases with smoking or use of drugs, including mind-altering drugs, muscle relaxants, antihypertensives, tranquilizers, sleep inducers, insulin, sedatives, beta-adrenergic blockers or corticosteroids.

HOW TO PREVENT
● Build your strength with a good conditioning program before beginning regular athletic practice or competition. Increased muscle mass helps protect bones and underlying tissue.
● If you have had an arm injury, use padded arm splints when participating in contact sports.

WHAT TO EXPECT

APPROPRIATE HEALTH CARE
● Doctor's treatment.
● Hospitalization (sometimes) for anesthesia and surgery to set the fracture.
● Whirlpool, ultrasound, or massage to displace excess fluid from the injury area.

DIAGNOSTIC MEASURES
● Your own observation of symptoms.
● Medical history and exam by a doctor.
● X-rays of injured areas, including joints above and below the primary injury site.

POSSIBLE COMPLICATIONS
At the time of injury:
● Shock.
● Pressure on or injury to nearby nerves,

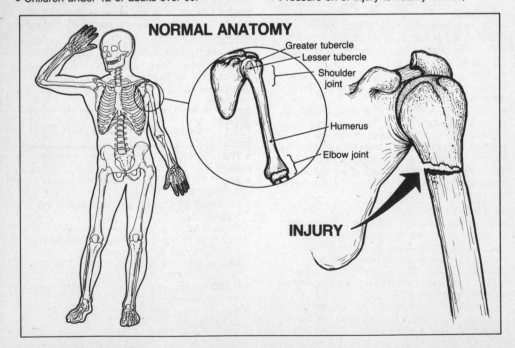

NORMAL ANATOMY

Greater tubercle
Lesser tubercle
Shoulder joint
Humerus
Elbow joint

INJURY

ligaments, tendons, muscles, blood vessels or connective tissues.

After treatment or surgery:
- Delayed union or non-union of the fracture.
- Impaired blood supply to the fracture site.
- Avascular necrosis (death of bone cells) due to interruption of the blood supply.
- Arrest of normal bone growth in children.
- Infection in open fractures (skin broken over the fracture), or at the incision following surgery.
- Shortening of the injured humerus.
- Unstable or arthritic shoulder or elbow joint following repeated injury.
- Prolonged healing time if activity is resumed too soon.
- Proneness to repeated arm injury.
- Problems caused by casts. See Appendix 2 (Care of Casts).

PROBABLE OUTCOME—The average healing time for this fracture is 6 to 8 weeks. Healing is considered complete when there is no motion at the fracture site and when X-rays show complete bone union.

HOW TO TREAT

NOTE—Follow your doctor's instructions. These instructions are supplemental.

FIRST AID
- Keep the person warm with blankets to decrease the possibility of shock.
- Cut away clothing, if possible, but don't move the injured arm to do so.
- Follow instructions for R.I.C.E., the first letters of *rest, ice, compression* and *elevation*. See Appendix 1 for details.
- The doctor will realign the broken bones with surgery or, if possible, without. This manipulation should be done as soon as possible after injury. Six or more hours after the fracture, bleeding and displacement of body fluids may lead to shock. Also, many tissues lose their elasticity and become difficult to return to a normal position.

CONTINUING CARE
- Immobilization will be necessary. It can take several forms, depending on the fracture:
  (1) Placement of surgical nails or pins to hold bone fragments together for fractures of tubercles. Usually only minimal external immobilization is necessary after surgery.
  (2) Hanging cast for fractures of the neck of the humerus. A hanging cast is one placed on the lower arm to provide weight to overcome muscle spasms so the fractured bones will realign themselves.
  (3) Shoulder-to-wrist rigid cast for uncomplicated shaft fractures.
- If a cast is not necessary, continue R.I.C.E. instructions for 48 hours.

- After 48 hours, apply heat. Localized heat promotes healing by increasing blood circulation in the injured area. If no cast is necessary, use hot baths, showers, compresses, heating ointments and liniments, or whirlpools. If a cast is necessary, use a heat lamp or heating pad so heat can penetrate the cast.
- After the cast is removed, use frequent ice massage. Fill a large Styrofoam cup with water and freeze. Tear a small amount of foam from the top so ice protrudes. Massage firmly over the injured area in a circle about the size of a baseball. Do this for 15 minutes at a time, 3 or 4 times a day.

MEDICATION—Your doctor may prescribe:
- General anesthesia, local anesthesia, or muscle relaxants to make bone manipulation and fixation of bone fragments possible.
- Narcotic or synthetic narcotic pain relievers for severe pain.
- Acetaminophen for mild pain.
- Stool softeners to prevent constipation due to inactivity.

ACTIVITY
- Actively exercise all muscle groups not immobilized. These muscle contractions promote fracture alignment and hasten healing.
- Begin reconditioning the arm after clearance from your doctor.
- Resume your normal activities gradually after treatment. Don't drive until healing is complete.

DIET
- Drink only water before manipulation or surgery to treat the fracture. Solid food in your stomach makes vomiting while under anesthesia more hazardous.
- During recovery, eat a well-balanced diet that includes extra protein, such as meat, fish, poultry, cheese, milk and eggs. Increase fiber and fluid intake to prevent constipation.

REHABILITATION—Begin daily rehabilitation exercises when movement is comfortable. Use ice massage for 10 minutes prior to exercise. See page 465 for rehabilitation exercises.

CALL YOUR DOCTOR IF

- You have symptoms of a fractured arm.
- Any of the following occurs after surgery or other treatment:
  Blue or gray skin color beyond the cast, particularly under the fingernails.
  Loss of feeling below the fracture site.
  Increased pain, swelling or drainage in the surgical area.
  Signs of infection (headache, muscle aches, dizziness, or a general ill feeling and fever).
  Swelling above or below the cast.
  Nausea or vomiting.
  Constipation.

ARM & SHOULDER TENOSYNOVITIS, BICEPS-TENDON SHEATH

 ## GENERAL INFORMATION

DEFINITION—Inflammation of the lining of the biceps-tendon sheath in the upper arm and shoulder. This lining secretes a fluid that lubricates the tendon. When the lining becomes inflamed, the tendon cannot glide smoothly in its covering.

BODY PARTS INVOLVED
● Biceps tendon, which attaches the biceps muscle to the shoulder.
● Lining and covering of the biceps tendon.
● Soft tissue in the surrounding area, including blood vessels, nerves, ligaments, periosteum (covering to bone) and connective tissue.

SIGNS & SYMPTOMS
● Constant pain or pain with motion.
● Limited motion of the shoulder and elbow.
● Crepitation (a "crackling" sound when the tendon moves or is touched).
● Heat and redness over the inflamed tendon.
● Restriction of movement followed by a sudden painful snap, if the tendon breaks away from its attachment to bone.

CAUSES
● Strain from unusual use or overuse of the biceps muscle.
● Direct blow or injury to the shoulder.
Tenosynovitis becomes more likely with repeated injury to the biceps muscle-tendon unit.
● Infection introduced through broken skin at the time of injury or through a surgical incision after injury.

RISK INCREASES WITH
● Contact sports.
● Throwing sports.
● Gymnastics.
● Weight-lifting.
● If surgery is needed, surgical risk increases with smoking, poor nutrition, alcoholism or drug abuse, and recent or chronic illness.

HOW TO PREVENT
● Engage in a vigorous program of physical conditioning before beginning regular sports participation.
● Warm up adequately before practice or competition.
● Wear protective gear appropriate for your sport.
● Learn proper moves and techniques for your sport.

 ## WHAT TO EXPECT

APPROPRIATE HEALTH CARE
● Doctor's examination and diagnosis.
● Surgery (sometimes) to enlarge the tunnel of the tendon covering and restore a smooth

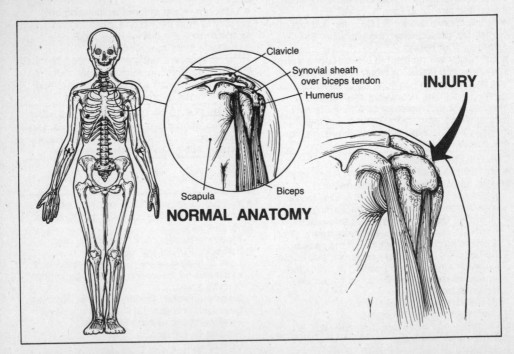

Clavicle
Synovial sheath over biceps tendon
Humerus
Scapula
Biceps

NORMAL ANATOMY

INJURY

gliding motion. The surgical procedure under general anesthesia is performed in an outpatient surgical facility or hospital operating room.

DIAGNOSTIC MEASURES
- Your own observation of symptoms and signs.
- Medical history and physical examination by your doctor.
- X-rays of the area to rule out other abnormalities.
- Laboratory studies:
  Blood and urine studies before surgery.
  Tissue examination after surgery.

POSSIBLE COMPLICATIONS
- Prolonged healing time if activity is resumed too soon.
- Proneness to repeated injury of the biceps tendon.
- Adhesive tenosynovitis: The tendon and its covering become bound together. Loss of motion may be complete or partial. Surgery is necessary to remove the covering or transfer the tendon to a new area.
- Constrictive tenosynovitis: The walls of the covering thicken and narrow the opening, preventing the tendon from sliding through. Surgery is necessary to cut away part of the covering.
- Rupture of the tendon, if motion is forced when the tendon and its covering are bound together.

PROBABLE OUTCOME—Tenosynovitis is usually curable in about 6 weeks with heat treatments, corticosteroid injections and rest of the inflamed area. Recovery is usually quicker if the inflammation is caused by a direct blow rather than by a strain or sprain.

 HOW TO TREAT

NOTE—Follow your doctor's instructions. These instructions are supplemental.

FIRST AID—None. This problem develops slowly.

CONTINUING CARE
- Wrap the shoulder with an elasticized bandage or use a sling until healing is complete.
- Apply heat frequently. Use heat lamps, hot soaks, hot showers, heating pads, or heat liniments and ointments.

MEDICATION—You may use non-prescription drugs, such as acetaminophen, for minor pain. Your doctor may prescribe:
- Stronger pain relievers. Don't take prescription pain medication longer than 4 to 7 days. Use only as much as you need.
- Injection of the unruptured tendon covering with a combination of a long-acting local anesthetic and a non-absorbable corticosteroid such as triamcinolone.

ACTIVITY—Resume normal activities slowly.

DIET—During recovery, eat a well-balanced diet that includes extra protein, such as meat, fish, poultry, cheese, milk and eggs. Increase fiber and fluid intake to prevent constipation that may result from decreased activity.

REHABILITATION
- Begin daily rehabilitation exercises when supportive wrapping is no longer needed.
- Use ice massage for 10 minutes before and after exercise. Fill a large Styrofoam cup with water and freeze. Tear a small amount of foam from the top so ice protrudes. Massage firmly over the injured area in a circle about the size of a softball.
- See page 465 for rehabilitation exercises.

 CALL YOUR DOCTOR IF

- You have symptoms of biceps tenosynovitis.
- Any of the following occur after surgery:
  Increased pain, swelling, redness, drainage or bleeding in the surgical area.
  Signs of infection (headache, muscle aches, dizziness, or a general ill feeling and fever).
  New, unexplained symptoms. Drugs used in treatment may produce side effects.

ARM STRAIN, BICEPS

GENERAL INFORMATION

DEFINITION—Injury to the biceps muscle or tendon. The biceps muscle is a large muscle in the front of the upper arm. The muscle, tendon and attached bone comprise a unit. The unit stabilizes the elbow and shoulder joints and allows their motion. A strain occurs at the weakest part of a unit. Strains are of 3 types:
● Mild (Grade I)—Slightly pulled muscle without tearing of muscle or tendon fibers. There is no loss of strength.
● Moderate (Grade II)—Tearing of fibers in a muscle, tendon or at the attachment to bone. Strength is diminished.
● Severe (Grade III)—Rupture of the muscle-tendon-bone attachment with separation of fibers. Severe strain requires surgical repair. Chronic strains are caused by overuse. Acute strains are caused by direct injury or overstress.

BODY PARTS INVOLVED
● Biceps muscle.
● Biceps tendon.
● Humerus and bones of the shoulder.
● Soft tissue surrounding the strain, including nerves, periosteum (covering to bone), blood vessels and lymph vessels.

SIGNS & SYMPTOMS
● Pain when moving or stretching the biceps muscle.
● Muscle spasm.
● Swelling around the injury.
● Loss of strength (moderate or severe strain).
● Crepitation ("crackling") feeling and sound when pressed with fingers.
● Calcification of the muscle or tendon (visible with X-rays).
● Inflammation of the sheath covering the tendon.

CAUSES
● Prolonged overuse of muscle-tendon units in the biceps of the upper arm.
● Single violent blow or force applied to the biceps.

RISK INCREASES WITH
● Contact sports such as boxing or wrestling.
● Throwing sports.
● Weight-lifting.
● Any cardiovascular medical problem that results in decreased circulation.
● Medical history of any bleeding disorder.
● Obesity.
● Poor nutrition.
● Previous upper-arm injury.
● Poor muscle conditioning.

HOW TO PREVENT
● Participate in a strengthening and conditioning program appropriate for your sport.
● Warm up before practice or competition.
● Wear proper protective equipment.

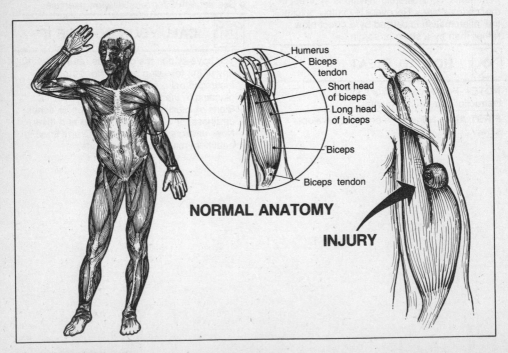

Humerus
Biceps tendon
Short head of biceps
Long head of biceps
Biceps
Biceps tendon

NORMAL ANATOMY

INJURY

WHAT TO EXPECT

APPROPRIATE HEALTH CARE
- Doctor's diagnosis.
- Application of tape, plaster splints or casts (sometimes).
- Self-care during rehabilitation.
- Physical therapy (moderate or severe strain).
- Surgery (severe strain).

DIAGNOSTIC MEASURES
- Your own observation of symptoms.
- Medical history and exam by a doctor.
- X-rays of the shoulder, arm and elbow to rule out fractures.

POSSIBLE COMPLICATIONS
- Prolonged healing time if activity is resumed too soon.
- Proneness to repeated injury.
- Unstable or arthritic shoulder or elbow following repeated injury.
- Inflammation at the attachment to bone (periostitis).
- Prolonged disability (sometimes).

PROBABLE OUTCOME—If this is a first-time injury, proper care and sufficient healing time before resuming activity should prevent permanent disability. Torn ligaments and tendons require as long to heal as fractured bones. Average healing times are:
- Mild strain—2 to 10 days.
- Moderate strain—10 days to 6 weeks.
- Severe strain—6 to 10 weeks.

If this is a repeat injury, complications listed above are more likely to occur.

 HOW TO TREAT

NOTE—Follow your doctor's instructions. These instructions are supplemental.

FIRST AID—Use instructions for R.I.C.E., the first letters of *rest, ice, compression* and *elevation.* See Appendix 1 for details.

CONTINUING CARE
- Use ice massage 3 or 4 times a day for 15 minutes at a time. Fill a large Styrofoam cup with water and freeze. Tear a small amount of foam from the top so ice protrudes. Massage firmly over the injured area in a circle about the size of a softball.
- After the first 24 hours, apply heat instead of ice, if it feels better. Use heat lamps, hot soaks, hot showers, heating pads, or heat liniments and ointments.
- Take whirlpool treatments, if available.
- Wrap the injured arm with an elasticized bandage between treatments.
- Massage gently and often to provide comfort and decrease swelling.

MEDICATION
- For minor discomfort, you may use:
  Aspirin, acetaminophen or ibuprofen.
  Topical liniments and ointments.
- Your doctor may prescribe:
  Stronger pain relievers.
  Injection of a long-acting local anesthetic to reduce pain.
  Injections of a corticosteroid, such as triamcinolone, to reduce inflammation.

ACTIVITY
- For a moderate or severe strain, use a sling for at least 72 hours—longer with a cast or splints.
- Resume your normal activities gradually.

DIET—Eat a well-balanced diet that includes extra protein, such as meat, fish, poultry, cheese, milk and eggs. Increase fiber and fluid intake to prevent constipation that may result from decreased activity.

REHABILITATION
- Begin daily rehabilitation exercises when supportive wrapping is no longer needed. Use ice massage for 10 minutes prior to exercise.
- See page 465 for rehabilitation exercises.
- Begin a supervised weight-lifting program.

 CALL YOUR DOCTOR IF

- You have symptoms of a moderate or severe biceps strain, or a mild strain persists longer than 10 days.
- Pain or swelling worsens despite treatment.
- The following occurs with a cast or splints:
  Pain, numbness or coldness below the injury.
  Dusky, blue or gray fingernails.

ARM STRAIN, FOREARM

GENERAL INFORMATION

DEFINITION—Injury to the muscles or tendons connected to the bones in the lower arm. Forearm strain is common because of the many tendons that glide together in the same or separate sheaths. Muscles, tendons and bones comprise units. These units stabilize the elbow and wrist joints and allow their motion. A strain occurs at the weakest part of a unit. Strains are of 3 types:
● Mild (Grade I)—Slightly pulled muscle without tearing of muscle or tendon fibers. There is no loss of strength.
● Moderate (Grade II)—Tearing of fibers in a muscle, tendon or at the attachment to bone. Strength is diminished.
● Severe (Grade III)—Rupture of the muscle-tendon-bone attachment with separation of fibers. Severe strain requires surgical repair. Chronic strains are caused by overuse. Acute strains are caused by direct injury or overstress.

BODY PARTS INVOLVED
● Muscles and tendons of the forearm.
● Ulna and radius, the bones attached to lower-arm muscles and tendons.
● Soft tissue surrounding the strain including nerves, periosteum (covering to bone), blood vessels and lymph vessels.

SIGNS & SYMPTOMS
● Pain when moving or stretching the forearm.
● Muscle spasm in the forearm.
● Swelling over the injury.
● Loss of strength (moderate or severe strain).
● Crepitation ("crackling") feeling and sound when the injured area is pressed with fingers.
● Calcification of the muscle or tendon (visible with X-rays).
● Inflammation of the sheath covering the tendon.

CAUSES
● Prolonged overuse of muscle-tendon units in the forearm and wrist.
● Single violent injury or force applied to the lower arm.

RISK INCREASES WITH
● Contact sports such as football, wrestling or hockey.
● Any cardiovascular medical problem that results in decreased circulation.
● Medical history of any bleeding disorder.
● Obesity.
● Poor nutrition.
● Previous injury to the forearm, wrist or elbow.
● Poor muscle conditioning.

HOW TO PREVENT
● Participate in a strengthening and conditioning program appropriate for your sport.
● Warm up before practice or competition.

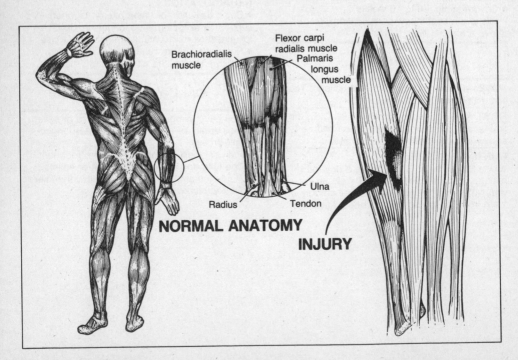

Brachioradialis muscle

Flexor carpi radialis muscle

Palmaris longus muscle

Radius

Ulna

Tendon

NORMAL ANATOMY

INJURY

- Decrease repetitive forearm and hand movements when pain or soreness begins.
- Use proper protective equipment.

 WHAT TO EXPECT

APPROPRIATE HEALTH CARE
- Doctor's diagnosis.
- Application of tape, plaster splints or casts (sometimes).
- Self-care during rehabilitation.
- Physical therapy (moderate or severe strain).
- Surgery (severe strain).

DIAGNOSTIC MEASURES
- Your own observation of symptoms.
- Medical history and exam by a doctor.
- X-rays of the forearm, wrist and elbow to rule out fractures.

POSSIBLE COMPLICATIONS
- Prolonged healing time if activity is resumed too soon.
- Proneness to repeated injury.
- Unstable or arthritic elbow or wrist following repeated injury.
- Inflammation at the attachment to bone (periostitis).
- Prolonged disability (sometimes).

PROBABLE OUTCOME—If this is a first-time injury, proper care and sufficient healing time before resuming activity should prevent permanent disability. Torn ligaments and tendons require as long to heal as fractured bones do. Average healing times are:
- Mild strain—2 to 10 days.
- Moderate strain—10 days to 6 weeks.
- Severe strain—6 to 10 weeks.

If this is a repeat injury, complications listed above are more likely to occur.

 HOW TO TREAT

NOTE—Follow your doctor's instructions. These instructions are supplemental.

FIRST AID—Follow instructions for R.I.C.E., the first letters of *rest, ice, compression* and *elevation*. See Appendix 1 for details.

CONTINUING CARE
If casts or splints are necessary:
- Keep fingers free and exercise them frequently.
- Begin daily rehabilitation exercises when casts or splints are no longer needed. Use ice massage for 10 minutes prior to exercise.

- See Appendix 2 (Care of Casts).

If cast or splints are not necessary:
- Use ice massage 3 or 4 times a day for 15 minutes at a time. Fill a large Styrofoam cup with water and freeze. Tear a small amount of foam from the top so ice protrudes. Massage firmly over the injured area in a circle about the size of a softball.
- After the first 24 hours, apply heat instead of ice, if it feels better. Use heat lamps, hot soaks, hot showers, heating pads, or heat liniments and ointments.
- Take whirlpool treatments, if available.
- Wrap the injured forearm with an elasticized bandage between treatments.
- Begin daily rehabilitation exercises when supportive wrapping is no longer needed. Use ice massage for 10 minutes prior to exercise.
- Massage gently and often to provide comfort and decrease swelling.

MEDICATION
- For minor discomfort, you may use:
  Aspirin, acetaminophen or ibuprofen.
  Topical liniments and ointments.
- Your doctor may prescribe:
  Stronger pain relievers.
  Injection of a long-acting local anesthetic to reduce pain (rare).
  Injections of a corticosteroid, such as triamcinolone, to reduce inflammation (rare).

ACTIVITY
- For a moderate or severe strain, use a sling for at least 72 hours—longer with a cast or splints.
- Resume your normal activities gradually.

DIET—Eat a well-balanced diet that includes extra protein, such as meat, fish, poultry, cheese, milk and eggs. Increase fiber and fluid intake to prevent constipation that may result from decreased activity.

REHABILITATION—See pages 455 and 474 for rehabilitation exercises.

 CALL YOUR DOCTOR IF

- You have symptoms of a moderate or severe forearm strain, or a mild strain persists longer than 10 days.
- Pain or swelling worsens despite treatment.
- The following occurs with a cast or splints:
  Pain, numbness or coldness below the injury.
  Dusky, blue or gray fingernails.

ARM STRAIN, TRICEPS

GENERAL INFORMATION

DEFINITION—Injury to the triceps muscle or tendon. The triceps muscle is the large muscle at the back of the upper arm. The muscle, tendon and attached bone comprise a unit. The unit stabilizes the elbow and shoulder joints and allows their motion. A strain occurs at the weakest part of a unit. Strains are of 3 types:
● Mild (Grade I)—Slightly pulled muscle without tearing of muscle or tendon fibers. There is no loss of strength.
● Moderate (Grade II)—Tearing of fibers in a muscle, tendon or at the attachment to bone. Strength is diminished.
● Severe (Grade III)—Rupture of the muscle-tendon-bone attachment with separation of fibers. Severe strain requires surgical repair. Chronic strains are caused by overuse. Acute strains are caused by direct injury or overstress.

BODY PARTS INVOLVED
● Triceps muscle.
● Tendon of the triceps.
● Bones in the shoulder and arm.
● Soft tissue surrounding the strain, including nerves, periosteum (covering to bone), blood vessels and lymph vessels.

SIGNS & SYMPTOMS
● Pain with motion or stretching, especially forceful extension of the forearm at the elbow joint.
● Muscle spasm.
● Swelling around the injury.
● Loss of strength (moderate or severe strain).
● Crepitation ("crackling") feeling and sound when the injured area is pressed with fingers.
● Calcification of the muscle or tendon (visible with X-rays).
● Inflammation of the sheath covering the tendon.

CAUSES
● Prolonged overuse of muscle-tendon units in the arm and elbow.
● Single violent injury or force applied to the upper arm and elbow.

RISK INCREASES WITH
● Contact sports such as football, baseball or boxing.
● Throwing sports.
● Weight-lifting.
● Any cardiovascular medical problem that results in decreased circulation.
● Medical history of any bleeding disorder.
● Obesity.
● Poor nutrition.
● Previous upper-arm injury.
● Poor muscle conditioning.

HOW TO PREVENT
● Participate in a strengthening and conditioning program appropriate for your sport.
● Warm up before practice, competition or stretching.

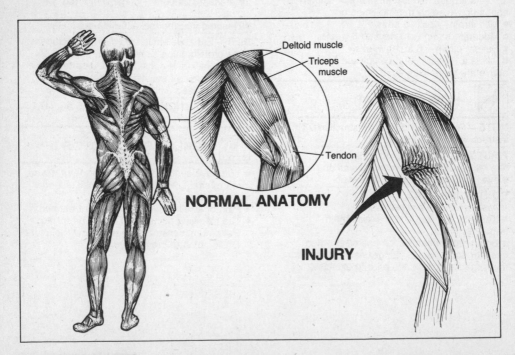

Deltoid muscle

Triceps muscle

Tendon

NORMAL ANATOMY

INJURY

- Use proper protective equipment such as shoulder pads.

WHAT TO EXPECT

APPROPRIATE HEALTH CARE
- Doctor's diagnosis.
- Application of tape, plaster splints or casts (sometimes).
- Self-care during rehabilitation.
- Physical therapy (moderate or severe strain).
- Surgery (severe strain).

DIAGNOSTIC MEASURES
- Your own observation of symptoms.
- Medical history and exam by a doctor.
- X-rays of the shoulder, arm and elbow to rule out fractures.

POSSIBLE COMPLICATIONS
- Prolonged healing time if activity is resumed too soon.
- Proneness to repeated injury.
- Unstable or arthritic shoulder or elbow following repeated injury.
- Inflammation at the attachment to bone (periostitis).
- Prolonged disability (sometimes).

PROBABLE OUTCOME—If this is a first-time injury, proper care and sufficient healing time before resuming activity should prevent permanent disability. Torn ligaments and tendons require as long to heal as fractured bones. Average healing times are:
- Mild strain—2 to 10 days.
- Moderate strain—10 days to 6 weeks.
- Severe strain—6 to 10 weeks.
If this is a repeat injury, complications listed above are more likely to occur.

HOW TO TREAT

NOTE—Follow your doctor's instructions. These instructions are supplemental.

FIRST AID—Use instructions for R.I.C.E., the first letters of *rest, ice, compression* and *elevation*. See Appendix 1 for details.

CONTINUING CARE
- Use ice massage 3 or 4 times a day for 15 minutes at a time. Fill a large Styrofoam cup with water and freeze. Tear a small amount of foam from the top so ice protrudes. Massage firmly over the injured area in a circle about the size of a softball.
- After the first 24 hours, apply heat instead of ice, if it feels better. Use heat lamps, hot soaks, hot showers, heating pads, or heat liniments and ointments.
- Take whirlpool treatments, if available.
- Wrap the injured arm with an elasticized bandage between treatments.
- Massage gently and often to provide comfort and decrease swelling.

MEDICATION
- For minor discomfort, you may use:
  Aspirin, acetaminophen or ibuprofen.
  Topical liniments and ointments.
- Your doctor may prescribe:
  Stronger pain relievers.
  Injection of a long-acting local anesthetic to reduce pain (rare).
  Injections of corticosteroids, such as triamcinolone, to reduce inflammation (rare).

ACTIVITY
- For a moderate or severe strain, use a sling for at least 72 hours—longer with a cast or splints.
- Resume your normal activities gradually.

DIET—Eat a well-balanced diet that includes extra protein, such as meat, fish, poultry, cheese, milk and eggs. Increase fiber and fluid intake to prevent constipation that may result from decreased activity.

REHABILITATION—Begin daily rehabilitation exercises when supportive wrapping is no longer needed. Use ice massage for 10 minutes prior to exercise. See pages 455 and 465 for rehabilitation exercises.

CALL YOUR DOCTOR IF

- You have symptoms of a moderate or severe triceps strain, or a mild strain persists longer than 10 days.
- Pain or swelling worsens despite treatment.
- The following occurs with a cast or splints:
  Pain, numbness or coldness below the injury.
  Dusky, blue or gray fingernails.

ARM STRAIN, UPPER ARM

GENERAL INFORMATION

DEFINITION—Injury to the muscles or tendons connected to the humerus, the bone in the upper arm. Muscles, tendons and bone comprise units. These units stabilize the elbow and shoulder joints and allow their motion. A strain occurs at the weakest part of a unit. Strains are of 3 types:
- Mild (Grade I)—Slightly pulled muscle without tearing of muscle or tendon fibers. There is no loss of strength.
- Moderate (Grade II)—Tearing of fibers in a muscle, tendon or at the attachment to bone. Strength is diminished.
- Severe (Grade III)—Rupture of the muscle-tendon-bone attachment with separation of fibers. Severe strain requires surgical repair. Chronic strains are caused by overuse. Acute strains are caused by direct injury or overstress.

BODY PARTS INVOLVED
- Muscles of the upper arm.
- Tendons of the upper-arm muscles.
- Humerus, the bone of the upper arm.
- Soft tissue surrounding the strain, including nerves, periosteum (covering to bone), blood vessels and lymph vessels.

SIGNS & SYMPTOMS
- Pain when moving or stretching the upper arm.
- Muscle spasm of the injured muscles.
- Swelling in the upper arm.
- Loss of strength in the upper arm (moderate or severe strain).
- Crepitation ("crackling") feeling and sound when the injured area is pressed with fingers.
- Calcification of the muscle or its tendon (visible with X-rays).
- Inflammation of the tendon sheath.

CAUSES
- Prolonged overuse of muscle-tendon units in the upper arm.
- Single violent injury or force applied to the upper arm.

RISK INCREASES WITH
- Contact sports.
- Throwing sports.
- Any cardiovascular medical problem that results in decreased circulation.
- Medical history of any bleeding disorder.
- Obesity.
- Poor nutrition.
- Previous elbow, upper-arm or shoulder injury.
- Poor muscle conditioning or muscle overuse.

HOW TO PREVENT
- Participate in a strengthening and conditioning program appropriate for your sport.
- Warm up before practice or competition.
- Use proper protective equipment such as shoulder pads.

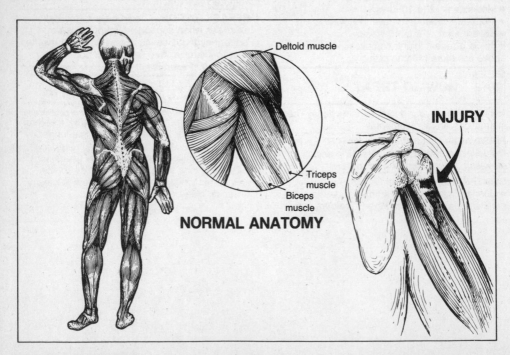

Deltoid muscle

Triceps muscle

Biceps muscle

NORMAL ANATOMY

INJURY

WHAT TO EXPECT

APPROPRIATE HEALTH CARE
- Doctor's diagnosis.
- Application of tape, plaster splints or casts (sometimes).
- Self-care during rehabilitation.
- Physical therapy (moderate or severe strain).
- Surgery (severe strain).

DIAGNOSTIC MEASURES
- Your own observation of symptoms.
- Medical history and exam by a doctor.
- X-rays of the elbow, arm and shoulder to rule out fractures.

POSSIBLE COMPLICATIONS
- Prolonged healing time if activity is resumed too soon.
- Proneness to repeated injury.
- Unstable or arthritic shoulder or elbow following repeated injury.
- Inflammation at the attachment to bone (periostitis).
- Prolonged disability (sometimes).

PROBABLE OUTCOME—If this is a first-time injury, proper care and sufficient healing time before resuming activity should prevent permanent disability. Torn ligaments and tendons require as long to heal as fractured bones do. Average healing times are:
- Mild strain—2 to 10 days.
- Moderate strain—10 days to 6 weeks.
- Severe strain—6 to 10 weeks.

If this is a repeat injury, complications listed above are more likely to occur.

 HOW TO TREAT

NOTE—Follow your doctor's instructions. These instructions are supplemental.

FIRST AID—Use instructions for R.I.C.E., the first letters of *rest, ice, compression* and *elevation.* See Appendix 1 for details.

CONTINUING CARE
- Use ice massage 3 or 4 times a day for 15 minutes at a time. Fill a large Styrofoam cup with water and freeze. Tear a small amount of foam from the top so ice protrudes. Massage firmly over the injured area in a circle about the size of a softball.
- After the first 24 hours, apply heat instead of ice, if it feels better. Use heat lamps, hot soaks, hot showers, heating pads, or heat liniments and ointments.
- Take whirlpool treatments, if available.
- Wrap the injured arm with an elasticized bandage between treatments.
- Massage gently and often to provide comfort and decrease swelling.

MEDICATION
- For minor discomfort, you may use:
  Aspirin, acetaminophen or ibuprofen.
  Topical liniments and ointments.
- Your doctor may prescribe:
  Stronger pain relievers.
  Injection of a long-acting local anesthetic to reduce pain.
  Injection of a corticosteroid, such as triamcinolone, to reduce inflammation.

ACTIVITY
- For a moderate or severe strain, use a sling for at least 72 hours—longer with a cast or splints.
- Resume your normal activities gradually.

DIET—Eat a well-balanced diet that includes extra protein, such as meat, fish, poultry, cheese, milk and eggs. Increase fiber and fluid intake to prevent constipation that may result from decreased activity.

REHABILITATION—Begin daily rehabilitation exercises when supportive wrapping is no longer needed. Use ice massage for 10 minutes prior to exercise. See page 465 for rehabilitation exercises.

 CALL YOUR DOCTOR IF

- You have symptoms of a moderate or severe upper-arm strain, or a mild strain persists longer than 10 days.
- Pain or swelling worsens despite treatment.
- The following occurs with a cast or splints:
  Dusky, blue or gray fingernails.
  Pain, numbness or coldness below the injury.

BACK, RUPTURED DISK
(Herniated Disk; Slipped Disk;
Herniated Nucleus Pulposus)

 ## GENERAL INFORMATION

DEFINITION—Sudden or gradual break in the supportive ligaments surrounding a spinal disk (a cushion separating bony spinal vertebrae).

BODY PARTS INVOLVED—Disks of the neck or lower spine are the most common sites, especially between the 4th and 5th lumbar vertebrae.

SIGNS & SYMPTOMS
In the lower back:
- Severe pain in the low back or in the back of one leg, buttock or foot (sciatica). Pain usually affects one side and worsens with movement, coughing, sneezing, lifting or straining.
- Weakness, numbness or muscular wasting of the affected leg.
In the neck:
- Pain in the neck, shoulder or down one arm. Pain worsens with movement.
- Weakness, numbness or muscular wasting of the affected arm.

CAUSES—Weakening and rupture of the disk material, creating pressure on nearby spinal nerves. Rupture of the disk is caused by sudden injury or chronic stress, such as from constant lifting or obesity.

RISK INCREASES WITH
- Any sport in which movement causes downward or twisting pressure on the neck or spine. The most common include bowling, tennis, jogging, track, football, racquetball, weight-lifting or gymnastics.
- Poor muscle conditioning and inadequate warm-up.
- Family history of low-back pain or disk disorders. Genetic factors apparently play a poorly understood role in increasing risk.
- Pre-existing spondylolisthesis.

HOW TO PREVENT
- Practice proper posture when lifting.
- Exercise regularly to maintain good muscle tone.
- If previously injured, avoid any vigorous physical activity that requires twisting of the body under uncontrollable conditions.

 ## WHAT TO EXPECT

APPROPRIATE HEALTH CARE
- Self-care after diagnosis.
- Doctor's treatment. *(Warning:* Violent chiropractic adjustments may be hazardous.)
- Traction at home or in the hospital (sometimes).

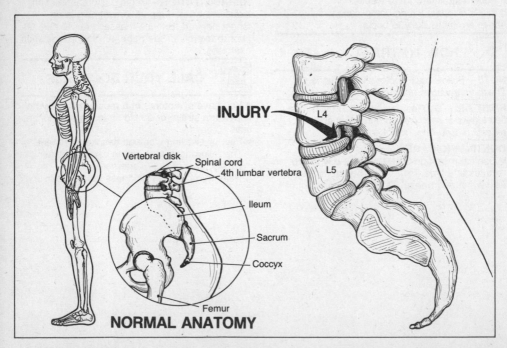

INJURY — L4

L5

Vertebral disk
Spinal cord
4th lumbar vertebra
Ileum
Sacrum
Coccyx
Femur

NORMAL ANATOMY

- Surgery to relieve nerve pressure if bed rest does not relieve symptoms and special studies confirm the diagnosis and location of a protruding, ruptured disk.
- Injection of chymopapain enzymes into the disk (sometimes).
- Rehabilitation to strengthen muscles.
- Psychotherapy, counseling or biofeedback training to learn coping methods for enduring pain when pain persists despite treatment.

DIAGNOSTIC MEASURES
- Your own observation symptoms.
- Medical history and physical exam by a doctor.
- X-rays of the neck or lower spine, including myelogram (see Glossary).
- CAT scan (see Glossary).

POSSIBLE COMPLICATIONS
- Loss of bladder and bowel function.
- Paralysis of the arm (neck disk rupture) or leg (lower-back disk rupture).
- Muscle wasting and weakness.
- Decreased sexual function.
- Surgical-wound infection if surgery is required.

PROBABLE OUTCOME—Spontaneous recovery in many cases. Bed rest for at least 2 weeks should be tried before considering other therapy (unless complications occur). When necessary, surgery with or without spinal fusion may cure the problem.

 # HOW TO TREAT

NOTE—Follow your doctor's instructions. These instructions are supplemental.

FIRST AID
- Don't move any person with a neck or back injury unless his or her life is at risk. Don't twist the back, neck or head. Support the whole back and neck with splints of any sort.
- Keep the person warm with blankets to decrease the possibility of shock.
- Seek emergency medical help immediately.

CONTINUING CARE—Apply ice packs to the painful area during the first 72 hours and occasionally thereafter, if they provide relief. Alternately, try to relieve pain with a heat lamp, hot showers, hot baths, warm compresses or a heating pad.

MEDICATION
- For minor discomfort, you may use non-prescription drugs such as aspirin or ibuprofen.
- Your doctor may prescribe:
  Pain relievers.
  Muscle relaxants.
  Non-steroidal anti-inflammatory drugs to reduce inflammation around the rupture.
  Laxatives or stool softeners to prevent constipation.

ACTIVITY—Rest in bed at least 2 weeks during the acute phase. You may read or watch TV. Resume your normal activities when symptoms improve or after recovery from surgery. Resume athletic activities after clearance from your doctor.

REHABILITATION—See pages 448, 451 or 464 for rehabilitation exercises, depending on the area of injury. Begin rehabilitation after clearance from your doctor.

DIET—No special diet. Increase consumption of dietary fiber and drink at least 8 glasses of fluid a day to prevent constipation or fecal impaction due to decreased physical activity during treatment.

 # CALL YOUR DOCTOR IF

- You have symptoms of a ruptured disk.
- The following occurs during treatment:
  Increased pain or weakness in the extremities.
  Loss of bladder or bowel control.
  New, unexplained symptoms. Drugs used in treatment may produce side effects.
- After treatment, weakness, numbness or pain in the back, buttock, legs or arms returns.

BACK SPRAIN, LUMBO-DORSAL REGION

 GENERAL INFORMATION

DEFINITION—Violent overstretching of one or more ligaments in the lumbo-dorsal vertebrae of the spine. This is the most stable section of the vertebral column. Sprains involving two or more ligaments cause considerably more disability than single-ligament sprains. When the ligament is overstretched, it becomes tense and gives way at its weakest point, either where it attaches to bone or within the ligament itself. If the ligament pulls loose a fragment of bone, it is called a *sprain-fracture.* There are 3 types of sprains:
● Mild (Grade I)—Tearing of some ligament fibers and associated muscle spasm. There is no loss of function.
● Moderate (Grade II)—Rupture of a portion of the ligament, resulting in some loss of function.
● Severe (Grade III)—Complete rupture of the ligament or complete separation of ligament from bone. There is total loss of function. A severe sprain requires surgical repair.

BODY PARTS INVOLVED
● Any of the many ligaments connecting the vertebrae in the lumbo-dorsal spine.
● Tissue surrounding the sprain, including blood vessels, tendons, bone, periosteum (covering of bone) and muscles.

SIGNS & SYMPTOMS
● Severe pain at the time of injury.
● Popping or feeling of tearing in the back.
● Tenderness at the injury site.
● Swelling in the back.
● Bruising that appears soon after injury.

CAUSES—Stress on a ligament that temporarily forces the lumbo-dorsal vertebrae out of their normal location. A sprain of the lumbo-dorsal vertebrae will frequently occur when a stressful act is performed when the athlete is off-balance, or during repeated stressful activity involving muscles in the lumbo-dorsal area.

RISK INCREASES WITH
● Contact, throwing and lifting sports.
● Gymnastics or diving.
● Previous spine injury.
● Obesity.
● Poor muscle conditioning.

HOW TO PREVENT
● Build your strength with a conditioning program appropriate for your sport.
● Warm up before practice or competition.
● Tape vulnerable joints before practice or competition to prevent reinjury.

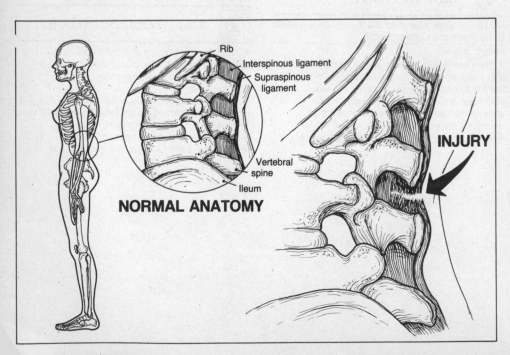

Rib
Interspinous ligament
Supraspinous ligament
Vertebral spine
Ileum

NORMAL ANATOMY

INJURY

WHAT TO EXPECT

APPROPRIATE HEALTH CARE
- Doctor's diagnosis.
- Application of tape, cast (rare) or elastic bandage.
- Self-care during rehabilitation.
- Physical therapy (moderate or severe sprain).
- Hospitalization (rare) for traction.
- Surgery (severe sprain).

DIAGNOSTIC MEASURES
- Your own observation of symptoms.
- Medical history and exam by a doctor.
- X-rays of the the spine to rule out fractures.

POSSIBLE COMPLICATIONS
- Prolonged healing time if usual activities are resumed too soon.
- Proneness to repeated back injury.
- Inflammation at the ligament attachment to bone (periostitis).
- Prolonged disability (sometimes).
- Unstable or arthritic spine following repeated injury.

PROBABLE OUTCOME
If this is a first-time injury, proper care and sufficient healing time before resuming activity should prevent permanent disability. Ligaments have a poor blood supply, and torn ligaments require as much healing time as fractures. Average healing times are:
- Mild sprains—2 to 6 weeks.
- Moderate sprains—6 to 8 weeks.
- Severe sprains—8 to 10 weeks.

 # HOW TO TREAT

NOTE—Follow your doctor's instructions. These instructions are supplemental.

FIRST AID—Use instructions for R.I.C.E., the first letters of *rest, ice, compression* and *elevation*. See Appendix 1 for details.

CONTINUING CARE—If your doctor does not apply a cast, tape or elastic bandage:
- Continue using an ice pack 3 or 4 times a day. Place ice chips or cubes in a plastic bag. Wrap the bag in a moist towel, and place it over the injured area. Use for 20 minutes at a time.
- Wrap the injured area from the top of the hip to the lower rib cage with an elasticized bandage between ice treatments.
- After 72 hours, apply heat instead of ice if it feels better. Use heat lamps, hot soaks, hot showers, heating pads, or heat liniments or ointments.
- Take whirlpool treatments, if available.
- Massage gently and often to provide comfort and decrease swelling.
- Ask your doctor about the advisability of using a special corset.

MEDICATION
- For minor discomfort, you may use:
  Aspirin, acetaminophen or ibuprofen.
  Topical liniments and ointments.
- Your doctor may prescribe:
  Stronger pain relievers.
  Injection of a long-acting local anesthetic to reduce pain.
  Injection of a corticosteroid, such as triamcinolone, to reduce inflammation.

ACTIVITY—Resume your normal activities gradually after clearance from your doctor.

DIET—During recovery, eat a well-balanced diet that includes extra protein, such as meat, fish, poultry, cheese, milk and eggs. Increase fiber and fluid intake to prevent constipation that may result from decreased activity.

REHABILITATION
- Begin daily rehabilitation exercises when the cast or supportive wrapping is no longer necessary.
- Use ice massage for 10 minutes before and after exercise. Fill a large Styrofoam cup with water and freeze. Tear a small amount of foam from the top so ice protrudes. Massage firmly over the injured area in a circle about the size of a softball.
- See pages 448 and 457 for rehabilitation exercises.

 # CALL YOUR DOCTOR IF

- You have symptoms of a moderate or severe lumbo-dorsal back sprain, or a mild sprain persists longer than 2 weeks.
- Pain, swelling or bruising worsens despite treatment.
- Pain develops in the leg.
- Any of the following occur after surgery:
  Increased pain, swelling, redness, drainage or bleeding in the surgical area.
  Signs of infection (headache, muscle aches, dizziness, or a general ill feeling with fever).
- New, unexplained symptoms develop. Drugs used in treatment may produce side effects.

BACK SPRAIN, SACROILIAC REGION

GENERAL INFORMATION

DEFINITION—Violent overstretching of one or more ligaments in the sacroiliac region of the spine. When the ligament is overstretched, it becomes tense and gives way at its weakest point, either where it attaches to bone or within the ligament itself. There are 3 types of sprains:
● Mild (Grade I)—Tearing of some ligament fibers and associated muscle spasm. There is no loss of function.
● Moderate (Grade II)—Rupture of a portion of the ligament, resulting in some loss of function.
● Severe (Grade III)—Complete rupture of the ligament or complete separation of ligament from bone. There is total loss of function. A severe sprain requires surgical repair.

BODY PARTS INVOLVED
● Ligaments of the sacroiliac region.
● Sacrum (spinal region) and ilium (bones of the pelvis).
● Tissue surrounding the sprain, including blood vessels, tendons, bone, periosteum (covering of bone) and muscles.

SIGNS & SYMPTOMS
● Severe back pain at the time of injury.
● A feeling of popping or tearing in the sacroiliac area.
● Tenderness and swelling at the injury site.
● Bruising (sometimes) that appears soon after injury.

CAUSES—Direct blow or stress on a ligament that temporarily forces or pries the sacroiliac joint out of its normal configuration.

RISK INCREASES WITH
● Contact sports such as football or wrestling.
● Weight-lifting.
● Sudden movement while one leg is in front and the other is behind.
● Previous back injury.
● Obesity.
● Poor muscle conditioning.
● Inadequate protection from equipment.

HOW TO PREVENT
● Build your strength with a conditioning program appropriate for your sport.
● Warm up before practice or competition.
● Tape vulnerable joints before practice or competition if you have been previously injured.

WHAT TO EXPECT

APPROPRIATE HEALTH CARE
● Doctor's care.
● Physical therapy (moderate or severe sprain).

DIAGNOSTIC MEASURES
● Your own observation of symptoms.
● Medical history and exam by a doctor.
● X-rays of the lower spine, hip and pelvis to rule out fractures.

POSSIBLE COMPLICATIONS
● Prolonged healing time if usual activities are

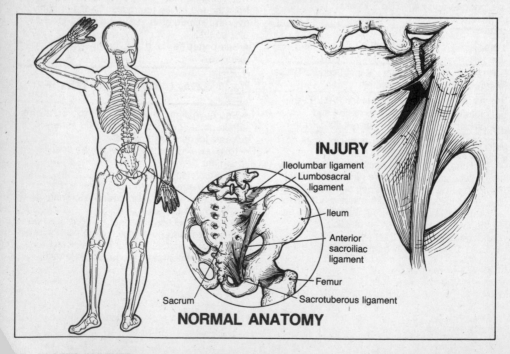

INJURY

Ileolumbar ligament
Lumbosacral ligament
Ileum
Anterior sacroiliac ligament
Femur
Sacrum
Sacrotuberous ligament

NORMAL ANATOMY

resumed too soon.
- Proneness to repeated sacroiliac injury.
- Inflammation at the ligament attachment to bone (periostitis).
- Prolonged disability (sometimes).
- Unstable or arthritic sacroiliac joint following repeated injury.

PROBABLE OUTCOME—If this is a first-time injury, proper care and sufficient healing time before resuming activity should prevent permanent disability. Ligaments have a poor blood supply, and torn ligaments require as much healing time as fractures. Average healing times are:
- Mild sprains—2 to 6 weeks.
- Moderate sprains—6 to 8 weeks.
- Severe sprains—8 to 10 weeks.

HOW TO TREAT

NOTE—Follow your doctor's instructions. These instructions are supplemental.

FIRST AID
- Use instructions for R.I.C.E., the first letters of *rest, ice, compression* and *elevation* (if possible). See Appendix 1 for details.
- Don't move the person until a litter or spineboard can be obtained for safe transport.
- Don't allow the person to walk until the diagnosis is confirmed. The spinal cord may be injured with movement.

CONTINUING CARE—If the doctor does not apply tape or an elastic bandage:
- Use an ice pack 3 or 4 times a day. Place ice chips or cubes in a plastic bag. Wrap the bag in a moist towel, and place it over the injured area. Use for 20 minutes at a time.
- Wrap the lower abdomen and hips with an elasticized bandage between ice treatments.
- After 72 hours, apply heat instead of ice, if it feels better. Use heat lamps, hot soaks, hot showers or heating pads.
- Take whirlpool treatments, if available.

MEDICATION
- For minor discomfort, you may use:
  Aspirin, acetaminophen or ibuprofen.
  Topical liniments and ointments.
- Your doctor may prescribe:
  Stronger pain relievers.
  Injection of a long-acting local anesthetic to reduce pain.
  Injection of a corticosteroid, such as triamcinolone, to reduce inflammation.

ACTIVITY—Resume your normal activities gradually after clearance from your doctor. The following exercises are safe to do while back pain is present:
- While lying on your back, bring one knee up to the chest. Lower it slowly, but do not straighten the leg. Relax. Repeat with each leg 10 times.
- Bring both knees slowly up to the chest. Tighten the abdominal muscles and press the back flat against the bed. Hold knees to chest 20 seconds, then lower slowly. Relax. Repeat 5 times.
- Clasp knees and bring them up to the chest. At the same time, come up to a sitting position. Rock back and forth.

DIET—During recovery, eat a well-balanced diet that includes extra protein, such as meat, fish, poultry, cheese, milk and eggs. Increase fiber and fluid intake to prevent constipation that may result from decreased activity.

REHABILITATION—Begin daily rehabilitation exercises when pain subsides and supportive wrapping is no longer needed. Use ice massage for 10 minutes before and after workouts. (Fill a large Styrofoam cup with water and freeze. Tear a small amount of foam from the top so ice protrudes. Massage firmly in a circle over the injured area.)
  Do the following exercises whenever you have a spare moment during the day, both to reduce tension and improve the tone of important muscle groups:
- Rotate your shoulders forward and backward.
- Turn your head slowly from side to side.
- Turn your head down and to the right as if stretching to see your right armpit. Stretch your neck slowly up, around and down, switching to see your left armpit. Repeat, starting on the left side.
- Slowly touch your left ear to your left shoulder, then your right ear to your right shoulder. Raise both shoulders to touch the ears, then drop them as far down as possible.
- As often as you remember, pull in the abdominal muscles, tighten and hold them for the count of 8 without breathing. Relax slowly. Increase the count gradually after the first week, and practice breathing normally with the abdomen flat and contracted. Do this while sitting, standing and walking.
- See pages 448 and 457 for additional rehabilitation exercises.

CALL YOUR DOCTOR IF

- You have symptoms of a moderate or severe sacroiliac sprain, or a mild sprain persists longer than 2 weeks.
- Pain, swelling or bruising worsens despite treatment.
- You experience pain, numbness or coldness in the legs.
- New, unexplained symptoms develop. Drugs used in treatment may produce side effects.

BACK STRAIN, DORSAL- OR THORACIC-SPINE REGION

GENERAL INFORMATION

DEFINITION—Injury to muscles or tendons that attach to the vertebral column at the dorsal or thoracic region of the back. The dorsal or thoracic spine is that part where ribs attach to surround the lungs. Muscles, tendons and vertebrae comprise units. The units stabilize the spine and allow its motion. A strain occurs at the weakest part of a unit. Strains are of 3 types:
● Mild (Grade I)—Slightly pulled muscle without tearing of muscle or tendon fibers. There is no loss of strength.
● Moderate (Grade II)—Tearing of fibers in a muscle, tendon or at the attachment to bone. Strength is diminished.
● Severe (Grade III)—Rupture of the muscle-tendon-bone attachment with separation of fibers.
Chronic strains are caused by overuse. Acute strains are caused by direct injury or overstress.

BODY PARTS INVOLVED
● Tendons and muscles of the dorsal or thoracic spine.
● One or more vertebral bones.
● Soft tissue surrounding the strain, including nerves, periosteum (covering to bone), blood vessels and lymph vessels.

SIGNS & SYMPTOMS
● Pain with motion or stretching of the back, or generalized pain in the back.
● Muscle spasm when moving the back.
● Swelling along a muscle of the back.
● Loss of strength (moderate or severe strain).
● Crepitation ("crackling") feeling and sound when the injured area is pressed with fingers.
● Calcification of the muscle or its tendon (visible with X-rays).
● Inflammation of the tendon sheath.

CAUSES
● Prolonged overuse or stretching of muscle-tendon units in the back.
● Single violent injury or force applied to the dorsal region of the back.

RISK INCREASES WITH
● Major exertion in an off-balance position, such as a shotputter throwing from an imperfect stance.
● Sports such as gymnastics, weight-lifting or diving.
● Any cardiovascular medical problem that results in decreased circulation.
● Medical history of any bleeding disorder.
● Obesity.
● Poor nutrition.
● Previous back injury.
● Poor muscle conditioning.

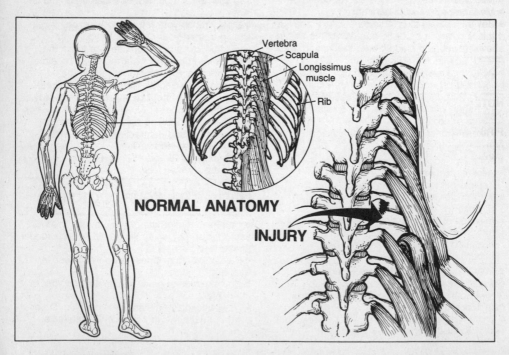

Vertebra
Scapula
Longissimus muscle
Rib

NORMAL ANATOMY

INJURY

HOW TO PREVENT

- Participate in a strengthening and conditioning program appropriate for your sport.
- Warm up before practice or competition.

 # WHAT TO EXPECT

APPROPRIATE HEALTH CARE

- Doctor's diagnosis.
- Application of tape (sometimes).
- Self-care during rehabilitation.
- Physical therapy (moderate or severe strain).

DIAGNOSTIC MEASURES

- Your own observation of symptoms.
- Medical history and exam by a doctor.
- X-rays of the back to rule out fractures.

POSSIBLE COMPLICATIONS

- Prolonged healing time if activity is resumed too soon.
- Proneness to repeated injury.
- Chronically painful or arthritic back following repeated injury.
- Inflammation at the attachment to bone (periostitis).
- Prolonged disability (sometimes).

PROBABLE OUTCOME—If this is a first-time injury, proper care and sufficient healing time before resuming activity should prevent permanent disability. Torn ligaments and tendons require as long to heal as fractured bones. Average healing times are:

- Mild strain—2 to 10 days.
- Moderate strain—10 days to 6 weeks.
- Severe strain—6 to 10 weeks.

If this is a repeat injury, complications listed above are more likely to occur.

 # HOW TO TREAT

NOTE—Follow your doctor's instructions. These instructions are supplemental.

FIRST AID—Use instructions for R.I.C.E., the first letters of *rest, ice, compression* and *elevation*. See Appendix 1 for details.

CONTINUING CARE

- Use ice massage 3 or 4 times a day for 15 minutes at a time. Fill a large Styrofoam cup with water and freeze. Tear a small amount of foam from the top so ice protrudes. Massage firmly over the injured area in a circle about the size of a softball.
- After the first 24 hours, apply heat instead of ice, if it feels better. Use heat lamps, hot soaks, hot showers, heating pads, or heat liniments and ointments.
- Take whirlpool treatments, if available.
- Wrap the injured back with an elasticized bandage between treatments.
- Massage gently and often to provide comfort and decrease swelling.

MEDICATION

- For minor discomfort, you may use:
  Aspirin, acetaminophen or ibuprofen.
  Topical liniments and ointments.
- Your doctor may prescribe:
  Stronger pain relievers.
  Muscle relaxants.
  Tranquilizers.
  Injection of a long-acting local anesthetic to reduce pain.
  Injection of a corticosteroid, such as triamcinolone, to reduce inflammation.

ACTIVITY—Rest in bed until pain improves. Resume your normal activities gradually after treatment.

DIET—Eat a well-balanced diet that includes extra protein, such as meat, fish, poultry, cheese, milk and eggs. Increase fiber and fluid intake to prevent constipation that may result from decreased activity.

REHABILITATION—Begin daily rehabilitation exercises when supportive wrapping is no longer needed. See pages 448 and 451 for rehabilitation exercises.

 # CALL YOUR DOCTOR IF

- You have symptoms of a moderate or severe back strain, or a mild strain persists longer than 10 days.
- Pain or swelling worsens despite treatment.

BACK STRAIN, LUMBAR-SPINE REGION

GENERAL INFORMATION

DEFINITION—Injury to muscles or tendons that attach to the vertebral column at the lumbar (lower midportion) spine. Muscles, tendons and vertebrae comprise units. The units stabilize the spine and allow its motion. A strain occurs at the weakest part of a unit. Strains are of 3 types:
- Mild (Grade I)—Slightly pulled muscle without tearing of muscle or tendon fibers. There is no loss of strength.
- Moderate (Grade II)—Tearing of fibers in a muscle, tendon or at the attachment to bone. Strength is diminished.
- Severe (Grade III)—Rupture of the muscle-tendon-bone attachment with separation of fibers. Severe strain requires surgical repair. Chronic strains are caused by overuse. Acute strains are caused by direct injury or overstress.

BODY PARTS INVOLVED
- Tendons and muscles of the lower midspine.
- One or more vertebral bones or bones of the pelvis.
- Soft tissue surrounding the strain, including nerves, periosteum (covering to bone), blood vessels and lymph vessels.

SIGNS & SYMPTOMS
- Pain with motion or stretching of the lower back.
- Muscle spasm in the lower back.
- Swelling along muscles of the back.
- Loss of strength (moderate or severe strain).
- Crepitation ("crackling") feeling and sound when the injured area is pressed with fingers.
- Calcification of the muscle or tendon (visible with X-rays).

CAUSES
- Prolonged overuse of muscle-tendon units in the lower back.
- Single violent injury or force applied to the lower back.

RISK INCREASES WITH
- Contact sports, especially football or hockey.
- Gymnastics or diving.
- Improper lifting of heavy objects.
- Any cardiovascular medical problem that results in decreased circulation.
- Medical history of any bleeding disorder.
- Obesity.
- Poor nutrition.
- Previous back injury, especially if it resulted in loss of back mobility.
- Poor muscle conditioning.

HOW TO PREVENT
- Participate in a strengthening and conditioning program appropriate for your sport. Include exercises to promote back flexibility.
- Warm up before practice or competition.
- Use proper lifting techniques. Don't bend over to lift. Squat to lift, and rise using leg muscles.

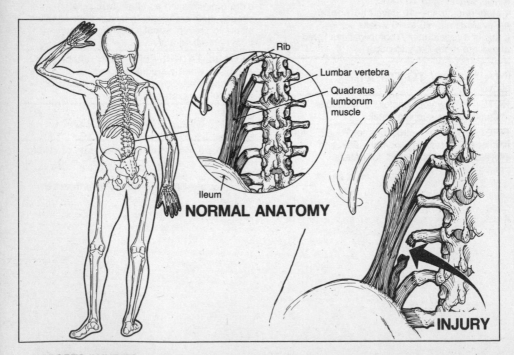

Rib

Lumbar vertebra

Quadratus lumborum muscle

Ileum

NORMAL ANATOMY

INJURY

- Wear proper protective devices, such as a back brace or taping, to prevent a recurrence after you recover.

 WHAT TO EXPECT

APPROPRIATE HEALTH CARE
- Doctor's diagnosis.
- Application of a cast (rare), brace or corset (sometimes).
- Self-care during rehabilitation.
- Physical therapy (moderate or severe strain).
- Surgery (severe strain).

DIAGNOSTIC MEASURES
- Your own observation of symptoms.
- Medical history and exam by a doctor.
- X-rays of the lumbar spine to rule out fractures or dislocations.

POSSIBLE COMPLICATIONS
- Prolonged healing time if activity is resumed too soon.
- Proneness to repeated lumbar-spine injury.
- Unstable or arthritic vertebrae following repeated injury.
- Inflammation at the attachment to bone (periostitis).
- Prolonged disability (sometimes).

PROBABLE OUTCOME—If this is a first-time injury, proper care and sufficient healing time before resuming activity should prevent permanent disability. Recurrence is likely without adequate healing time. Torn ligaments and tendons require as long to heal as fractured bones. Average healing times are:
- Mild strain—2 to 10 days.
- Moderate strain—10 days to 6 weeks.
- Severe strain—6 to 10 weeks.
If this is a repeat injury, complications listed above are more likely to occur.

 HOW TO TREAT

NOTE—Follow your doctor's instructions. These instructions are supplemental.

FIRST AID
- Rest the injured area at the first sign of severe symptoms. Rest in bed until pain decreases. Use a firm mattress.
- Use ice to help stop internal bleeding. Prepare an ice pack of ice cubes or chips wrapped in plastic or in a container. Place a towel over the injured area to prevent skin damage. Apply ice for 20 minutes, then rest 10 minutes. Repeat applications for 24 to 48 hours after injury.

CONTINUING CARE
- When bed rest is discontinued, you may need a cast or brace to allow the strain to heal completely. Later, a special corset may be used.
- Use ice massage 3 or 4 times a day for 15 minutes at a time. Fill a large Styrofoam cup with water and freeze. Tear a small amount of foam from the top so ice protrudes. Massage firmly over the injured area in a circle about the size of a softball.
- After 24 to 48 hours, apply heat instead of ice, if it feels better. Use heat lamps, hot soaks, heating pads, or heat liniments and ointments.
- Take whirlpool treatments, if available.
- Massage gently and often to provide comfort and decrease swelling.

MEDICATION
- For minor discomfort, you may use:
  Aspirin, acetaminophen or ibuprofen.
  Topical liniments and ointments.
- Your doctor may prescribe:
  Stronger pain relievers.
  Injection of a long-acting local anesthetic to reduce pain.
  Oral dose or injection of a corticosteroid, such as triamcinolone, to reduce inflammation.

ACTIVITY—Rest in bed until pain subsides. If activities are resumed too early, recurrence is likely.

DIET—Eat a well-balanced diet that includes extra protein, such as meat, fish, poultry, cheese, milk and eggs. Increase fiber and fluid intake to prevent constipation that may result from decreased activity.

REHABILITATION—Begin daily rehabilitation exercises when supportive devices are no longer needed. Use ice massage for 10 minutes prior to exercise. See pages 448 and 457 for rehabilitation exercises.

 CALL YOUR DOCTOR IF

- You have persistent back pain.
- Pain or swelling worsens despite treatment.

BLADDER OR URETHRA INJURY

GENERAL INFORMATION

DEFINITION—Damage to the urinary bladder (the organ that stores urine manufactured by the kidneys) or the urethra (the tube through which urine travels from the bladder to the outside).

BODY PARTS INVOLVED
- Bladder.
- Urethra.
- Muscles, tendons, blood vessels, nerves and connective tissue of the pelvic floor.

SIGNS & SYMPTOMS
- Severe abdominal pain and tenderness over the bladder.
- Shock (sweating; faintness; nausea; panting; rapid pulse; pale, cold, moist skin).
- Bloody discharge from the urethra or blood in the urine.

CAUSES—Fracture of a pelvic bone that punctures or bruises the bladder or urethra (usually).

RISK INCREASES WITH
- Contact sports such as football, rugby, soccer or hockey.
- Full bladder during sports activities.
- Repeated injury to the lower pelvis.

HOW TO PREVENT
- Wear adequate protective equipment.
- Keep bladder empty during exercise or competitive sports.

WHAT TO EXPECT

APPROPRIATE HEALTH CARE
- Doctor's treatment.
- Hospitalization or emergency-room care.
- Surgery (usually) to repair a punctured bladder. A damaged urethra may heal without surgery.

DIAGNOSTIC MEASURES
- Your own observation of symptoms.
- Medical history and physical exam by a doctor.
- Laboratory urine studies.
- X-rays of the urinary tract.

POSSIBLE COMPLICATIONS
- Internal bleeding.
- Rupture of the bladder (rare).
- Urine leakage into the abdomen, causing abdominal inflammation or infection.
- Recurrent infections from scars in the urethra that narrow the urinary passage.

PROBABLE OUTCOME—A punctured bladder or urethra requires emergency hospital

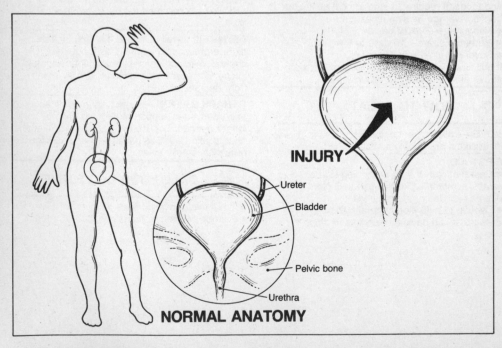

INJURY

Ureter
Bladder

Pelvic bone

Urethra

NORMAL ANATOMY

treatment. Most bladder and urethra injuries heal completely with bed rest, time, supportive treatment or surgery.

 ## HOW TO TREAT

NOTE—Follow your doctor's instructions. These instructions are supplemental.

FIRST AID
● Keep the person warm with blankets to decrease the possibility of shock.
● Immobilize the person on a stretcher or spineboard.
● Elevate the lower extremities with pillows or blocks.
● Take the patient to the nearest emergency facility.

CONTINUING CARE—No specific instructions except those under other headings. If surgery is required, your surgeon will supply postoperative instructions.

MEDICATION—Your doctor may prescribe antibiotics to prevent infection.

ACTIVITY—Stay as active as your strength allows. Allow 1 month for recovery. Don't return to work, exercise, competitive sports, or resume sexual relations until healing is complete.

DIET
● No food or water before surgery.
● Drink 6 to 8 glasses of fluid daily.
● Don't drink alcohol.
● During recovery, eat a well-balanced diet that includes extra protein, such as meat, fish, poultry, cheese, milk and eggs. Increase fiber and fluid intake to prevent constipation that may result from decreased activity.

REHABILITATION—Rehabilitation exercises must be individualized. Follow your doctor's or surgeon's directions.

 ## CALL YOUR DOCTOR IF

● You have any symptoms of bladder or urethra injury.
● During or after treatment, you develop chills and fever of 101F (38.3C) or higher.
● New, unexplained symptoms develop. Drugs used in treatment may produce side effects.

BREAST CONTUSION

 GENERAL INFORMATION

DEFINITION—Bruising of skin and underlying tissues of the breast or nipple. Contusions cause bleeding from ruptured small capillaries that allow blood to infiltrate fatty tissue, muscles, tendons, nerves or other soft tissue.

BODY PARTS INVOLVED
- Male or female breast.
- Skin, nipple, subcutaneous fatty tissue, blood vessels (both large vessels and capillaries), muscles and connective tissue.

SIGNS & SYMPTOMS
- Local swelling of the breast—either superficial or deep.
- Pain in the breast or nipple.
- Feeling of firmness when pressure is exerted on the injury area.
- Tenderness.
- Discoloration under the skin, beginning with redness and progressing to the characteristic "black and blue" bruise.
- Hard, tender ring surrounding the nipple.

CAUSES—Direct blow to the breast, usually by a blunt object.

RISK INCREASES WITH
- Contact sports such as wrestling, baseball, softball or boxing, especially if the breast area has inadequate protection.
- Medical history of any bleeding disorder such as hemophilia.
- Poor nutrition.
- Obesity.

HOW TO PREVENT
- Wear appropriate protective gear for the chest during competition or other athletic activity if there is risk of contusion.
- Women should wear breast support—a sport brassiere, elasticized binder or both—for participation in contact sports.

 WHAT TO EXPECT

APPROPRIATE HEALTH CARE
- Doctor's care unless the contusion is quite small.
- Self-care during recovery.

DIAGNOSTIC MEASURES
- Your own observation of symptoms.
- Physical exam and medical history by a doctor for all except minor injuries. Total extent of the injury may not be apparent for 48 to 72 hours following injury.

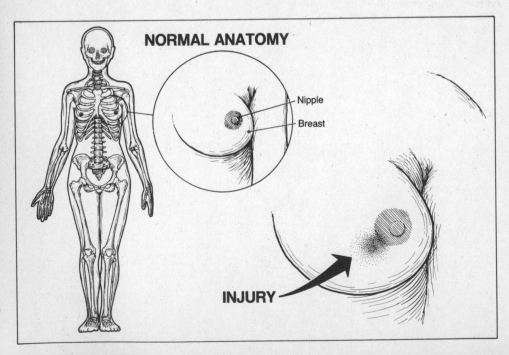

NORMAL ANATOMY

Nipple

Breast

INJURY

- X-rays of injured area to assess total injury to soft tissue and to rule out the possibility of underlying fracture.
- Follow-up exam to make sure that any lumps remaining 3 months after injury do not represent possible malignancy.

POSSIBLE COMPLICATIONS
- Excessive bleeding leading to disability. Infiltrative-type bleeding can (rarely) lead to calcification.
- Prolonged healing time if usual activities are resumed too soon.
- Infection if skin over the injury is broken.

PROBABLE OUTCOME—Healing time varies from 2 to 6 weeks, depending on the extent of injury.

 # HOW TO TREAT

NOTE—Follow your doctor's instructions. These instructions are supplemental.

FIRST AID—Use instructions for R.I.C.E., the first letters of *rest, ice, compression* and *elevation.* See Appendix 1 for details.

CONTINUING CARE
- Continue to use ice massage. Fill a large Styrofoam cup with water and freeze. Tear a small amount of foam from the top so ice protrudes. Massage firmly over the injured area in a circle about the size of a softball. Do this for 15 minutes at a time, 3 or 4 times a day, and before workouts or competition.
- After 48 hours, apply heat instead of ice if it feels better. Use heat lamps, hot soaks, hot showers, heating pads, or heat liniments or ointments.
- Take whirlpool treatments, if available.
- Protect the injured area with pads or an elasticized-bandage wrap between treatments.

MEDICATIONS
- For minor discomfort, you may use non-prescription medicines such as acetaminophen or ibuprofen (available under many different brand names). Do not use aspirin for injuries involving bleeding.
- Your doctor may prescribe stronger medicine for pain, if needed.

ACTIVITY—Begin activities slowly and stop exercise as soon as pain begins. Increase activity as healing progresses.

DIET—Eat a well-balanced diet that includes extra protein, such as meat, fish, poultry, cheese, milk and eggs. Increase fiber and fluid intake to prevent constipation that may result from decreased activity.

REHABILITATION—None.

 # CALL YOUR DOCTOR IF

- A breast contusion doesn't improve within a day or two.
- Signs of infection (drainage from skin, headache, muscle aches, dizziness, fever or a general ill feeling) occur if skin was broken.
- Firm nodules that appear following injury do not disappear in 3 months.

BREASTBONE (STERNUM) SPRAIN AT THE COLLARBONE (CLAVICLE)
(Sterno-Clavicular Sprain)

GENERAL INFORMATION

DEFINITION—Violent overstretching of one or more ligaments in the sterno-clavicular joint where the collarbone meets the breastbone. Sprains involving two or more ligaments cause considerably more disability than single-ligament sprains. When the ligament is overstretched, it becomes tense and gives way at its weakest point, either where it attaches to bone or within the ligament itself. If the ligament pulls loose a fragment of bone, it is called a *sprain-fracture*. There are 3 types of sprains:
- Mild (Grade I)—Tearing of some ligament fibers. There is no loss of function.
- Moderate (Grade II)—Rupture of a portion of the ligament, resulting in some loss of function.
- Severe (Grade III)—Complete rupture of the ligament or complete separation of ligament from bone. There is total loss of function. A severe sprain requires surgical repair.

BODY PARTS INVOLVED
- Ligaments of the sterno-clavicular joint.
- Tissue surrounding the sprain, including blood vessels, tendons, bone, periosteum (covering of bone) and muscles.

SIGNS & SYMPTOMS
- Severe pain at the time of injury.
- A feeling of popping or tearing in the collarbone area.
- Tenderness at the injury site.
- Swelling in the collarbone area.
- Bruising that appears soon after injury.

CAUSES
- Stress on a ligament by a force that thrusts the shoulder sharply forward, temporarily forcing the sterno-clavicular joint out of its normal location.
- Falling on an outstretched hand.

RISK INCREASES WITH
- Contact sports such as boxing or football.
- Weight-lifting.
- Previous breastbone or collarbone injury.
- Obesity.
- Poor muscle conditioning.
- Inadequate protection from equipment.

HOW TO PREVENT
- Warm up before practice or competition.
- Wear proper protective equipment, such as shoulder and chest pads.

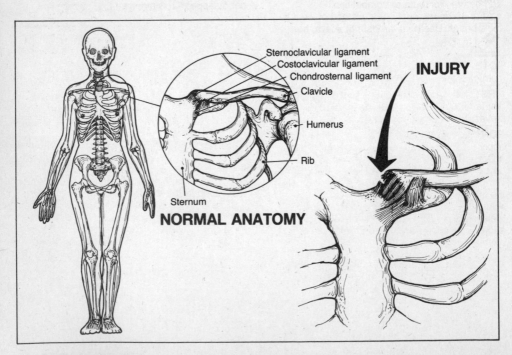

Sternoclavicular ligament
Costoclavicular ligament
Chondrosternal ligament
Clavicle
Humerus
Rib
Sternum

NORMAL ANATOMY

INJURY

WHAT TO EXPECT

APPROPRIATE HEALTH CARE
- Doctor's diagnosis.
- Application of a cast, tape, elastic bandage or special brace.
- Self-care during rehabilitation.
- Physical therapy (moderate or severe sprain).
- Surgery (severe sprain).

DIAGNOSTIC MEASURES
- Your own observation of symptoms.
- Medical history and exam by a doctor.
- X-rays of the the shoulder, chest and clavicle to rule out fractures.

POSSIBLE COMPLICATIONS
- Prolonged healing time if usual activities are resumed too soon.
- Proneness to repeated injury.
- Inflammation at the ligament attachment to bone (periostitis).
- Prolonged disability (sometimes).
- Unstable or arthritic joint following repeated injury.

PROBABLE OUTCOME—If this is a first-time injury, proper care and sufficient healing time before resuming activity should prevent permanent disability. Ligaments have a poor blood supply, and torn ligaments require as much healing time as fractures. Average healing times are:
- Mild sprains—2 to 6 weeks.
- Moderate sprains—6 to 8 weeks.
- Severe sprains—8 to 10 weeks.

 HOW TO TREAT

NOTE—Follow your doctor's instructions. These instructions are supplemental.

FIRST AID—Use instructions for R.I.C.E., the first letters of *rest, ice, compression* and *elevation.* See Appendix XX for details.

CONTINUING CARE—If the doctor does not apply a cast, tape or elastic bandage:
- Continue using an ice pack 3 or 4 times a day. Place ice chips or cubes in a plastic bag. Wrap the bag in a moist towel, and place it over the injured area. Use for 20 minutes at a time.
- After 72 hours, apply heat instead of ice if it feels better. Use heat lamps, hot soaks, hot showers, heating pads, or heat liniments or ointments.

- Take whirlpool treatments, if available.
- Massage gently and often to provide comfort and decrease swelling.

MEDICATION
- For minor discomfort, you may use:
  Aspirin, acetaminophen or ibuprofen.
  Topical liniments and ointments.
- Your doctor may prescribe:
  Stronger pain relievers.
  Injection of a long-acting local anesthetic to reduce pain.
  Injection of a corticosteroid, such as triamcinolone, to reduce inflammation.

ACTIVITY—Resume your normal activities gradually after clearance from your doctor.

DIET—During recovery, eat a well-balanced diet that includes extra protein, such as meat, fish, poultry, cheese, milk and eggs. Increase fiber and fluid intake to prevent constipation that may result from decreased activity.

REHABILITATION
- Begin daily rehabilitation exercises when pain subsides.
- Use ice massage for 10 minutes before and 10 minutes after exercise. Fill a large Styrofoam cup with water and freeze. Tear a small amount of foam from the top so ice protrudes. Massage firmly over the injured area in a circle about the size of a softball.
- See pages 451 and 465 for rehabilitation exercises.

 CALL YOUR DOCTOR IF

- You have symptoms of a moderate or severe sterno-clavicular sprain, or a mild sprain persists longer than 2 weeks.
- Pain, swelling or bruising worsens despite treatment.
- You experience pain, numbness or coldness in the shoulder, arm or below the injury site.
- Skin turns blue, gray or a dusky color beyond the cast or sling.
- The collarbone moves backward out of normal position.
- Any of the following occur after surgery:
  Increased pain, swelling, redness, drainage or bleeding in the surgical area.
  Signs of infection (headache, muscle aches, dizziness, or a general ill feeling with fever).
- New, unexplained symptoms develop. Drugs used in treatment may produce side effects.

BUTTOCK CONTUSION

GENERAL INFORMATION

DEFINITION—Bruising of skin and underlying tissues of the buttock caused by a direct blow. Contusions cause bleeding from ruptured small capillaries that allow blood to infiltrate muscles, tendons, nerves or other soft tissue.

BODY PARTS INVOLVED
- Buttocks.
- Skin, subcutaneous tissue, tendons, ligaments, blood vessels (both large vessels and capillaries), periosteum (the outside lining of bone), muscles and connective tissue.

SIGNS & SYMPTOMS
- Swelling and a hard lump in the injured buttock—either superficial or deep.
- Pain and tenderness in the buttock.
- Feeling of firmness when pressure is exerted on the buttock.
- Discoloration under the skin, beginning with redness and progressing to the characteristic "black and blue" bruise.

CAUSES—Direct blow to the buttock, usually by a blunt object.

RISK INCREASES WITH
- Contact sports, especially football, ice hockey, basketball and baseball (sliding).
- Sports that make falling from a height likely, such as high-jumping, pole-vaulting, skating or gymnastics.
- Medical history of any bleeding disorder such as hemophilia.
- Poor nutrition.
- Inadequate protection of exposed areas during contact sports.
- Obesity.

HOW TO PREVENT
- Wear protective equipment such as hip pads, when appropriate.
- Build adequate muscle strength and achieve good coordination prior to exercise, athletic practice or competition.

WHAT TO EXPECT

APPROPRIATE HEALTH CARE
- Doctor's care for precise diagnosis unless the injury is quite small.
- Self-care for minor contusions and during rehabilitation for serious contusions.
- Physical therapy for serious contusions.

DIAGNOSTIC MEASURES
- Your own observation of symptoms.
- Physical exam and medical history by a doctor for all except minor injuries.
- X-rays of the buttocks to assess total injury to soft tissue and to rule out the possibility of underlying fracture. The total extent of injury may not be apparent for 48 to 72 hours following injury.

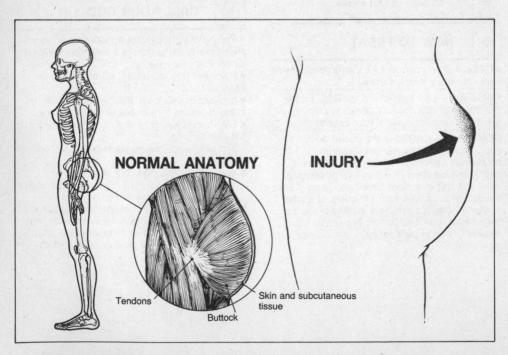

NORMAL ANATOMY

INJURY

Tendons

Buttock

Skin and subcutaneous tissue

POSSIBLE COMPLICATIONS
- Excessive bleeding into the buttock leading to disability. Infiltrative-type bleeding can (rarely) lead to calcification and impaired function of injured muscle.
- Prolonged healing time if usual activities are resumed too soon.
- Infection if skin over the injury site is broken.
- Fracture of the underlying pelvic bone (frequent complication of buttock contusion).
- Injury to the sciatic nerve.

PROBABLE OUTCOME—Healing time varies from 1 to 4 weeks, depending on the extent of injury.

 ## HOW TO TREAT

NOTE—Follow your doctor's instructions. These instructions are supplemental.

FIRST AID—Use instructions for R.I.C.E., the first letters of *rest, ice, compression* and *elevation* (if possible). See Appendix 1 for details.

CONTINUING CARE
- Continue ice massage. Fill a large Styrofoam cup with water and freeze. Tear a small amount of foam from the top so ice protrudes. Massage firmly over the injured area in a circle about the size of a softball. Do this for 15 minutes at a time, 3 or 4 times a day, and before workouts or competition.
- After 48 hours, apply heat instead of ice if it feels better. Use heat lamps, hot soaks, hot showers, heating pads, or heat liniments or ointments.
- Take whirlpool treatments, if available.
- Protect the injured area with pads or an elasticized bandage wrap between treatments.
- Massage gently and often to provide comfort and decrease swelling.

MEDICATIONS
- For minor discomfort, you may use non-prescription medicines such as acetaminophen or ibuprofen (available under many different brand names). Do not use aspirin for injuries involving bleeding.
- Your doctor may prescribe stronger medicine for pain, if needed.

ACTIVITY—Begin activities slowly and stop exercise as soon as pain begins. Increase activity as healing progresses.

DIET—Eat a well-balanced diet that includes extra protein, such as meat, fish, poultry, cheese, milk and eggs. Increase fiber and fluid intake to prevent constipation that may result from decreased activity.

REHABILITATION—Rehabilitation exercises must be individualized. Follow your doctor's or surgeon's directions.

 ## CALL YOUR DOCTOR IF

- A buttock contusion doesn't improve within a day or two.
- Signs of infection (drainage from skin, headache, muscle aches, dizziness, fever or a general ill feeling) occur if skin was broken.

CHEST-MUSCLE STRAIN

GENERAL INFORMATION

DEFINITION—Injury to the muscles and tendons that attach to the sternum (breastbone). Muscles, tendons and bone comprise units. The units stabilize the breastbone and ribs and allow their motion. A strain occurs at the weakest part of a unit. Strains are of 3 types:
- Mild (Grade I)—Slightly pulled muscle without tearing of muscle or tendon fibers. There is no loss of strength.
- Moderate (Grade II)—Tearing of fibers in a muscle, tendon or at the attachment to a rib. Strength is diminished.
- Severe (Grade III)—Rupture of the muscle-tendon-rib attachment with separation of fibers. Severe strain requires surgical repair. Chronic strains are caused by overuse. Acute strains are caused by direct injury or overstress.

BODY PARTS INVOLVED
- Muscle and tendons that attach the ribs to the sternum.
- Sternum.
- Soft tissue surrounding the strain, including nerves, periosteum (covering to bone), blood vessels and lymph vessels.

SIGNS & SYMPTOMS
- Pain when moving or stretching, especially "pushing" movements of the arms.
- Muscle spasm.
- Swelling around the injury.
- Loss of strength (moderate or severe strain).
- Crepitation ("crackling") feeling and sound when the injured area is pressed with fingers.
- Calcification of muscles or tendons (visible with X-rays).

CAUSES
- Prolonged overuse of muscle-tendon units attached to the sternum and ribs.
- Single violent injury or force applied to the muscle-tendon units around the sternum and ribs.

RISK INCREASES WITH
- Contact sports.
- Weight-lifting.
- Any cardiovascular medical problem that results in decreased circulation.
- Medical history of any bleeding disorder.
- Obesity.
- Poor nutrition.
- Previous sternum or rib injury.
- Poor muscle conditioning.

HOW TO PREVENT
- Participate in a strengthening and conditioning program appropriate for your sport.
- Warm up before practice or competition.
- Wear proper protective chest padding.

WHAT TO EXPECT

APPROPRIATE HEALTH CARE
- Doctor's diagnosis.

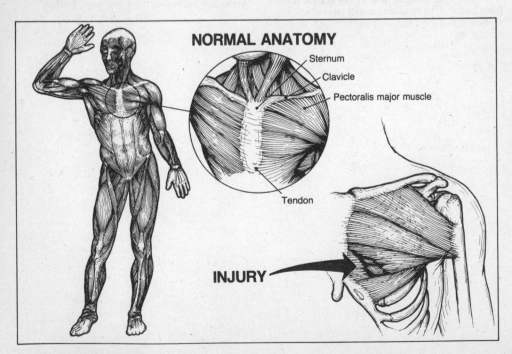

NORMAL ANATOMY

Sternum

Clavicle

Pectoralis major muscle

Tendon

INJURY

- Application of tape (sometimes).
- Self-care during rehabilitation.
- Physical therapy (moderate or severe strain).
- Surgery (severe strain).

DIAGNOSTIC MEASURES
- Your own observation of symptoms.
- Medical history and exam by a doctor.
- X-rays of the chest to rule out fractures.

POSSIBLE COMPLICATIONS
- Prolonged healing time if activity is resumed too soon.
- Proneness to repeated injury.
- Inflammation at the attachment to bone (periostitis).
- Prolonged disability (sometimes).

PROBABLE OUTCOME—If this is a first-time injury, proper care and sufficient healing time before resuming activity should prevent permanent disability. Torn ligaments and tendons require as long to heal as fractured bones do. Average healing times are:
- Mild strain—2 to 10 days.
- Moderate strain—10 days to 6 weeks.
- Severe strain—6 to 10 weeks.

If this is a repeat injury, complications listed above are more likely to occur.

 ## HOW TO TREAT

NOTE—Follow your doctor's instructions. These instructions are supplemental.

FIRST AID—Use instructions for R.I.C.E., the first letters of *rest, ice, compression* and *elevation*. See Appendix 1 for details.

CONTINUING CARE
- Use ice massage 3 or 4 times a day for 15 minutes at a time. Fill a large Styrofoam cup with water and freeze. Tear a small amount of foam from the top so ice protrudes. Massage firmly over the injured area in a circle about the size of a softball.
- After the first 24 hours, apply heat instead of ice, if it feels better. Use heat lamps, hot soaks, hot showers, heating pads, or heat liniments and ointments.
- Take whirlpool treatments, if available.
- Wrap the chest with an elasticized bandage between treatments.
- Massage gently and often to provide comfort and decrease swelling.

MEDICATION
- For minor discomfort, you may use:
  Aspirin, acetaminophen or ibuprofen.
  Topical liniments and ointments.
- Your doctor may prescribe:
  Stronger pain relievers.
  Injection of a long-acting local anesthetic to reduce pain.
  Injections of corticosteroids, such as triamcinolone, to reduce inflammation.

ACTIVITY—Resume your normal activities gradually.

DIET—Eat a well-balanced diet that includes extra protein, such as meat, fish, poultry, cheese, milk and eggs. Increase fiber and fluid intake to prevent constipation that may result from decreased activity.

REHABILITATION—Begin a supervised weight-lifting program after clearance from your doctor.

 ## CALL YOUR DOCTOR IF

- You have symptoms of a moderate or severe chest-muscle strain, or a mild strain persists longer than 10 days.
- Pain or swelling worsens despite treatment.

COLLARBONE-AREA STRAIN, DELTOID MUSCLE

GENERAL INFORMATION

DEFINITION—Injury to the deltoid muscle or tendon that attaches to the collarbone (clavicle). Muscle, tendon and bone comprise a unit. The unit stabilizes the shoulder and allows its motion. A strain occurs at the unit's weakest part. Strains are of 3 types:
● Mild (Grade I)—Slightly pulled muscle without tearing of muscle or tendon fibers. There is no loss of strength.
● Moderate (Grade II)—Tearing of fibers in the muscle, tendon or at the attachment to bone. Strength is diminished.
● Severe (Grade III)—Rupture of the muscle-tendon-bone attachment with separation of fibers. Severe strain requires surgical repair.

BODY PARTS INVOLVED
● Deltoid muscle and deltoid tendon in the collarbone area.
● Collarbone (clavicle).
● Soft tissue surrounding the strain, including nerves, periosteum (covering to bone), blood vessels and lymph vessels.

SIGNS & SYMPTOMS
● Pain with motion or stretching, particularly throwing.
● Muscle spasm.
● Swelling in the collarbone area.
● Loss of strength (moderate or severe strain).
● Crepitation ("crackling") feeling and sound when the injured area is pressed with fingers.
● Calcification of the muscle or tendon (visible with X-rays).
● Inflammation of the tendon sheath.

CAUSES
● Prolonged overuse of the deltoid muscle-tendon unit.
● Single violent injury or force applied to the collarbone area.

RISK INCREASES WITH
● Contact sports.
● Weight-lifting.
● Throwing sports.
● Any cardiovascular medical problem that results in decreased circulation.
● Medical history of any bleeding disorder.
● Obesity.
● Poor nutrition.
● Previous shoulder or collarbone injury.
● Poor muscle conditioning.

HOW TO PREVENT
● Participate in a strengthening and conditioning program appropriate for your sport.
● Warm up before practice or competition.
● Use proper protective equipment, such as shoulder pads, when appropriate.

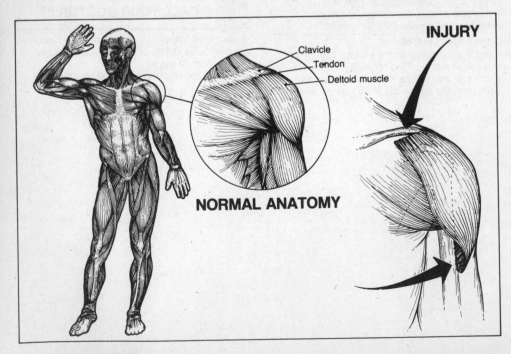

Clavicle
Tendon
Deltoid muscle

INJURY

NORMAL ANATOMY

WHAT TO EXPECT

APPROPRIATE HEALTH CARE
- Doctor's diagnosis.
- Self-care during rehabilitation.
- Physical therapy (moderate or severe strain).
- Surgery (severe strain).

DIAGNOSTIC MEASURES
- Your own observation of symptoms.
- Medical history and exam by a doctor.
- X-rays of the collarbone area to rule out fractures.

POSSIBLE COMPLICATIONS
- Prolonged healing time if activity is resumed too soon.
- Proneness to repeated injury.
- Unstable or arthritic shoulder following repeated injury.
- Inflammation at the attachment to bone (periostitis).
- Prolonged disability (sometimes).

PROBABLE OUTCOME—If this is a first-time injury, proper care and sufficient healing time before resuming activity should prevent permanent disability. Torn ligaments and tendons require as long to heal as fractured bones. Average healing times are:
- Mild strain—2 to 10 days.
- Moderate strain—10 days to 6 weeks.
- Severe strain—6 to 10 weeks.

If this is a repeat injury, complications listed above are more likely to occur.

 HOW TO TREAT

NOTE—Follow your doctor's instructions. These instructions are supplemental.

FIRST AID—Use instructions for R.I.C.E., the first letters of *rest, ice, compression* and *elevation*. See Appendix 1 for details.

CONTINUING CARE
- Use ice massage 3 or 4 times a day for 15 minutes at a time. Fill a large Styrofoam cup with water and freeze. Tear a small amount of foam from the top so ice protrudes. Massage firmly over the injured area in a circle about the size of a baseball.
- After the first 24 hours, apply heat instead of ice, if it feels better. Use heat lamps, hot soaks, hot showers, heating pads, or heat liniments and ointments.
- Massage gently and often to provide comfort and decrease swelling.

MEDICATION
- For minor discomfort, you may use:
  Aspirin, acetaminophen or ibuprofen.
  Topical liniments and ointments.
- Your doctor may prescribe:
  Stronger pain relievers.
  Injection of a long-acting local anesthetic to reduce pain.
  Injections of corticosteroids, such as triamcinolone, to reduce inflammation.

ACTIVITY
- For a moderate or severe strain, use a sling for at least 72 hours.
- Resume your normal activities gradually.

DIET—Eat a well-balanced diet that includes extra protein, such as meat, fish, poultry, cheese, milk and eggs. Increase fiber and fluid intake to prevent constipation that may result from decreased activity.

REHABILITATION—Begin daily rehabilitation exercises when pain subsides. Use ice massage for 10 minutes prior to exercise. See page 465 for rehabilitation exercises.

 CALL YOUR DOCTOR IF

- You have symptoms of a moderate or severe deltoid strain, or a mild strain persists longer than 10 days.
- Pain or swelling worsens despite treatment.

COLLARBONE (CLAVICLE) CONTUSION

 ## GENERAL INFORMATION

DEFINITION—Bruising of skin and underlying tissues at the clavicle (collarbone) caused by a direct blow. Contusions cause bleeding from ruptured small capillaries that allow blood to infiltrate muscles, tendons or other soft tissue. A collarbone contusion is usually accompanied by injury to the sternum (breastbone) or shoulder joint.

BODY PARTS INVOLVED—Tissue over the clavicle, shoulder and breastbone, including blood vessels, muscles, tendons, nerves, covering to bone (periosteum) and connective tissue.

SIGNS & SYMPTOMS
- Local swelling—either superficial or deep.
- Tenderness over the injury, but no additional pain when moving.
- Feeling of firmness when pressure is exerted at the injury site.
- Discoloration under the skin, beginning with redness and progressing to the characteristic "black and blue" bruise.
- Restricted shoulder and chest activity proportional to the extent of injury.

CAUSES—Direct blow to the clavicle, usually from a blunt object.

RISK INCREASES WITH
- Contact sports such as football, wrestling, ice hockey and basketball, especially if the shoulders and chest are not adequately protected.
- Medical history of any bleeding disorder such as hemophilia.
- Poor nutrition, including vitamin deficiency.
- Use of anticoagulants or aspirin.

HOW TO PREVENT—Wear appropriate protective shoulder and chest pads during competition or other athletic activity if there is risk of a clavicle contusion.

 ## WHAT TO EXPECT

APPROPRIATE HEALTH CARE
- Doctor's care unless the contusion is quite small.
- Self-care for minor contusions, or for serious contusions during rehabilitation.
- Physical therapy for serious contusions.

DIAGNOSTIC MEASURES
- Your own observation of symptoms.
- Medical history and physical exam by a doctor for all except minor injuries.
- X-rays of the clavicle, shoulder and sternum to assess total injury to soft tissue and to rule out the possibility of an underlying fracture or

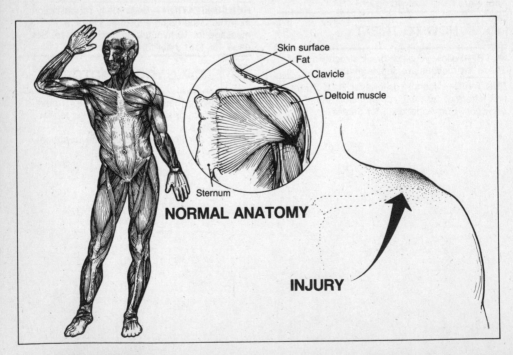

Skin surface
Fat
Clavicle
Deltoid muscle
Sternum

NORMAL ANATOMY

INJURY

shoulder dislocation. The total extent of injury may not be apparent for 48 to 72 hours.

POSSIBLE COMPLICATIONS
● Excessive bleeding leading to disability. Infiltrative-type bleeding can (rarely) lead to calcification and impaired function of injured muscle.
● Prolonged healing time if usual activities are resumed too soon.
● Infection if skin over the contusion is broken.
● Unstable or arthritic joint following repeated injury.

PROBABLE OUTCOME—Healing time varies with the extent of injury, but all but the most serious contusions should heal in 6 to 10 days.

 # HOW TO TREAT

NOTE—Follow your doctor's instructions. These instructions are supplemental.

FIRST AID—Use instructions for R.I.C.E., the first letters of *rest, ice, compression* and *elevation.* See Appendix 1 for details.

CONTINUING CARE
● Use a sling if it makes you more comfortable.
● Continue ice massage. Fill a large Styrofoam cup with water and freeze. Tear a small amount of foam from the top so ice protrudes. Massage gently over the injured area in a circle about the size of a softball. Do this for 15 minutes at a time, 3 or 4 times a day, and before workouts or competition.

● After 72 hours, apply heat instead of ice if it feels better. Use heat lamps, hot soaks, hot showers, heating pads, heat liniments or ointments, or whirlpool treatments.
● Massage gently and often to provide comfort and decrease swelling.

MEDICATION
● For minor discomfort, you may use:
  Acetaminophen or ibuprofen.
  Topical liniments and ointments.
● Your doctor may prescribe stronger medicine for pain.

ACTIVITY—Begin activities slowly and stop exercise as soon as pain begins. Increase activity as healing progresses.

DIET—During recovery, eat a well-balanced diet that includes extra protein, such as meat, fish, poultry, cheese, milk and eggs. Your doctor may prescribe vitamin and mineral supplements to promote healing.

REHABILITATION
● Begin daily rehabilitation exercises when movement is comfortable and a sling is no longer necessary.
● See page 465 for rehabilitation exercises.

 # CALL YOUR DOCTOR IF

● You have a clavicle contusion that doesn't improve in 1 or 2 days.
● Skin is broken and signs of infection (drainage, increasing pain, fever, headache, muscle aches, dizziness or a general ill feeling) occur.

COLLARBONE (CLAVICLE) DISLOCATION AT SHOULDER JOINT
(Clavicle-Acromion Dislocation)

 ## GENERAL INFORMATION

DEFINITION—An injury in which adjoining bones of the clavicle (collarbone) are displaced from their normal position and no longer touch each other. A minor dislocation is called a *subluxation.*

BODY PARTS INVOLVED
- Clavicle, sternum (breastbone) and scapula (shoulder blade).
- Ligaments that hold the clavicle to the sternum and the scapula.
- Soft tissue in the injury area, including nerves, periosteum (covering of bone), blood vessels and muscles.

SIGNS & SYMPTOMS
- Excruciating pain in the collarbone-shoulder area at the time of injury.
- Loss of shoulder function.
- Severe pain when attempting to move the tip of the shoulder.
- Visible deformity if the dislocated bones have locked in the dislocated position. Bones may spontaneously reposition themselves and leave no deformity, but damage is the same.
- Tenderness over the dislocation.
- Swelling and bruising over the injury.
- Numbness or paralysis in the arm below the

dislocation caused by pressure on blood vessels or nerves.

CAUSES
- Direct fall on the tip of the shoulder.
- Pulling or jerking on the arm.
- Falling on an outstretched hand or flexed elbow (common in football and polo).
- End result of a severe clavicle sprain.

RISK INCREASES WITH
- Contact sports.
- Previous shoulder-clavicle dislocation or sprain.
- Repeated shoulder injury of any type.
- Arthritis of any type (rheumatoid, gout).
- Poor muscle conditioning.

HOW TO PREVENT
- Build your overall strength and muscle tone with a conditioning program appropriate for your sport.
- Warm up adequately before physical activity.
- Wear shoulder pads during contact sports to protect the shoulder-clavicle area from injury.
- Avoid contact sports if treatment does not restore a strong, stable shoulder.

 ## WHAT TO EXPECT

APPROPRIATE HEALTH CARE
- Doctor's treatment, which includes

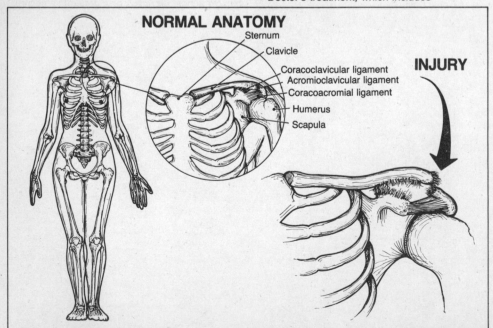

NORMAL ANATOMY

Sternum

Clavicle

Coracoclavicular ligament
Acromioclavicular ligament
Coracoacromial ligament

Humerus

Scapula

INJURY

manipulating the joint to reposition the bones or fitting a sling for traction during healing.
• Surgery (sometimes) to restore the joint to its normal position and repair torn ligaments and tendons. Acute or recurring dislocations may require surgical reconstruction or replacement of the joint.

DIAGNOSTIC MEASURES
• Your own observation of symptoms.
• Medical history and exam by a doctor.
• X-rays of the shoulder.

POSSIBLE COMPLICATIONS
At the time of injury:
• Shock.
• Pressure on or injury to nearby nerves, ligaments, tendons, muscles, blood vessels or connective tissue.
After treatment or surgery:
• Excessive internal bleeding.
• Impaired blood supply to the dislocated area.
• Death of bone cells due to interruption of the blood supply.
• Infection introduced during surgical treatment.
• Recurrent dislocations.
• Prolonged healing if activity is resumed too soon.
• Unstable or arthritic shoulder joint following repeated injury.

PROBABLE OUTCOME—After the dislocation has been corrected, the shoulder may require immobilization with a semirigid dressing and sling for 2 to 3 weeks. Injured ligaments require a minimum of 6 weeks to heal, but range-of-motion exercises and general body conditioning can begin earlier.

 HOW TO TREAT

NOTE—Follow your doctor's instructions. These instructions are supplemental.

FIRST AID
• Use instructions for R.I.C.E., the first letters of *rest, ice, compression* and *elevation*. See Appendix 1 for details.
• The doctor will manipulate the dislocated clavicle to return it to its normal position. Manipulation should occur within 6 hours of injury, or shock may result. Also, many tissues lose their elasticity and may become difficult to return to their normal position.

CONTINUING CARE
• At home, continue ice massage 3 or 4 times a day for 15 minutes at a time. Fill a large Styrofoam cup with water and freeze. Tear a small amount of foam from the top so ice protrudes. Massage firmly over the injured area in a circle about the size of a softball.
• After 24 to 48 hours, apply heat instead of

ice, if it feels better. Use heat lamps, hot soaks, hot showers or heating pads.
• Massage gently and often to provide comfort and decrease swelling.
• Wrap the injured shoulder with an elasticized bandage between treatments.

MEDICATION—Your doctor may prescribe:
• General anesthesia or muscle relaxants to make joint manipulation possible.
• Acetaminophen to relieve moderate pain.
• Narcotic pain relievers for severe pain.
• Stool softeners to prevent constipation due to decreased activity.
• Antibiotics to fight infection if surgery is necessary.

ACTIVITY
• If surgery is not necessary, resume your normal conditioning program after clearance from your doctor.
• If surgery is necessary, resume activity gradually under your doctor's supervision.
• Don't drive until healing is complete enough to allow full movement of the arm and shoulder.

DIET
• Drink only water before surgery or manipulation to correct the dislocation. Solid food in your stomach makes vomiting while under general anesthesia more hazardous.
• During recovery, eat a well-balanced diet that includes extra protein, such as meat, fish, poultry, cheese, milk and eggs. Increase fiber and fluid intake to prevent constipation that may result from decreased activity.

REHABILITATION—Begin daily rehabilitation exercises when pain subsides. Use ice massage for 10 minutes prior to exercise. See page 465 for rehabilitation exercises.

 CALL YOUR DOCTOR IF

• You have symptoms of a dislocated clavicle.
• Any of the following occur after injury or treatment:
  Numbness, loss of feeling, paleness or coldness in the arm. This is an emergency!
  Nausea or vomiting.
  Blue or gray skin color below the shoulder, especially under the fingernails.
  Swelling above or below the dressing or sling.
  Constipation.
• Any of the following occur after surgery:
  Increasing pain, swelling or drainage in the surgical area.
  Signs of infection (headache, muscle aches, dizziness, or a general ill feeling and fever).
• New, unexplained symptoms develop. Drugs used in treatment may produce side effects.
• Collarbone dislocations occur repeatedly that you can "pop" back into normal position.

COLLARBONE (CLAVICLE) FRACTURE, OUTER END

GENERAL INFORMATION

DEFINITION—A complete or incomplete break in the outer third of the clavicle (collarbone). Frequently, this fracture extends into the shoulder joint and is associated with rupture of the shoulder ligaments.

BODY PARTS INVOLVED
- Clavicle (collarbone).
- Shoulder joint.
- Joint between the shoulder and collarbone.
- Soft tissue surrounding the fracture site, including nerves, tendons, ligaments, blood vessels and bone attached to ligaments.

SIGNS & SYMPTOMS
- Severe pain at the fracture site.
- Swelling around the fracture.
- Visible deformity if the fracture is complete and bone fragments separate enough to distort normal contours.
- Tenderness to the touch.
- Numbness or coldness in the shoulder and arm on the affected side, if the blood supply is impaired.

CAUSES—Direct blow or indirect stress to the bone. Indirect stress may be caused by twisting or a violent muscle contraction.

RISK INCREASES WITH
- Contact sports such as football or soccer.
- History of bone or joint disease, especially osteoporosis.
- Obesity.
- Poor nutrition, especially calcium deficiency.
- If surgery or anesthesia are needed, surgical risk increases with smoking and use of drugs, including mind-altering drugs, muscle relaxants, antihypertensives, tranquilizers, sleep inducers, insulin, sedatives, beta-adrenergic blockers or corticosteroids.

HOW TO PREVENT
- Build adequate muscle strength and achieve good conditioning prior to exercise, athletic practice or competition. Increased muscle mass helps protect bones and underlying tissue.
- Use protective equipment such as shoulder pads, when appropriate.

WHAT TO EXPECT

APPROPRIATE HEALTH CARE
- Doctor's treatment.
- Hospitalization (sometimes) for anesthesia and surgery to set the fracture.
- Special shoulder harness to promote healing (sometimes).

DIAGNOSTIC MEASURES
- Your own observation of symptoms.
- Medical history and exam by a doctor.
- X-rays of injured areas, including the shoulder

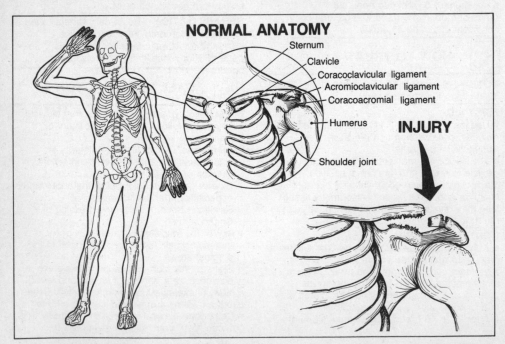

NORMAL ANATOMY

Sternum
Clavicle
Coracoclavicular ligament
Acromioclavicular ligament
Coracoacromial ligament
Humerus

INJURY

Shoulder joint

joint and joint between shoulder and clavicle.

POSSIBLE COMPLICATIONS

At the time of injury:
- Shock.
- Pressure on or injury to nearby nerves, ligaments, tendons, muscles, blood vessels or connective tissues.

After treatment or surgery:
- Delayed union or non-union of the fracture. This is frequent in fractures of the clavicle because of its naturally poor blood supply.
- Avascular necrosis (death of bone cells) due to interruption of the blood supply.
- Excessive scar tissue at the fracture site, causing compression on nerves and blood vessels in the neck. This may lead to pain, numbness and tingling in the neck, shoulder, arms and hands.
- Arrest of normal bone growth in children.
- Infection in open fractures (skin broken over fracture site), or at the incision if surgical setting was necessary.
- Shortening of the injured bones.
- Proneness to repeated collarbone injury.
- Unstable or arthritic joint following repeated injury.
- Prolonged healing time if activity is resumed too soon.

PROBABLE OUTCOME—Plates and screws implanted in surgery may be in place for a year or more. However, try to resume full function and normal range of motion within 3 or 4 weeks. Healing is complete when there is no motion at the fracture site and when X-rays show complete bone union.

 ## HOW TO TREAT

NOTE—Follow your doctor's instructions. These instructions are supplemental.

FIRST AID
- Keep the person warm with blankets to decrease the possibility of shock.
- Cut away clothing, if possible. Don't move the injured area to remove clothing.
- Follow instructions for R.I.C.E., the first letters of *rest, ice, compression* and *elevation*. See Appendix 1 for details.
- The doctor will realign and set the broken bones with surgery or, if possible, without. Manipulation should be done as soon as possible after injury. Six or more hours after the fracture, bleeding and displacement of body fluids may lead to shock. Also, many tissues lose their elasticity and become difficult to return to a normal position.

CONTINUING CARE
- Immobilization will be necessary. For this fracture, a sling usually works quite well.

- Use frequent ice massage. Fill a large Styrofoam cup with water and freeze. Tear a small amount of foam from the top so ice protrudes. Massage firmly over the injured area in a circle about the size of a baseball. Do this for 15 minutes at a time, 3 or 4 times a day, and before workouts or competition.
- After 48 hours, localized heat promotes healing by increasing blood circulation in the injured area. Use a heating pad, hot soaks, hot showers, heating pads, or heat liniments and ointments.

MEDICATION—Your doctor may prescribe:
- General anesthesia, local anesthesia, or muscle relaxants to make bone manipulation and fixation of bone fragments possible.
- Narcotic or synthetic narcotic pain relievers for severe pain.
- Stool softeners to prevent constipation due to inactivity.
- Acetaminophen or aspirin for mild pain.

ACTIVITY
- Actively exercise all muscle groups not immobilized. These muscle contractions promote fracture alignment and hasten healing.
- Resume normal activities gradually after treatment. Don't drive until healing is complete.

DIET
- Drink only water before manipulation or surgery to treat the fracture. Solid food in your stomach makes vomiting while under anesthesia more hazardous.
- During recovery, eat a well-balanced diet that includes extra protein, such as meat, fish, poultry, cheese, milk and eggs. Increase fiber and fluid intake to prevent constipation that may result from decreased activity.

REHABILITATION
- Circumduction exercises (see Glossary) should begin the first day after surgery.
- Begin reconditioning the injured area after clearance from your doctor.
- See page 465 for rehabilitation exercises.

 ## CALL YOUR DOCTOR IF

- You have symptoms of a collarbone fracture.
- Any of the following occur after surgery or other treatment:
  Increased pain, swelling or drainage in the surgical area.
  Signs of infection (headache, muscle aches, dizziness, or a general ill feeling and fever).
  Blue or gray skin color beyond the sling, especially under the fingernails.
  Loss of feeling below the fracture site.
  Nausea or vomiting.
  Constipation.

COLLARBONE (CLAVICLE) FRACTURE, SHAFT MIDPORTION

GENERAL INFORMATION

DEFINITION—A complete or incomplete break in the middle third of the clavicle (collarbone). This is the most common collarbone fracture.

BODY PARTS INVOLVED
- Clavicle (collarbone).
- Shoulder joint.
- Soft tissue surrounding the fracture site, including nerves, tendons, ligaments, blood vessels and bone attached to ligaments.

SIGNS & SYMPTOMS
- Severe pain at the fracture site.
- Swelling around the fracture.
- Visible deformity if the fracture is complete and bone fragments separate enough to distort normal body contours.
- Tenderness to the touch.
- Numbness or coldness in the shoulder and arm on the affected side, if the blood supply is impaired.

CAUSES—Direct blow or indirect stress to the clavicle, either at the shoulder or at the collarbone midpoint.

RISK INCREASES WITH
- Contact sports such as football or hockey.
- History of bone or joint disease, especially osteoporosis.
- Poor nutrition, especially calcium deficiency.
- Children.
- Obesity.
- If surgery is needed, surgical risk increases with smoking and use of drugs, including mind-altering drugs, muscle relaxants, antihypertensives, tranquilizers, sleep inducers, insulin, sedatives, beta-adrenergic blockers or corticosteroids.

HOW TO PREVENT
- Build adequate muscle strength and achieve good conditioning prior to exercise, athletic practice or competition. Increased muscle mass helps protect bones and underlying tissue.
- Use appropriate protective equipment when participating in contact sports.

? WHAT TO EXPECT

APPROPRIATE HEALTH CARE
- Doctor's treatment.
- Hospitalization (sometimes) for anesthesia and surgery to set the fracture.

DIAGNOSTIC MEASURES
- Your own observation of symptoms.
- Medical history and exam by a doctor.
- X-rays of injured areas, including the shoulder joint and joint between shoulder and clavicle.

POSSIBLE COMPLICATIONS
At the time of injury:
- Shock.

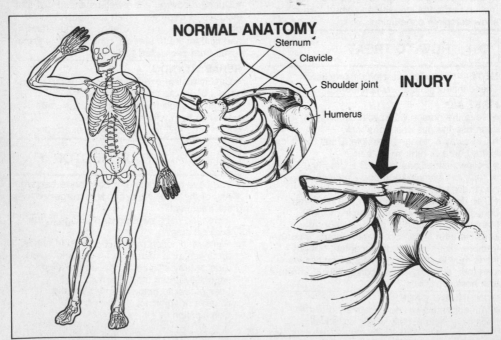

NORMAL ANATOMY

Sternum

Clavicle

Shoulder joint

INJURY

Humerus

• Pressure on or injury to nearby nerves, ligaments, tendons, muscles, blood vessels or connective tissues.

After treatment or surgery:

• Delayed union or non-union of the fracture. This is common in fractures of the clavicle because of its naturally poor blood supply.

• Avascular necrosis (death of bone cells) due to interruption of the blood supply.

• Excessive scar tissue at the fracture site, causing compression on nerves and blood vessels in the neck. This may lead to pain, numbness and tingling in the neck, shoulder, arms and hands.

• Arrest of normal bone growth in children.

• Infection in open fractures (skin broken over fracture site), or at the incision if surgical setting was necessary.

• Shortening of the injured bones.

• Proneness to repeated collarbone injury if healing is incomplete.

• Unstable or arthritic joint following repeated injury.

• Prolonged healing time if activity is resumed too soon.

PROBABLE OUTCOME—Plates and screws implanted in surgery may be in place for a year or more. However, try to resume full function and normal range of motion by 3 or 4 weeks. Healing is complete when there is no motion at the fracture site and when X-rays show complete bone union.

HOW TO TREAT

NOTE—Follow your doctor's instructions. These instructions are supplemental.

FIRST AID

• Keep the person warm with blankets to decrease the possibility of shock.

• Cut away clothing, if possible. Don't move the injured area to remove clothing.

• Use instructions for R.I.C.E., the first letters of *rest, ice, compression* and *elevation.* See Appendix 1 for details.

• Use a sling to immobilize the injured area and surrounding joints before taking the injured person to a medical facility.

CONTINUING CARE

• The doctor will realign and set the broken bones with surgery or, if possible, without. Children rarely require surgery. Manipulation should be done as soon as possible after injury. Six or more hours after the fracture, bleeding and displacement of body fluids may lead to shock. Also, many tissues lose their elasticity and become difficult to return to normal.

• Immobilization will be necessary. For this fracture, a sling usually works quite well.

• After 48 hours, localized heat promotes

healing by increasing blood circulation in the injured area. Use heat lamps, hot soaks, hot showers or heating pads.

• Use frequent ice massage. Fill a large Styrofoam cup with water and freeze. Tear a small amount of foam from the top so ice protrudes. Massage firmly over the injured area in a circle about the size of a baseball. Do this for 15 minutes at a time, 3 or 4 times a day.

• Take whirlpool treatments, if available.

MEDICATION—Your doctor may prescribe:

• General anesthesia, local anesthesia, or muscle relaxants to make bone manipulation and fixation of bone fragments possible.

• Narcotic or synthetic narcotic pain relievers for severe pain.

• Stool softeners to prevent constipation due to inactivity.

• Acetaminophen for moderate pain.

ACTIVITY

• Actively exercise all muscle groups not immobilized. These muscle contractions promote fracture alignment and hasten healing.

• Resume normal activities gradually after treatment. Don't drive until healing is complete.

• Begin reconditioning the injured area after clearance from your doctor.

DIET

• Drink only water before manipulation or surgery to treat the fracture. Solid food in your stomach makes vomiting while under anesthesia more hazardous.

• During recovery, eat a well-balanced diet that includes extra protein, such as meat, fish, poultry, cheese, milk and eggs. Increase fiber and fluid intake to prevent constipation that may result from decreased activity.

REHABILITATION

• Circumduction exercises (see Glossary) should begin the first day after surgery.

• Begin daily rehabilitation exercises when movement is comfortable. Use ice massage for 10 minutes following exercise.

• See page 465 for rehabilitation exercises.

CALL YOUR DOCTOR IF

• You have signs or symptoms of a collarbone fracture.

• Any of the following occur after surgery or other treatment:

Increased pain, swelling or drainage in the surgical area.

Signs of infection (headache, muscle aches, dizziness, or a general ill feeling and fever).

Change in skin color beyond the sling to blue or gray, particularly under the fingernails.

Loss of feeling below the fracture site.

Nausea or vomiting.

Constipation.

EAR INJURY

 GENERAL INFORMATION

DEFINITION—Ear injuries may include:
- Contusion (bruising).
- Laceration from a sharp instrument.
- Injury to the eardrum or internal ear.

BODY PARTS INVOLVED
- Skin of the ear.
- Cartilage of the ear.
- Perichondrium (thin membrane layer between the cartilage and skin).
- Nerves, blood vessels and connective tissue.
- Parts of the internal ear—eardrum, middle ear, inner ear.

SIGNS & SYMPTOMS
- Contusion or laceration: Pain, swelling, bleeding and bruising of skin around the ear.
- Internal injury: Loss of hearing, ringing in the ear, loss of equilibrium or bleeding from a ruptured eardrum.

CAUSES
- Direct blow to the ear.
- Accidental insertion of a sharp object into the ear.
- Sudden, excessive changes in pressure.

RISK INCREASES WITH
- Contact sports, especially wrestling or boxing.
- Diving.

HOW TO PREVENT—Wear protective headgear for contact sports. Some ear injuries cannot be prevented.

 WHAT TO EXPECT

APPROPRIATE HEALTH CARE
- Doctor's examination and treatment.
- Emergency-room care for laceration or internal-ear injury.
- Self-care during healing.

DIAGNOSTIC MEASURES
- Your own observation of symptoms.
- Medical history and physical exam by a doctor, including consultation with an ear specialist or plastic surgeon if necessary.
- X-rays of the skull to detect an accompanying skull fracture.

POSSIBLE COMPLICATIONS
- Chronic infection of the injured ear if the skin is broken from laceration or contusion.
- "Cauliflower ear," resulting from repeated contusions with bleeding through soft tissues. The tissues under the skin and the lining of the ear cartilage thicken permanently. (There is no treatment for this condition—only prevention.)
- Infection from contusion, laceration or other injury to the eardrum or other internal ear structures.
- Temporary or permanent hearing loss.

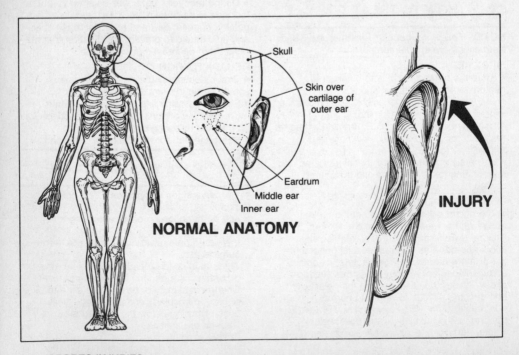

Skull

Skin over cartilage of outer ear

Eardrum

Middle ear

Inner ear

NORMAL ANATOMY

INJURY

PROBABLE OUTCOME—Contusions and lacerations may require 10 to 14 days to heal. Sutures from lacerations are usually removed in about 10 days. Other types of ear injuries usually heal without complications if they are diagnosed and treated quickly. In some cases, hearing loss after injury is permanent.

 ## HOW TO TREAT

NOTE—Follow your doctor's instructions. These instructions are supplemental.

FIRST AID
• Don't try to stop bleeding from inside the ear.
• Don't allow the injured person to hit or thump the head to try to restore hearing.
• Cover the external ear with a clean cloth or sterile bandage.
• Apply an ice pack of ice cubes or chips in a plastic bag or moist towel.
• Compress the area loosely with an elastic wrap. Don't wrap too tightly.
• Keep the injured person in a partial reclining position while transporting him or her to an emergency facility.

CONTINUING CARE
For contusions:
• The doctor will aspirate blood between the skin and ear cartilage if needed. If swelling persists, multiple small incisions may prevent a cauliflower ear from developing.
• Use ice packs or warm compresses to relieve discomfort.
• Sleep with the head elevated with 2 pillows until symptoms subside.
• Change bulky bandages often to keep them soft and protective.

For lacerations:
• Your doctor must carefully repair the cut to prevent deformity.
• Keep the wound dry and covered for 48 hours.
• After 48 hours, replace the bandage when it gets wet.
• When you change the bandage, apply a small amount of petroleum jelly or non-prescription antibiotic ointment to the bandage.
• Ignore small amounts of bleeding. Control heavier bleeding by firmly pressing a facial tissue or clean cloth to the bleeding spot for 10 minutes.

MEDICATION—Your doctor may prescribe:
• Antibiotics to treat infection.
• Pain relievers.

ACTIVITY—Resume your normal activities as soon as you are able.

DIET—During recovery, eat a well-balanced diet that includes extra protein, such as meat, fish, poultry, cheese, milk and eggs.

REHABILITATION—None.

 ## CALL YOUR DOCTOR IF

• You have any ear injury.
• Any of the following occur after treatment:
  Increased pain or pain that persists longer than 2 days.
  Hearing loss.
  Increased bleeding or swelling.
  Signs of infection (headache, muscle aches, dizziness, fever, general ill feeling).
  New, unexplained symptoms. Drugs used in treatment may produce side effects.

ELBOW BURSITIS, RADIO-HUMERAL

GENERAL INFORMATION

DEFINITION—Inflammation of the radio-humeral bursa in the elbow. Bursitis may vary in degree from mild irritation to an abscess formation that causes excruciating pain. In acute bursitis at the elbow, blood from an injury usually causes the inflammation. Bursitis will continue until the blood is removed or reabsorbed. Chronic bursitis results from undertreated acute bursitis and usually requires surgery to repair.

BODY PARTS INVOLVED
- Bursa between the radius and humerus (arm bones) where they meet in the elbow. This bursa is a soft sac filled with lubricating fluid that facilitates motion between the radius and humerus.
- Soft tissue surrounding the elbow, including nerves, tendons, ligaments, blood vessels (both large vessels and capillaries), periosteum (the outside lining of bone) and muscles.

SIGNS & SYMPTOMS
- Pain at the elbow.
- Tenderness.
- Swelling.
- Redness (sometimes) over the affected bursa.
- Fever, if infection is present.
- Limited elbow movement.

CAUSES
- Direct blow to the elbow or forearm.
- Acute or chronic infection.
- Arthritis.
- Gout.
- Unknown (frequently).

RISK INCREASES WITH
- Participating in competitive athletics, particularly contact sports.
- Previous history of bursitis in any joint.
- Exposure to cold weather.
- Poor conditioning and inadequate warmup before exercise.
- Inadequate protective equipment in contact sports.

HOW TO PREVENT
- Use protective elbow pads for contact sports.
- Wear warm clothing in cold weather.
- To prevent recurrence, continue to wear extra protection over the elbow until healing is complete.

WHAT TO EXPECT

APPROPRIATE HEALTH CARE
- Doctor's treatment.
- Surgery (sometimes), particularly for a frozen elbow or for a severely infected joint that drains to the outside.

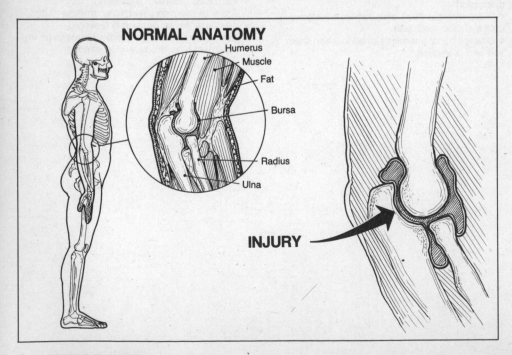

NORMAL ANATOMY

Humerus
Muscle
Fat
Bursa
Radius
Ulna

INJURY

DIAGNOSTIC MEASURES
- Your own observation of symptoms.
- Medical history and physical exam by a doctor.
- X-rays of the elbow and wrist.

POSSIBLE COMPLICATIONS
- Temporary or permanent limitation of elbow's normal mobility.
- Prolonged healing time if activity is resumed too soon.
- Proneness to repeated flare-ups.
- Unstable or arthritic elbow following repeated episodes of bursitis.
- Spontaneous rupture of bursa if severe infection is present.

PROBABLE OUTCOME—Radio-humeral bursitis is a common problem. Symptoms usually subside in 3 to 4 weeks with treatment. If serious infection occurs and surgery is needed, allow 6 to 8 weeks for healing.

 ## HOW TO TREAT

NOTE—Follow your doctor's instructions. These instructions are supplemental.

FIRST AID—None. This problem develops slowly.

CONTINUING CARE
- Use frequent ice massage. Fill a large Styrofoam cup with water and freeze. Tear a small amount of foam from the top so ice protrudes. Massage firmly over the injured area in a circle about the size of a softball. Do this for 15 minutes at a time, 3 or 4 times a day, and before workouts or competition.
- After 72 hours, apply heat instead of ice, if it feels better. Use heat lamps, hot soaks, hot showers, heating pads, or heat liniments and ointments.
- Take whirlpool treatments, if available.
- Use a sling to support the elbow joint, if needed. Don't exercise the elbow with the palm turned up or down.
- Elevate the elbow above the level of the heart to reduce swelling and prevent accumulation of fluid. Use pillows for propping.

- Massage gently and often to provide comfort and decrease swelling.

MEDICATION—Your doctor may prescribe:
- Non-steroidal anti-inflammatory drugs.
- Corticosteroid injections into the bursa to reduce inflammation.
- Prescription pain relievers for severe pain. Use non-prescription acetaminophen or ibuprofen (available under many trade names) for mild pain.
- Injection into the inflamed bursa of a long-lasting local anesthetic mixed with a corticosteroid drug, such as triamcinolone.
- Antibiotics if the bursa is infected.

ACTIVITY—Rest the inflamed area as much as possible. If you must resume normal activity immediately, wear a sling until the pain becomes more bearable. To prevent a frozen elbow, begin normal, slow joint movement as soon as possible.

DIET—Eat a well-balanced diet that includes extra protein, such as meat, fish, poultry, cheese, milk and eggs. Increase fiber and fluid intake to prevent constipation that may result from decreased activity. Your doctor may suggest vitamin and mineral supplements to promote healing.

REHABILITATION—See page 455 for rehabilitation exercises.

 ## CALL YOUR DOCTOR IF

- You have symptoms of elbow bursitis.
- Pain increases despite treatment.
- Any of the following occur after surgery:
  Pain, swelling, tenderness, drainage or bleeding increases in the surgical area.
  You develop signs of infection (headache, muscle aches, dizziness or a general ill feeling and fever).
  New, unexplained symptoms develop. Drugs used in treatment may produce side effects.

ELBOW CONTUSION

GENERAL INFORMATION

DEFINITION—Bruising of the skin and underlying tissues of the elbow due to a direct blow. Contusions cause bleeding from ruptured small capillaries that allow blood to infiltrate muscles, tendons or other soft tissue. Because skin is so close to bone in this area, contusion of the elbow is a common injury to athletes.

BODY PARTS INVOLVED—Elbow tissues, including blood vessels, muscles, tendons, nerves, olecranon bursa, connective tissue and covering to bone (periosteum). Periosteum injury is particularly common in elbow contusions.

SIGNS & SYMPTOMS
● Swelling in the elbow—either superficial or deep.
● Pain and tenderness over the elbow.
● Feeling of firmness when pressure is exerted at the injury site.
● Discoloration under the skin, beginning with redness and progressing to the characteristic "black and blue" bruise.
● Restricted elbow activity proportional to the extent of injury.

CAUSES
● Direct blow to the elbow, usually from a blunt object.

● Falling on the elbow.

RISK INCREASES WITH
● Contact sports such as football, hockey, basketball or soccer, especially if the elbows are not adequately protected.
● Medical history of any bleeding disorder such as hemophilia.
● Poor nutrition, including vitamin deficiency.
● Use of anticoagulants or aspirin.

HOW TO PREVENT—Wear appropriate protective gear and equipment, such as elbow pads, during competition or other athletic activity if there is risk of an elbow contusion.

WHAT TO EXPECT

APPROPRIATE HEALTH CARE
● Doctor's care unless the contusion is quite small.
● Self-care for minor contusions, or for serious contusions during rehabilitation.
● Physical therapy for serious elbow contusions.

DIAGNOSTIC MEASURES
● Your own observation of symptoms.
● Medical history and physical exam by a doctor for all except minor injuries.
● X-rays of the elbow, wrist and shoulder to assess total injury to soft tissue and to rule out the possibility of underlying fractures. The total

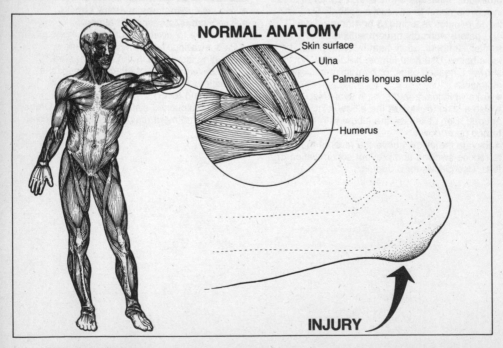

NORMAL ANATOMY

Skin surface
Ulna
Palmaris longus muscle
Humerus

INJURY

extent of injury may not be apparent for 48 to 72 hours.

POSSIBLE COMPLICATIONS
- Excessive bleeding leading to disability. Infiltrative-type bleeding can (rarely) lead to calcification and impaired function of injured muscle.
- Prolonged healing time if usual activities are resumed too soon.
- Infection if skin over the contusion is broken.

PROBABLE OUTCOME—Complete healing without complications. Most elbow contusions will heal in 6 to 10 days.

HOW TO TREAT

NOTE—Follow your doctor's instructions. These instructions are supplemental.

FIRST AID—Use instructions for R.I.C.E., the first letters of *rest, ice, compression* and *elevation.* See Appendix 1 for details.

CONTINUING CARE
- Wrap an elasticized bandage over a felt pad on the injured area. Keep the area compressed for about 72 hours.
- Immobilize the arm in a sling.
- Use ice soaks 3 or 4 times a day. Fill a bucket with ice water, and soak the injured area for 20 minutes at a time.
- After 72 hours, apply heat instead of ice if it feels better. Use heat lamps, hot soaks, hot showers, heating pads, heat liniments or ointments, or whirlpool treatments.
- Massage gently and often from wrist toward shoulder to provide comfort and decrease swelling.

MEDICATION
- For minor discomfort, you may use: Acetaminophen or ibuprofen. Topical liniments and ointments.
- Your doctor may prescribe stronger medicine.

ACTIVITY—Begin activities slowly and stop exercise as soon as pain begins. Increase activity as healing progresses.

DIET—During recovery, eat a well-balanced diet that includes extra protein, such as meat, fish, poultry, cheese, milk and eggs. Your doctor may prescribe vitamin and mineral supplements to promote healing.

REHABILITATION
- Begin daily rehabilitation exercises when supportive wrapping is no longer needed.
- Use ice massage for 10 minutes before and after workouts. Fill a large Styrofoam cup with water and freeze. Tear a small amount of foam from the top so ice protrudes. Massage firmly over the injured area in a circle about the size of a softball.
- See page 455 for rehabilitation exercises.

CALL YOUR DOCTOR IF

- You have an elbow contusion that doesn't improve in 1 or 2 days.
- Skin is broken and signs of infection (drainage, increasing pain, fever, headache, muscle aches, dizziness or a general ill feeling) occur.

ELBOW CONTUSION, ULNAR NERVE
("Crazybone" or "Crazy Nerve" Contusion)

 GENERAL INFORMATION

DEFINITION—Bruising injury from a direct blow to the ulnar nerve where it lies close to the surface at the elbow. Contusions cause bleeding from ruptured small capillaries that allow blood to infiltrate the nerve. Direct injury to the nerve causes damage even if bleeding of capillaries is not a factor.

BODY PARTS INVOLVED
- Ulnar nerve.
- Ulnar groove in the elbow portion of the humerus (bone of the upper arm).

SIGNS & SYMPTOMS
- Swelling in the elbow—either superficial or deep.
- Immediate pain in the elbow.
- Shocking, electric sensations extending down to the ring fingers and little fingers.
- Gradually increasing numbness and pain along the route of the ulnar nerve in the forearm and hand.
- Atrophy of muscles in the hand.

CAUSES
- Direct blow to the elbow area from a blunt object.
- Falling on the elbow.

RISK INCREASES WITH
- Contact sports such as football, soccer or hockey, especially when elbows are not adequately protected.
- Medical history of any bleeding disorder such as hemophilia.
- Poor nutrition, including vitamin deficiency.

HOW TO PREVENT—Wear appropriate protective gear, such as elbow pads, during competition or other athletic activity if there is risk of an elbow injury.

 WHAT TO EXPECT

APPROPRIATE HEALTH CARE
- Doctor's care unless the contusion is quite small.
- Surgery to treat the contused nerve. This usually involves transferring and transplanting the nerve into muscle where it is sutured in place.
- Self-care for minor contusions or during rehabilitation following surgery for serious ulnar-nerve contusions.
- Physical therapy following surgery.

DIAGNOSTIC MEASURES
- Your own observation of symptoms.
- Medical history and physical exam by a doctor for all except minor injuries.

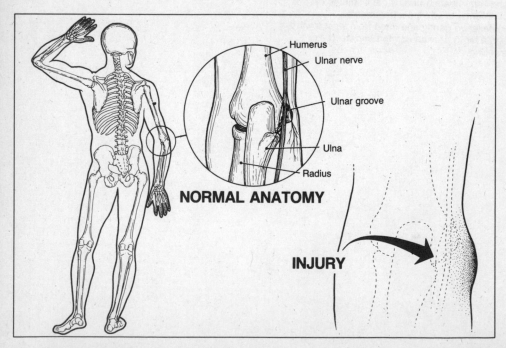

Humerus
Ulnar nerve
Ulnar groove
Ulna
Radius

NORMAL ANATOMY

INJURY

- X-rays of the elbow to assess total injury to soft tissue and to rule out the possibility of underlying fractures. The total extent of injury may not be apparent for 48 to 72 hours.

POSSIBLE COMPLICATIONS
- Permanent damage to the ulnar nerve, leading to disability in the forearm and hand.
- Prolonged healing time if usual activities are resumed too soon.
- Infection if skin over the contusion is broken.

PROBABLE OUTCOME—Healing time varies from 2 to 6 weeks, depending on the extent of injury and whether surgery is required or not. In a few cases, some symptoms may be permanent.

HOW TO TREAT

NOTE—Follow your doctor's instructions. These instructions are supplemental.

FIRST AID—Use instructions for R.I.C.E., the first letters of *rest, ice, compression* and *elevation.* See Appendix 1 for details.

CONTINUING CARE
- Wrap an elasticized bandage over a felt pad on the injured area. Keep the area compressed for about 72 hours.
- Immobilize the arm in a sling.
- Use ice soaks 3 or 4 times a day. Fill a bucket with ice water, and soak the injured area for 20 minutes at a time.
- After 72 hours, apply heat instead of ice if it feels better. Use heat lamps, hot soaks, hot showers, heating pads, heat liniments or ointments, or whirlpool treatments.
- Massage gently and often from the fingers upward to the shoulder to provide comfort and decrease swelling.

MEDICATION
- For minor discomfort, you may use: Acetaminophen or ibuprofen. Topical liniments and ointments.
- Your doctor may prescribe stronger medicine for pain.

ACTIVITY—Begin activities slowly and stop exercise as soon as pain begins. Increase activity as healing progresses.

DIET—During recovery, eat a well-balanced diet that includes extra protein, such as meat, fish, poultry, cheese, milk and eggs. Your doctor may prescribe vitamin and mineral supplements to promote healing.

REHABILITATION
- Begin daily rehabilitation exercises when movement is comfortable and sling is no longer needed.
- Use ice massage for 10 minutes before and after workouts. Fill a large Styrofoam cup with water and freeze. Tear a small amount of foam from the top so ice protrudes. Massage firmly over the injured area in a circle about the size of a softball.
- See page 455 for rehabilitation exercises.

CALL YOUR DOCTOR IF

- You have symptoms of an elbow or ulnar-nerve contusion.
- Any of the following occur after surgery:
  Increasing pain, swelling, redness, drainage or bleeding in the surgical area.
  Signs of infection: headache, muscle aches, dizziness, fever, or a general ill feeling.
  Nausea or vomiting.
  Constipation.
- New, unexplained symptoms develop. Drugs used in treatment may produce side effects.

ELBOW DISLOCATION

GENERAL INFORMATION

DEFINITION—An injury to the elbow joint so that adjoining bones are displaced from their normal position and no longer touch each other. An elbow dislocation is usually a surgical emergency because damage to nerves and blood vessels is common and severe.

BODY PARTS INVOLVED
- Elbow joint.
- Adjoining arm bones (ulna, radius and humerus).
- Collateral ligament of the elbow.
- Soft tissue surrounding the dislocation, including nerves, tendons, muscles and blood vessels.

SIGNS & SYMPTOMS
- Excruciating pain at the time of injury.
- Loss of elbow function.
- Severe pain when attempting to move the elbow.
- Visible deformity if the dislocated bones have locked in the dislocated position. Bones may spontaneously reposition themselves and leave no deformity, but damage is the same.
- Tenderness over the dislocation.
- Swelling and bruising around the elbow.
- Numbness or paralysis in the arm below the dislocation caused by pressure on blood vessels or nerves.

- Decreased or absent pulse at the wrist because of blood-vessel damage.

CAUSES
- Direct blow to the elbow.
- Fall onto an outstretched hand.
- End result of a severe elbow sprain.
- Congenital elbow abnormality, such as shallow or malformed joint surfaces.
- Powerful muscle contractions.

RISK INCREASES WITH
- Contact sports such as football, soccer or basketball.
- Field or track events that involve jumping, such as the high jump or pole vault.
- Previous elbow dislocations or sprains.
- Repeated elbow injury of any kind.
- Arthritis of any type (rheumatoid, gout).
- Poor muscle conditioning.

HOW TO PREVENT
- Build your overall strength and muscle tone with a long-term conditioning program appropriate for your sport.
- Wear elbow pads for contact sports.

WHAT TO EXPECT

APPROPRIATE HEALTH CARE
- Doctor's treatment to aspirate blood from the dislocated elbow and to reposition the bones with manipulation under general anesthesia.

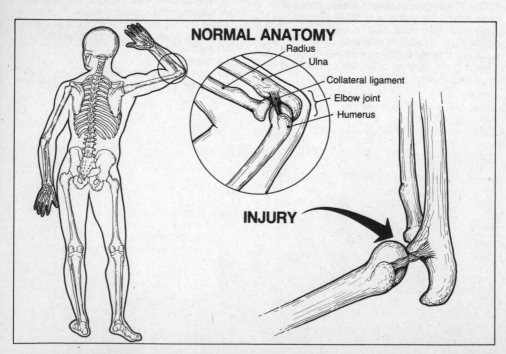

NORMAL ANATOMY

Radius
Ulna
Collateral ligament
Elbow joint
Humerus

INJURY

• Surgery (sometimes) to restore the elbow to its normal position and repair tendons and collateral ligament. Acute or recurring dislocations may require surgical reconstruction or replacement of the elbow.
• Application of splints or cast and a sling.

DIAGNOSTIC MEASURES
• Your own observation of symptoms.
• Medical history and exam by a doctor.
• X-rays of the elbow and adjacent bones.

POSSIBLE COMPLICATIONS
• Damage to nearby nerves or major blood vessels.
• Excessive internal bleeding.
• Shock or loss of consciousness.
• Recurrent dislocations, particularly if a previous dislocation has not healed completely.
• Proneness to repeated injury.
• Unstable or arthritic elbow following repeated injury.

PROBABLE OUTCOME—After the dislocation has been corrected, the elbow will require immobilization with anterior and posterior splints and a sling for 3 to 5 weeks. There will be marked stiffness after all elbow dislocations, but with competent medical care, motion should be unrestricted after 2 to 6 months. Injured ligaments require a minimum of 6 weeks to heal.

 HOW TO TREAT

NOTE—Follow your doctor's instructions. These instructions are supplemental.

FIRST AID
• Keep the person warm with blankets to decrease the possibility of shock.
• Cut away clothing if possible, but don't move the injured area to do so.
• Immobilize the elbow, shoulder and wrist with padded splints in the position they are in. Don't try to manipulate the elbow.
• Follow instructions for R.I.C.E., the first letters of *rest, ice, compression* and *elevation*. See Appendix 1 for details.
• The doctor will manipulate and realign the dislocated bones. Surgery may be required to do this. Manipulation should occur within 6 hours of injury or shock may occur. Also, many tissues lose their elasticity and may become difficult to return to a normal functional position.

CONTINUING CARE
• Splints will be necessary to immobilize the elbow, and a sling will be necessary to immobilize the entire arm. The posterior (hind) splint is usually removed 2 weeks after injury, and the anterior (front) splint is removed 1 week later. A sling is used for another week.
• Use ice soaks 3 or 4 times a day. Fill a bucket with ice water, and soak the injured area

for 20 minutes at a time.
• Use heat applications if heat feels better. Use heat lamps, hot showers or heating pads.
• Take whirlpool treatments, if available.

MEDICATION—Your doctor may prescribe:
• General anesthesia or muscle relaxants to make joint manipulation possible.
• Acetaminophen to relieve moderate pain.
• Narcotic pain relievers for severe pain.
• Antibiotics to fight infection if surgery is necessary.

ACTIVITY
• Actively exercise all muscle groups not immobilized. The muscle contractions promote proper bone alignment and hasten healing.
• Resume your normal activities gradually.
• Don't drive until all symptoms disappear.

DIET
• Drink only water before manipulation or surgery to correct the dislocation. Solid food in your stomach makes vomiting under general anesthesia more hazardous.
• Eat a well-balanced diet that includes extra protein, such as meat, fish, poultry, cheese, milk and eggs. Increase fiber and fluid intake to prevent constipation due to decreased activity.

REHABILITATION
• Begin daily rehabilitation exercises when supportive wrapping is no longer needed.
• Use ice massage for 10 minutes before and after workouts. Fill a large Styrofoam cup with water and freeze. Tear a small amount of foam from the top so ice protrudes. Massage firmly in a circle over the injured area.
• See page 455 for rehabilitation exercises.

 CALL YOUR DOCTOR IF

• Any of the following occur after injury:
  Numbness, paleness or coldness in the elbow. This is an emergency!
  Elbow deformity.
  Difficulty moving the elbow joint.
  Nausea or vomiting.
  Numbness or complete loss of feeling below the elbow.
• Any of the following occur after treatment:
  Swelling above or below the splints.
  Blue or gray skin color under the fingernails.
  Constipation.
• Any of the following occur after surgery:
  Increased pain, swelling or drainage in the surgical area.
  Signs of infection (headache, muscle aches, dizziness, or a general ill feeling and fever).
• New, unexplained symptoms develop. Drugs used in treatment may cause side effects.
• Elbow dislocations that you can "pop" back into normal position occur repeatedly.

ELBOW FRACTURE, CORONOID PROCESS

GENERAL INFORMATION

DEFINITION—A complete or incomplete break in the coronoid process of the ulna (a part of a bone in the forearm). It usually accompanies an elbow dislocation.

BODY PARTS INVOLVED
- Elbow joint.
- Coronoid process of the ulna, a curved portion of the bone that forms part of the joint.
- Soft tissue surrounding the fracture site, including nerves, tendons, ligaments, blood vessels, cartilage and muscle.

SIGNS & SYMPTOMS
- Severe pain at the fracture site.
- Swelling around the fracture.
- Visible deformity if the fracture is complete and bone fragments separate enough to distort normal body contours.
- Tenderness to the touch.
- Numbness or coldness in the lower arm and hand, if the blood supply is impaired.

CAUSES
- Direct blow to the elbow.
- Indirect injury due to falling on an outstretched hand with the elbow stiff, or any injury that causes dislocation of the elbow.

RISK INCREASES WITH
- Activities such as gymnastics or cheerleading.
- History of bone or joint disease, especially osteoporosis.
- Children under 12 and adults over 60.
- Obesity.
- If surgery is necessary, surgical risk increases with smoking and use of drugs, including mind-altering drugs, muscle relaxants, antihypertensives, tranquilizers, sleep inducers, insulin, sedatives, beta-adrenergic blockers or corticosteroids.

HOW TO PREVENT
- Build adequate muscle strength and achieve good conditioning prior to exercise, athletic practice or competition. Increased muscle mass helps protect bones and underlying tissue.
- Use appropriate protective equipment, such as padded elbow pads, when participating in contact sports.

WHAT TO EXPECT

APPROPRIATE HEALTH CARE
- Doctor's treatment to aspirate blood from the elbow joint and to remove the coronoid process surgically or to reattach it to its normal position.
- Hospitalization for surgery to set the fracture and repair soft tissues of the elbow.
- Whirlpool, ultrasound or massage (to displace excess fluid from the injured joint space).

DIAGNOSTIC MEASURES
- Your own observation of symptoms.

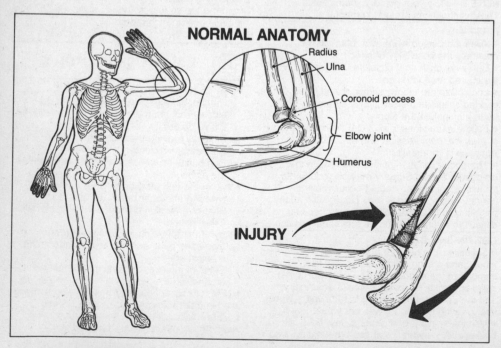

NORMAL ANATOMY

Radius
Ulna
Coronoid process
Elbow joint
Humerus

INJURY

- Medical history and exam by a doctor.
- X-rays of injured areas, including joints above and below the primary injury site.
- Repeat X-rays after approximately 1 week, if first X-rays were negative and pain continues.

POSSIBLE COMPLICATIONS
At the time of injury:
- Shock.
- Pressure on or injury to nearby nerves, ligaments, tendons, muscles, blood vessels or connective tissues.

After treatment or surgery:
- Delayed union or non-union of the fracture.
- Impaired blood supply to the fracture site.
- Arrest of normal bone growth in children.
- Infection in open fractures (skin broken over fracture site), or at the incision if surgical setting was necessary.
- Shortening of the injured bones.
- Unstable or arthritic joint following repeated injury.
- Proneness to repeated injury.
- Prolonged healing time if activity is resumed too soon.
- Problems caused by casts. See Appendix 2 (Care of Casts).

PROBABLE OUTCOME—The average time for healing of this fracture is 6 to 8 weeks in adults and 4 to 6 weeks in children. Healing is considered to be complete when there is no motion at the fracture site and when X-rays show complete bone union.

 ## HOW TO TREAT

NOTE—Follow your doctor's instructions. These instructions are supplemental.

FIRST AID
- Keep the person warm with blankets to decrease the possibility of shock.
- Cut away clothing, if possible. Don't move the injured elbow to remove clothing.
- Use instructions for R.I.C.E., the first letters of *rest, ice, compression* and *elevation*. See Appendix 1 for details.

CONTINUING CARE
- The doctor will set the broken bones and repair soft tissue with surgery. Surgery is necessary to ensure normal rotation of the forearm after healing is complete. Manipulation should be done as soon as possible after injury. Six or more hours after the fracture, bleeding and displacement of body fluids may lead to shock. Also, many tissues lose elasticity and become difficult to return to a normal position.
- Immobilization will be necessary with rigid splints around the injured area to immobilize the joints above and below the fracture site.

- After 48 hours, localized heat promotes healing by increasing blood circulation in the injured area. Use heat lamps or heating pads so heat can penetrate splints.
- After splints are removed, use frequent ice massage. Fill a large Styrofoam cup with water and freeze. Tear a small amount of foam from the top so ice protrudes. Massage firmly over the injured area in a circle about the size of a baseball. Do this for 15 minutes at a time, 3 or 4 times a day.
- Apply heat instead of ice, if it feels better. Use heat lamps, hot soaks, hot showers, heating pads, or heat liniments or ointments.
- Take whirlpool treatments, if available.

MEDICATION—Your doctor may prescribe:
- General anesthesia for surgery.
- Narcotic or synthetic narcotic pain relievers for severe pain.
- Stool softeners to prevent constipation due to inactivity.
- Acetaminophen (available without prescription) for mild pain after initial treatment.

ACTIVITY
- Resume normal activities gradually after treatment. Don't drive until healing is complete.
- Begin reconditioning the injured area after clearance from your doctor.

DIET
- Drink only water before manipulation or surgery to treat the fracture. Solid food in your stomach makes vomiting while under anesthesia more hazardous.
- During recovery, eat a well-balanced diet that includes extra protein, such as meat, fish, poultry, cheese, milk and eggs. Increase fiber and fluid intake to prevent constipation.

REHABILITATION—Begin daily rehabilitation exercises when movement is comfortable. Use ice massage for 10 minutes prior to exercise. See page 455 for rehabilitation exercises.

 ## CALL YOUR DOCTOR IF

- You have signs or symptoms of an elbow fracture.
- Any of the following occur after surgery or other treatment:
   Increased pain, swelling or drainage in the surgical area.
   Signs of infection (headache, muscle aches, dizziness, or a general ill feeling and fever).
   Swelling above or below the splints.
   Blue or gray skin color, particularly under the fingernails.
   Numbness or complete loss of feeling below the fracture site.
   Nausea or vomiting.
   Constipation.

ELBOW FRACTURE, EPICONDYLE

GENERAL INFORMATION

DEFINITION—A complete or incomplete break in the epicondyle of the humerus (the large bone in the arm between the elbow and shoulder). The epicondyle is located on the outside of the humerus at its lower end and forms a part of the elbow joint. This fracture is often accompanied by elbow dislocation.

BODY PARTS INVOLVED
- Epicondyle of the humerus.
- Elbow joint.
- Soft tissue around the fracture site, including nerves, tendons, ligaments, joint membranes and blood vessels.

SIGNS & SYMPTOMS
- Severe elbow pain at the time of injury.
- Swelling of soft tissue around the fracture.
- Visible deformity if the fracture is complete and the bone fragments separate enough to distort normal arm contours.
- Tenderness to the touch.
- Numbness and coldness in the hand and lower arm if the blood supply is impaired.

CAUSES—Direct blow or indirect stress to the elbow. Indirect stress may be caused by twisting or violent muscle contraction.

RISK INCREASES WITH
- Contact sports such as football or hockey.
- History of bone or joint disease, especially osteoporosis.
- Children under 12 or adults over 60.
- Obesity.
- If surgery or anesthesia is needed, surgical risk increases with smoking and use of drugs, including mind-altering drugs, muscle relaxants, antihypertensives, tranquilizers, sleep inducers, insulin, sedatives, beta-adrenergic blockers or corticosteroids.

HOW TO PREVENT
- Build your strength with a good conditioning program before beginning regular athletic practice or competition. Increased muscle mass helps protect bones and underlying tissue.
- Use appropriate protective equipment, such as foam-rubber elbow pads, during participation in contact sports.

WHAT TO EXPECT

APPROPRIATE HEALTH CARE
- Doctor's treatment.
- Hospitalization (sometimes) for surgical setting of the fracture.
- Whirlpool, ultrasound or massage (to displace excess fluid from the injured joint space).

DIAGNOSTIC MEASURES
- Your own observation of symptoms.
- Medical history and exam by a doctor.
- X-rays of the arm from shoulder to wrist.

POSSIBLE COMPLICATIONS
At the time of injury:
- Shock.

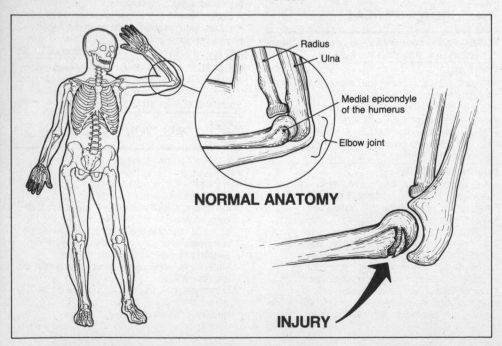

Radius
Ulna
Medial epicondyle of the humerus
Elbow joint

NORMAL ANATOMY

INJURY

• Pressure on or injury to nearby nerves, ligaments, tendons, muscles, blood vessels or connective tissues.
After treatment or surgery:
• Delayed union or non-union of the fracture.
• Impaired blood supply to the fracture site.
• Avascular necrosis (death of bone cells) due to interruption of the blood supply.
• Arrest of normal bone growth in children.
• Infection in open fractures (skin broken over fracture site), or at the incision if surgical setting was necessary.
• Shortening of the injured bones.
• Problems caused by casts. See Appendix 2 (Care of Casts).
• Prolonged healing time if activity is resumed too soon.
• Proneness to repeated elbow injury.
• Unstable or arthritic elbow following repeated injury.

PROBABLE OUTCOME—The average healing time for this fracture is 6 to 8 weeks in adults and 4 to 6 weeks in children. Healing is complete when there is no motion at the fracture site and when X-rays show complete bone union.

HOW TO TREAT

NOTE—Follow your doctor's instructions. These Instructions are supplemental.

FIRST AID
• Keep the person warm with blankets to decrease the possibility of shock.
• Cut away clothing, if possible, but don't move the injured elbow to do so.
• Follow instructions for R.I.C.E., the first letters of *rest, ice, compression* and *elevation.* See Appendix 1 for details.
• The doctor will set the broken bones with surgery or, if possible, without. The setting lines up the broken bones as close to their normal position as possible. Manipulation should be done as soon as possible after injury. Six or more hours after the fracture, bleeding and displacement of body fluids may lead to shock. Also, many tissues lose their elasticity and become difficult to return to a normal position.

CONTINUING CARE
• Immobilization will be necessary, usually with plaster splints around the injured area to immobilize the elbow and wrist.
• After 48 hours, localized heat promotes healing by increasing blood circulation in the injured area. Use a heat lamp or a heating pad for 30 minutes at a time so heat can penetrate the cast or splints.
• After the cast or splints are removed, use frequent ice massage. Fill a large Styrofoam cup with water and freeze. Tear a small amount of foam from the top so ice protrudes. Massage firmly over the injured area in a circle about the size of a baseball. Do this for 15 minutes at a time, 3 or 4 times a day.
• Apply heat instead of ice, if it feels better. Use heat lamps, hot soaks, hot showers, heating pads, or heat liniments and ointments.
• Take whirlpool treatments, if available.

MEDICATION—Your doctor may prescribe:
• General anesthesia, local anesthesia or muscle relaxants to make bone manipulation and fixation of bone fragments possible.
• Narcotic or synthetic narcotic pain relievers for severe pain.
• Stool softeners to prevent constipation due to inactivity.
• Acetaminophen for mild pain.

ACTIVITY
• Actively exercise all muscle groups not immobilized. These muscle contractions promote fracture alignment and hasten healing.
• Begin reconditioning the elbow area after clearance from your doctor.
• Resume normal activities gradually after treatment. Don't drive until healing is complete.

DIET
• Drink only water before manipulation or surgery to treat the fracture. Solid food in your stomach makes vomiting while under anesthesia more hazardous.
• During recovery, eat a well-balanced diet that includes extra protein, such as meat, fish, poultry, cheese, milk and eggs. Increase fiber and fluid intake to prevent constipation that may result from decreased activity.

REHABILITATION—Begin daily rehabilitation exercises when movement is comfortable. Use ice massage for 10 minutes prior to exercise. See page 455 for rehabilitation exercises.

CALL YOUR DOCTOR IF

• You have signs and symptoms of an elbow fracture.
• Any of the following occur after surgery or other treatment:
  Increased pain, swelling or drainage in the surgical area.
  Signs of infection (headache, muscle aches, dizziness, or a general ill feeling and fever).
  Swelling above or below the cast or splints.
  Blue or gray skin color beyond the cast or splints, particularly under the fingernails.
  Numbness or complete loss of feeling below the fracture site.
  Nausea or vomiting.
  Constipation.

ELBOW FRACTURE, LOWER HUMERUS

GENERAL INFORMATION

DEFINITION—A complete or incomplete break in the lower end of the humerus at the elbow joint.

BODY PARTS INVOLVED
- Lower end of the humerus (upper arm bone).
- Elbow joint.
- Soft tissue surrounding the fracture site, including nerves, tendons, ligaments, blood vessels, cartilage and muscles.

SIGNS & SYMPTOMS
- Severe elbow and arm pain at the time of injury.
- Swelling around the fracture.
- Visible deformity if the fracture is complete and bone fragments separate enough to distort normal body contours.
- Tenderness to the touch.
- Numbness or coldness in the elbow, lower arm and hand, if the blood supply is impaired.

CAUSES
- Direct blow to the elbow.
- Indirect stress due to falling on an outstretched hand with the elbow locked.

RISK INCREASES WITH
- Contact sports such as football.
- Children under 10 years.
- History of bone or joint disease, especially osteoporosis.
- Obesity.

- Surgical risk increases with smoking and use of drugs, including mind-altering drugs, muscle relaxants, antihypertensives, tranquilizers, sleep inducers, insulin, sedatives, beta-adrenergic blockers or corticosteroids.

HOW TO PREVENT
- Build adequate muscle strength and achieve good conditioning prior to exercise, athletic practice or competition. Increased muscle mass helps protect bones and underlying tissue.
- Use appropriate protective equipment, such as padded elbow pads for contact sports.

WHAT TO EXPECT

APPROPRIATE HEALTH CARE
- Doctor's treatment to aspirate blood from the elbow joint, manipulate the broken bones and repair soft tissue of the elbow.
- Hospitalization for anesthesia and surgery to set the fracture and repair soft tissues.
- Whirlpool, ultrasound or massage (to displace excess fluid from the injured joint space).

DIAGNOSTIC MEASURES
- Your own observation of symptoms.
- Medical history and exam by a doctor.
- X-rays of injured areas, including joints above and below the primary injury site.

POSSIBLE COMPLICATIONS
At the time of injury:
- Shock.

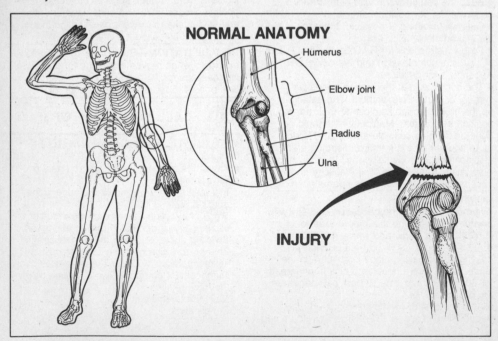

NORMAL ANATOMY

Humerus

Elbow joint

Radius

Ulna

INJURY

- Pressure on or injury to nearby nerves, ligaments, tendons, muscles, blood vessels or connective tissues.

After treatment or surgery:
- Delayed union or non-union of the fracture.
- Impaired blood supply to the fracture site.
- Avascular necrosis (death of bone cells) due to interruption of the blood supply.
- Arrest of normal bone growth in children.
- Infection in open fractures (skin broken over fracture site), or at the incision if surgical setting was necessary.
- Shortening of the injured bones.
- Unstable or arthritic joint following repeated injury.
- Prolonged healing time if activity is resumed too soon.
- Proneness to repeated injury.
- Problems caused by casts. See Appendix 2 (Care of Casts).
- Atrophy of muscles and poor hand control due to damage to blood vessels, nerves, cartilage, tendons, muscle, ligaments and fascia (thin covering of muscles).

PROBABLE OUTCOME—The average healing time for this fracture is 6 to 8 weeks in adults and 4 to 6 weeks in children. Healing is considered complete when there is no motion at the fracture site and when X-rays show complete bone union.

HOW TO TREAT

NOTE—Follow your doctor's instructions. These instructions are supplemental.

FIRST AID
- Keep the person warm with blankets to decrease the possibility of shock.
- Cut away clothing, if possible. Don't move the injured area to remove clothing.
- Follow instructions for R.I.C.E., the first letters of *rest, ice, compression* and *elevation.* See Appendix 1 for details.
- The doctor will realign and set the broken bones either with surgery or, if possible, without. Manipulation should be done as soon as possible after injury. Six or more hours after the fracture, bleeding and displacement of body fluids may lead to shock. Also, many tissues lose their elasticity and become difficult to return to a normal position.

CONTINUING CARE
- Immobilization will be necessary, usually with rigid splints around the elbow and wrist.
- After 48 hours, localized heat promotes healing by increasing blood circulation in the injured area. Use a heating pad or heat lamp for 30 minutes at a time so heat can penetrate the splints.

- After the splints are removed, use frequent ice massage. Fill a large Styrofoam cup with water and freeze. Tear a small amount of foam from the top so ice protrudes. Massage firmly over the injured area in a circle about the size of a baseball. Do this for 15 minutes at a time, 3 or 4 times a day.
- Apply heat instead of ice if it feels better. Use heat lamps, hot soaks, hot showers or heating pads.
- Take whirlpool treatments, if available.

MEDICATION—Your doctor may prescribe:
- General anesthesia for surgery.
- Narcotic or synthetic narcotic pain relievers for severe pain.
- Stool softeners to prevent constipation due to inactivity.
- Acetaminophen for mild pain.

ACTIVITY
- Actively exercise all muscle groups not immobilized. These muscle contractions promote fracture alignment and hasten healing.
- Resume normal activities gradually after treatment. Don't drive until healing is complete.
- Begin reconditioning the injured area after clearance from your doctor.

DIET
- Drink only water before manipulation or surgery to treat the fracture. Solid food in your stomach makes vomiting while under anesthesia more hazardous.
- During recovery, eat a well-balanced diet that includes extra protein, such as meat, fish, poultry, cheese, milk and eggs. Increase fiber and fluid intake to prevent constipation that may result from decreased activity.

REHABILITATION—Begin daily rehabilitation exercises when movement is comfortable. Use ice massage for 10 minutes prior to exercise. See page 455 for rehabilitation exercises.

CALL YOUR DOCTOR IF

- You have signs or symptoms of an elbow fracture.
- Any of the following occur after surgery or other treatment:
    Increased pain, swelling or drainage in the surgical area.
    Signs of infection (headache, muscle aches, dizziness, or a general ill feeling and fever).
    Swelling above or below the cast.
    Blue or gray skin color beyond the cast, particularly under the fingernails.
    Numbness or complete loss of feeling below the fracture site.
    Nausea or vomiting.
    Constipation.

ELBOW FRACTURE, RADIUS

GENERAL INFORMATION

DEFINITION—A complete or incomplete break in the head of the radius, one of the bones of the forearm.

BODY PARTS INVOLVED
● Head of the radius.
● Elbow joint.
● Soft tissue surrounding the fracture site, including nerves, tendons, ligaments, blood vessels, cartilage and muscles.

SIGNS & SYMPTOMS
● Severe pain at the fracture site.
● Swelling around the fracture.
● Visible deformity if the fracture is complete and bone fragments separate enough to distort normal arm contours.
● Tenderness to the touch.
● Numbness and coldness in the lower arm and hand, if the blood supply is impaired.

CAUSES
● Direct blow to the elbow.
● Indirect injury due to falling on an outstretched hand with the elbow stiff, or any injury that causes dislocation of the elbow.

RISK INCREASES WITH
● Contact sports such as football.
● History of bone or joint disease, especially osteoporosis.
● Poor nutrition, especially calcium deficiency.
● Children under 12 or adults over 60.

● Obesity.
● If surgery is necessary, surgical risk increases with smoking and use of drugs, including mind-altering drugs, muscle relaxants, antihypertensives, tranquilizers, sleep inducers, insulin, sedatives, beta-adrenergic blockers or corticosteroids.

HOW TO PREVENT
● Build adequate muscle strength and achieve good conditioning prior to exercise, athletic practice or competition. Increased muscle mass helps protect bones and underlying tissue.
● Use appropriate protective equipment, such as padded elbow pads, when participating in contact sports.

WHAT TO EXPECT

APPROPRIATE HEALTH CARE
● Doctor's treatment to aspirate blood from the elbow joint and to remove the radial head surgically if it is shattered beyond repair.
● Hospitalization for surgery to set the fracture and repair soft tissue of the elbow.
● Whirlpool, ultrasound or massage (to displace excess fluid from the injured joint space).

DIAGNOSTIC MEASURES
● Your own observation of symptoms.
● Medical history and exam by a doctor.
● X-rays of injured areas, including joints above and below the primary injury site.
● Additional X-rays a week later if pain persists

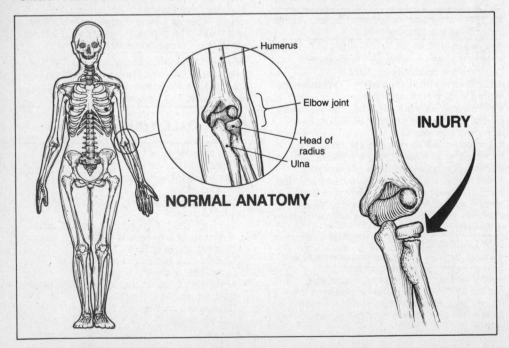

Humerus

Elbow joint

Head of radius

Ulna

NORMAL ANATOMY

INJURY

despite a normal X-ray immediately following the injury.

POSSIBLE COMPLICATIONS

At the time of injury:
- Shock.
- Pressure on or injury to nearby nerves, ligaments, tendons, muscles, blood vessels, cartilage or connective tissues.

After treatment or surgery:
- Delayed union or non-union of the fracture.
- Impaired blood supply to the fracture site.
- Avascular necrosis (death of bone cells) due to interruption of the blood supply.
- Arrest of normal bone growth in children.
- Infection in open fractures (skin broken over fracture site), or at the incision if surgical setting was necessary.
- Shortening of the injured bones.
- Proneness to repeated elbow injury.
- Unstable or arthritic elbow following repeated injury.
- Prolonged healing time if activity is resumed too soon.
- Problems caused by casts or plaster splints. See Appendix 2 (Care of Casts).

PROBABLE OUTCOME—The average healing time for this fracture is 6 to 8 weeks in adults and 4 to 6 weeks in children. Healing is considered complete when there is no motion at the fracture site and when X-rays show complete bone union.

 HOW TO TREAT

NOTE—Follow your doctor's instructions. These instructions are supplemental.

FIRST AID
- Keep the person warm with blankets to decrease the possibility of shock.
- Cut away clothing, if possible. Don't move the injured area to remove clothing.
- Use instructions for R.I.C.E., the first letters of *rest, ice, compression* and *elevation*. See Appendix 1 for details.
- The doctor will realign and set the broken bones and repair damaged soft tissue with surgery. Surgery is necessary for this injury to ensure normal rotation of the forearm after healing is complete. Manipulation should be done as soon as possible after injury. Six or more hours after the fracture, bleeding and displacement of body fluids may lead to shock. Also, many tissues lose their elasticity and become difficult to return to a normal position.

CONTINUING CARE
- Immobilization of the elbow with rigid splints will be necessary.
- After 48 hours, localized heat promotes healing by increasing blood circulation in the injured area. Use a heating pad or heat lamp so heat can penetrate the splints.
- After splints are removed, use an ice pack 3 or 4 times a day. Place ice chips or cubes in a plastic bag, and wrap the bag in a moist towel. Place it over the injured area for 20 minutes at a time.
- Apply heat instead of ice, if it feels better. Use heat lamps, hot soaks, hot showers, heating pads, or heat liniments and ointments.
- Take whirlpool treatments, if available.

MEDICATION—Your doctor may prescribe:
- General anesthesia for surgery.
- Narcotic or synthetic narcotic pain relievers for severe pain.
- Stool softeners to prevent constipation due to inactivity.
- Acetaminophen for mild pain.

ACTIVITY
- Actively exercise all muscle groups not immobilized. These muscle contractions promote fracture alignment and hasten healing.
- Resume normal activities gradually after treatment. Don't drive until healing is complete.

DIET
- Drink only water before manipulation or surgery to treat the fracture. Solid food in your stomach makes vomiting while under anesthesia more hazardous.
- During recovery, eat a well-balanced diet that includes extra protein, such as meat, fish, poultry, cheese, milk and eggs. Increase fiber and fluid intake to prevent constipation that may result from decreased activity.

REHABILITATION
- Begin reconditioning the injured area after clearance from your doctor.
- Use ice massage for 10 minutes before and after workouts. Fill a large Styrofoam cup with water and freeze. Tear a small amount of foam from the top so ice protrudes. Massage firmly in a circle over the injured area.
- See page 455 for rehabilitation exercises.

 CALL YOUR DOCTOR IF

- You have signs or symptoms of an elbow fracture.
- Any of the following occur after surgery or other treatment:
  Increased pain, swelling or drainage in the surgical area.
  Signs of infection (headache, muscle aches, dizziness, or a general ill feeling and fever).
  Swelling above or below the splints.
  Blue or gray skin color beyond the splints, particularly under the fingernails.
  Loss of feeling below the fracture site.
  Nausea or vomiting.
  Constipation.

ELBOW FRACTURE, ULNA

GENERAL INFORMATION

DEFINITION—A complete or incomplete break in the head of the ulna (one of the bones of the forearm). This fracture is often associated with an elbow dislocation.

BODY PARTS INVOLVED
- Head of the ulna that forms part of the elbow.
- Elbow joint.
- Soft tissue surrounding the fracture site, including nerves, tendons, ligaments, blood vessels, cartilage and muscles.

SIGNS & SYMPTOMS
- Severe pain at the fracture site.
- Swelling around the fracture.
- Visible deformity if the fracture is complete and bone fragments separate enough to distort normal arm contours.
- Tenderness to the touch.
- Numbness or coldness in the lower arm and hand, if the blood supply is impaired.

CAUSES
- Direct blow to the elbow.
- Indirect stress due to falling on an outstretched hand with the elbow stiff, or any injury that causes dislocation of the elbow.

RISK INCREASES WITH
- Contact sports such as football.
- Anterior (backward) dislocation of the elbow joint.
- History of bone or joint disease, especially osteoporosis.
- Poor nutrition, especially calcium deficiency.
- Children under 12 or adults over 60.
- Obesity.
- If surgery is necessary, surgical risk increases with smoking and use of drugs, including mind-altering drugs, muscle relaxants, antihypertensives, tranquilizers, sleep inducers, insulin, sedatives, beta-adrenergic blockers or corticosteroids.

HOW TO PREVENT
- Build adequate muscle strength and achieve good conditioning prior to exercise, athletic practice or competition. Increased muscle mass helps protect bones and underlying tissue.
- Use appropriate protective equipment, such as padded elbow pads for contact sports.

WHAT TO EXPECT

APPROPRIATE HEALTH CARE
- Doctor's treatment to aspirate blood from the elbow joint and to remove the olecranon process surgically (if it is shattered), or to reattach it to its normal position.
- Hospitalization for surgery to set the fracture and repair soft tissues of the elbow.
- Whirlpool, ultrasound or massage (to displace excess fluid from the injured joint space).

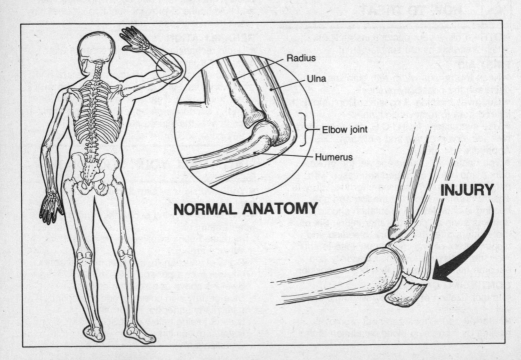

Radius
Ulna
Elbow joint
Humerus

NORMAL ANATOMY

INJURY

DIAGNOSTIC MEASURES
- Your own observation of symptoms.
- Medical history and exam by a doctor.
- X-rays of injured areas, including joints above and below the primary injury site.
- Repeat X-rays after approximately 1 week, if first X-rays were normal but pain continues.

POSSIBLE COMPLICATIONS
At the time of injury:
- Shock.
- Pressure on or injury to nearby nerves, ligaments, tendons, muscles, blood vessels or connective tissues.

After treatment or surgery:
- Delayed union or non-union of the fracture.
- Impaired blood supply to the fracture site.
- Avascular necrosis (death of bone cells) due to interruption of the blood supply.
- Arrest of normal bone growth in children.
- Infection in open fractures (skin broken over fracture site), or at the incision if surgical setting was necessary.
- Shortening of the injured bones.
- Proneness to repeated elbow injury.
- Unstable or arthritic joint following repeated injury.
- Prolonged healing time if activity is resumed too soon.

PROBABLE OUTCOME—The average healing time for this fracture is 6 to 8 weeks in adults and 4 to 6 weeks in children. Healing is considered complete when there is no motion at the fracture site and when X-rays show complete bone union.

HOW TO TREAT

NOTE—Follow your doctor's instructions. These instructions are supplemental.

FIRST AID
- Keep the person warm with blankets to decrease the possibility of shock.
- Cut away clothing, if possible. Don't move the injured area to remove clothing.
- Use instructions for R.I.C.E., the first letters of *rest, ice, compression* and *elevation.* See Appendix 1 for details.
- The doctor will realign and set the broken bones and repair damaged soft tissues with surgery. Surgery is necessary to ensure normal rotation of the forearm after healing is complete. Manipulation should be done as soon as possible after injury. Six or more hours after the fracture, bleeding and displacement of body fluids may lead to shock. Also, many tissues lose their elasticity and become difficult to return to a normal position.

CONTINUING CARE
- Immobilization will be necessary. Rigid splints

are used to immobilize the elbow and wrist.
- After 48 hours, localized heat promotes healing by increasing blood circulation in the injured area. Use a heating pad or heat lamp so heat can penetrate the splints.
- After the splints are removed, use frequent ice massage. Fill a large Styrofoam cup with water and freeze. Tear a small amount of foam from the top so ice protrudes. Massage firmly over the injured area in a circle about the size of a baseball. Do this for 15 minutes at a time, 3 or 4 times a day, and before workouts or competition.
- Apply heat instead of ice, if it feels better. Use heat lamps, hot soaks, hot showers, heating pads, or heat liniments and ointments.
- Take whirlpool treatments, if available.

MEDICATION—Your doctor may prescribe:
- General anesthesia for surgery.
- Narcotic or synthetic narcotic pain relievers.
- Stool softeners to prevent constipation due to inactivity.
- Acetaminophen for mild pain.

ACTIVITY
- Actively exercise all muscle groups not immobilized. These muscle contractions promote fracture alignment and hasten healing.
- Resume normal activities gradually after treatment. Don't drive until healing is complete.

DIET
- Drink only water before manipulation or surgery to treat the fracture. Solid food in your stomach makes vomiting while under anesthesia more hazardous.
- During recovery, eat a well-balanced diet that includes extra protein, such as meat, fish, poultry, cheese, milk and eggs. Increase fiber and fluid intake to prevent constipation that may result from decreased activity.

REHABILITATION—Begin reconditioning the injured area after clearance from your doctor. See page 455 for rehabilitation exercises.

CALL YOUR DOCTOR IF

- You have signs or symptoms of an elbow fracture.
- Any of the following occur after surgery or other treatment:
    Increased pain, swelling or drainage in the surgical area.
    Signs of infection (headache, muscle aches, dizziness, or a general ill feeling and fever).
    Swelling above or below the splints.
    Blue or gray skin color beyond the splints, particularly under the fingernails.
    Loss of feeling below the fracture site.
    Nausea or vomiting.
    Constipation.

ELBOW SPRAIN

GENERAL INFORMATION

DEFINITION—Violent overstretching of one or more ligaments in the elbow joint. Elbow sprains are relatively uncommon. Sprains involving two or more ligaments cause considerably more disability than single-ligament sprains. When the ligament is overstretched, it becomes tense and gives way at its weakest point, either where it attaches to bone or within the ligament itself. If the ligament pulls loose a fragment of bone, it is called a *sprain-fracture*. There are 3 types of sprains:
● Mild (Grade I)—Tearing of some ligament fibers. There is no loss of function.
● Moderate (Grade II)—Rupture of a portion of the ligament, resulting in some loss of function.
● Severe (Grade III)—Complete rupture of the ligament or complete separation of ligament from bone. There is total loss of function. A severe sprain requires surgical repair.

BODY PARTS INVOLVED
● Ligaments of the elbow joint.
● Tissue surrounding the sprain, including blood vessels, tendons, bone, periosteum (covering of bone) and muscles.

SIGNS & SYMPTOMS
● Severe pain at the time of injury.
● A feeling of popping or tearing inside the elbow.
● Tenderness at the injury site.
● Swelling around the elbow.
● Bruising that appears soon after injury.

CAUSES—Sharp force that bends the elbow sideways or backward, causing stress on a ligament and temporarily forcing or prying the elbow joint out of its normal location.

RISK INCREASES WITH
● Contact sports such as football, basketball, hockey and soccer.
● Previous elbow injury.
● Obesity.
● Poor muscle conditioning.

HOW TO PREVENT
● Long-term strengthening and conditioning appropriate for sport.
● Warm up before practice or competition.
● Tape vulnerable joints before practice or competition.

WHAT TO EXPECT

APPROPRIATE HEALTH CARE
● Doctor's diagnosis.
● Application of a cast, tape, elastic bandage or sling.
● Self-care during rehabilitation.
● Physical therapy (moderate or severe sprain).
● Surgery (severe sprain).

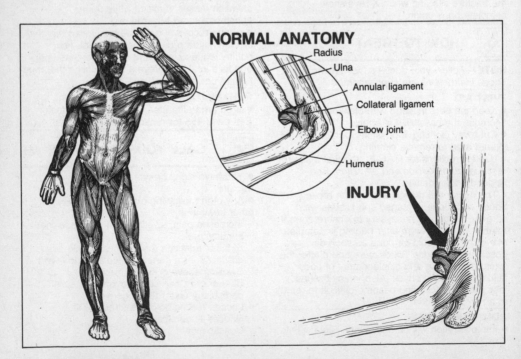

NORMAL ANATOMY

Radius
Ulna
Annular ligament
Collateral ligament
Elbow joint
Humerus

INJURY

DIAGNOSTIC MEASURES
- Your own observation of symptoms.
- Medical history and exam by a doctor.
- X-rays of the the elbow, wrist and shoulder to rule out fractures.

POSSIBLE COMPLICATIONS
- Prolonged healing time if usual activities are resumed too soon.
- Proneness to repeated injury.
- Inflammation at the ligament attachment to bone (periostitis).
- Prolonged disability (sometimes).
- Unstable or arthritic elbow following repeated injury.

PROBABLE OUTCOME—If this is a first-time injury, proper care and sufficient healing time before resuming activity should prevent permanent disability. Ligaments have a poor blood supply, and torn ligaments require as much healing time as fractures. Average healing times are:
- Mild sprains—2 to 6 weeks.
- Moderate sprains—6 to 8 weeks.
- Severe sprains—8 to 10 weeks.

 ## HOW TO TREAT

NOTE—Follow your doctor's instructions. These instructions are supplemental.

FIRST AID—Use instructions for R.I.C.E., the first letters of *rest, ice, compression* and *elevation*. See Appendix XX for details.

CONTINUING CARE—If the doctor does not apply a cast, tape or elastic bandage:
- Continue using an ice pack 3 or 4 times a day. Place ice chips or cubes in a plastic bag. Wrap the bag in a moist towel, and place it over the injured area. Use for 20 minutes at a time.
- Wrap the elbow with an elasticized bandage between ice treatments.
- After 72 hours, apply heat instead of ice if it feels better. Use heat lamps, hot soaks, hot showers, heating pads, or heat liniments or ointments.
- Take whirlpool treatments, if available.
- Massage gently and often to provide comfort and decrease swelling.

MEDICATION
- For minor discomfort, you may use:
  Aspirin, acetaminophen or ibuprofen.
  Topical liniments and ointments.
- Your doctor may prescribe:
  Stronger pain relievers.
  Injection of a long-acting local anesthetic to reduce pain.
  Injection of a corticosteroid, such as triamcinolone, to reduce inflammation.
  Other oral non-steroidal anti-inflammatory medications.

ACTIVITY—Resume your normal activities gradually after clearance from your doctor.

DIET—During recovery, eat a well-balanced diet that includes extra protein, such as meat, fish, poultry, cheese, milk and eggs. Increase fiber and fluid intake to prevent constipation that may result from decreased activity.

REHABILITATION
- Begin daily rehabilitation exercises when the cast or supportive wrapping is no longer necessary.
- Use ice massage for 10 minutes before and after exercise. Fill a large Styrofoam cup with water and freeze. Tear a small amount of foam from the top so ice protrudes. Massage firmly over the injured area in a circle about the size of a softball.
- See page 455 for rehabilitation exercises.

 ## CALL YOUR DOCTOR IF

- You have symptoms of a moderate or severe elbow sprain, or a mild sprain persists longer than 2 weeks.
- Pain, swelling or bruising worsens despite treatment.
- Any of the following occur after casting or splinting:
  Pain, numbness or coldness below the elbow.
  Blue, gray or dusky fingernails.
- Any of the following occur after surgery:
  Increased pain, swelling, redness, drainage or bleeding in the surgical area.
  Signs of infection (headache, muscle aches, dizziness, or a general ill feeling with fever).
- New, unexplained symptoms develop. Drugs used in treatment may produce side effects.

ELBOW STRAIN

GENERAL INFORMATION

DEFINITION—Injury to the muscles or tendons that attach to bones in the elbow. Muscles, tendons and bones comprise units. These units stabilize the elbow joint and allow its motion. A strain occurs at a unit's weakest part. Strains are of 3 types:
- Mild (Grade I)—Slightly pulled muscle without tearing of muscle or tendon fibers. There is no loss of strength.
- Moderate (Grade II)—Tearing of fibers in a muscle, tendon or at the attachment to bone. Strength is diminished.
- Severe (Grade III)—Rupture of the muscle-tendon-bone attachment with separation of fibers. Severe strain requires surgical repair. Chronic strains are caused by overuse. Acute strains are caused by direct injury or overstress.

BODY PARTS INVOLVED
- Tendons and muscles around the elbow.
- Bones in the elbow region.
- Soft tissue surrounding the strain, including nerves, periosteum (covering to bone), blood vessels and lymph vessels.

SIGNS & SYMPTOMS
- Pain when moving or stretching the elbow.
- Muscle spasm in the elbow area.
- Swelling over the injury.
- Loss of strength (moderate or severe strain).

- Crepitation ("crackling") feeling and sound when the injured area is pressed with fingers.
- Calcification of muscles or tendons (visible with X-rays).
- Inflammation of a tendon sheath.

CAUSES
- Prolonged overuse of muscle-tendon units in the elbow.
- Sudden, forceful hyperextension of the elbow.
- Single violent injury or force applied to the elbow.

RISK INCREASES WITH
- Contact sports.
- Racket sports.
- Throwing sports.
- Any cardiovascular medical problem that results in decreased circulation.
- Medical history of any bleeding disorder.
- Obesity.
- Poor nutrition.
- Previous elbow injury.
- Poor muscle conditioning.

HOW TO PREVENT
- Participate in a strengthening and conditioning program appropriate for your sport.
- Warm up before practice or competition. Include adequate stretching.
- Tape the elbow area before practice or competition to prevent recurrence of injury.
- Wear proper protective equipment, such as elbow pads, for participation in contact sports.

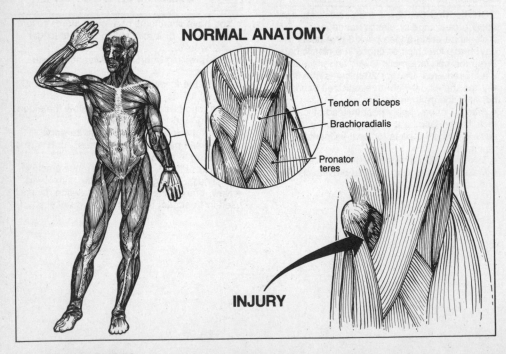

NORMAL ANATOMY

Tendon of biceps

Brachioradialis

Pronator teres

INJURY

WHAT TO EXPECT

APPROPRIATE HEALTH CARE
- Doctor's diagnosis.
- Application of tape, plaster splints or casts (sometimes).
- Self-care during rehabilitation.
- Physical therapy (moderate or severe strain).
- Surgery (severe strain).

DIAGNOSTIC MEASURES
- Your own observation of symptoms.
- Medical history and exam by a doctor.
- X-rays of the elbow and wrist to rule out fractures.

POSSIBLE COMPLICATIONS
- Prolonged healing time if activity is resumed too soon.
- Proneness to repeated elbow injury.
- Unstable or arthritic elbow following repeated injury.
- Inflammation at the attachment to bone (periostitis).
- Prolonged disability (sometimes).

PROBABLE OUTCOME—If this is a first-time injury, proper care and sufficient healing time before resuming activity should prevent permanent disability. Torn ligaments and tendons require as long to heal as fractured bones. Average healing times are:
- Mild strain—2 to 10 days.
- Moderate strain—10 days to 6 weeks.
- Severe strain—6 to 10 weeks.
If this is a repeat injury, complications listed above are more likely to occur.

HOW TO TREAT

NOTE—Follow your doctor's instructions. These instructions are supplemental.

FIRST AID—Use instructions for R.I.C.E., the first letters of *rest, ice, compression* and *elevation*. See Appendix 1 for details.

CONTINUING CARE
If cast or splints are used:
- Be sure to keep fingers free and exercise them frequently.
- See Appendix 2 (Care of Casts).

If casts or splints are not used:
- Use ice massage 3 or 4 times a day for 15 minutes at a time. Fill a large Styrofoam cup with water and freeze. Tear a small amount of foam from the top so ice protrudes. Massage firmly over the injured area in a circle about the size of a softball.
- After the first 24 hours, apply heat instead of ice, if it feels better. Use heat lamps, hot soaks, hot showers, heating pads, or heat liniments and ointments.
- Take whirlpool treatments, if available.
- Wrap the injured elbow with an elasticized bandage between treatments.
- Massage gently and often to provide comfort and decrease swelling.

MEDICATION
- For minor discomfort, you may use:
  Aspirin, acetaminophen or ibuprofen.
  Topical liniments and ointments.
- Your doctor may prescribe:
  Stronger pain relievers.
  Injection of a long-acting local anesthetic to reduce pain.
  Injections of corticosteroids, such as triamcinolone, to reduce inflammation.

ACTIVITY
- For a moderate or severe strain, use a sling for at least 72 hours—longer with a cast or splints.
- Resume your normal activities gradually.

DIET—Eat a well-balanced diet that includes extra protein, such as meat, fish, poultry, cheese, milk and eggs. Increase fiber and fluid intake to prevent constipation that may result from decreased activity.

REHABILITATION—Begin daily rehabilitation exercises when supportive wrapping is no longer needed. Use ice massage for 10 minutes prior to exercise. See page 455 for rehabilitation exercises.

CALL YOUR DOCTOR IF

- You have symptoms of a moderate or severe elbow strain, or a mild strain persists longer than 10 days.
- Pain or swelling worsens despite treatment.
- The following occurs with a cast or splints:
  Pain, numbness or coldness below the injury.
  Dusky, blue or gray fingernails.

ELBOW TENDINITIS OR EPICONDYLITIS
(Tennis Elbow)

GENERAL INFORMATION

DEFINITION—Inflammation of muscles, tendons, bursa, or covering to bones (periosteum) at the elbow.

BODY PARTS INVOLVED—Elbow muscles, tendons and one or both of the epicondyles (bony prominences on the sides of the elbow where muscles of the forearm attach to the bone of the upper arm).

SIGNS & SYMPTOMS
● Pain and tenderness over the epicondyles. Pain worsens with gripping or rotation of the forearm.
● Weak grip.
● Pain when twisting the hand and arm, as when playing tennis, throwing a ball with a twist, bowling, golfing, pushing off while skiing or using a screwdriver.

CAUSES—Partial tear of the tendon and attached covering of the bone caused by:
● Chronic stress on the tissues that attach the forearm muscles to the elbow area.
● Sudden stress on the forearm.
● Wrist snap when serving balls in racket sports.

● Incorrect grip.
● Incorrect hitting position.
● Using a racket or club that is too heavy.
● Using an oversize grip.

RISK INCREASES WITH
● Participation in sports that require strenuous forearm movement, such as tennis and racquetball.
● Poor conditioning of forearm muscles prior to vigorous exercise.
● Inadequate warmup before competing.
● Returning to activity before healing is complete.

HOW TO PREVENT
● Don't play sports, such as tennis, for long periods until your forearm muscles are strong and limber. Take frequent rest periods.
● Do forearm conditioning exercises to build your strength gradually.
● Warm up slowly and completely before participating in sports—especially before competition.
● Get lessons from a professional if you are a novice.
● Use a tennis-elbow strap when you resume normal activity after treatment.

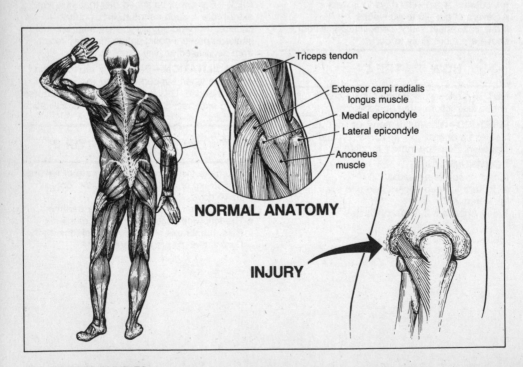

Triceps tendon
Extensor carpi radialis longus muscle
Medial epicondyle
Lateral epicondyle
Anconeus muscle

NORMAL ANATOMY

INJURY

WHAT TO EXPECT

APPROPRIATE HEALTH CARE
- Self-care after diagnosis.
- Doctor's treatment.
- Physical therapy.
- Surgery (rare).

DIAGNOSTIC MEASURES
- Your own observation of symptoms.
- Medical history and physical exam by a doctor.
- X-rays of the elbow.

POSSIBLE COMPLICATIONS
- Complete ligament tear, requiring surgery to repair.
- Slow healing.
- Frequent recurrences.

PROBABLE OUTCOME—Tennis elbow usually heals with heat treatments, corticosteroid injections and rest of the elbow. Treatment may require 3 to 6 months.

 # HOW TO TREAT

NOTE—Follow your doctor's instructions. These instructions are supplemental.

FIRST AID—None. This problem develops slowly.

CONTINUING CARE
- Use heat to relieve pain. Use warm soaks, a heating pad or a heat lamp. You may receive diathermy or ultrasound (see Glossary), whirlpool or massage treatments in your doctor's office or a physical-therapy facility. These may bring quicker symptom relief and healing.
- You may need to wear a forearm splint to immobilize the elbow.

MEDICATION—Your doctor may prescribe:
- Non-steroidal anti-inflammatory drugs to reduce inflammation.
- Injections of anesthetics to temporarily relieve pain.
- Injections of corticosteroids to reduce inflammation. *Caution:* Repeated injections may weaken the muscle tendon.

ACTIVITY—Don't repeat the activity that caused tennis elbow until symptoms disappear. Then resume your normal activities gradually after proper conditioning.

DIET—During recovery, eat a well-balanced diet that includes extra protein, such as meat, fish, poultry, cheese, milk and eggs.

REHABILITATION
- Do the following exercise 3 or 4 times a day while wearing the splint: Stretch your arm, flex your wrist, then press the back of your hand against a wall. Hold for 1 minute.
- See page 455 for additional rehabilitation exercises. Begin rehabilitation after pain disappears.

 # CALL YOUR DOCTOR IF

- You have symptoms of tennis elbow.
- Symptoms don't improve in 2 weeks, despite treatment.

EYE INJURY

GENERAL INFORMATION

DEFINITION—Injuries to the eye include:
- Contusions and fractures of bones that form the eye socket or orbit.
- Contusions and lacerations of the eyelids.
- Abrasion of the cornea (the transparent covering of the pupil of the eye) or other injury to the eyeball.

BODY PARTS INVOLVED
- Bones that form the orbit.
- Eyelids.
- Eyeball: cornea, conjunctiva (white of the eye), iris (colored part of the eye) and aqueous humor (fluid in the eyeball).
- Muscles, tendons, periosteum (covering to bone), nerves, blood vessels, skin and connective tissue in the vicinity of the eye.

SIGNS & SYMPTOMS
Injury to the orbit:
- Pain.
- Swollen lids.
- Protruding eyeball if bleeding occurs in back of the eye.
- Numbness around the eye.
- Inability to move the eye normally.
- Decreased vision.

Injury to the lids:
- Pain.
- A cut, laceration or contusion with swelling, redness, tenderness, pain, bleeding or bruising ("black eye") in or around the eye.
- Change in ability to see clearly.

Injury to the eyeball:
- Eye pain.
- Sensitivity to bright light.
- Eyelid spasm.
- Tearing.
- Blurred vision.
- Redness in the white of the eye.
- Irregular size of pupils.

CAUSES
- Direct blow in the vicinity of the eye.
- Irritation from many different materials, such as pesticides on grass, lime used for lines, or gravel or dust.
- Foreign body imbedded in the eye, such as a small piece of gravel, sand or glass.
- Scratching of the cornea, either by a fingernail or a rough foreign body.

RISK INCREASES WITH
- Contact sports such as football or soccer.
- Racket sports.
- Windy weather.
- Rough terrain for workouts or competition.

HOW TO PREVENT
- Wear a face mask for contact sports.
- Wear protective glasses for racket sports.
- Avoid areas that contain substances to which you are allergic, if possible.

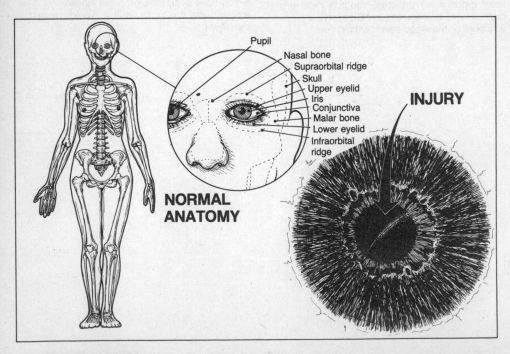

Pupil
Nasal bone
Supraorbital ridge
Skull
Upper eyelid
Iris
Conjunctiva
Malar bone
Lower eyelid
Infraorbital ridge

NORMAL ANATOMY

INJURY

WHAT TO EXPECT

APPROPRIATE HEALTH CARE
- Doctor's examination and treatment.
- Emergency-room care.
- Hospitalization for repair of facial bones that affect the orbit.

DIAGNOSTIC MEASURES
- Your own observation of symptoms.
- Medical history and physical exam by a doctor (usually an ophthalmologist, eye specialist or a surgeon specializing in facial injury).
- X-rays of the skull to detect possible fractures.

POSSIBLE COMPLICATIONS
- Infection, especially when imbedded foreign bodies are not completely removed from the cornea.
- Permanent (sometimes total) loss of vision if infection penetrates the eyeball from the cornea.
- Bleeding into the eye as a result of a blunt injury.
- Scarring if eyelid lacerations are unattended.

PROBABLE OUTCOME
- Cornea injury with infection: This serious eye problem is usually curable in 2 to 3 weeks with special care from an ophthalmologist.
- Eyelid injury: Eyelid lacerations usually heal in 1 to 2 weeks if they are carefully closed surgically. Sutures are usually removed in 7 to 10 days.
- Orbit (bone) injury: Facial surgery by a cosmetic surgeon usually improves appearance. Bones require 6 to 8 weeks to heal.
- Injuries due to foreign bodies: These injuries heal easily if the foreign body is removed and antibiotic medication is used to fight infection.

 # HOW TO TREAT

NOTE—Follow your doctor's instructions. These instructions are supplemental.

FIRST AID
- Don't try to remove contact lenses.
- Don't rub the eye.
- Don't wash the eye.
- Cover both eyes with loose cloth pads. Eyes move together, so both eyes must be covered to prevent movement of the injured eye.
- Apply crushed ice in a soft cloth bag or a towel—not a heavy ice bag.
- Avoid any pressure on the eye. Bleeding from eyelids is usually inconsequential but pressure can cause further damage.
- Keep the injured person in a partial reclining position while en route to an emergency facility.

CONTINUING CARE
After emergency treatment:
- Protect eyes from bright light or sunlight by wearing dark glasses.
- Use ice packs or warm moist compresses to relieve discomfort. Prepare a compress by folding a clean cloth in several layers. Dip in warm water, wring out slightly, and apply to the eye. Dip the compress often to keep it moist. Apply the compress for an hour, rest an hour and repeat.
- Sleep with the head elevated with 2 pillows until symptoms subside.
- Don't rub the eye.

For lacerations after suturing:
- Keep the wound dry and covered for 48 hours.
- If you change the bandage, apply a small amount of petroleum jelly or non-prescription antibiotic ointment to the bandage.
- After 48 hours, replace the bandage if it gets wet.
- Ignore small amounts of bleeding. Control heavier bleeding by firmly pressing a facial tissue or clean cloth to the bleeding spot, avoiding pressure on the eyeball itself.

MEDICATION—Your doctor may prescribe:
- Antibiotic eyedrops or ointment to prevent infection.
- Pain relievers.
- Local anesthetic eyedrops or drops to dilate the pupil and rest the eye muscle.

ACTIVITY—Resume your normal activities gradually after treatment.

DIET—Eat a well-balanced diet that includes extra protein, such as meat, fish, poultry, cheese, milk and eggs.

REHABILITATION—Rehabilitation exercises must be individualized. Follow your doctor's or surgeon's directions.

 # CALL YOUR DOCTOR IF

- You have a foreign body in the eye.
- You have a cut or other eye injury.
- The following occurs during or after treatment:
  Pain increases or does not disappear in 2 days.
  Your vision changes.
  You cannot move the eye up and down normally.
  You have a fever over 101F (38.3C).
  You experience pain that is not relieved by acetaminophen.
  New, unexplained symptoms develop. Drugs used in treatment may produce side effects.

FACE CONTUSION

GENERAL INFORMATION

DEFINITION—Bruising of skin and underlying tissues of the face caused by a direct blow. Contusions cause bleeding from ruptured small capillaries that allow blood to infiltrate muscles, tendons or other soft tissue. The face is particularly vulnerable to contusion because skin is so close to hard, underlying bone. (Note: Contusions and other injuries of the eyes, nose and ears require special considerations and care. They are addressed separately in this book.)

BODY PARTS INVOLVED—Face tissues, including blood vessels, muscles, tendons, nerves, covering to bone (periosteum) and connective tissue.

SIGNS & SYMPTOMS
● Local swelling at the contusion site. The swelling may be round or egg-shaped and superficial or deep.
● Pain and tenderness over the injury.
● Feeling of firmness when pressure is exerted on the injured area.
● Discoloration under the skin, beginning with redness and progressing to the characteristic "black and blue" bruise.

CAUSES—Direct blow to the skin, usually from a blunt object.

RISK INCREASES WITH
● Violent contact sports such as boxing or hockey, especially if the face is not adequately protected. Also common in baseball and fencing.
● Racket sports.
● Medical history of any bleeding disorder such as hemophilia.
● Poor nutrition, including vitamin deficiency.
● Use of anticoagulants or aspirin.

HOW TO PREVENT—Wear an appropriate face mask during competition or other athletic activity if a face contusion is likely.

? WHAT TO EXPECT

APPROPRIATE HEALTH CARE
● Doctor's care unless the contusion is quite small.
● Self-care for minor contusions.

DIAGNOSTIC MEASURES
● Your own observation of symptoms.
● Medical history and physical exam by a doctor for all except minor injuries.
● X-rays of the facial area to rule out the

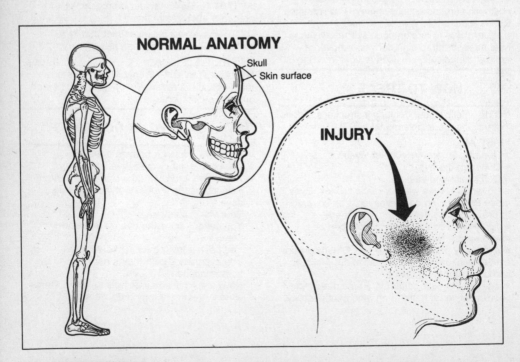

NORMAL ANATOMY

Skull
Skin surface

INJURY

possibility of underlying fracture. The total extent of injury may not be apparent for 48 to 72 hours.

POSSIBLE COMPLICATIONS

● Excessive bleeding. Infiltrative-type bleeding can (rarely) lead to calcification and impaired function, and facial disfiguration.
● Prolonged healing time if usual activities are resumed too soon.
● Infection if skin over the contusion is broken.

PROBABLE OUTCOME—Healing time varies with the extent of injury, but all but the most serious face contusions should heal in 6 to 10 days.

 # HOW TO TREAT

NOTE—Follow your doctor's instructions. These instructions are supplemental.

FIRST AID—Use instructions for R.I.C.E., the first letters of *rest, ice, compression* and *elevation.* See Appendix 1 for details.

CONTINUING CARE

● Use an ice pack 3 or 4 times a day. Wrap ice chips or cubes in a plastic bag, and wrap the bag in a moist towel. Place it over the injured area for 20 minutes at a time.
● After 72 hours, apply heat instead of ice if it feels better. Use heat lamps, hot soaks, hot showers, heating pads, or heat liniments and ointments.
● Massage gently and often to provide comfort and decrease swelling.

MEDICATION

● For minor discomfort, you may use:
  Acetaminophen or ibuprofen.
  Topical liniments and ointments.
● Your doctor may prescribe stronger medicine for pain.

ACTIVITY—Begin activities slowly and stop exercise as soon as pain begins. Increase activity as healing progresses.

DIET—During recovery, eat a well-balanced diet that includes extra protein, such as meat, fish, poultry, cheese, milk and eggs. Your doctor may prescribe vitamin and mineral supplements to promote healing.

REHABILITATION—Rehabilitation exercises must be individualized. Follow your doctor's or surgeon's directions.

 # CALL YOUR DOCTOR IF

● You have a face contusion that doesn't improve in 1 or 2 days.
● Skin is broken and signs of infection (drainage, increasing pain, fever, headache, muscle aches, dizziness or a general ill feeling) occur.

FACIAL-BONE FRACTURE

GENERAL INFORMATION

DEFINITION—A complete or incomplete break in one or several bones in the face.

BODY PARTS INVOLVED
- Facial bones: upper jaw (maxilla), cheek bones, malar and other bones that form the eye sockets (orbits), and nose. (See also Jaw Fracture, page 218.)
- Joints between bones listed above.
- Teeth.
- Eyes and nose.
- Soft tissue around the fracture site, including nerves, tendons, ligaments, periosteum (covering to bone), blood vessels and connective tissue.

SIGNS & SYMPTOMS
- Severe pain at the injury site.
- Swelling and bruising of soft tissue around the fracture, including black eyes.
- Visible deformity if the fracture is complete and bone fragments separate enough to distort normal facial contours.
- Tenderness to the touch.
- Numbness around the fracture site.
- Bleeding from the nose or eye.

CAUSES—Direct blow to the face.

RISK INCREASES WITH
- Contact sports, especially boxing, wrestling and baseball.
- Cycling.
- Poor nutrition, especially calcium deficiency.
- If surgery or anesthesia are needed, surgical risk increases with smoking and use of drugs, including mind-altering drugs, muscle relaxants, antihypertensives, tranquilizers, sleep inducers, insulin, sedatives, beta-adrenergic blockers or corticosteroids.

HOW TO PREVENT—Wear protective face masks and headgear when cycling or competing in contact sports. The use of protective equipment has significantly decreased the incidence of facial fractures.

WHAT TO EXPECT

APPROPRIATE HEALTH CARE
- Doctor's treatment. A plastic surgeon, oral surgeon, ophthalmologist, or ear, nose and throat specialist may be consulted.
- Surgery (sometimes) to realign fractured bones and reconstruct normal facial contours.
- Self-care during rehabilitation.

DIAGNOSTIC MEASURES
- Your own observation of symptoms.
- Medical history and physical exam by a doctor.
- X-rays of the skull and facial bones.
- Laboratory studies to measure blood loss.
- CAT scan (see Glossary) to rule out brain injury.
- Vision examination.

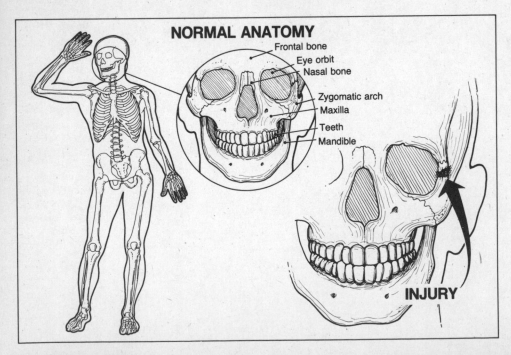

NORMAL ANATOMY

Frontal bone
Eye orbit
Nasal bone
Zygomatic arch
Maxilla
Teeth
Mandible

INJURY

POSSIBLE COMPLICATIONS

At the time of fracture:
- Shock.
- Pressure on or injury to eyes, nose, nearby nerves, ligaments, tendons, blood vessels or connective tissues.
- Breathing obstruction.

After treatment or surgery:
- Excessive bleeding.
- Impaired blood supply to the healing bone.
- Avascular necrosis (death of bone cells) due to interruption of the blood supply.
- Infection introduced during surgical treatment.
- Unstable or arthritic jaw or neck joints following repeated injury.

PROBABLE OUTCOME
- Surgery usually restores normal features and facial function.
- Teeth that have been knocked out can sometimes be replanted (see Tooth Injury & Loss, page 356). Speech will be changed while the wires are in place, but it should return to normal when they are removed.
- Normal vision should return if the eye is not injured.
- Recovery usually takes about 6 weeks. Healing is considered complete when there is no pain at the fracture site and when X-rays show complete bone union.

HOW TO TREAT

NOTE—Follow your doctor's instructions. These instructions are supplemental.

FIRST AID
- If the victim is wearing a face mask, cut it away.
- Check for excessive bleeding and swelling that may cause breathing obstruction. If the victim is not breathing, administer cardiopulmonary resuscitation (CPR).
- Apply ice packs to the face to decrease swelling and pain.
- Elevate the upper body so the face is above the level of the heart. This reduces swelling and prevents accumulation of excess fluid. Use pillows to prop the head if you are sure there is no neck injury.
- Keep the person warm with blankets to decrease the possibility of shock.

CONTINUING CARE
- A broken jaw is corrected by securing the teeth with wire or plastic splints so the jaw heals in its proper position.
- Surgery is frequently necessary to realign facial bones and restore a normal appearance. For best results it should be done as soon as possible after injury.

During convalescence:
- Don't exercise to the point that you must pant for breath, because breathing may be difficult for a while.
- Protect the face from pressure. Sleep on your back.
- Don't blow your nose hard or use makeup until healing is complete.
- If your jaws are wired, learn how to release them quickly in case of emergency, such as severe coughing or vomiting.

MEDICATION—Your doctor may prescribe:
- Pain relievers.
- Antibiotics to fight infection if necessary.

ACTIVITY—Rest quietly for about 2 days, then resume your normal activities as strength returns.

DIET
- Drink only water before manipulation or surgery to treat the fracture. Solid food in your stomach makes vomiting while under anesthesia more hazardous.
- Eat a high-protein, liquid diet for several days. If your jaw is wired, a liquid diet will be necessary for up to 8 weeks. Add soft solid foods as you are able.

REHABILITATION—None.

CALL YOUR DOCTOR IF

- You or someone else have signs or symptoms of a facial-bone fracture.
- The following occurs after treatment:
  Fever.
  Impaired vision.
  Severe headache.
  Loss of sensation in the face.
  Intolerable pain.
  Upper-respiratory illness of any kind during healing. This increases the danger of infection.
  Loosening of wires or splints.
  New, unexplained symptoms. Drugs used in treatment may produce side effects.

FINGER DISLOCATION

GENERAL INFORMATION

DEFINITION—Injury to any finger joint so that adjoining bones are displaced from their normal position and no longer touch each other. Fractures and ligament sprains frequently accompany this dislocation. Finger dislocations are a common problem for athletes.

BODY PARTS INVOLVED
- Any of the many finger bones.
- Ligaments that hold finger bones in place.
- Soft tissue surrounding the dislocation site, including periosteum (covering to bone), nerves, tendons, blood vessels and connective tissue.

SIGNS & SYMPTOMS
- Excruciating pain in the finger at the time of injury.
- Loss of function in the dislocated joint.
- Severe pain when attempting to move the injured finger.
- Visible deformity if the dislocated finger has locked in the dislocated position. Bones may spontaneously reposition themselves and leave no deformity, but damage is the same.
- Tenderness over the dislocation.
- Swelling and bruising at the injury site.
- Numbness or paralysis beyond the dislocation from pinching, cutting or pressure on blood vessels or nerves.

CAUSES
- Direct or indirect blow to the hand, finger or thumb.
- End result of a severe finger sprain.
- Congenital abnormality, such as a shallow or malformed joint surface.

RISK INCREASES WITH
- Contact sports, especially basketball, baseball and soccer.
- Previous finger or hand dislocation or sprain.
- Repeated injury to any part of the hand.
- Arthritis of any type (rheumatoid, gout).
- Poor muscle conditioning in the hand.

HOW TO PREVENT
- To prevent a recurrence, protect vulnerable joints after healing with protective devices or tape.
- Develop a high level of muscle strength and conditioning, including the hand area.

WHAT TO EXPECT

APPROPRIATE HEALTH CARE
- Doctor's treatment. This will include manipulating the joint to reposition the bones.
- Surgery (sometimes) to restore the joint to its normal position and repair torn ligaments and tendons. Acute or recurring dislocations may require surgical reconstruction or eventual replacement of the joint.
- Self-care during rehabilitation.

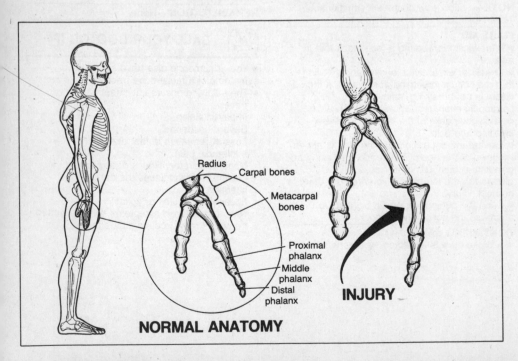

Radius
Carpal bones
Metacarpal bones
Proximal phalanx
Middle phalanx
Distal phalanx

INJURY

NORMAL ANATOMY

DIAGNOSTIC MEASURES
- Your own observation of symptoms.
- Medical history and exam by a doctor.
- X-rays of the hand and wrist.

POSSIBLE COMPLICATIONS
At the time of injury:
- Shock.
- Pressure on or injury to nearby nerves, ligaments, tendons, muscles, blood vessels and connective tissue.

After treatment or surgery:
- Impaired blood supply to the dislocated area.
- Death of bone cells due to interruption of the blood supply.
- Infection introduced during surgical treatment.
- Excessive bleeding around the dislocation site.
- Continuing recurrent dislocations with progressively less severe injuries.
- Prolonged healing if activity is resumed too soon.
- Unstable or arthritic joint following repeated injury or surgery.

PROBABLE OUTCOME—After the dislocation has been corrected, the hand may require immobilization with a cast or splint for 2 to 3 weeks. Complete healing of injured ligaments requires a minimum of 6 weeks.

HOW TO TREAT

NOTE—Follow your doctor's instructions. These instructions are supplemental.

FIRST AID
- Use instructions for R.I.C.E., the first letters of *rest, ice, compression* and *elevation.* See Appendix 1 for details.
- The doctor will manipulate the dislocated finger to return bones to their normal position. Manipulation should be done within 6 hours of injury. If not, many tissues lose their elasticity and become difficult to return to a normal position.

CONTINUING CARE—After removal of the splint or cast:
- Use ice soaks 3 or 4 times a day. Fill a bucket with ice water, and soak the injured area for 20 minutes at a time.
- Apply heat if it feels better. Use heat lamps, hot soaks, hot showers, heating pads, or heat liniments and ointments.
- Tape the injured finger to adjacent fingers.
- Massage gently and often to provide comfort and decrease swelling.

MEDICATION—Your doctor may prescribe:
- General anesthesia or local anesthesia to make joint manipulation possible.
- Acetaminophen or aspirin to relieve moderate pain.
- Narcotic pain relievers for severe pain.
- Antibiotics to fight infection, if surgery is necessary.

ACTIVITY
- If surgery is not necessary, activity is not restricted except for limitations imposed by immobilization of the hand.
- If surgery is necessary, resume normal activities and reconditioning gradually.

DIET
- Drink only water before manipulation or surgery to correct the dislocation. Solid food in your stomach makes vomiting while under general anesthesia more hazardous.
- During recovery, eat a well-balanced diet that includes extra protein, such as meat, fish, poultry, cheese, milk and eggs.

REHABILITATION
- Begin daily rehabilitation exercises when supportive wrapping is no longer needed.
- Use ice massage for 10 minutes before and after workouts. Fill a large Styrofoam cup with water and freeze. Tear a small amount of foam from the top so ice protrudes. Massage firmly over the injured area in a circle about the size of a softball.
- Rehabilitation exercises must be individualized. Follow your doctor's or surgeon's directions.

 CALL YOUR DOCTOR IF

- You have signs or symptoms of a dislocated finger.
- Any of the following occur after treatment:
  Numbness, paleness or coldness in the finger. This is an emergency!
  Swelling above or below the splint or cast.
  Blue or gray skin color, particularly under the fingernails.
- Any of the following occur after surgery:
  Increased pain, swelling or drainage in the surgical area.
  Signs of infection: headache, muscle aches, dizziness, or a general ill feeling and fever.
- New, unexplained symptoms develop. Drugs used in treatment may produce side effects.
- Finger dislocations that you can "pop" back into normal position occur repeatedly.

FINGER FRACTURE

GENERAL INFORMATION

DEFINITION—A complete or incomplete break in a finger bone.

BODY PARTS INVOLVED
- Any of the bones of a finger, but usually the bone closest to the hand.
- Any of the joints of the fingers, or the joints between the fingers and the hand.
- Soft tissue surrounding the fracture site, including nerves, tendons, ligaments and blood vessels.

SIGNS & SYMPTOMS
- Severe pain at the fracture site.
- Swelling of soft tissue surrounding the fracture.
- Visible deformity if the fracture is complete and bone fragments separate enough to distort normal finger contours.
- Tenderness to the touch.
- Numb or cold finger or fingertip, if the blood supply is impaired.

CAUSES—Direct blow or indirect stress on the finger bones.

RISK INCREASES WITH
- Dislocation of a finger joint or of a joint between finger and hand.
- Contact sports such as boxing or baseball.
- History of bone or joint disease, especially osteoporosis.
- Poor nutrition, especially calcium deficiency.
- If surgery or anesthesia are needed, surgical risk increases with smoking and use of drugs, including mind-altering drugs, muscle relaxants, antihypertensives, tranquilizers, sleep inducers, insulin, sedatives, beta-adrenergic blockers or corticosteroids.

HOW TO PREVENT—If you have had a previous finger injury, use tape or padding to protect the finger when participating in contact sports.

WHAT TO EXPECT

APPROPRIATE HEALTH CARE
- Doctor's treatment to manipulate the broken bones.
- Hospitalization (sometimes) for anesthesia and surgery to set the fracture.
- Self-care during rehabilitation.
- Whirlpool, ultrasound or massage (to displace excess fluid from the injured joint space).

DIAGNOSTIC MEASURES
- Your own observation of symptoms.
- Medical history and physical exam by a doctor.
- X-rays of injured areas, including joints above and below the primary injury site.

POSSIBLE COMPLICATIONS
- Pressure on or injury to nearby nerves,

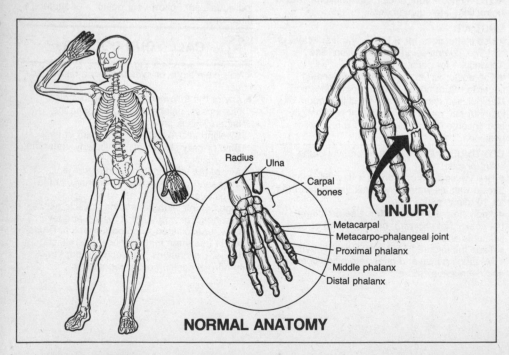

Radius Ulna

Carpal bones

Metacarpal
Metacarpo-phalangeal joint
Proximal phalanx
Middle phalanx
Distal phalanx

INJURY

NORMAL ANATOMY

ligaments, tendons, muscles, blood vessels or connective tissues.
- Delayed union or non-union of the fracture.
- Impaired blood supply to the fracture site.
- Avascular necrosis (death of bone cells) due to interruption of the blood supply.
- Arrest of normal bone growth in children.
- Infection in open fractures (skin broken over fracture site), or at the incision if surgical setting was necessary.
- Shortening of the injured bones.
- Proneness to repeated finger injury.
- Unstable or arthritic joint following repeated injury.
- Prolonged healing time if activity is resumed too soon.

PROBABLE OUTCOME—It is impossible to predict exactly how long it will take for any fracture to heal. Variable factors include age, sex, and previous state of health and conditioning. The average healing time for this fracture is 6 to 8 weeks. Healing is considered complete when there is no motion at the fracture site and when X-rays show complete bone union.

 HOW TO TREAT

NOTE—Follow your doctor's instructions. These instructions are supplemental.

FIRST AID
- Use a padded splint or sling to immobilize the hand and wrist before transporting the injured person to the doctor's office or emergency facility.
- Use instructions for R.I.C.E., the first letters of *rest, ice, compression* and *elevation*. See Appendix 1 for details.
- The doctor will realign and set the broken bones either with surgery or, if possible, without. Manipulation should be done as soon as possible after injury. Six or more hours after the fracture, bleeding and displacement of body fluids may lead to shock. Also, many tissues lose their elasticity and become difficult to return to a normal position.

CONTINUING CARE
- Immobilization will be necessary. A splint is placed on the injured finger, extending beyond the finger-hand joint.
- After 48 hours, localized heat promotes healing by increasing blood circulation in the injured area. Use a heating pad or heat lamp.
- After the splint is removed, use ice soaks 3 or 4 times a day. Fill a bucket with ice water, and soak the injured area for 20 minutes at a time.
- Apply heat instead of ice, if it feels better. Use heat lamps, hot soaks, hot showers, heating pads, or heat liniments or ointments.
- Take whirlpool treatments, if available.

MEDICATION—Your doctor may prescribe:
- General anesthesia, local anesthesia, or muscle relaxants to make bone manipulation possible.
- Narcotic or synthetic narcotic pain relievers for severe pain.
- Acetaminophen (available without prescription) for mild pain after initial treatment.

ACTIVITY
- Actively exercise all muscle groups not immobilized. These muscle contractions in the hand and arm promote fracture alignment and hasten healing.
- Resume normal activities gradually after treatment.
- Begin reconditioning the injured area after clearance from your doctor.

DIET
- Drink only water before manipulation or surgery to treat the fracture. Solid food in your stomach makes vomiting while under anesthesia more hazardous.
- During recovery, eat a well-balanced diet that includes extra protein, such as meat, fish, poultry, cheese, milk and eggs.

REHABILITATION—Begin daily rehabilitation exercises when movement is comfortable. Use ice soaks for 10 minutes prior to exercise. See pages 457 and 474 for rehabilitation exercises.

 CALL YOUR DOCTOR IF

- You have signs or symptoms of a finger fracture.
- Any of the following occur after surgery or other treatment:
    Increased pain, swelling or drainage in the surgical area.
    Signs of infection (headache, muscle aches, dizziness, or a general ill feeling and fever).
    Nausea or vomiting.
    Swelling or irritation above or below the splint.
    Blue or gray skin color beyond the splint, particularly in the fingertip or under the fingernails.
    Numbness or complete loss of feeling in the injured finger.

FINGER SPRAIN

GENERAL INFORMATION

DEFINITION—Violent overstretching of one or more ligaments that hold the finger joints together. Sprains involving two or more ligaments cause considerably more disability than single-ligament sprains. When the ligament is overstretched, it becomes tense and gives way at its weakest point, either where it attaches to bone or within the ligament itself. There are 3 types of sprains:
• Mild (Grade I)—Tearing of some ligament fibers. There is no loss of function.
• Moderate (Grade II)—Rupture of a portion of the ligament, resulting in some loss of function.
• Severe (Grade III)—Complete rupture of the ligament or complete separation of ligament from bone. There is total loss of function. A severe sprain requires surgical repair.

BODY PARTS INVOLVED
• Ligaments holding the joints of the fingers together.
• Tissue surrounding the sprain, including blood vessels, tendons, bone, periosteum (covering of bone) and muscles.

SIGNS & SYMPTOMS
• Severe pain at the time of injury.
• A feeling of popping or tearing inside a finger or fingers.
• Tenderness at the injury site.
• Swelling in the finger.
• Bruising that appears soon after injury.

CAUSES—Stress on a ligament that temporarily forces or pries finger joints out of their normal location. Finger sprains occur frequently in football, baseball, basketball and other exercise or sports activities.

RISK INCREASES WITH
• Contact sports, especially "catching" and "throwing" sports.
• Previous hand injury.
• Poor muscle conditioning.
• Inadequate protection from equipment.

HOW TO PREVENT—Tape vulnerable joints before practice or competition.

WHAT TO EXPECT

APPROPRIATE HEALTH CARE
• Doctor's diagnosis.
• Application of a splint, tape or elastic bandage.
• Self-care during rehabilitation.
• Physical therapy (moderate or severe sprain).
• Surgery (severe sprain).

DIAGNOSTIC MEASURES
• Your own observation of symptoms.

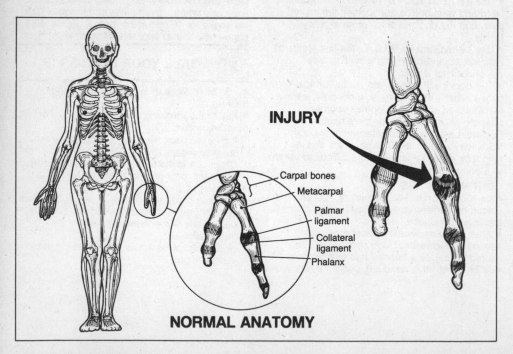

INJURY

Carpal bones
Metacarpal
Palmar ligament
Collateral ligament
Phalanx

NORMAL ANATOMY

- Medical history and exam by a doctor.
- X-rays of the hand and wrist to rule out fractures.

POSSIBLE COMPLICATIONS
- Prolonged healing time if usual activities are resumed too soon.
- Proneness to repeated finger injury.
- Inflammation at the ligament attachment to bone (periostitis).
- Prolonged disability (sometimes).
- Unstable or arthritic finger following repeated injury.

PROBABLE OUTCOME—If this is a first-time injury, proper care and sufficient healing time before resuming activity should prevent permanent disability. Ligaments have a poor blood supply, and torn ligaments require as much healing time as fractures. Average healing times are:
- Mild sprains—2 to 6 weeks.
- Moderate sprains—6 to 8 weeks.
- Severe sprains—8 to 10 weeks.

 ## HOW TO TREAT

NOTE—Follow your doctor's instructions. These instructions are supplemental.

FIRST AID—Use instructions for R.I.C.E., the first letters of *rest, ice, compression* and *elevation*. See Appendix 1 for details.

CONTINUING CARE—If the doctor does not apply a splint, tape or elastic bandage:
- Continue using an ice pack 3 or 4 times a day. Put ice chips or cubes in a plastic bag. Wrap the bag in a moist towel, and place it over the injured area. Use for 20 minutes at a time.
- After 72 hours, apply heat instead of ice, if it feels better. Use heat lamps, hot soaks, hot showers, heating pads, or heat liniments or ointments.
- Take whirlpool treatments, if available.
- Massage gently and often to provide comfort and decrease swelling.

MEDICATION
- For minor discomfort, you may use:
  Aspirin, acetaminophen or ibuprofen.
  Topical liniments and ointments.
- Your doctor may prescribe:
  Stronger pain relievers.
  Injection of a long-acting local anesthetic to reduce pain.
  Injection of a corticosteroid such as triamcinolone to reduce inflammation.

ACTIVITY—Resume your normal activities gradually after clearance from your doctor.

DIET—During recovery, eat a well-balanced diet that includes extra protein, such as meat, fish, poultry, cheese, milk and eggs.

REHABILITATION
- Begin daily rehabilitation exercises when the splint or supportive wrapping is no longer necessary.
- Use ice soaks 3 or 4 times a day. Fill a bucket with ice water, and soak the injured area for 20 minutes at a time.
- See page 457 for hand and finger exercises.

 ## CALL YOUR DOCTOR IF

- You have symptoms of a moderate or severe finger sprain, or a mild sprain persists longer than 2 weeks.
- Pain, swelling or bruising worsens despite treatment.
- Any of the following occur after splinting:
  Pain, numbness or coldness in the finger.
  Blue, gray or dusky fingernail.
- Any of the following occur after surgery:
  Increased pain, swelling, redness, drainage or bleeding in the surgical area.
  Signs of infection (headache, muscle aches, dizziness, or a general ill feeling with fever).
- New, unexplained symptoms develop. Drugs used in treatment may produce side effects.

FINGERTIP INJURY

GENERAL INFORMATION

DEFINITION—Fingertip injuries include:
- Contusion or bruise with hemorrhage under the fingernail or in the tip of the finger.
- Lacerated fingernail.
- Avulsion injury (tearing away of part of the fingertip).

BODY PARTS INVOLVED
- Last phalanx (section of bone) of any finger or thumb.
- Skin on finger.
- Fingernail.
- Blood vessels, nerves, tendons, ligaments, subcutaneous tissue and connective tissue.

SIGNS & SYMPTOMS—Fingertip injuries may include any of these signs:
- Pain in the fingertip.
- Torn fingernail.
- Jagged cut in the tip of the finger.
- Tearing away (avulsion of a part) of the fingertip.
- Crushed or broken bone in the fingertip.
- Numbness if the nerve is damaged.
- Bleeding under the fingernail or external bleeding.
- Swelling of the fingertip.
- Bruising of the injured fingertip.

CAUSES
- Direct violence to the fingertip.
- Crushing blow to the fingertip.
- Jamming of the fingertip, as happens when catching balls.

RISK INCREASES WITH
- Contact sports such as football or baseball.
- Sports with bats or balls moving at high speed.

HOW TO PREVENT—No preventive measures.

WHAT TO EXPECT

APPROPRIATE HEALTH CARE
- Self-care for mild injury.
- Doctor's treatment for serious injuries.

DIAGNOSTIC MEASURES
- Your own observation of symptoms.
- Description of circumstances of injury to a doctor for serious injuries.
- Physical exam by doctor to establish a diagnosis. Your doctor will need a description of the circumstances of injury.
- X-rays of the hand to disclose the extent of injury and to rule out fractures.

POSSIBLE COMPLICATIONS
- Excessive bleeding.
- Loss of function in the fingertip from damage to tissue, the fingernail, nerve endings or bone.
- Arthritic changes in any finger joint injured simultaneously.
- Prolonged disability if the injured finger is used before healing is complete.

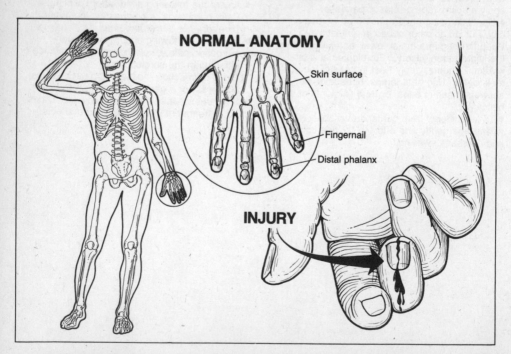

NORMAL ANATOMY

Skin surface

Fingernail

Distal phalanx

INJURY

• Inflammation at the tendon's attachment to bone (periostitis).

PROBABLE OUTCOME
• Contusions: Complete healing in 2 to 3 weeks.
• Lacerated fingernails: Injured nail usually requires surgical removal in a hospital or hospital outpatient facility. Expect complete healing in about 3 weeks if no complications occur.
• Avulsion injuries: Probably requires surgical repair or skin grafting. Allow 6 weeks for healing.

 ## HOW TO TREAT

NOTE—Follow your doctor's instructions. These instructions are supplemental.

FIRST AID—Use instructions for R.I.C.E., the first letters of *rest, ice, compression* and *elevation*. See Appendix 1 for details.

CONTINUING CARE
Care after surgery to repair a damaged fingertip:
• Keep the hand elevated to relieve pain and throbbing.
• Change bandages frequently. Keep bandages dry between baths. If the bandage gets wet, change it promptly.
If a cast is required:
• Do not allow pressure on any part of the cast until it is completely dry. Drying time varies, depending on the thickness of the cast, temperature and humidity.
• If the cast gets wet and a soft area appears, return to your doctor's office to have it repaired.
• Whenever possible, raise the hand. Propping on pillows will keep swelling and discomfort at a minimum.

MEDICATION—Your doctor may prescribe:
• Pain relievers. Don't take prescription pain medication longer than 4 to 7 days. Use only as much as you need.
• Antibiotics to fight infection.
• You may use non-prescription drugs such as acetaminophen for minor pain.

ACTIVITY
• Resume work and normal activity as soon as possible.
• Avoid vigorous exercise for 6 weeks following surgery.
• Resume driving when your doctor determines that healing is complete.

DIET—During recovery from surgery, eat a well-balanced diet that includes extra protein, such as meat, fish, poultry, cheese, milk and eggs.

REHABILITATION—See pages 457 and 474 for rehabilitation exercises.

 ## CALL YOUR DOCTOR IF

Any of the following occurs:
• Severe, persistent pain under the cast.
• Color change, coldness or numbness in tissues beyond the cast.
• Tissue swelling greater than before the cast was applied.
• Signs of infection (headache, muscle aches, dizziness or a general ill feeling and fever).
• Pain, swelling, redness, drainage or bleeding in the surgical area.
• New, unexplained symptoms. Drugs used in treatment may produce side effects.

FOOT BURSITIS

GENERAL INFORMATION

DEFINITION—Inflammation of one of the bursas in the foot. Bursitis may vary in degree from mild irritation to an abscess formation that causes excruciating pain. The most significant bursas to become inflamed are in the heel bone, the Achilles' tendon where it meets the heel bone, or the joint where the big toe meets the foot.

BODY PARTS INVOLVED
● Foot bursas (soft sacs filled with lubricating fluid that facilitate motion in the foot).
● Soft tissue surrounding the joints in the foot, including nerves, tendons, ligaments, blood vessels (both large vessels and capillaries), periosteum (the outside lining of bone) and muscles.

SIGNS & SYMPTOMS
● Pain.
● Tenderness.
● Swelling.
● Redness (sometimes) over the affected bursa.
● Fever, if infection is present.
● Restriction of motion of the foot.

CAUSES
● Direct blow or other injury to a foot joint.
● Acute or chronic infection.
● Arthritis.
● Gout.
● Unknown (frequently).

RISK INCREASES WITH
● Participating in competitive athletics, particularly contact sports such as football, soccer or hockey.
● Previous history of bursitis in any joint.
● Exposure to cold weather.
● Poor conditioning and inadequate warmup.
● Inadequate protective equipment in contact sports.

HOW TO PREVENT
● Wear well-fitting athletic shoes for contact sports.
● Warm up adequately before athletic practice or competition.
● Wear warm socks in cold weather.
● To prevent recurrence, continue to wear extra protection over the involved bursa in the foot until healing is complete.

WHAT TO EXPECT

APPROPRIATE HEALTH CARE
● Doctor's diagnosis and treatment.
● Surgery (sometimes), particularly for a frozen foot joint or chronic pain.

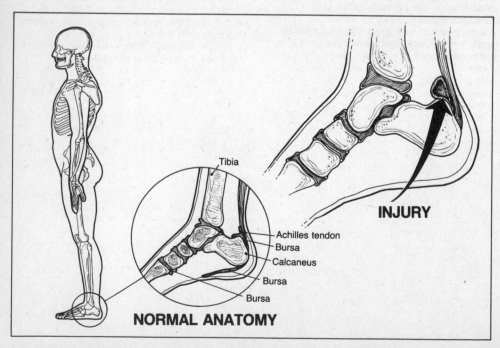

Tibia

Achilles tendon
Bursa
Calcaneus

Bursa

Bursa

INJURY

NORMAL ANATOMY

DIAGNOSTIC MEASURES
- Your own observation of symptoms.
- Medical history and physical exam by a doctor.
- X-rays of the foot and ankle.

POSSIBLE COMPLICATIONS
- Frozen foot joint.
- Permanent limitation of the joint's normal mobility.
- Prolonged healing time if activity is resumed too soon.
- Proneness to repeated flare-ups.
- Unstable or arthritic joint following repeated episodes of foot bursitis.
- Spontaneous rupture of the bursa if severe infection is present.

PROBABLE OUTCOME—Foot bursitis is a common—but usually not serious—problem. Symptoms usually subside in 7 to 14 days with treatment if there is no infection present. Infection or the need for surgery may dictate 6 to 8 weeks to heal.

 ## HOW TO TREAT

NOTE—Follow your doctor's instructions. These instructions are supplemental.

FIRST AID—None. This problem develops slowly.

CONTINUING CARE
- Use frequent ice massage. Fill a large Styrofoam cup with water and freeze. Tear a small amount of foam from the top so ice protrudes. Massage firmly over the injured area in a circle about the size of a softball. Do this for 15 minutes at a time, 3 or 4 times a day, and before workouts or competition.
- After 72 hours, apply heat instead of ice, if it feels better. Use heat lamps, hot soaks, hot showers, heating pads, or heat liniments or ointments.
- Take whirlpool treatments, if available.
- Use crutches to prevent weight-bearing, if needed.

- Elevate the foot above the level of the heart to reduce swelling and prevent accumulation of fluid. Use pillows for propping or elevate the foot of the bed.
- Gentle massage will frequently provide comfort and decrease swelling.

MEDICATION—Your doctor may prescribe:
- Non-steroidal anti-inflammatory drugs.
- Antibiotics if the bursa is infected.
- Prescription pain relievers for severe pain. Use non-prescription acetaminophen or ibuprofen (available under many trade names) for mild pain.
- Injection with a long-lasting local anesthetic mixed with a corticosteroid drug, such as triamcinolone.

ACTIVITY—Rest the inflamed area as much as possible. If you must resume normal activity immediately, use crutches until the pain becomes more bearable. To prevent a frozen joint, begin normal, slow joint movement as soon as possible.

DIET—Eat a well-balanced diet that includes extra protein, such as meat, fish, poultry, cheese, milk and eggs. Increase fiber and fluid intake to prevent constipation that may result from decreased activity. Your doctor may suggest vitamin and mineral supplements to promote healing.

REHABILITATION—See pages 446 and 455 for rehabilitation exercises.

 ## CALL YOUR DOCTOR IF

- You have symptoms of foot bursitis.
- Pain increases, despite treatment.
- Pain, swelling, tenderness, drainage or bleeding increases in the surgical area.
- You develop signs of infection (headache, muscle aches, dizziness or a general ill feeling and fever).
- New, unexplained symptoms develop. Drugs used in treatment may produce side effects.

FOOT CONTUSION

GENERAL INFORMATION

DEFINITION—Bruising of the skin and underlying tissues of the foot caused by a direct blow. Contusions cause bleeding from ruptured small capillaries that allow blood to infiltrate muscles, tendons or other soft tissue.

BODY PARTS INVOLVED—Foot tissues, including blood vessels, muscle, tendons, nerves, covering to bone (periosteum) and connective tissue.

SIGNS & SYMPTOMS
- Local swelling—either superficial or deep.
- Pain and tenderness over the injury.
- Feeling of firmness when pressure is exerted at the injury site.
- Discoloration under the skin, beginning with redness and progressing to the characteristic "black and blue" bruise.
- Restricted foot activity proportional to the extent of injury.

CAUSES
- Direct blow to the foot, usually from a blunt object.
- Wearing a shoe that has faulty cleats or spikes or wearing a wrinkled sock. This will cause a "stone bruise."

RISK INCREASES WITH
- Contact sports such as football, basketball or baseball, especially if the foot is not adequately protected.
- Medical history of any bleeding disorder such as hemophilia.
- Poor nutrition, including vitamin deficiency.
- Use of anticoagulants or aspirin.

HOW TO PREVENT—Wear appropriate protective footgear during competition or other athletic activity.

WHAT TO EXPECT

APPROPRIATE HEALTH CARE
- Doctor's care.
- Injections with long-acting local anesthetics and corticosteroids, unless the injury is quite small.
- Self-care for minor contusions, or for serious contusions during rehabilitation.
- Physical therapy for serious contusions.

DIAGNOSTIC MEASURES
- Your own observation of symptoms.
- Medical history and physical exam by a doctor for all except minor injuries.
- X-rays of the foot and ankle to assess total injury to soft tissue and to rule out the possibility of underlying fractures. The total extent of injury may not be apparent for 48 to 72 hours.

POSSIBLE COMPLICATIONS
- Excessive bleeding leading to disability. Infiltrative-type bleeding can (rarely) lead to

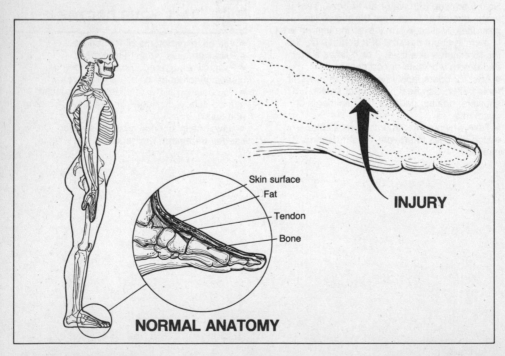

Skin surface
Fat
Tendon
Bone

INJURY

NORMAL ANATOMY

calcification and impaired function of injured muscle.

● Prolonged healing time if usual activities are resumed too soon.

● Infection if skin over the contusion is broken.

PROBABLE OUTCOME—Healing time varies with the extent of injury, but average healing time for foot contusions is 1 to 2 weeks.

 ## HOW TO TREAT

NOTE—Follow your doctor's instructions. These instructions are supplemental.

FIRST AID—Use instructions for R.I.C.E., the first letters of *rest, ice, compression* and *elevation*. See Appendix 1 for details.

CONTINUING CARE

● Wrap an elasticized bandage over a sponge-rubber pad on the injured area. Keep the area compressed for about 72 hours.

● Continue ice massage. Fill a large Styrofoam cup with water and freeze. Tear a small amount of foam from the top so ice protrudes. Massage gently over the injured area in a circle about the size of a softball. Do this for 15 minutes at a time, 3 or 4 times a day, and before workouts or competition.

● After 72 hours, apply heat instead of ice if it feels better. Use heat lamps, hot soaks, hot showers, heating pads, heat liniments or ointments, or whirlpool treatments.

● Massage gently and often to provide comfort and decrease swelling.

MEDICATION

● For minor discomfort, you may use:
Acetaminophen or ibuprofen.
Topical liniments and ointments.

● Your doctor may prescribe stronger medicine for pain.

ACTIVITY—Begin activities slowly and stop exercise as soon as pain begins. Increase activity as healing progresses.

DIET—During recovery, eat a well-balanced diet that includes extra protein, such as meat, fish, poultry, cheese, milk and eggs. Your doctor may prescribe vitamin and mineral supplements to promote healing.

REHABILITATION

● Begin daily rehabilitation exercises when supportive wrapping is no longer needed.

● See page 455 for rehabilitation exercises.

 ## CALL YOUR DOCTOR IF

● You have a foot contusion that doesn't improve in 1 or 2 days.

● Skin is broken and signs of infection (drainage, increasing pain, fever, headache, muscle aches, dizziness or a general ill feeling) occur.

FOOT DISLOCATION, SUBTALAR

GENERAL INFORMATION

DEFINITION—Injury to a joint in the foot below the talus so that adjoining bones are displaced from their normal position and no longer touch each other. A minor dislocation is called a *subluxation*. Joint surfaces still touch, but not in normal relation to each other.

BODY PARTS INVOLVED
- Any of the foot bones below the talus.
- Ligaments that hold foot bones in place.
- Soft tissue surrounding the dislocated bones, including nerves, tendons, muscles and blood vessels.

SIGNS & SYMPTOMS
- Excruciating pain at the time of injury.
- Inability to bear weight and walk.
- Severe pain when attempting to move the foot.
- Tenderness over the dislocation.
- Swelling and bruising at the injury site.
- Numbness or paralysis below the dislocation from pinching, cutting or pressure on blood vessels or nerves.

CAUSES
- Direct blow to the foot.
- End result of a severe foot sprain.
- Congenital abnormality, such as a shallow or malformed joint surface.

RISK INCREASES WITH
- Participation in contact sports.
- Running or fast walking.
- Exercise on uneven terrain or surfaces.
- Previous foot sprains or dislocations.
- Repeated injury to any joint in the foot.
- Arthritis of any type (rheumatoid, gout).
- Poor muscle conditioning.

HOW TO PREVENT
- For participation in contact sports, protect vulnerable joints with supportive devices, such as wrapped elastic bandages, tape or high-top athletic shoes.
- Warm up adequately before physical activity.
- Build your overall strength and muscle tone with a long-term conditioning program appropriate for your sport.
- Avoid irregular surfaces for running, fast walking, or track and field events.

WHAT TO EXPECT

APPROPRIATE HEALTH CARE
- Doctor's treatment, which includes manipulation of the joint to reposition the bones.
- Surgery (sometimes) to restore the joint to its normal position and repair torn ligaments and tendons.
- Self-care during rehabilitation.

DIAGNOSTIC MEASURES
- Your own observation of symptoms.
- Medical history and exam by a doctor.
- X-rays of the foot, ankle and adjacent bones.

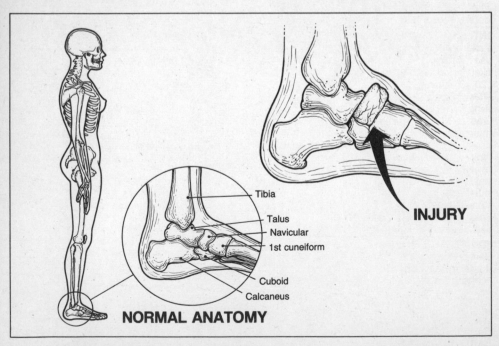

Tibia
Talus
Navicular
1st cuneiform
Cuboid
Calcaneus

NORMAL ANATOMY

INJURY

POSSIBLE COMPLICATIONS
- Damage to nearby nerves or major blood vessels.
- Death of bone cells caused by interruption of the blood supply.
- Excessive internal bleeding at the dislocation site.
- Shock or loss of consciousness.
- Prolonged healing if activity is resumed too soon.
- Recurrent dislocations, particularly if a previous dislocation has not healed completely.
- Unstable or arthritic joint following repeated injury.

PROBABLE OUTCOME—After the dislocation has been corrected, the joint may require immobilization for 6 to 8 weeks with a cast from knee to toes. Complete healing of injured ligaments requires a minimum of 6 weeks.

 HOW TO TREAT

NOTE—Follow your doctor's instructions. These instructions are supplemental.

FIRST AID
- Keep the person warm with blankets to decrease the possibility of shock.
- Cut away clothing and shoe, if possible, but don't move the injured area to do so.
- Immobilize the foot and ankle with padded splints.
- Follow instructions for R.I.C.E., the first letters of *rest, ice, compression* and *elevation*. See Appendix 1 for details.

CONTINUING CARE
If a cast is not necessary:
- Use ice soaks 3 or 4 times a day. Fill a bucket with ice water, and soak the injured area for 20 minutes at a time.
- After 48 hours, localized heat promotes healing by increasing blood circulation in the injured area. Use hot baths, showers, compresses, heat lamps, heating pads, heat ointments and liniments, or whirlpools.
- Wrap the foot with an elasticized bandage between treatments.
- Massage gently and often to provide comfort and decrease swelling.
If a cast is necessary:
- See Appendix 2 (Care of Casts).
- See Appendix 3 (Safe Use of Crutches).

MEDICATION—Your doctor may prescribe:
- General anesthesia or muscle relaxants to make joint manipulation possible.
- Acetaminophen or aspirin to relieve moderate pain.
- Narcotic pain relievers for severe pain.
- Stool softeners to prevent constipation due to decreased activity.
- Antibiotics to fight infection.

ACTIVITY
If surgery is not necessary:
- Resume sports participation after clearance from your doctor.
If surgery is necessary:
- Avoid vigorous exercise for 6 weeks after surgery. Then resume normal activities gradually.
- Don't drive until healing is complete.

DIET
- Drink only water before manipulation or surgery to correct the dislocation. Solid food in your stomach makes vomiting under general anesthesia more hazardous.
- During recovery, eat a well-balanced diet that includes extra protein, such as meat, fish, poultry, cheese, milk and eggs. Increase fiber and fluid intake to prevent constipation that may result from decreased activity.

REHABILITATION
- Begin daily rehabilitation exercises when supportive wrapping is no longer needed.
- Use ice massage for 10 minutes before and after workouts. Fill a large Styrofoam cup with water and freeze. Tear a small amount of foam from the top so ice protrudes. Massage firmly over the injured area in a circle about the size of a softball.
- See page 455 for rehabilitation exercises.

 CALL YOUR DOCTOR IF

- Any of the following occur after injury:
  Numbness, paleness or coldness in the foot. This is an emergency!
  Foot deformity.
  Difficulty moving the foot.
  Nausea or vomiting.
- Any of the following occur after treatment:
  Swelling above or below the cast.
  Blue or gray skin color, particularly under the toenails.
  Constipation.
- Any of the following occur after surgery:
  Increased pain, swelling or drainage in the surgical area.
  Signs of infection: headache, muscle aches, dizziness, or a general ill feeling and fever.
- New, unexplained symptoms develop. Drugs used in treatment may cause side effects.
- Foot dislocations that you can "pop" back into normal position occur repeatedly.

FOOT DISLOCATION, TALUS

GENERAL INFORMATION

DEFINITION—Injury and displacement of the talus so it no longer touches adjoining bones. Fractures and ligament sprains frequently accompany this dislocation.

BODY PARTS INVOLVED
- Talus and adjacent foot bones (tibia, navicular, calcaneus).
- Ligaments that hold foot bones together.
- Soft tissue surrounding the dislocation site, including periosteum (covering to bone), nerves, tendons, blood vessels and connective tissue.

SIGNS & SYMPTOMS
- Excruciating pain in the foot at the time of injury.
- Loss of function in the foot and ankle, and severe pain when attempting to move them.
- Visible deformity if the dislocated bones have locked in the dislocated position. Bones may spontaneously reposition themselves and leave no deformity, but damage is the same.
- Tenderness over the dislocation.
- Swelling and bruising at the injury site.
- Numbness or paralysis below the dislocation from pressure on, pinching or cutting of blood vessels or nerves.

CAUSES
- Direct or indirect blow to the foot and ankle.
- End result of a severe foot sprain.
- Congenital abnormality, such as abnormal arches or shallow or malformed joint surfaces.

RISK INCREASES WITH
- Contact sports.
- Running and jumping events.
- Exercise on uneven surfaces.
- Previous foot dislocation or sprain.
- Repeated injury to any joint in the foot.
- Arthritis of any type (rheumatoid, gout).
- Poor muscle conditioning.

HOW TO PREVENT
- For participation in contact sports or activities involving running and jumping, protect vulnerable joints. Wear protective devices, such as high-top athletic shoes, and use tape.
- Avoid irregular surfaces for running, fast walking, and track and field events.
- Warm up adequately before physical activity.
- Build your overall strength and muscle tone with a long-term conditioning program.
- Avoid contact sports if treatment does not restore a strong, stable foot and ankle.

? WHAT TO EXPECT

APPROPRIATE HEALTH CARE
- Doctor's treatment. This will include manipulating the joint to reposition the bones.
- Surgery (sometimes) to restore the joint to its normal position and repair torn ligaments and tendons. Acute or recurring dislocations may require surgical reconstruction or replacement of the joint.

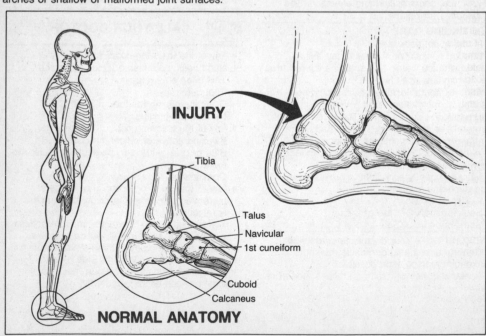

INJURY

Tibia

Talus

Navicular

1st cuneiform

Cuboid

Calcaneus

NORMAL ANATOMY

DIAGNOSTIC MEASURES
- Your own observation of symptoms.
- Medical history and exam by a doctor.
- X-rays of the foot, ankle and adjacent bones.

POSSIBLE COMPLICATIONS
At the time of injury:
- Shock.
- Pressure on or injury to nearby nerves, ligaments, tendons, muscles, blood vessels and connective tissue.

After treatment or surgery:
- Excessive internal bleeding.
- Impaired blood supply to the dislocated area.
- Death of bone cells due to interruption of the blood supply.
- Infection introduced during surgical treatment.
- Prolonged healing if activity is resumed too soon.
- Recurrent dislocations.
- Unstable or arthritic joint following repeated injury.

PROBABLE OUTCOME—After the dislocation has been corrected, the joint may require immobilization with a cast or splint covering the foot and ankle for 2 to 3 weeks. Injured ligaments require a minimum of 6 weeks to heal.

 ## HOW TO TREAT

NOTE—Follow your doctor's instructions. These instructions are supplemental.

FIRST AID
- Keep the person warm with blankets to decrease the possibility of shock.
- Cut away clothing and shoe, if possible, but don't move the injured area to do so.
- Immobilize the foot and ankle with padded splints.
- Follow instructions for R.I.C.E., the first letters of *rest, ice, compression* and *elevation.* See Appendix 1 for details.

CONTINUING CARE
If a cast is not necessary:
- Use ice soaks 3 or 4 times a day. Fill a bucket with ice water, and soak the injured area for 20 minutes at a time.
- After 48 hours, localized heat promotes healing by increasing blood circulation in the injured area. Use hot baths, showers, compresses, heat lamps, heating pads, heat ointments and liniments, or whirlpools.
- Wrap the foot and ankle with an elasticized bandage between treatments.
- Massage gently and often to provide comfort and decrease swelling.
If a cast is necessary:
- See Appendix 2 (Care of Casts).
- See Appendix 3 (Safe Use of Crutches).

MEDICATION—Your doctor may prescribe:
- General anesthesia or muscle relaxants to make joint manipulation possible.
- Acetaminophen to relieve moderate pain.
- Narcotic pain relievers for severe pain.
- Stool softeners to prevent constipation due to decreased activity.
- Antibiotics to fight infection.

ACTIVITY
If surgery is not necessary:
- Resume sports participation after clearance from your doctor.
If surgery is necessary:
- Avoid vigorous exercise for 6 weeks after surgery. Then resume normal activities gradually. Don't drive until healing is complete.

DIET
- Drink only water before manipulation or surgery to correct the dislocation. Solid food in your stomach makes vomiting while under general anesthesia more hazardous.
- During recovery, eat a well-balanced diet that includes extra protein, such as meat, fish, poultry, cheese, milk and eggs. Increase fiber and fluid intake to prevent constipation that may result from decreased activity.

REHABILITATION
- Begin daily rehabilitation exercises when supportive wrapping is no longer needed.
- Use ice massage for 10 minutes before and after workouts. Fill a large Styrofoam cup with water and freeze. Tear a small amount of foam from the top so ice protrudes. Massage firmly in a circle over the injured area.
- See page 455 for rehabilitation exercises.

 ## CALL YOUR DOCTOR IF

- Any of the following occur after injury:
  Foot deformity.
  Difficulty moving the foot.
  Numbness, paleness or coldness in the foot. This is an emergency!
  Nausea or vomiting.
- Any of the following occur after treatment:
  Swelling above or below the cast.
  Blue or gray skin color under the toenails.
  Constipation.
- Any of the following occur after surgery:
  Increased pain, swelling or drainage in the surgical area.
  Signs of infection (headache, muscle aches, dizziness, or a general ill feeling and fever).
- New, unexplained symptoms develop. Drugs used in treatment may cause side effects.
- Foot dislocations that you can "pop" back into normal position occur repeatedly.

FOOT FRACTURE

GENERAL INFORMATION

DEFINITION—A complete or incomplete break in bones of the foot. The many bones of the central and front portions of the foot are the most susceptible to fracture.

BODY PARTS INVOLVED
- Bones of the foot.
- Ankle joint and the many joints of the foot.
- Soft tissue surrounding the fracture site, including nerves, tendons, ligaments and blood vessels.

SIGNS & SYMPTOMS
- Severe foot pain at the time of injury.
- Swelling of soft tissue surrounding the fracture.
- Visible deformity if the fracture is complete and bone fragments separate enough to distort normal foot contours.
- Tenderness to the touch.
- Numbness and coldness in the foot and toes, if the blood supply is impaired.

CAUSES—Direct blow or indirect stress to the bone. Indirect stress may be caused by twisting or violent muscle contraction, such as kicking.

RISK INCREASES WITH
- Contact sports, especially football and soccer.
- History of bone or joint disease, especially osteoporosis.
- Obesity.
- Poor nutrition, especially calcium deficiency.
- If surgery or anesthesia are needed, surgical risk increases with smoking and use of drugs such as mind-altering drugs, muscle relaxants, antihypertensives, tranquilizers, sleep inducers, insulin, sedatives, beta-adrenergic blockers or corticosteroids.

HOW TO PREVENT—Use athletic shoes especially designed for the sport in which you are involved.

WHAT TO EXPECT

APPROPRIATE HEALTH CARE
- Doctor's treatment to manipulate and set the broken bones.
- Hospitalization (sometimes) for anesthesia and surgery to set the fracture.
- Self-care during rehabilitation.
- Whirlpool, ultrasound or massage (to displace fluid from the injured joint space).

DIAGNOSTIC MEASURES
- Your own observation of symptoms.
- Medical history and physical exam by a doctor.
- X-rays of injured areas, including joints above and below the primary injury site.

POSSIBLE COMPLICATIONS
At the time of injury:
- Shock.
- Pressure on or injury to nearby nerves,

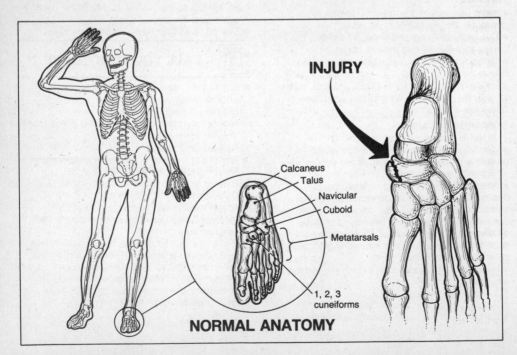

INJURY

Calcaneus
Talus
Navicular
Cuboid
Metatarsals
1, 2, 3 cuneiforms

NORMAL ANATOMY

ligaments, tendons, muscles, blood vessels or connective tissues.

After treatment or surgery:
- Delayed union or non-union of the fracture.
- Impaired blood supply to the fracture site.
- Avascular necrosis (death of bone cells) due to interruption of the blood supply.
- Arrest of normal bone growth in children.
- Infection in open fractures (skin broken over fracture site), or at the incision if surgical setting was necessary.
- Shortening of the injured bones.
- Proneness to repeated foot injury.
- Unstable or arthritic joint following repeated injury.
- Prolonged healing time if activity is resumed too soon.
- Problems caused by casts. See Appendix 2 (Care of Casts).

PROBABLE OUTCOME—It is impossible to predict exactly how long it will take for any fracture to heal. Variable factors include age, sex and previous state of health and conditioning. The average healing time for this fracture is 6 to 8 weeks. Healing is considered complete when there is no motion at the fracture site and when X-rays show complete bone union.

 HOW TO TREAT

NOTE—Follow your doctor's instructions. These instructions are supplemental.

FIRST AID
- Keep the person warm with blankets to decrease the possibility of shock.
- Use instructions for R.I.C.E., the first letters of *rest, ice, compression* and *elevation.* See Appendix 1 for details.
- The doctor will probably realign and set the broken bones in the following manner:
  Hind-portion fracture: Large fragments are repositioned surgically. Otherwise the fracture is treated as a moderate sprain.
  Central-portion fracture: These uncommon compression fractures require surgery.
  Front-portion fracture: These are treated like toe fractures (see Toe Fracture).
Manipulation should be done as soon as possible after injury. Six or more hours after the fracture, bleeding and displacement of body fluids may lead to shock. Also, many tissues lose their elasticity and become difficult to return to a normal position.

CONTINUING CARE
- Immobilization is usually necessary. If so, a rigid cast covers the entire foot and extends to just below the knee.
- After cast removal, use frequent ice massage. Fill a large Styrofoam cup with water and freeze.

Tear a small amount of foam from the top so ice protrudes. Massage firmly over the injured area in a circle about the size of a softball. Do this for 15 minutes at a time, 3 or 4 times a day, and before workouts or competition.
- Apply heat instead of ice if it feels better. Use heat lamps, hot soaks, hot showers, heating pads, or heat liniments and ointments.
- Take whirlpool treatments, if available.

MEDICATION—Your doctor may prescribe:
- General anesthesia, local anesthesia, or muscle relaxants to make bone manipulation and fixation of bone fragments possible.
- Narcotic or synthetic narcotic pain relievers for severe pain.
- Stool softeners to prevent constipation due to inactivity.
- Acetaminophen (available without prescription) for mild pain after initial treatment.

ACTIVITY
- Actively exercise all muscle groups not immobilized. The resulting muscle contractions promote fracture alignment and hasten healing.
- Resume normal activities gradually after treatment. Don't drive until healing is complete.
- Begin reconditioning the injured area after clearance from your doctor.

DIET
- Drink only water before manipulation or surgery to treat the fracture. Solid food in your stomach makes vomiting while under anesthesia more hazardous.
- During recovery, eat a well-balanced diet that includes extra protein, such as meat, fish, poultry, cheese, milk and eggs. Increase fiber and fluid intake to prevent constipation that may result from decreased activity.

REHABILITATION—Begin daily rehabilitation exercises when supportive wrapping is no longer needed. Use ice massage for 10 minutes prior to exercise. See pages 446 and 455 for rehabilitation exercises.

 CALL YOUR DOCTOR IF

- You have signs or symptoms of a foot fracture.
- Any of the following occur after surgery or other treatment:
  Increased pain, swelling or drainage in the surgical area.
  Signs of infection (headache, muscle aches, dizziness, or a general ill feeling and fever).
  Swelling above or below the cast.
  Change in skin color beyond the cast to blue or gray, particularly under the toenails.
  Numbness or complete loss of feeling beyond the fracture site.
  Nausea or vomiting.
  Constipation.

FOOT GANGLION
(Synovial Hernia; Synovial Cyst)

 GENERAL INFORMATION

DEFINITION—A small, usually hard nodule lying directly over a tendon or a joint capsule on the top or bottom of the foot. Occasionally the nodule may become quite large. Sometimes a foot ganglion may regress and disappear altogether, only to reappear later.

BODY PARTS INVOLVED
- Top or sole of the foot.
- Tendon sheath (a thin membranous covering to any tendon).
- Any of many joint spaces in the foot.

SIGNS & SYMPTOMS
- Hard lump over a tendon or joint capsule in the foot. The nodule "yields" to heavy pressure because it is not solid.
- No pain usually, but overuse of the foot may cause mild pain and aching.
- Tenderness if the lump is pressed hard.
- Discomfort with extremes of motion (flexing or extending) and with repetition of the exercise that produced the ganglion.

CAUSES
- Mild or chronic sprains in a foot joint, causing weakness of the joint capsule.
- Defect in the fibrous sheath of the joint or tendon, permitting part of the underlying

synovium (thin membrane that lines the tendon sheath) to protrude through. Irritation of the protruding synovium causes it to fill with fluid. Continued irritation makes it enlarge and harden, forming the ganglion.

RISK INCREASES WITH
- Repeated injury, especially mild sprains. Foot ganglions frequently occur in runners, jumpers, skiiers and participants in contact sports.
- Inadequate warmup prior to practice or competition.
- Poor muscle strength or conditioning.
- If surgery is necessary, surgical risk increases with smoking, poor nutrition, alcoholism, and recent or chronic illness.

HOW TO PREVENT
- Build your strength in a long-term conditioning program appropriate for your sport.
- Warmup before practice or competition.

 WHAT TO EXPECT

APPROPRIATE HEALTH CARE
- Doctor's care for diagnosis and possible injections of local anesthetic or corticosteroids.
- Surgery (usually). Surgery will be conducted under general or local anesthesia in an outpatient surgical facility or hospital operating room.

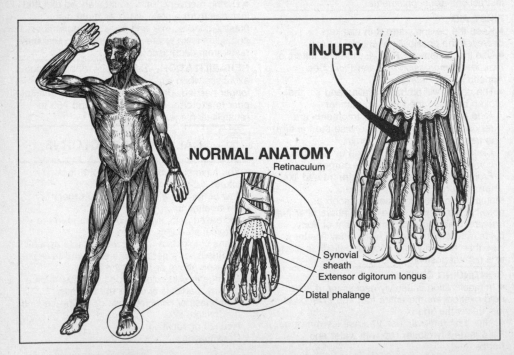

INJURY

NORMAL ANATOMY

Retinaculum

Synovial sheath

Extensor digitorum longus

Distal phalange

DIAGNOSTIC MEASURES
- Your own observation of signs and symptoms.
- Medical history and physical examination by a doctor.
- X-rays of the area.

POSSIBLE COMPLICATIONS
- After surgery:
  Excessive bleeding.
  Surgical-wound infection.
  Recurrence if surgical removal is incomplete.
- Calcification of ganglion (rare).

PROBABLE OUTCOME—Ganglions sometimes disappear spontaneously, only to recur later. Surgery is usually necessary. After surgery, allow about 3 weeks for recovery if no complications occur.

 HOW TO TREAT

NOTE—Follow your doctor's instructions. These instructions are supplemental.

FIRST AID—None. This condition develops gradually.

CONTINUING CARE
Immediately after surgery:
- The affected area is usually immobilized in a splint for 1 to 2 weeks following surgery.
- If the wound bleeds during the first 24 hours after surgery, press a clean tissue or cloth to it for 10 minutes.
- A hard ridge should form along the incision. As it heals, the ridge will recede gradually.
- Use an electric heating pad, a heat lamp, or a warm compress to relieve incisional pain.
- Bathe and shower as usual. You may wash the incision gently with mild unscented soap.
- Between baths, keep the wound dry with a bandage for the first 2 or 3 days after surgery. If a bandage gets wet, change it promptly.
- Apply non-prescription antibiotic ointment to the wound before applying new bandages.
- Wrap the foot with an elasticized bandage until healing is complete.
After the incision has healed:
- Use an ice pack 3 or 4 times a day. Wrap ice chips or cubes in a plastic bag, and wrap the

bag in a moist towel. Place it over the injured area for 20 minutes at a time.
- You may apply heat instead of ice if it feels better. Use heat lamps, hot soaks, hot showers, heating pads, or heat liniments and ointments.
- Take whirlpool treatments, if available.

MEDICATION
- Your doctor may prescribe pain relievers. Don't take prescription pain medication longer than 4 to 7 days. Use only as much as you need.
- You may use non-prescription drugs, such as acetaminophen, for minor pain.

ACTIVITY
- Return to work and normal activity as soon as possible. This reduces postoperative depression and irritability, which are common.
- Avoid vigorous exercise for 3 weeks after surgery.
- Resume driving when healing is complete.

DIET—During recovery, eat a well-balanced diet that includes extra protein, such as meat, fish, poultry, cheese, milk and eggs. Increase fiber and fluid intake to prevent constipation that may result from decreased activity.

REHABILITATION
- Begin daily rehabilitation exercises when supportive wrapping is no longer needed.
- Use ice massage for 10 minutes before and after workouts. Fill a large Styrofoam cup with water and freeze. Tear a small amount of foam from the top so ice protrudes. Massage firmly over the injured area in a circle about the size of a softball.
- See page 455 for rehabilitation exercises.

 CALL YOUR DOCTOR IF

- You have signs or symptoms of a foot ganglion.
- Any of the following occur after surgery:
  Increased pain, swelling, redness, drainage or bleeding in the surgical area.
  Signs of infection (headache, muscle aches, dizziness, or a general ill feeling and fever).
  New, unexplained symptoms. Drugs used in treatment may produce side effects.

FOOT HEMATOMA

GENERAL INFORMATION

DEFINITION—A collection of pooled blood within constricted space on the top of the foot (dorsum) or bottom of the foot (plantar area).

BODY PARTS INVOLVED
- Dorsum or plantar area.
- Soft tissue surrounding the hematoma, including nerves, tendons, ligaments, muscles and blood vessels.

SIGNS & SYMPTOMS
- Swelling over the injured area.
- Fluctuance (feeling of tenseness to the touch, like pushing on an overinflated balloon).
- Tenderness.
- Redness that progresses through several color changes—purple, green-yellow, yellow—before it completely heals.

CAUSES—Direct injury, usually from a blunt object or from landing on a hard surface. Bleeding into tissues then causes the surrounding tissue to be pushed away.

RISK INCREASES WITH
- Contact sports, especially if the foot is not adequately protected.
- Medical history of any bleeding disorder, such as hemophilia.
- Poor nutrition, including vitamin deficiency.
- Use of anticoagulants or aspirin.

HOW TO PREVENT—Wear appropriate, well-designed shoes during competition or other athletic activity to decrease the risk of foot injury.

WHAT TO EXPECT

APPROPRIATE HEALTH CARE
- Doctor's care unless the hematoma is very small.
- Needle aspiration of blood from the hematoma, if the hematoma is accessible. At the same time hyaluronidase (an enzyme) can be injected into the hematoma space. Hyaluronidase hastens absorption of the blood.
- Self-care for minor hematomas, or following serious hematomas during the rehabilitation phase.
- Physical therapy following serious hematomas.

DIAGNOSTIC MEASURES
- Your own observation of symptoms.
- Physical exam and medical history by a doctor for all except minor injuries.
- X-rays of the injured area to assess total injury to the foot and to rule out the possibility of an underlying bone fracture. Total extent of the injury may not be apparent for 48 to 72 hours.

POSSIBLE COMPLICATIONS
- Infection introduced through a break in the

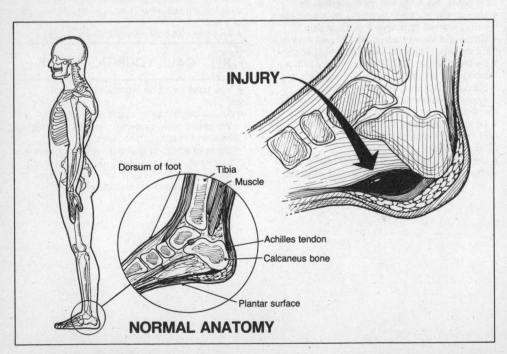

INJURY

Dorsum of foot

Tibia

Muscle

Achilles tendon

Calcaneus bone

Plantar surface

NORMAL ANATOMY

skin at the time of injury or during aspiration of the hematoma.
- Prolonged healing time if activity is resumed too soon.
- Calcification of the blood remaining in the hematoma if the blood is not completely removed or absorbed.

PROBABLE OUTCOME—Average healing time is 2 weeks to 2 months unless the blood is removed with aspiration. Healing time is much less with this treatment.

HOW TO TREAT

NOTE—Follow your doctor's instructions. These instructions are supplemental.

FIRST AID—Use instructions for R.I.C.E., the first letters of *rest, ice, compression* and *elevation*. See Appendix 1 for details.

CONTINUING CARE
- Continue ice massage 3 or 4 times a day for 15 minutes at a time. Fill a large Styrofoam cup with water and freeze. Tear a small amount of foam from the top so ice protrudes. Massage firmly over the injured area in a circle about the size of a softball.
- After 48 hours, localized heat promotes healing by increasing blood circulation in the injured area. Use hot baths, showers, compresses, heat lamps, heating pads, heat ointments and liniments, or whirlpools.
- Don't massage the foot. You may trigger bleeding again.

MEDICATION
- For minor discomfort, you may use:

Non-prescription medicines such as acetaminophen or ibuprofen.
Topical liniments and ointments.
- Your doctor may prescribe stronger medicine for pain, if needed.

ACTIVITY—Begin activities slowly and stop exercise as soon as pain begins. Increase activity as healing progresses. To prevent a delay in healing, protect the hematoma area against excessive motion soon after injury. Motion breaks down the clot and causes irritation throughout the foot, leading to possible scar formation, calcification and restricted movement after healing.

DIET—During recovery, eat a well-balanced diet that includes extra protein, such as meat, fish, poultry, cheese, milk and eggs. Increase fiber and fluid intake to prevent constipation that may result from decreased activity.

REHABILITATION
- Begin daily rehabilitation exercises when supportive wrapping is no longer needed. Use gentle ice massage for 10 minutes prior to exercise.
- See page 455 for rehabilitation exercises.

CALL YOUR DOCTOR IF

- You have signs or symptoms of a foot hematoma that doesn't begin to improve in 1 or 2 days.
- Skin is broken and signs of infection (drainage, increasing pain, fever, headache, muscle aches, dizziness or a general ill feeling) occur.

FOOT SPRAIN

GENERAL INFORMATION

DEFINITION—Violent overstretching of one or more ligaments in the foot. Sprains involving two or more ligaments cause considerably more disability than single-ligament sprains. When the ligament is overstretched, it becomes tense and gives way at its weakest point, either where it attaches to bone or within the ligament itself. If the ligament pulls loose a fragment of bone, it is called a *sprain-fracture.* There are 3 types of sprains:
- Mild (Grade I)—Tearing of some ligament fibers. There is no loss of function.
- Moderate (Grade II)—Rupture of a portion of the ligament, resulting in some loss of function.
- Severe (Grade III)—Complete rupture of the ligament or complete separation of ligament from bone. There is total loss of function. A severe sprain requires surgical repair.

BODY PARTS INVOLVED
- Any ligament in the foot.
- Tissue surrounding the sprain, including blood vessels, tendons, bone, periosteum (covering of bone) and muscles.

SIGNS & SYMPTOMS
- Severe pain at the time of injury.
- A feeling of popping or tearing inside the foot.
- Tenderness at the injury site.
- Swelling in the foot.
- Bruising that appears soon after injury.

CAUSES—Stress on a ligament that temporarily forces or pries a joint in the foot out of its normal location.

RISK INCREASES WITH
- Runners, walkers and those who jump in such sports as basketball, soccer, volleyball, skiing, distance jumping or high jumping. These athletes often accidentally land on the side of the foot.
- Previous foot injury.
- Poor muscle strength or conditioning.
- Inadequate protection from equipment.

HOW TO PREVENT
- Build your strength with a conditioning program appropriate for your sport.
- Warm up before practice or competition.
- Tape vulnerable joints before practice or competition.
- Use protective equipment, such as appropriate shoes with good support.

WHAT TO EXPECT

APPROPRIATE HEALTH CARE
- Doctor's care.
- Application of a cast, tape or elastic bandage.
- Surgery (sometimes) to repair severe sprains.
- Physical therapy for rehabilitation.
- Self-care during and after rehabilitation.

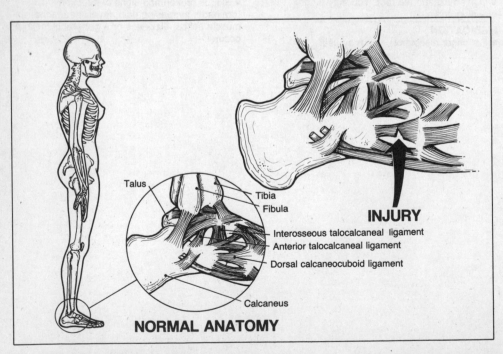

Talus

Tibia
Fibula

INJURY

Interosseous talocalcaneal ligament
Anterior talocalcaneal ligament
Dorsal calcaneocuboid ligament

Calcaneus

NORMAL ANATOMY

DIAGNOSTIC MEASURES
- Your own observation of symptoms.
- Medical history and exam by a doctor.
- X-rays of the foot and ankle to rule out fractures.

POSSIBLE COMPLICATIONS
- Prolonged healing time if usual activities are resumed too soon.
- Proneness to repeated foot injury.
- Inflammation at the ligament attachment to bone (periostitis).
- Prolonged disability (sometimes).
- Unstable or permanently arthritic foot joints following repeated injury.

PROBABLE OUTCOME—If this is a first-time injury, proper care and sufficient healing time before resuming activity should prevent permanent disability. Ligaments have a poor blood supply, and torn ligaments require as much healing time as fractures. Average healing times are:
- Mild sprains—2 to 6 weeks.
- Moderate sprains—6 to 8 weeks.
- Severe sprains—8 to 10 weeks.

HOW TO TREAT

NOTE—Follow your doctor's instructions. These instructions are supplemental.

FIRST AID—Use instructions for R.I.C.E., the first letters of *rest, ice, compression* and *elevation.* See Appendix 1 for details.

CONTINUING CARE—If the doctor does not apply a cast, tape or elastic bandage:
- Continue using an ice pack 3 or 4 times a day. Place ice chips or cubes in a plastic bag. Wrap the bag in a moist towel, and place it over the injured area. Use for 20 minutes at a time.
- Wrap the injured foot with an elasticized bandage between ice treatments.
- After 72 hours, apply heat instead of ice if it feels better. Use heat lamps, hot soaks, hot showers, heating pads, or heat liniments and ointments.
- Take whirlpool treatments, if available.
- Massage the foot gently and often to provide comfort and decrease swelling.

MEDICATION
- For minor discomfort, you may use:
  Aspirin, acetaminophen or ibuprofen.
  Topical liniments and ointments.
- Your doctor may prescribe:
  Stronger pain relievers.
  Injection of a long-acting local anesthetic to reduce pain.
  Injection of a corticosteroid, such as triamcinolone, to reduce inflammation.

ACTIVITY—Resume your normal activities gradually after clearance from your doctor.

DIET—During recovery, eat a well-balanced diet that includes extra protein, such as meat, fish, poultry, cheese, milk and eggs. Increase fiber and fluid intake to prevent constipation that may result from decreased activity.

REHABILITATION
- Begin daily rehabilitation exercises when the cast or supportive wrapping is no longer necessary.
- Use ice massage for 10 minutes before and after exercise. Fill a large Styrofoam cup with water and freeze. Tear a small amount of foam from the top so ice protrudes. Massage firmly over the injured area in a circle about the size of a softball.
- See page 455 for rehabilitation exercises.

CALL YOUR DOCTOR IF

- You have symptoms of a moderate or severe foot sprain, or a mild sprain persists longer than 2 weeks.
- Pain, swelling or bruising worsens despite treatment.
- Any of the following occur after casting or splinting:
  Pain, numbness or coldness below the cast or splint.
  Blue, gray or dusky toenails.
- Any of the following occur after surgery:
  Increased pain, swelling, redness, drainage or bleeding in the surgical area.
  Signs of infection (headache, muscle aches, dizziness, or a general ill feeling with fever).
- New, unexplained symptoms develop. Drugs used in treatment may produce side effects.

FOOT STRAIN

GENERAL INFORMATION

DEFINITION—Injury to the muscles or tendons that surround the foot. Muscles, tendons and bones comprise units. These units stabilize the foot and allow its motion. A strain occurs at the weakest part of a unit. Strains are of 3 types:
- Mild (Grade I)—Slightly pulled muscle without tearing of muscle or tendon fibers. There is no loss of strength.
- Moderate (Grade II)—Tearing of fibers in a muscle, tendon or at the attachment to bone. Strength is diminished.
- Severe (Grade III)—Rupture of the muscle-tendon-bone attachment with separation of fibers. Severe strain requires surgical repair. Chronic strains are caused by overuse. Acute strains are caused by direct injury or overstress.

BODY PARTS INVOLVED
- Tendons and muscles of the foot.
- Foot bones.
- Soft tissue surrounding the strain, including nerves, periosteum (covering to bone), blood vessels and lymph vessels.

SIGNS & SYMPTOMS
- Pain when moving or stretching the foot.
- Muscle spasm in the foot.
- Tenderness and swelling at the injury site.
- Loss of strength (moderate or severe strain).
- Crepitation ("crackling") feeling and sound when the injured area is pressed with fingers.

- Calcification of the muscle or its tendon (visible with X-ray).
- Inflammation of the tendon sheath.

CAUSES
- Prolonged overuse of muscle-tendon units in the ankle or foot.
- Single violent injury or force applied to the foot or ankle.

RISK INCREASES WITH
- Contact sports such as football, soccer or hockey.
- Sports that require quick starts, such as starting a race.
- Any cardiovascular medical problem that results in decreased circulation.
- Medical history of any bleeding disorder.
- Obesity.
- Poor nutrition.
- Previous foot or ankle injury.
- Poor muscle conditioning.

HOW TO PREVENT
- Participate in a strengthening and conditioning program appropriate for your sport.
- Warm up before practice or competition.
- Wear well-fitting athletic shoes appropriate for your sport.

WHAT TO EXPECT

APPROPRIATE HEALTH CARE
- Doctor's diagnosis.

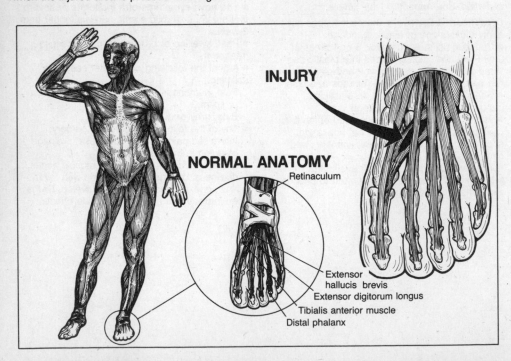

INJURY

NORMAL ANATOMY

Retinaculum

Extensor hallucis brevis
Extensor digitorum longus
Tibialis anterior muscle
Distal phalanx

- Application of tape, plaster splints or casts (sometimes).
- Self-care during rehabilitation.
- Physical therapy (moderate or severe strain).
- Surgery (severe strain).

DIAGNOSTIC MEASURES
- Your own observation of symptoms.
- Medical history and exam by a doctor.
- X-rays of the foot and ankle to rule out fractures.

POSSIBLE COMPLICATIONS
- Prolonged healing time if activity is resumed too soon.
- Proneness to repeated injury.
- Unstable or arthritic foot joints following repeated injury.
- Inflammation at the attachment to bone (periostitis).
- Prolonged disability (sometimes).

PROBABLE OUTCOME—If this is a first-time injury, proper care and sufficient healing time before resuming activity should prevent permanent disability. Torn ligaments and tendons require as long to heal as fractured bones. Average healing times are:
- Mild strain—2 to 10 days.
- Moderate strain—10 days to 6 weeks.
- Severe strain—6 to 10 weeks.

If this is a repeat injury, complications listed above are more likely to occur.

 ## HOW TO TREAT

NOTE—Follow your doctor's instructions. These instructions are supplemental.

FIRST AID—Use instructions for R.I.C.E., the first letters of *rest, ice, compression* and *elevation*. See Appendix 1 for details.

CONTINUING CARE—If a cast or splints are used, leave toes free and exercise them occasionally. If a cast or splints are not used:
- Use ice massage 3 or 4 times a day for 15 minutes at a time. Fill a large Styrofoam cup with water and freeze. Tear a small amount of foam from the top so ice protrudes. Massage firmly over the injured area in a circle about the size of a softball.

- After the first 24 hours, apply heat instead of ice, if it feels better. Use heat lamps, hot soaks, hot showers, heating pads, or heat liniments and ointments.
- Take whirlpool treatments, if available.
- Wrap the injured ankle with an elasticized bandage between treatments.
- Massage gently and often to provide comfort and decrease swelling.

MEDICATION
- For minor discomfort, you may use:
  Aspirin, acetaminophen or ibuprofen.
  Topical liniments and ointments.
- Your doctor may prescribe:
  Stronger pain relievers.
  Injection of a long-acting local anesthetic to reduce pain.
  Injection of a corticosteroid, such as triamcinolone, to reduce inflammation.

ACTIVITY
- For a moderate or severe strain, walk with crutches for at least 72 hours—longer with a cast or splints. See Appendix 3 (Safe Use of Crutches).
- Resume normal activities gradually after pain has subsided.

DIET—Eat a well-balanced diet that includes extra protein, such as meat, fish, poultry, cheese, milk and eggs. Increase fiber and fluid intake to prevent constipation that may result from decreased activity.

REHABILITATION—Begin daily rehabilitation exercises when supportive wrapping is no longer needed. See page 455 for rehabilitation exercises.

 ## CALL YOUR DOCTOR IF

- You have symptoms of a moderate or severe foot strain, or a mild strain persists longer than 10 days.
- Pain or swelling worsens despite treatment.
- The following occurs with casts or splints:
  Pain, numbness or coldness below the injury site.
  Dusky, blue or gray toenails.

FOOT STRESS-FRACTURE
(March Fracture; Fatigue Fracture)

GENERAL INFORMATION

DEFINITION—A complete or incomplete hairline break in a foot (metatarsal) bone. The term *march fracture* arose during World War I when many young soldiers, not conditioned for stress, were put into ill-fitting shoes and required to take long hikes over rough terrain. The X-ray appearance may be similar to a bone tumor. Stress fractures may not appear clearly for several weeks after pain begins in the foot.

BODY PARTS INVOLVED
- Metatarsal bones of the foot.
- Metatarsal joints.
- Soft tissue around the fracture site, including muscles, nerves, tendons, ligaments, periosteum (covering to bone), blood vessels and connective tissue.

SIGNS & SYMPTOMS
- Pain in the foot when walking or running. Pain diminishes or disappears when the load is taken off the feet.
- Tenderness to the touch in the fracture area.

CAUSES—Fatigue of the foot bone(s) caused by repeated overload, as with marching, walking, running or jogging.

RISK INCREASES WITH
- Adults over age 60.
- Walking, running, jogging or standing for prolonged periods.
- History of bone or joint disease, especially osteoporosis.
- Obesity.
- Poor nutrition, especially calcium deficiency.

HOW TO PREVENT
- Heed early warnings of an impending stress fracture, such as foot pain after extended standing or walking. Adjust activities before a fracture occurs.
- Ensure an adequate calcium intake (1000mg to 1500mg a day) with milk and milk products or calcium supplements.

WHAT TO EXPECT

APPROPRIATE HEALTH CARE
- Doctor's diagnosis and care.
- Physical therapy and rehabilitation.
- Self-care during rehabilitation.

DIAGNOSTIC MEASURES
- Your own observation of symptoms.
- Medical history and physical exam by a doctor.

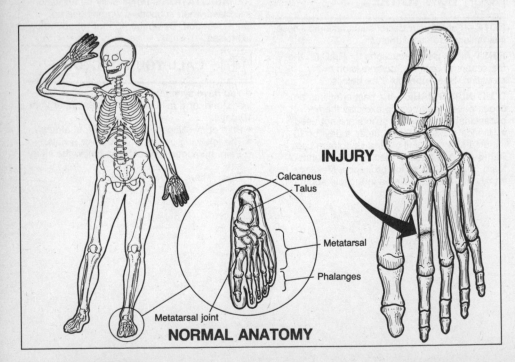

Calcaneus
Talus

INJURY

Metatarsal

Phalanges

Metatarsal joint

NORMAL ANATOMY

- X-rays of both feet and ankles. X-rays are often normal for the first 10 to 24 days after symptoms begin.
- Radioactive technetium 99 scan (see Glossary), if symptoms are typical but X-rays are negative.

POSSIBLE COMPLICATIONS
- Complete fracture from continued stress on the foot after symptoms begin.
- Pressure on or injury to nearby nerves, ligaments, tendons, blood vessels or connective tissues.
- Problems arising from plaster casts, splints or other immobilizing materials. See Appendix 2 (Care of Casts).
- Unstable or arthritic joint following repeated injury.

PROBABLE OUTCOME—It is impossible to predict exactly how long it will take for any fracture to heal. Variable factors include age, sex and previous state of health and conditioning. The average healing time for this fracture is 6 to 8 weeks with adequate treatment. Healing is considered complete when there is no pain at the fracture site and when X-rays show complete bone union.

 HOW TO TREAT

NOTE—Follow your doctor's instructions. These instructions are supplemental.

FIRST AID—None. This injury develops gradually.

CONTINUING CARE
- This fracture does not require setting (realignment) because the fractured bone is not displaced.
- Immobilization may be necessary. If so, a rigid walking cast will be placed around the foot, ankle and lower leg for 3 weeks, followed by a supportive shoe. Sometimes a stiff-soled shoe provides enough support and immobilization to allow healing.
- Use frequent ice massage after the cast is removed. Fill a large Styrofoam cup with water

and freeze. Tear a small amount of foam from the top so ice protrudes. Massage firmly over the injured area in a circle about the size of a baseball. Do this for 15 minutes at a time, 3 or 4 times a day, and before workouts or competition.
- Apply heat instead of ice, if it feels better. Use heat lamps, hot soaks, hot showers, heating pads, or heat liniments or ointments.
- Take whirlpool treatments, if available.
- Massage gently and often to provide comfort and decrease swelling.

MEDICATION—Your doctor may prescribe:
- Narcotic or synthetic narcotic pain relievers for severe pain.
- Stool softeners to prevent constipation due to inactivity.
- Acetaminophen or ibuprofen (available without prescription) for mild pain after initial treatment.

ACTIVITY
- Don't bear weight on the injured foot. Learn to walk with crutches, and use them through the first week with your walking cast. See Appendix 3 (Safe Use of Crutches). Prop your foot up whenever possible.
- Begin reconditioning and rehabilitation after clearance from your doctor.
- Resume normal daily activities gradually after treatment.

DIET—During recovery, eat a well-balanced diet that includes extra protein, such as meat, fish, poultry, cheese, milk and eggs. Increase fiber and fluid intake to prevent constipation that may result from decreased activity.

REHABILITATION—Begin daily rehabilitation exercises when movement is comfortable. Use ice massage for 10 minutes prior to exercise. See page 455 for rehabilitation exercises.

 CALL YOUR DOCTOR IF

- You have unexplained foot pain.
- Toes become dark, blue, cold or numb while the cast is on.

FOOT TENOSYNOVITIS

GENERAL INFORMATION

DEFINITION—Inflammation of the lining of a tendon sheath in the foot. This lining secretes a fluid that lubricates the tendon. When the lining becomes inflamed, the tendon cannot glide smoothly in its covering.

BODY PARTS INVOLVED
- Any foot-tendon lining.
- Soft tissue in the surrounding area, including blood vessels, nerves, ligaments, periosteum (covering to bone) and connective tissue.

SIGNS & SYMPTOMS
- Constant pain or pain with motion.
- Limited motion of the foot and ankle.
- Crepitation (a "crackling" sound when the tendon moves or is touched).
- Redness and tenderness over the inflamed tendon.

CAUSES
- Strain from unusual use or overuse of muscles and tendons in the foot.
- Direct blow or injury to the foot. Tenosynovitis becomes more likely with repeated injury to the ankle or foot.
- Infection introduced through broken skin at the time of injury or through a surgical incision after injury.

RISK INCREASES WITH
- Contact sports, especially "kicking" sports such as soccer or football.
- Skiing.
- If surgery is needed, surgical risk increases with smoking, poor nutrition, alcoholism or drug abuse, and recent or chronic illness.

HOW TO PREVENT
- Engage in a vigorous program of physical conditioning before beginning regular sports participation.
- Warm up adequately before practice or competition.
- Wear protective gear appropriate for your sport.
- Learn proper moves and techniques for your sport.

WHAT TO EXPECT

APPROPRIATE HEALTH CARE
- Doctor's examination and diagnosis.
- Surgery (sometimes) to enlarge the tendon's covering and restore a smooth gliding motion. The surgical procedure under general anesthesia is performed in an outpatient surgical facility or hospital operating room.

DIAGNOSTIC MEASURES
- Your own observations of symptoms and signs.

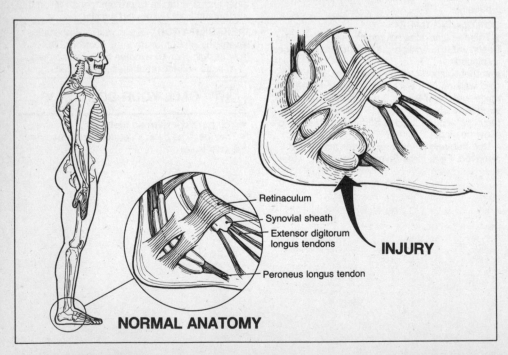

Retinaculum

Synovial sheath

Extensor digitorum longus tendons

Peroneus longus tendon

INJURY

NORMAL ANATOMY

- Medical history and physical examination by your doctor.
- X-rays of the area to rule out other abnormalities.
- Laboratory studies:
  Blood and urine studies before surgery.
  Tissue examination after surgery.

POSSIBLE COMPLICATIONS
- Prolonged healing time if activity is resumed too soon.
- Proneness to repeated injury of foot tendons.
- Adhesive tenosynovitis: The tendon and its covering become bound together. Restriction of motion may be complete or partial. Surgery is necessary to remove the covering or transfer the tendon to a less constrictive area.
- Constrictive tenosynovitis: The walls of the covering thicken and narrow its opening, preventing the tendon from sliding through. Surgery is necessary to cut away part of the covering.

PROBABLE OUTCOME—Tenosynovitis is usually curable in about 6 weeks with heat treatments, corticosteroid injections and rest of the inflamed area. Recovery is usually quicker if the inflammation is caused by a direct blow rather than by a strain or sprain.

 ## HOW TO TREAT

NOTE—Follow your doctor's instructions. These instructions are supplemental.

FIRST AID—None. This problem develops slowly.

CONTINUING CARE
- Wrap the foot and ankle with an elasticized bandage until healing is complete.
- Apply heat frequently. Use heat lamps, hot soaks, hot showers, heating pads, or heat liniments and ointments.

- Take whirlpool treatments, if available.

MEDICATION—You may use non-prescription drugs such as acetaminophen, for minor pain. Your doctor may prescribe:
- Stronger pain relievers. Don't take prescription pain medication longer than 4 to 7 days. Use only as much as you need.
- Injection of the tendon's covering with a combination of a long-acting local anesthetic and a non-absorbable corticosteroid to relieve pain and inflammation.

ACTIVITY—Resume normal activity slowly.

DIET—During recovery, eat a well-balanced diet that includes extra protein, such as meat, fish, poultry, cheese, milk and eggs. Increase fiber and fluid intake to prevent constipation that may result from decreased activity. Your doctor may suggest vitamin and mineral supplements to promote healing.

REHABILITATION
- Begin daily rehabilitation exercises when supportive wrapping is no longer needed.
- Use ice massage for 10 minutes before and after exercise. Fill a large Styrofoam cup with water and freeze. Tear a small amount of foam from the top so ice protrudes. Massage firmly over the injured area in a circle about the size of a softball.
- See page 455 for rehabilitation exercises.

 ## CALL YOUR DOCTOR IF

- You have symptoms of foot tenosynovitis.
- Any of the following occur after surgery:
  Increased pain, swelling, redness, drainage or bleeding in the surgical area.
  Signs of infection (headache, muscle aches, dizziness, or a general ill feeling and fever).
  New, unexplained symptoms. Drugs used in treatment may produce side effects.

GENITAL CONTUSION

GENERAL INFORMATION

DEFINITION—Bruising of the skin and underlying tissues of the external genitals of the male or female due to a direct blow. Contusions cause bleeding from ruptured small capillaries that allow blood to infiltrate skin, scrotum, vaginal lips or other soft tissue.

BODY PARTS INVOLVED—Genitals, including penis, scrotum, spermatic cord and testicles, or vaginal lips and clitoris, urethra, blood vessels and covering to bones (periosteum) in the pelvis.

SIGNS & SYMPTOMS
- Local swelling in the genital area—either superficial or deep.
- Pain and tenderness over the injury.
- Feeling of firmness when pressure is exerted at the injury site.
- Discoloration under the skin, beginning with redness and progressing to the characteristic "black and blue" bruise.
- Restricted activity in the genital area in proportion to the extent of injury.

CAUSES—Direct blow to the genitals, usually from a blunt object.

RISK INCREASES WITH
- Contact sports.
- Gymnastics.
- Bicycling.
- Horseback riding.
- Medical history of any bleeding disorder such as hemophilia.
- Poor nutrition, including vitamin deficiency.

HOW TO PREVENT—Wear appropriate protective gear, such as a padded athletic supporter, during competition or other athletic activity if there is risk of a genital contusion.

WHAT TO EXPECT

APPROPRIATE HEALTH CARE
- Doctor's care unless the contusion is quite small. A doctor should evaluate *any* testicle injury.
- Self-care for minor contusions.
- Ultrasound studies to evaluate testicle injuries.

DIAGNOSTIC MEASURES
- Your own observation of symptoms.
- Medical history and physical exam by a doctor for all except minor injuries.
- X-rays of injured area to assess total injury to soft tissue and to rule out the possibility of

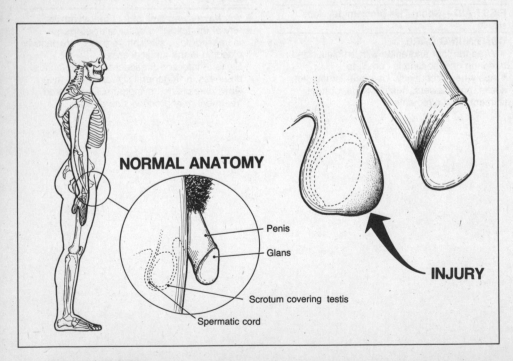

NORMAL ANATOMY

Penis

Glans

Scrotum covering testis

Spermatic cord

INJURY

underlying fractures. The total extent of injury may not be apparent for 48 to 72 hours.

POSSIBLE COMPLICATIONS
- Excessive internal bleeding.
- Loss of testicle from injury.
- Prolonged healing time if usual activities are resumed too soon.
- Infection if skin over the contusion is broken.

PROBABLE OUTCOME—Despite severe pain at the time of injury, most genital contusions heal without complications. Reproductive capacity is rarely affected. Healing time varies with the extent of injury from 3 to 14 days.

HOW TO TREAT

NOTE—Follow your doctor's instructions. These instructions are supplemental.

FIRST AID—Use instructions for R.I.C.E., the first letters of *rest, ice, compression* and *elevation* (if possible). See Appendix 1 for details.

CONTINUING CARE
- Keep the area compressed for 72 hours. Use an athletic supporter for compression for males and sanitary pads for females.
- Use an ice pack 3 or 4 times a day. Wrap ice chips or cubes in a plastic bag, and wrap the bag in a moist towel. Place it over the injured area for 20 minutes at a time.
- After 72 hours, apply heat instead of ice if it feels better. Use heat lamps, hot soaks, hot showers, heating pads, heat liniments or ointments, or whirlpool treatments.

- Use crutches for a few days to avoid weight-bearing if the contusion is severe and hurts worse when walking.

MEDICATION
- For minor discomfort, you may use:
  Acetaminophen or ibuprofen.
  Topical liniments and ointments.
- Your doctor may prescribe stronger medicine for pain.

ACTIVITY
- Avoid sexual intercourse and sexual excitement until healing is complete.
- Begin activities slowly and stop exercise as soon as pain begins. Increase activity as healing progresses.
- Avoid contact sports if the function of one testicle is lost.

DIET—During recovery, eat a well-balanced diet that includes extra protein, such as meat, fish, poultry, cheese, milk and eggs. Your doctor may prescribe vitamin and mineral supplements to promote healing.

REHABILITATION—None.

CALL YOUR DOCTOR IF

- You have a genital contusion that doesn't improve in 1 or 2 days.
- Skin is broken and signs of infection (drainage, increasing pain, fever, headache, muscle aches, dizziness or a general ill feeling) occur.

GROIN STRAIN

GENERAL INFORMATION

DEFINITION—Injury to the muscles or tendons in the area of the groin where the abdomen meets the thigh. Muscles, tendons and bones comprise units. These units stabilize the pelvis and allow its motion. A strain occurs at a unit's weakest part. Strains are of 3 types:
- Mild (Grade I)—Slightly pulled muscle without tearing of muscle or tendon fibers. There is no loss of strength.
- Moderate (Grade II)—Tearing of fibers in a muscle, tendon or at the attachment to bone. Strength is diminished.
- Severe (Grade III)—Rupture of the muscle-tendon-bone attachment with separation of fibers. Severe strain requires surgical repair. Chronic strains are caused by overuse. Acute strains are caused by direct injury or overstress.

BODY PARTS INVOLVED
- Tendons and muscles of the groin area, including abdominal, pelvic and thigh muscles.
- Bones of the groin area, including the pelvis, spine and upper-leg bone (femur).
- Soft tissue surrounding the strain, including nerves, periosteum (covering to bone), blood vessels and lymph vessels.

SIGNS & SYMPTOMS
- Pain in the groin with motion or stretching the leg at the hip joint.
- Muscle spasm in the abdomen or thigh.
- Swelling in the groin.
- Loss of strength (moderate or severe strain).
- Crepitation ("crackling") feeling and sound when the injured area is pressed with fingers.
- Calcification of a muscle or its tendon (visible with X-ray).

CAUSES
- Prolonged overuse of muscle-tendon units in the groin.
- Single violent injury or force applied to a groin muscle-tendon unit.

RISK INCREASES WITH
- Contact sports.
- Sports that require quick starts, such as the start of a race.
- Any cardiovascular medical problem that results in decreased circulation.
- Medical history of any bleeding disorder.
- Obesity.
- Poor nutrition.
- Previous groin injury.
- Poor muscle conditioning.

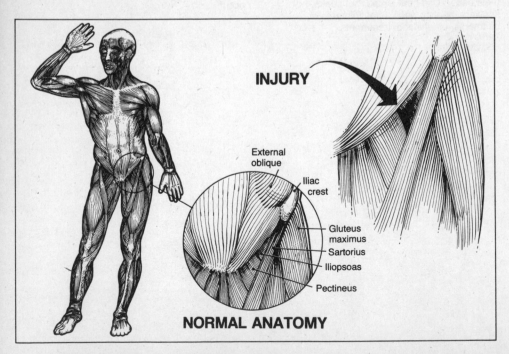

INJURY

External oblique

Iliac crest

Gluteus maximus

Sartorius

Iliopsoas

Pectineus

NORMAL ANATOMY

HOW TO PREVENT
- Participate in a strengthening and conditioning program appropriate for your sport.
- Warm up before practice or competition.

 ## WHAT TO EXPECT

APPROPRIATE HEALTH CARE
- Doctor's diagnosis.
- Self-care during rehabilitation.
- Physical therapy (moderate or severe strain).
- Surgery (severe strain).

DIAGNOSTIC MEASURES
- Your own observation of symptoms.
- Medical history and exam by a doctor.
- X-rays of the injured hip, thigh and pelvis to rule out possible fractures.

POSSIBLE COMPLICATIONS
- Prolonged healing time if activity is resumed too soon.
- Proneness to repeated injury.
- Unstable or arthritic hip following repeated injury.
- Inflammation at the attachment to bone (periostitis).
- Prolonged disability (sometimes).

PROBABLE OUTCOME—If this is a first-time injury, proper care and sufficient healing time before resuming activity should prevent permanent disability. Average healing times are:
- Mild strain—2 to 10 days.
- Moderate strain—10 days to 6 weeks.
- Severe strain—6 to 10 weeks.

If this is a repeat injury, complications listed above are more likely to occur.

 ## HOW TO TREAT

NOTE—Follow your doctor's instructions. These instructions are supplemental.

FIRST AID—Use instructions for R.I.C.E., the first letters of *rest, ice, compression* and *elevation* (if possible). See Appendix 1 for details.

CONTINUING CARE
- Use ice massage 3 or 4 times a day for 15 minutes at a time. Fill a large Styrofoam cup with water and freeze. Tear a small amount of foam from the top so ice protrudes. Massage firmly over the injured area in a circle about the size of a softball.
- After the first 24 hours, apply heat instead of ice, if it feels better. Use heat lamps, hot soaks, hot showers, heating pads, or heat liniments and ointments.
- Support the injured groin area with an elasticized bandage between treatments.

MEDICATION
- For minor discomfort, you may use:
  Aspirin, acetaminophen or ibuprofen.
  Topical liniments and ointments.
- Your doctor may prescribe:
  Stronger pain relievers.
  Injection of a long-acting local anesthetic to reduce pain.
  Injection of a corticosteroid, such as triamcinolone, to reduce inflammation.

ACTIVITY
- For a moderate or severe strain, walk with crutches for at least 72 hours. See Appendix 3 (Safe Use of Crutches).
- Resume your normal activities gradually.

DIET—Eat a well-balanced diet that includes extra protein, such as meat, fish, poultry, cheese, milk and eggs. Increase fiber and fluid intake to prevent constipation that may result from decreased activity.

REHABILITATION—Begin daily rehabilitation exercises when supportive wrapping is no longer needed. See page 457 for rehabilitation exercises.

 ## CALL YOUR DOCTOR IF

- You have symptoms of a groin strain.
- Pain or swelling worsens despite treatment.

HAND CONTUSION

GENERAL INFORMATION

DEFINITION—Bruising of the skin and underlying tissues of the hand due to a direct blow. Contusions cause bleeding from ruptured small capillaries that allow blood to infiltrate muscles, tendons or other soft tissue. The hand is especially vulnerable to contusions because of its exposure and use in almost all sports.

BODY PARTS INVOLVED—Hand tissues, including blood vessels, muscles, tendons, nerves, covering to bones (periosteum) and connective tissue.

SIGNS & SYMPTOMS
- Swelling on the back or in the palm of the hand. Swelling may be superficial or deep.
- Pain and tenderness over the injury.
- Feeling of firmness when pressure is exerted on the injured area.
- Discoloration under the skin, beginning with redness and progressing to the characteristic "black and blue" bruise.
- Restricted hand motion proportional to the extent of injury.

CAUSES—Direct blow to the hand, usually from a blunt object.

RISK INCREASES WITH
- Contact sports, especially when the hands are not adequately protected.

- Medical history of any bleeding disorder such as hemophilia.
- Poor nutrition, including vitamin deficiency.
- Use of anticoagulants or aspirin.

HOW TO PREVENT—If possible, wear appropriate protective padding during competition or other athletic activity. If you must compete before a hand contusion heals, use padding, tape or a cast.

WHAT TO EXPECT

APPROPRIATE HEALTH CARE
- Doctor's care, unless the injury is quite small.
- Self-care for minor contusions, and for serious contusions during the rehabilitation phase.
- Physical therapy for serious contusions.

DIAGNOSTIC MEASURES
- Your own observation of symptoms.
- Medical history and physical exam by a doctor for all except minor injuries.
- X-rays of the hand and wrist to assess total injury to soft tissue and to rule out the possibility of underlying fractures. The total extent of injury may not be apparent for 48 to 72 hours.

POSSIBLE COMPLICATIONS
- Excessive bleeding leading to disability. Infiltrative-type bleeding can (rarely) lead to calcification and impaired function of injured muscles or tendons.

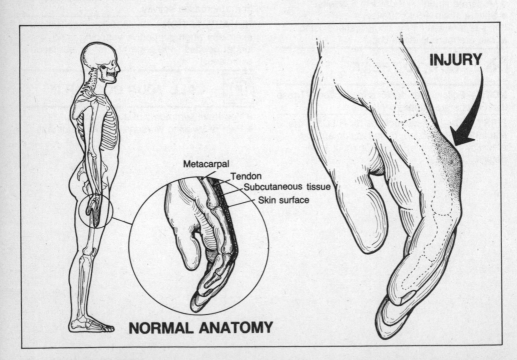

INJURY

Metacarpal
Tendon
Subcutaneous tissue
Skin surface

NORMAL ANATOMY

- Infection if skin over the contusion is broken.
- Infection of the tendon sheaths.
- Tendon rupture.

PROBABLE OUTCOME—Healing time varies with the extent of injury, but average healing time for hand contusions is 1 to 3 weeks.

 ## HOW TO TREAT

NOTE—Follow your doctor's instructions. These instructions are supplemental.

FIRST AID—Use instructions for R.I.C.E., the first letters of *rest, ice, compression* and *elevation*. See Appendix 1 for details.

CONTINUING CARE
- Wrap an elasticized bandage over a felt pad on the injured area. Keep the area compressed for about 72 hours.
- After 72 hours, apply heat instead of ice if it feels better. Use heat lamps, hot soaks, hot showers, heating pads, heat liniments or ointments, or whirlpool treatments.
- Massage gently and often with light lubricating oil to provide comfort and decrease swelling. Stroke from the fingers toward the shoulder.

MEDICATION
- For minor discomfort, you may use:
  Acetaminophen or ibuprofen.
  Topical liniments and ointments.

- Your doctor may prescribe stronger medicine for pain.

ACTIVITY—Begin activities slowly and stop exercise as soon as pain begins. Increase activity as healing progresses.

DIET—During recovery, eat a well-balanced diet that includes extra protein, such as meat, fish, poultry, cheese, milk and eggs. Your doctor may prescribe vitamin and mineral supplements to promote healing.

REHABILITATION
- Begin daily rehabilitation exercises when supportive wrapping is no longer needed.
- Use ice massage for 10 minutes before and after workouts. Fill a large Styrofoam cup with water and freeze. Tear a small amount of foam from the top so ice protrudes. Massage firmly over the injured area in a circle about the size of a softball.
- See pages 457 and 474 for rehabilitation exercises.

 ## CALL YOUR DOCTOR IF

- You have a hand contusion that doesn't improve in 1 or 2 days.
- Skin is broken and signs of infection (drainage, increasing pain, fever, headache, muscle aches, dizziness or a general ill feeling) occur.

HAND DISLOCATION

GENERAL INFORMATION

DEFINITION—Injury to the hand so that adjoining bones are displaced and no longer touch each other. The ulnar nerve is likely to be injured with this dislocation. If the ulnar nerve is involved, surgery is necessary to prevent permanent damage.

BODY PARTS INVOLVED
● Hand bones (carpal and metacarpal).
● Ligaments that hold the hand bones in the proper position.
● Soft tissue surrounding the dislocation site, including periosteum (covering to bone), tendons, blood vessels and connective tissue.
● Ulnar nerve.

SIGNS & SYMPTOMS
● Excruciating pain at the time of injury.
● Loss of normal hand function.
● Severe pain when attempting to move the hand.
● Visible deformity if the dislocated bones have locked in the dislocated position. Bones may spontaneously reposition themselves and leave no deformity, but damage is the same.
● Tenderness over the dislocation.
● Swelling and bruising at the injury site.
● Numbness or paralysis below the dislocation from pressure, pinching or cutting of blood vessels or nerves.

CAUSES
● Direct blow to the hand or falling on an outstretched hand (most common cause).
● End result of a severe hand sprain.

RISK INCREASES WITH
● Contact sports.
● Previous dislocation or sprain.
● Repeated injury to any hand joint.
● Arthritis of any type (rheumatoid, gout).
● Poor muscle conditioning.
● Congenital abnormality, such as shallow or malformed joint surfaces.

HOW TO PREVENT—Initial injury usually cannot be prevented. After healing, protect vulnerable hand joints with wrapped elastic bandages, tape wraps, felt or foam-rubber pads or plastic splints.

WHAT TO EXPECT

APPROPRIATE HEALTH CARE
● Doctor's treatment. This will include manipulating the joint to reposition the bones.
● Surgery (sometimes) to restore the joint to its normal position and repair torn ligaments and tendons. Acute or recurring dislocations may require surgical reconstruction or replacement of the joint. Ulnar-nerve involvement always requires surgery to salvage function in the muscles supplied by the ulnar nerve.

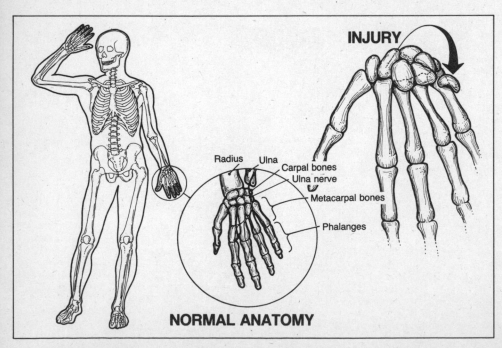

INJURY

Radius   Ulna   Carpal bones
Ulna nerve
Metacarpal bones
Phalanges

NORMAL ANATOMY

- Self-care during rehabilitation.

DIAGNOSTIC MEASURES
- Your own observation of symptoms.
- Medical history and exam by a doctor.
- X-rays of the wrist and hand.

POSSIBLE COMPLICATIONS
At the time of injury:
- Shock.
- Pressure on or injury to nearby nerves, ligaments, tendons, muscles, blood vessels or connective tissue.
After treatment or surgery:
- Excessive internal bleeding around the dislocation site.
- Impaired blood supply to the dislocated area.
- Death of bone cells due to interruption of the blood supply.
- Infection introduced during surgical treatment.
- Prolonged healing if activity is resumed too soon.
- Recurrent dislocations.
- Unstable or arthritic joint following repeated injury.

PROBABLE OUTCOME—After the dislocation has been corrected, the joint may require immobilization with a cast or splint for 2 to 8 weeks. Complete healing of injured ligaments requires a minimum of 6 weeks.

 # HOW TO TREAT

NOTE—Follow your doctor's instructions. These instructions are supplemental.

FIRST AID
- Use instructions for R.I.C.E., the first letters of *rest, ice, compression* and *elevation.* See Appendix 1 for details.
- The doctor will manipulate the dislocated bones in the hand to return them to their normal position. Anesthesia and traction on fingers and countertraction on a flexed elbow are usually necessary to correct this dislocation. Manipulation should be done within 6 hours of injury or many tissues will lose elasticity and become difficult to return to a normal position.

CONTINUING CARE
If a cast is necessary:
- See Appendix 2 (Care of Casts).
If a cast is not necessary:
- Use ice soaks 3 or 4 times a day. Fill a bucket with ice water, and soak the injured area for 20 minutes at a time.
- After 24 to 48 hours, apply heat instead of ice if it feels better. Use heat lamps, hot soaks, hot showers or heating pads.
- Take whirlpool treatments, if available.
- Wrap the hand with an elasticized bandage between treatments.
- Massage gently and often to provide comfort

and decrease swelling.

MEDICATION—Your doctor may prescribe:
- General anesthesia or muscle relaxants to make joint manipulation possible.
- Acetaminophen to relieve moderate pain.
- Narcotic pain relievers for severe pain.
- Stool softeners to prevent constipation due to decreased activity.
- Antibiotics to fight infection, if surgery is necessary.

ACTIVITY
If surgery is not necessary:
- Resume sports participation after clearance from your doctor.
If surgery is necessary:
- Resume normal activities gradually after surgery. Don't drive until healing is complete.

DIET
- Drink only water before manipulation or surgery to correct the dislocation. Solid food in your stomach makes vomiting while under general anesthesia more hazardous.
- During recovery, eat a well-balanced diet that includes extra protein, such as meat, fish, poultry, cheese, milk and eggs. Increase fiber and fluid intake to prevent constipation that may result from decreased activity.

REHABILITATION
- Begin daily rehabilitation exercises when supportive wrapping is no longer needed.
- Use ice massage for 10 minutes before and after workouts. Fill a large Styrofoam cup with water and freeze. Tear a small amount of foam from the top so ice protrudes. Massage firmly in a circle over the injured area.
- See pages 457 and 474 for rehabilitation exercises.

 # CALL YOUR DOCTOR IF

- You have symptoms of a dislocated hand. Call immediately if the hand becomes numb, pale or cold after injury. This is an emergency!
- Any of the following occurs after treatment:
  Swelling above or below the cast.
  Blue or gray skin color beyond the cast, particularly under the fingernails.
  Loss of feeling in the hand.
  Nausea or vomiting.
  Constipation.
- Any of the following occur after surgery:
  Increased pain, swelling or drainage in the surgical area.
  Signs of infection (headache, muscle aches, dizziness, or a general ill feeling and fever).
- New, unexplained symptoms develop. Drugs used in treatment may produce side effects.
- Hand dislocations that you can "pop" back into normal position occur repeatedly.

HAND FRACTURE, CARPAL

GENERAL INFORMATION

DEFINITION—A complete or incomplete break in any one of several bones of the hand.

BODY PARTS INVOLVED
● Any carpal bone in the hand.
● Wrist joint.
● Any of the joints between the hand and fingers.
● Soft tissue surrounding the fracture site, including nerves, tendons, ligaments and blood vessels.

SIGNS & SYMPTOMS
● Severe pain at the fracture site.
● Swelling of soft tissue surrounding the fracture.
● Tenderness to the touch.
● Numbness and coldness beyond the fracture site if the blood supply is impaired.

CAUSES—Direct blow or indirect stress to the bone. Indirect stress may be caused by twisting or violent muscle contraction.

RISK INCREASES WITH
● Contact sports, especially boxing.
● History of bone or joint disease, especially osteoporosis.
● Poor nutrition, especially calcium deficiency.

HOW TO PREVENT
● Use appropriate protective equipment, such as boxing gloves for boxing.

● If you have had a previous hand injury, protect the hand with taping and padding when participating in contact sports.

WHAT TO EXPECT

APPROPRIATE HEALTH CARE
● Doctor's treatment to immobilize the broken bones.
● Self-care during rehabilitation.

DIAGNOSTIC MEASURES
● Your own observation of symptoms.
● Medical history and physical exam by a doctor.
● X-rays of injured areas, including joints above and below the primary injury site.
● Repeat X-rays are frequently needed about 2 weeks after injury, if the original X-rays were negative and pain continues.

POSSIBLE COMPLICATIONS
At the time of injury:
● Misdiagnosis as a wrist sprain, delaying proper treatment.
● Shock.
● Pressure on or injury to nearby nerves, ligaments, tendons, muscles, blood vessels, or connective tissues.
After treatment or surgery:
● Delayed union or non-union of the fracture.
● Impaired blood supply to the fracture site.
● Arrest of normal bone growth in children.

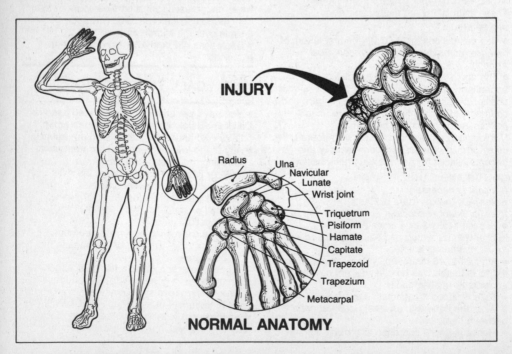

INJURY

Radius
Ulna
Navicular
Lunate
Wrist joint
Triquetrum
Pisiform
Hamate
Capitate
Trapezoid
Trapezium
Metacarpal

NORMAL ANATOMY

- Infection in open fractures (skin broken over fracture site).
- Shortening of the injured bones.
- Proneness to repeated hand injury.
- Unstable or arthritic joint following repeated injury.
- Prolonged healing time if activity is resumed too soon.
- Problems caused by casts. See Appendix 2 (Care of Casts).

PROBABLE OUTCOME—It is impossible to predict exactly how long it will take for any fracture to heal. Variable factors include age, sex, and previous state of health and conditioning. The average healing time for this fracture is 4 months. Healing is considered complete when there is no motion at the fracture site and when X-rays show complete bone union.

HOW TO TREAT

NOTE—Follow your doctor's instructions. These instructions are supplemental.

FIRST AID
- Use a padded splint or sling to immobilize the hand and wrist before transporting the injured person to the doctor's office or emergency facility.
- Keep the person warm with blankets to decrease the possibility of shock.
- Follow instructions for R.I.C.E., the first letters of *rest, ice, compression* and *elevation*. See Appendix 1 for details.

CONTINUING CARE
- Immobilization will be necessary. Rigid casts or splints are placed around the hand to immobilize the joint above and the joint below the fracture site. After the cast has been removed, the hand needs protection with taping or with a leather gauntlet.
- After 48 hours, localized heat promotes healing by increasing blood circulation in the injured area. Use a heating pad or heat lamp so heat can penetrate the cast.

- After the cast is removed, use frequent ice massage. Fill a large Styrofoam cup with water and freeze. Tear a small amount of foam from the top so ice protrudes. Massage firmly over the injured area in a circle about the size of a baseball. Do this for 15 minutes at a time, 3 or 4 times a day, and before workouts or competition.
- Apply heat instead of ice if it feels better. Use heat lamps, hot soaks, hot showers, heating pads, or heat liniments or ointments.
- Take whirlpool treatments, if available.

MEDICATION—Your doctor may prescribe:
- Narcotic or synthetic narcotic pain relievers for severe pain.
- Acetaminophen (available without prescription) for mild pain after initial treatment.

ACTIVITY
- Actively exercise all muscle groups not immobilized. These muscle contractions promote fracture alignment and hasten healing.
- Resume normal activities gradually after treatment. Don't drive until healing is complete.
- Begin reconditioning the injured area after clearance from your doctor.

DIET—During recovery, eat a well-balanced diet that includes extra protein, such as meat, fish, poultry, cheese, milk and eggs. Increase fiber and fluid intake to prevent constipation that may result from decreased activity.

REHABILITATION—Begin daily rehabilitation exercises when movement is comfortable. Use ice massage for 10 minutes prior to exercise. See page 474 for rehabilitation exercises.

CALL YOUR DOCTOR IF

- You have signs or symptoms of a hand fracture.
- Any of the following occur after treatment: Increased pain or swelling in the injured area. Swelling above or below the cast or splint. Change in skin color to blue or gray beyond the cast, particularly under the fingernails. Numbness or complete loss of feeling in the hand, fingers or thumb.

HAND FRACTURE, METACARPAL

GENERAL INFORMATION

DEFINITION—A complete or incomplete break in one of the metacarpal bones—the bones that connect the hand and wrist to the fingers.

BODY PARTS INVOLVED
- Metacarpal bones of the hand.
- Metacarpo-carpal joints and metacarpo-phalangeal joints.
- Soft tissue around the fracture site, including nerves, tendons, ligaments and blood vessels.

SIGNS & SYMPTOMS
- Severe hand pain at the time of injury.
- Swelling of soft tissue around the fracture.
- Visible deformity if the fracture is complete and the bone fragments separate enough to distort normal body contours.
- Tenderness to the touch.
- Numbness and coldness beyond the fracture site, if the blood supply is impaired.

CAUSES
- Direct blow, such as striking a blow with the fist.
- Indirect stress to the bone. Indirect stress may be caused by twisting or violent muscle contraction.

RISK INCREASES WITH
- Contact sports, especially football and boxing.
- History of bone or joint disease, especially osteoporosis.

- Poor nutrition, especially calcium deficiency.
- If surgery or anesthesia is needed, surgical risk increases with smoking and use of drugs, including mind-altering drugs, muscle relaxants, antihypertensives, tranquilizers, sleep inducers, insulin, sedatives, beta-adrenergic blockers or corticosteroids.

HOW TO PREVENT
- Use appropriate protective equipment, such as padded gloves for boxing and hand pads for football.
- If you have had a previous hand fracture, use tape and padding to protect your hands before participating in contact sports.

WHAT TO EXPECT

APPROPRIATE HEALTH CARE
- Doctor's treatment to manipulate the broken bones.
- Hospitalization (sometimes) for anesthesia and surgery to set the fracture.
- Self-care during rehabilitation.
- Whirlpool, ultrasound or massage (to displace excess fluid from the injured joint space).

DIAGNOSTIC MEASURES
- Your own observation of symptoms.
- Medical history and physical exam by a doctor.
- X-rays of injured areas, including joints above and below the primary injury site.

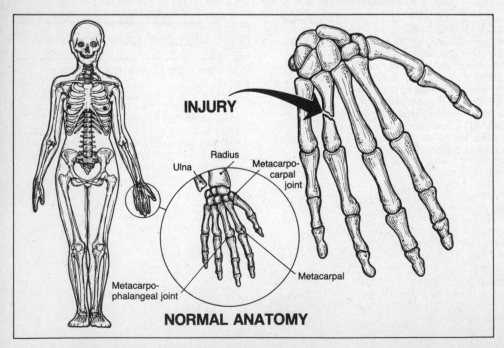

INJURY

Ulna

Radius

Metacarpo-carpal joint

Metacarpo-phalangeal joint

Metacarpal

NORMAL ANATOMY

POSSIBLE COMPLICATIONS

At the time of injury:
- Shock.
- Pressure on or injury to nearby nerves, ligaments, tendons, muscles, blood vessels or connective tissues.

After treatment or surgery:
- Delayed union or non-union of the fracture.
- Impaired blood supply to the fracture site.
- Avascular necrosis (death of bone cells) due to interruption of the blood supply.
- Arrest of normal bone growth in children.
- Infection in open fractures (skin broken over fracture site), or at the incision if surgical setting was necessary.
- Shortening of the injured bones.
- Proneness to repeated hand injury.
- Unstable or arthritic joint following repeated injury.
- Prolonged healing time if activity is resumed too soon.
- Problems caused by casts. See Appendix 2 (Care of Casts).

PROBABLE OUTCOME—It is impossible to predict exactly how long it will take for any fracture to heal. Variable factors include age, sex, and previous state of health and conditioning. The average healing time for this fracture is 6 to 8 weeks. Healing is considered complete when there is no motion at the fracture site and when X-rays show complete bone union.

 HOW TO TREAT

NOTE—Follow your doctor's instructions. These instructions are supplemental.

FIRST AID
- Keep the person warm with blankets to decrease the possibility of shock.
- Follow instructions for R.I.C.E., the first letters of *rest, ice, compression* and *elevation.* See Appendix 1 for details.
- Use a padded splint or sling to immobilize the hand and wrist before transporting the injured person to the doctor's office or emergency facility.
- The doctor will manipulate and set the broken bones with surgery or, if possible, without. Manipulation should be done as soon as possible after injury. Six or more hours after the fracture, bleeding and displacement of body fluids may lead to shock. Also, many tissues lose their elasticity and become difficult to return to a normal position.

CONTINUING CARE
- Immobilization will be necessary. A rigid cast is placed around the injured area to immobilize the fingers and wrist.

- After 48 hours, localized heat promotes healing by increasing blood circulation in the injured area. Use a heat lamp or heating pad so heat can penetrate the cast.
- After the cast is removed, use frequent ice massage. Fill a large Styrofoam cup with water and freeze. Tear a small amount of foam from the top so ice protrudes. Massage firmly over the injured area in a circle about the size of a baseball. Do this for 15 minutes at a time, 3 or 4 times a day, and before workouts or competition.

MEDICATION—Your doctor may prescribe:
- General anesthesia, local anesthesia, or muscle relaxants to make bone manipulation possible.
- Narcotic or synthetic narcotic pain relievers for severe pain.
- Acetaminophen (available without prescription) for mild pain after initial treatment.

ACTIVITY
- Actively exercise all muscle groups not immobilized. These muscle contractions promote fracture alignment and hasten healing.
- Begin reconditioning of the hand after clearance from your doctor.
- Resume normal activities gradually after treatment. Don't drive until healing is complete.

DIET
- Drink only water before manipulation or surgery to treat the fracture. Solid food in your stomach makes vomiting while under anesthesia more hazardous.
- During recovery, eat a well-balanced diet that includes extra protein, such as meat, fish, poultry, cheese, milk and eggs.

REHABILITATION—Begin daily rehabilitation exercises when movement is comfortable. Use ice massage for 10 minutes prior to exercise. See page 474 for rehabilitation exercises.

 CALL YOUR DOCTOR IF

- You have signs or symptoms of a hand fracture.
- Any of the following occurs after surgery or other treatment:
  Increased pain, swelling or drainage in the surgical area.
  Signs of infection (headache, muscle aches, dizziness, or a general ill feeling and fever).
  Swelling above or below the cast.
  Blue or gray skin color under the fingernails.
  Numbness or complete loss of feeling in the fingers of the affected hand.
  Nausea or vomiting.

HAND FRACTURE, NAVICULAR

GENERAL INFORMATION

DEFINITION—A complete or incomplete break in the navicular bone of the hand.

BODY PARTS INVOLVED
- Navicular (scaphoid) bone in the hand.
- Wrist joint.
- Soft tissue around the fracture site, including nerves, tendons, ligaments and blood vessels.

SIGNS & SYMPTOMS
- Severe pain at the fracture site.
- Swelling of soft tissue around the fracture.
- Tenderness to the touch.
- Numbness and coldness in the hand and fingers, if the blood supply is impaired.

CAUSES—Direct blow or indirect stress to the bone. The force is usually inflicted by a fall on an outstretched hand.

RISK INCREASES WITH
- Participation in contact sports, especially boxing, football and wrestling.
- History of bone or joint disease, especially osteoporosis.
- Obesity.
- If surgery or anesthesia is needed, surgical risk increases with smoking and use of drugs, including mind-altering drugs, muscle relaxants, antihypertensives, tranquilizers, sleep inducers, insulin, sedatives, beta-adrenergic blockers or corticosteroids.

HOW TO PREVENT
- Use appropriate protective equipment, such as boxing gloves for boxing.
- If you have had a previous injury, use tape and padding to protect your hand before participating in contact sports.

WHAT TO EXPECT

APPROPRIATE HEALTH CARE
- Doctor's treatment to manipulate the broken bones and immobilize the injured area.
- Hospitalization (sometimes) for anesthesia and surgery to set the fracture.
- Self-care during rehabilitation.
- Whirlpool, ultrasound or massage (to displace excess fluid from the injured joint space).

DIAGNOSTIC MEASURES
- Your own observation of symptoms.
- Medical history and physical exam by a doctor.
- X-rays of injured areas, including the wrist joint above and the bones in the hand.
- Repeat X-rays may be needed after 2 to 8 weeks if the first set shows no injury but symptoms continue. A third set is sometimes necessary because this injury may not appear on X-rays for several weeks.

POSSIBLE COMPLICATIONS
At the time of injury:
- Shock.

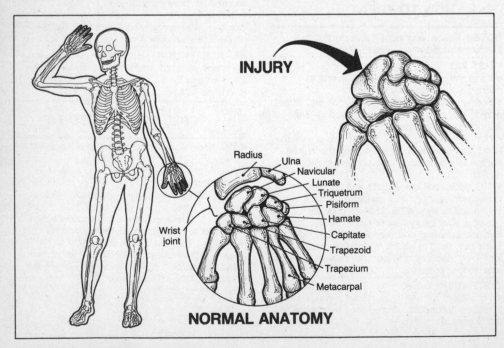

INJURY

Radius
Ulna
Navicular
Lunate
Triquetrum
Pisiform
Hamate
Capitate
Trapezoid
Trapezium
Metacarpal

Wrist joint

NORMAL ANATOMY

- Pressure on or injury to nearby nerves, ligaments, tendons, muscles, blood vessels or connective tissues.

After treatment or surgery:
- Delayed union or non-union of the fracture (frequently).
- Impaired blood supply to the fracture site.
- Arrest of normal bone growth in children.
- Infection in open fractures (skin broken over fracture site), or at the incision if surgical setting was necessary.
- Proneness to repeated hand injury.
- Unstable or arthritic joint following repeated injury.
- Prolonged healing time if activity is resumed too soon.
- Problems caused by casts. See Appendix 2 (Care of Casts).

PROBABLE OUTCOME—It is impossible to predict exactly how long it will take for any fracture to heal. Variable factors include age, sex, and previous state of health and conditioning. The average healing time for this fracture is 4 to 5 months (an unusually long time for a fracture to heal). Healing is considered complete when there is no motion at the fracture site and when X-rays show complete bone union. Sometimes this fracture never heals totally.

HOW TO TREAT

NOTE—Follow your doctor's instructions. These instructions are supplemental.

FIRST AID
- Keep the person warm with blankets to decrease the possibility of shock.
- Cut away clothing, if possible, but don't move the injured area to do so.
- Follow instructions for R.I.C.E., the first letters of *rest, ice, compression* and *elevation*. See Appendix 1 for details.
- Use a padded splint or sling to immobilize the hand and wrist before transporting the injured person to the doctor's office or emergency facility.
- The doctor will manipulate and set the broken bones with surgery or, if possible, without. A navicular fracture with separated bone fragments should be manipulated as soon as possible after injury. Six or more hours after the fracture, bleeding and displacement of body fluids may lead to shock. Also, many tissues lose their elasticity and become difficult to return to a normal position.

CONTINUING CARE
- Immobilization will be necessary. A rigid cast or plaster splints are placed around the injured area to immobilize the joint above and the joint below the fracture site.

- After 48 hours, localized heat promotes healing by increasing blood circulation in the injured area. Use a heat lamp or heating pad so heat can penetrate the cast.
- After the cast is removed, use frequent ice massage. Fill a large Styrofoam cup with water and freeze. Tear a small amount of foam from the top so ice protrudes. Massage firmly over the injured area in a circle about the size of a baseball. Do this for 15 minutes at a time, 3 or 4 times a day, and before workouts or competition.

MEDICATION—Your doctor may prescribe:
- General anesthesia, local anesthesia, or muscle relaxants to make bone manipulation possible.
- Narcotic or synthetic narcotic pain relievers for severe pain.
- Acetaminophen (available without prescription) for mild pain after initial treatment.

ACTIVITY
- Actively exercise all muscle groups not immobilized. Muscle contractions of the arm and hand promote fracture alignment and hasten healing.
- Begin reconditioning the hand after clearance from your doctor.
- Resume normal activities gradually after treatment. Don't drive until healing is complete.

DIET
- Drink only water before manipulation or surgery to treat the fracture. Solid food in your stomach makes vomiting while under anesthesia more hazardous.
- During recovery, eat a well-balanced diet that includes extra protein, such as meat, fish, poultry, cheese, milk and eggs.

REHABILITATION—Begin daily rehabilitation exercises when movement is comfortable. Use ice massage for 10 minutes prior to exercise. See page 474 for rehabilitation exercises.

CALL YOUR DOCTOR IF

- You have signs or symptoms of a hand fracture.
- Any of the following occurs after surgery or other treatment:
  Increased pain, swelling or drainage in the surgical area.
  Signs of infection (headache, muscle aches, dizziness, or a general ill feeling and fever).
  Swelling above or below the cast.
  Blue or gray skin color under the fingernails.
  Numbness or complete loss of feeling in the fingers of the affected hand.
  Nausea or vomiting.

HAND GANGLION
(Synovial Hernia; Synovial Cyst)

GENERAL INFORMATION

DEFINITION—A small, usually hard nodule lying directly over a tendon or a joint capsule on the back or palm of the hand. Occasionally the nodule may become quite large.

BODY PARTS INVOLVED
- Back or palm of the hand.
- Tendon sheath (a thin membranous covering to the tendon).
- Any of the joint spaces in the hand.

SIGNS & SYMPTOMS
- Hard lump over a tendon or joint capsule in the hand. The nodule "yields" to heavy pressure because it is not solid.
- No pain usually, but overuse of the hand may cause mild pain and aching.
- Tenderness if the lump is pressed hard.
- Discomfort with extremes of motion (flexing or extending) and with repetition of the exercise that produced the ganglion.

CAUSES
- Mild sprains and chronic sprains to a hand joint, causing weakness of the joint capsule.
- A defect in the fibrous sheath of the joint or tendon that permits a segment of underlying synovium (thin membrane that lines the tendon sheath) to herniate through it.

- Irritation accompanying the herniated synovium, causing continued secretion of fluid. The sac gradually fills, enlarges, and becomes hard, forming the ganglion.

RISK INCREASES WITH
- Repeated injury, especially mild sprains. Hand ganglions frequently occur in bowlers, tennis players, and handball, racquetball and squash players.
- Inadequate warmup prior to practice or competition.
- If surgery is necessary, surgical risk increases with smoking, poor nutrition, alcoholism, and recent or chronic illness.

HOW TO PREVENT
- Build your strength with a long-term conditioning program appropriate for your sport.
- Warm up before practice or competition.

WHAT TO EXPECT

APPROPRIATE HEALTH CARE
- Doctor's care for diagnosis and possible injections of local anesthetic or cortisone.
- Surgery (usually). Surgery will be conducted under local or general anesthesia in an outpatient surgical facility or hospital operating room.

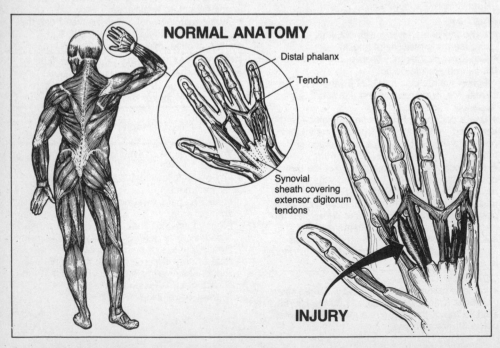

NORMAL ANATOMY

Distal phalanx

Tendon

Synovial sheath covering extensor digitorum tendons

INJURY

DIAGNOSTIC MEASURES
- Your own observation of signs and symptoms.
- Medical history and physical examination by a doctor.
- X-rays of the area.

POSSIBLE COMPLICATIONS
- After surgery:
  Excessive bleeding.
  Surgical-wound infection.
  Recurrence if surgical removal is incomplete.
- Calcification of ganglion (rare).

PROBABLE OUTCOME—Ganglions sometimes disappear spontaneously, only to recur later. Surgery is often the only treatment to guarantee cure. After surgery, allow about 3 weeks for recovery if no complications occur.

HOW TO TREAT

NOTE—Follow your doctor's instructions. These instructions are supplemental.

FIRST AID—None. This condition develops gradually.

CONTINUING CARE
Immediately after surgery:
- The affected area is usually immobilized in a splint for 1 to 2 weeks following surgery.
- If the wound bleeds during the first 24 hours after surgery, press a clean tissue or cloth to it for 10 minutes.
- A hard ridge should form along the incision. As it heals, the ridge will recede gradually.
- Use an electric heating pad, a heat lamp, or a warm compress to relieve incisional pain.
- Bathe and shower as usual. You may wash the incision gently with mild unscented soap.
- Between baths, keep the wound dry with a bandage for the first 2 or 3 days after surgery. If a bandage gets wet, change it promptly.
- Apply non-prescription antibiotic ointment to the wound before applying new bandages.
- Wrap the hand with an elasticized bandage until healing is complete.
After the incision has healed:
- Use ice soaks 3 or 4 times a day. Fill a bucket with ice water, and soak the injured area for 20 minutes at a time.

- You may apply heat instead of ice if it feels better. Use heat lamps, hot soaks, hot showers, heating pads, or heat liniments and ointments.
- Take whirlpool treatments, if available.

MEDICATION
- Your doctor may prescribe pain relievers. Don't take prescription pain medication longer than 4 to 7 days. Use only as much as you need.
- You may use non-prescription drugs, such as acetaminophen, for minor pain.

ACTIVITY
- Return to work and normal activity as soon as possible. This reduces postoperative depression and irritability, which are common.
- Avoid vigorous exercise for 3 weeks after surgery.
- Don't drive until healing is complete.

DIET—During recovery, eat a well-balanced diet that includes extra protein, such as meat, fish, poultry, cheese, milk and eggs. Increase fiber and fluid intake to prevent constipation that may result from decreased activity.

REHABILITATION
- Begin daily rehabilitation exercises when supportive wrapping is no longer needed.
- Use ice massage for 10 minutes before and after workouts. Fill a large Styrofoam cup with water and freeze. Tear a small amount of foam from the top so ice protrudes. Massage firmly over the injured area in a circle about the size of a softball.
- See pages 457 and 474 for rehabilitation exercises.

CALL YOUR DOCTOR IF

- You have signs or symptoms of a hand ganglion.
- Any of the following occur after surgery:
  Increased pain, swelling, redness, drainage or bleeding in the surgical area.
  Signs of infection (headache, muscle aches, dizziness, or a general ill feeling and fever).
  New, unexplained symptoms. Drugs used in treatment may produce side effects.

HAND HEMATOMA

GENERAL INFORMATION

DEFINITION—A collection of pooled blood in a small space on the back or palm of the hand.

BODY PARTS INVOLVED
- Back or palm of the hand.
- Soft tissue surrounding the hematoma, including nerves, tendons, ligaments, muscles and blood vessels.

SIGNS & SYMPTOMS
- Swelling over the injury site.
- Fluctuance (feeling of tenseness to the touch, like pushing on an overinflated balloon).
- Tenderness.
- Redness that progresses through several color changes—purple, green-yellow and yellow—before it completely heals.

CAUSES—Direct blow to the hand, usually with a blunt object. Bleeding into the tissue causes the surrounding tissue to be pushed away.

RISK INCREASES WITH
- Contact sports, especially if the hand is not adequately protected.
- Medical history of any bleeding disorder such as hemophilia.
- Poor nutrition, including vitamin deficiency.
- Use of anticoagulants or aspirin.

HOW TO PREVENT
- Protect the hand with padding if there is a risk of hand injury during participation in athletic activity.
- If you must compete before healing, use tape, padding, splints or a cast to prevent reinjury.

WHAT TO EXPECT

APPROPRIATE HEALTH CARE
- Doctor's care unless the hematoma is very small.
- Needle aspiration of blood from the hematoma if the hematoma is accessible. At the same time, hyaluronidase (an enzyme) can be injected into the hematoma space. Hyaluronidase hastens absorption of the blood.
- Self-care for minor hematomas, or during the rehabilitation phase following serious hematomas.
- Physical therapy for serious hematomas.

DIAGNOSTIC MEASURES
- Your own observation of symptoms.
- Physical exam and medical history by a doctor for all except minor injuries.
- X-rays of the injured area to assess the total injury and to rule out underlying bone fractures. Total extent of the injury may not be apparent for 48 to 72 hours.

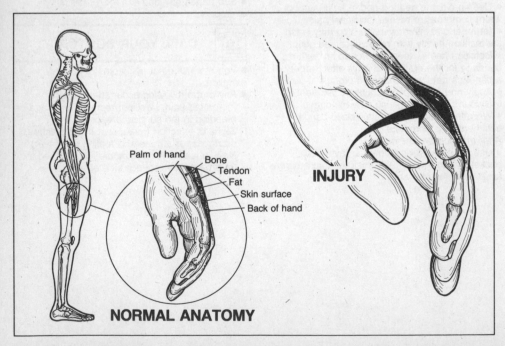

Palm of hand — Bone — Tendon — Fat — Skin surface — Back of hand

INJURY

NORMAL ANATOMY

POSSIBLE COMPLICATIONS

- Infection introduced through a break in the skin at the time of injury, or during aspiration of the hematoma by a doctor.
- Prolonged healing time if activity is resumed too soon.
- Calcification of the blood remaining in the hematoma, if blood has not been completely removed or absorbed.

PROBABLE OUTCOME—Average healing time is 2 weeks to 2 months unless blood is removed with aspiration. Healing time is much less with this treatment.

 HOW TO TREAT

NOTE—Follow your doctor's instructions. These instructions are supplemental.

FIRST AID—Use instructions for R.I.C.E., the first letters of *rest, ice, compression* and *elevation.* See Appendix 1 for details.

CONTINUING CARE

- Use ice soaks 3 or 4 times a day. Fill a bucket with ice water, and soak the injured area for 20 minutes at a time.
- After 48 hours, localized heat promotes healing by increasing blood circulation in the injured area. Use hot baths, showers, compresses, heat lamps, heating pads, heat ointments and liniments, or whirlpools.
- Don't massage the hand. You may trigger bleeding again.

MEDICATION

- For minor discomfort, you may use:
  Non-prescription medicines such as acetaminophen or ibuprofen.
  Topical liniments and ointments.

- Your doctor may prescribe stronger medicine for pain, if needed.

ACTIVITY—Begin activities slowly and stop exercise as soon as pain begins. Increase activity as healing progresses. To prevent delayed healing, protect the hematoma area against excessive motion soon after injury. Motion breaks down the clot and causes irritation throughout the hand, leading to possible scar formation, calcification and limited movement after healing.

DIET—During recovery, eat a well-balanced diet that includes extra protein, such as meat, fish, poultry, cheese, milk and eggs.

REHABILITATION

- Begin daily rehabilitation exercises when supportive wrapping is no longer needed.
- Use a gentle ice massage for 10 minutes before and after workouts. Fill a large Styrofoam cup with water and freeze. Tear a small amount of foam from the top so ice protrudes. Massage firmly over the injured area in a circle about the size of a softball.
- See pages 457 and 474 for rehabilitation exercises.

 CALL YOUR DOCTOR IF

- You have signs or symptoms of a hand hematoma that doesn't begin to improve in 1 or 2 days.
- Skin is broken and signs of infection (drainage, increasing pain, fever, headache, muscle aches, dizziness or a general ill feeling) occur.

HAND SPRAIN

GENERAL INFORMATION

DEFINITION—Violent overstretching of one or more ligaments in the hand. Sprains involving two or more ligaments cause considerably more disability than single-ligament sprains. When the ligament is overstretched, it becomes tense and gives way at its weakest point, either where it attaches to bone or within the ligament itself. If the ligament pulls loose a fragment of bone, it is called a *sprain-fracture*. There are 3 types of sprains:
- Mild (Grade I)—Tearing of some ligament fibers. There is no loss of function.
- Moderate (Grade II)—Rupture of a portion of the ligament, resulting in some loss of function.
- Severe (Grade III)—Complete rupture of the ligament or complete separation of ligament from bone. There is total loss of function. A severe sprain requires surgical repair.

BODY PARTS INVOLVED
- Ligaments connecting joints in the hand.
- Tissue surrounding the sprain, including blood vessels, tendons, bone, periosteum (covering of bone) and muscles.

SIGNS & SYMPTOMS
- Severe pain at the time of injury.
- A feeling of popping or tearing inside the hand.
- Tenderness at the injury site.
- Swelling in the hand.
- Bruising that appears soon after injury.

CAUSES—Stress on a ligament that temporarily forces or pries joints in the hand out of their normal location. Hand sprains occur frequently in contact sports or sports in which falling on an outstretched hand is likely.

RISK INCREASES WITH
- Contact sports, especially boxing.
- Gymnastics.
- Previous hand injury.
- Obesity.
- Poor muscle conditioning.
- Inadequate protection from equipment.

HOW TO PREVENT
- Build your strength with a conditioning program appropriate for your sport.
- Warm up before practice or competition.
- Tape vulnerable joints before practice or competition.

WHAT TO EXPECT

APPROPRIATE HEALTH CARE
- Doctor's diagnosis.
- Application of a cast, tape or elastic bandage.
- Self-care during rehabilitation.
- Physical therapy (moderate or severe sprain).
- Surgery (severe sprain).

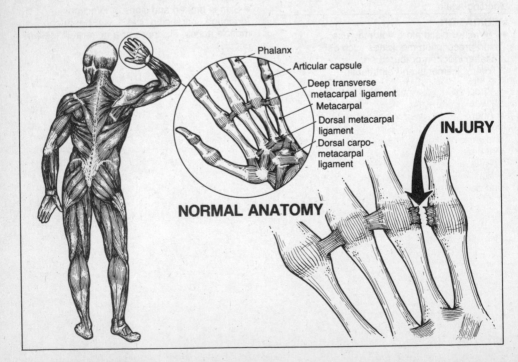

Phalanx
Articular capsule
Deep transverse metacarpal ligament
Metacarpal
Dorsal metacarpal ligament
Dorsal carpo-metacarpal ligament

NORMAL ANATOMY

INJURY

DIAGNOSTIC MEASURES
- Your own observation of symptoms.
- Medical history and exam by a doctor.
- X-rays of the hand and wrist to rule out fractures.

POSSIBLE COMPLICATIONS
- Prolonged healing time if usual activities are resumed too soon.
- Proneness to repeated injury.
- Inflammation at the ligament attachment to bone (periostitis).
- Prolonged disability (sometimes).
- Unstable or arthritic hand joints following repeated injury.

PROBABLE OUTCOME—If this is a first-time injury, proper care and sufficient healing time before resuming activity should prevent permanent disability. Ligaments have a poor blood supply, and torn ligaments require as much healing time as fractures. Average healing times are:
- Mild sprains—2 to 6 weeks.
- Moderate sprains—6 to 8 weeks.
- Severe sprains—8 to 10 weeks.

 ## HOW TO TREAT

NOTE—Follow your doctor's instructions. These instructions are supplemental.

FIRST AID—Use instructions for R.I.C.E., the first letters of *rest, ice, compression* and *elevation*. See Appendix 1 for details.

CONTINUING CARE—If the doctor does not apply a cast, tape or elastic bandage:
- Continue using an ice pack 3 or 4 times a day. Place ice chips or cubes in a plastic bag. Wrap the bag in a moist towel, and place it over the injured area. Use for 20 minutes at a time.
- Wrap the hand with an elasticized bandage between ice treatments.
- After 72 hours, apply heat instead of ice, if it feels better. Use heat lamps, hot soaks, hot showers, heating pads, or heat liniments or ointments.
- Take whirlpool treatments, if available.
- Massage gently and often to provide comfort and decrease swelling.

MEDICATION
- For minor discomfort, you may use:
  Aspirin, acetaminophen or ibuprofen.
  Topical liniments and ointments.
- Your doctor may prescribe:
  Stronger pain relievers.
  Injection of a long-acting local anesthetic to reduce pain.
  Injection of a corticosteroid, such as triamcinolone, to reduce inflammation.

ACTIVITY—Resume your normal activities gradually after clearance from your doctor.

DIET—During recovery, eat a well-balanced diet that includes extra protein, such as meat, fish, poultry, cheese, milk and eggs.

REHABILITATION
- Begin daily rehabilitation exercises when the cast or supportive wrapping is no longer necessary.
- Use ice massage for 10 minutes before and after exercise. Fill a large Styrofoam cup with water and freeze. Tear a small amount of foam from the top so ice protrudes. Massage firmly over the injured area.
- See pages 457 and 474 for rehabilitation exercises.

 ## CALL YOUR DOCTOR IF

- You have symptoms of a moderate or severe hand sprain, or a mild sprain persists longer than 2 weeks.
- Pain, swelling or bruising worsens despite treatment.
- Any of the following occur after casting or splinting:
  Pain, numbness or coldness in the hand.
  Blue, gray or dusky fingernails.
- Any of the following occur after surgery:
  Increased pain, swelling, redness, drainage or bleeding in the surgical area.
  Signs of infection (headache, muscle aches, dizziness, or a general ill feeling with fever).
- New, unexplained symptoms develop. Drugs used in treatment may produce side effects.

HAND STRAIN

GENERAL INFORMATION

DEFINITION—Injury to the muscles or tendons in the hand. Muscles, tendons and bones comprise units. The complex motions of the hand require many complex muscle-tendon units, so hand strains occur frequently. Strains are of 3 types:
● Mild (Grade I)—Slightly pulled muscle without tearing of muscle or tendon fibers. There is no loss of strength.
● Moderate (Grade II)—Tearing of fibers in a muscle, tendon or at the attachment to bone. Strength is diminished.
● Severe (Grade III)—Rupture of the muscle-tendon-bone attachment with separation of fibers. Severe strain requires surgical repair. Chronic strains are caused by overuse. Acute strains are caused by direct injury or overstress.

BODY PARTS INVOLVED
● Tendons and muscles of the hand.
● Bones of the hand where they attach to muscles and tendons.
● Soft tissue surrounding the strain, including nerves, periosteum (covering to bone), blood vessels and lymph vessels.

SIGNS & SYMPTOMS
● Cramping and fatigue of hand muscles.
● Pain with motion or stretching.

● Muscle spasm.
● Swelling.
● Loss of strength (moderate or severe strain).
● Crepitation ("crackling") feeling and sound when the injured area is pressed with fingers.
● Calcification of the muscle or tendon (visible with X-rays).
● Inflammation of the tendon sheath.

CAUSES
● Prolonged overuse of muscle-tendon units in the forearm, wrist or hand.
● Single violent injury or force applied to the forearm, wrist or hand.

RISK INCREASES WITH
● Contact sports such as wrestling.
● Sports that require constant gripping, such as rowing, tennis, golf or gymnastics.
● Any cardiovascular medical problem that results in decreased circulation.
● Medical history of any bleeding disorder.
● Poor nutrition.
● Previous hand injury.
● Poor muscle conditioning.

HOW TO PREVENT
● Participate in a strengthening and conditioning program appropriate for your sport.
● Warm up before practice or competition.
● Protect the hands with taping and appropriate protective gear during contact sports participation.

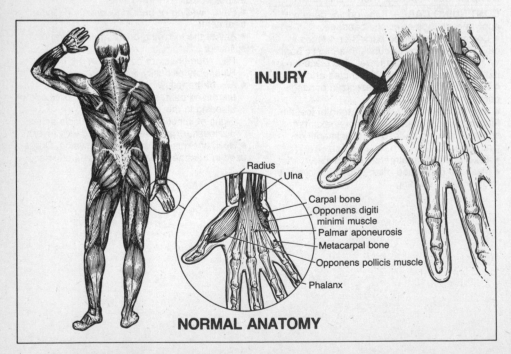

INJURY

Radius
Ulna
Carpal bone
Opponens digiti minimi muscle
Palmar aponeurosis
Metacarpal bone
Opponens pollicis muscle
Phalanx

NORMAL ANATOMY

WHAT TO EXPECT

APPROPRIATE HEALTH CARE
- Doctor's diagnosis.
- Self-care during rehabilitation.
- Physical therapy (moderate or severe strain).
- Surgery (severe strain).

DIAGNOSTIC MEASURES
- Your own observation of symptoms.
- Medical history and exam by a doctor.
- X-rays of the wrist, forearm and hand to rule out fractures.

POSSIBLE COMPLICATIONS
- Prolonged healing time if activity is resumed too soon.
- Proneness to repeated injury.
- Unstable or arthritic hand joints following repeated injury.
- Inflammation at the attachment to bone (periostitis).
- Prolonged disability (sometimes).

PROBABLE OUTCOME—If this is a first-time injury, proper care and sufficient healing time before resuming activity should prevent permanent disability. Torn ligaments and tendons require as long to heal as fractured bones. Average healing times are:
- Mild strain—2 to 10 days.
- Moderate strain—10 days to 6 weeks.
- Severe strain—6 to 10 weeks.

If this is a repeat injury, complications listed above are more likely to occur.

 HOW TO TREAT

NOTE—Follow your doctor's instructions. These instructions are supplemental.

FIRST AID—Follow instructions for R.I.C.E., the first letters of *rest, ice, compression* and *elevation.* See Appendix 1 for details.

CONTINUING CARE
- Use ice massage 3 or 4 times a day for 15 minutes at a time. Fill a large Styrofoam cup with water and freeze. Tear a small amount of foam from the top so ice protrudes. Massage firmly over the injured area in a circle about the size of a softball.
- After the first 24 hours, apply heat instead of ice, if it feels better. Use heat lamps, hot soaks, hot showers, heating pads, or heat liniments and ointments.
- Take whirlpool treatments, if available.
- Wrap the injured wrist and hand with an elasticized bandage between treatments.
- Massage gently and often to provide comfort and decrease swelling.

MEDICATION
- For minor discomfort, you may use:
  Aspirin, acetaminophen or ibuprofen.
  Topical liniments and ointments.
- Your doctor may prescribe:
  Stronger pain relievers.
  Injection of a long-acting local anesthetic to reduce pain (rare).
  Injections of corticosteroids, such as triamcinolone, to reduce inflammation (rare).

ACTIVITY
- For a moderate or severe strain, use a sling or splints for at least 72 hours.
- Resume your normal activities gradually.

DIET—Eat a well-balanced diet that includes extra protein, such as meat, fish, poultry, cheese, milk and eggs. Increase fiber and fluid intake to prevent constipation that may result from decreased activity.

REHABILITATION—Begin daily rehabilitation exercises when supportive wrapping is no longer needed. Use ice massage for 10 minutes prior to exercise. See page 474 for rehabilitation exercises.

 CALL YOUR DOCTOR IF

- You have symptoms of a moderate or severe hand strain, or a mild strain persists longer than 10 days.
- Pain or swelling worsens despite treatment.

HAND TENDINITIS & TENOSYNOVITIS

 GENERAL INFORMATION

DEFINITION—Inflammation of a tendon (tendinitis) or the lining of a tendon sheath (tenosynovitis) in the hand. This lining secretes a fluid that lubricates the tendon. When the lining becomes inflamed, the tendon cannot glide smoothly in its covering.

BODY PARTS INVOLVED
- Tendons in the hand.
- Lining and covering of the hand tendons.
- Soft tissue in the surrounding area, including blood vessels, nerves, ligaments, periosteum (covering to bone) and connective tissue.

SIGNS & SYMPTOMS
- Constant pain or pain with motion of the hand.
- Limited motion of the hand and wrist.
- Crepitation (a "crackling" sound when the tendon moves or is touched).
- Redness and tenderness over the injured tendon.

CAUSES
- Strain from unusual use or overuse of the wrist, hand or forearm.
- Direct blow or injury to the muscles and tendons of the wrist, hand or forearm. Tenosynovitis becomes more likely with repeated injury.
- Infection introduced through broken skin at the time of injury or through a surgical incision after injury.

RISK INCREASES WITH
- "Throwing" sports.
- Contact sports.
- If surgery is needed, surgical risk increases with smoking, poor nutrition, alcoholism or drug abuse, and recent or chronic illness.

HOW TO PREVENT
- Engage in a vigorous program of physical conditioning before beginning regular sports participation.
- Warm up adequately before practice or competition.
- Wear protective gear appropriate for your sport.
- Learn proper moves and techniques for your sport.

 WHAT TO EXPECT

APPROPRIATE HEALTH CARE
- Doctor's examination and diagnosis.
- Surgery (sometimes) to enlarge the tunnel of the tendon covering and restore a smooth gliding motion. The surgical procedure under general anesthesia is performed in an outpatient surgical facility or hospital operating room.

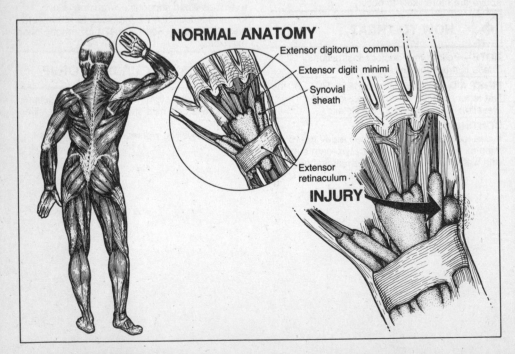

NORMAL ANATOMY

Extensor digitorum common

Extensor digiti minimi

Synovial sheath

Extensor retinaculum

INJURY

DIAGNOSTIC MEASURES
- Your own observations of symptoms and signs.
- Medical history and physical examination by your doctor.
- X-rays of the area to rule out other abnormalities.
- Laboratory studies:
  Blood and urine studies before surgery.
  Tissue examination after surgery.

POSSIBLE COMPLICATIONS
- Prolonged healing time if activity is resumed too soon.
- Proneness to repeated injury.
- Adhesive tenosynovitis: The tendon and its covering become bound together. Loss of motion may be complete or partial. Surgery is necessary to remove the covering or transfer the tendon to a new area.
- Constrictive tenosynovitis: The walls of the covering thicken and narrow the opening, preventing the tendon from sliding through. Surgery is necessary to cut away part of the covering.

PROBABLE OUTCOME—Tenosynovitis is usually curable in about 6 weeks with heat treatments, corticosteroid injections and rest of the inflamed area. Recovery is usually quicker if the inflammation is caused by a direct blow rather than by a strain or sprain.

 ## HOW TO TREAT

NOTE—Follow your doctor's instructions. These instructions are supplemental.

FIRST AID—None. This problem develops slowly.

CONTINUING CARE
- Wrap the hand and wrist with an elasticized bandage until healing is complete.
- Apply heat frequently. Use heat lamps, hot soaks, hot showers, heating pads, or heat liniments and ointments.
- Take whirlpool treatments, if available.

MEDICATION—You may use non-prescription drugs, such as acetaminophen, for minor pain. Your doctor may prescribe:
- Stronger pain relievers. Don't take prescription pain medication longer than 4 to 7 days. Use only as much as you need.
- Injection of the tendon covering with a combination of a long-acting local anesthetic and a non-absorbable corticosteroid such as triamcinolone.

ACTIVITY—Resume normal activities gradually.

DIET—During recovery, eat a well-balanced diet that includes extra protein, such as meat, fish, poultry, cheese, milk and eggs. Your doctor may suggest vitamin and mineral supplements to promote healing.

REHABILITATION
- Begin daily rehabilitation exercises after pain disappears when supportive wrapping is no longer needed.
- Use ice massage for 10 minutes before and after exercise. Fill a large Styrofoam cup with water and freeze. Tear a small amount of foam from the top so ice protrudes. Massage firmly over the injured area in a circle about the size of a baseball.
- See page 474 for rehabilitation exercises.

 ## CALL YOUR DOCTOR IF
- You have symptoms of hand tenosynovitis.
- Any of the following occur after surgery:
  Increased pain, swelling, redness, drainage or bleeding in the surgical area.
  Signs of infection (headache, muscle aches, dizziness, or a general ill feeling and fever).
  New, unexplained symptoms. Drugs used in treatment may produce side effects.

HEAD INJURY, CEREBRAL CONCUSSION

GENERAL INFORMATION

DEFINITION—A violent jar or shock to the brain that causes an immediate change in brain function, including possible loss of consciousness.

BODY PARTS INVOLVED
- Head.
- Skull.
- Brain.

SIGNS & SYMPTOMS
Mild concussion:
- Temporary loss of consciousness.
- Memory loss (amnesia).
- Emotional instability.

Severe concussion:
- Prolonged unconsciousness.
- Dilated pupils.
- Change in breathing.
- Disturbed vision.
- Disturbed equilibrium.
- Memory loss.

CAUSES—Blow to the head.

RISK INCREASES WITH
- Contact sports.
- Auto, motorcycle or bike racing.

HOW TO PREVENT—Wear a protective helmet for any activity at risk for a head injury.

WHAT TO EXPECT

APPROPRIATE HEALTH CARE
- Doctor's diagnosis and care.
- Hospitalization for a serious brain concussion.
- Home care if the initial evaluation doesn't dictate hospitalization.

DIAGNOSTIC MEASURES
- Your own observation of symptoms.
- Physical exam and medical history by a doctor. The total extent of injury may not be apparent for 48 to 72 hours.
- X-rays of the head and neck to assess total injury to soft tissue and to rule out the possibility of a skull fracture.
- CAT scan (see Glossary) of the head.
- Laboratory studies of blood and cerebrospinal fluid.

POSSIBLE COMPLICATIONS
- Permanent brain damage, depending on the extent of injury. Repeated concussions can cause slurred speech, slow movement, slow thought processes and tremor.
- Excessive cerebral bleeding, causing a clot that puts pressure on the brain.
- Prolonged healing time if usual activities are resumed too soon.
- Infection if skin over the concussion site is broken.

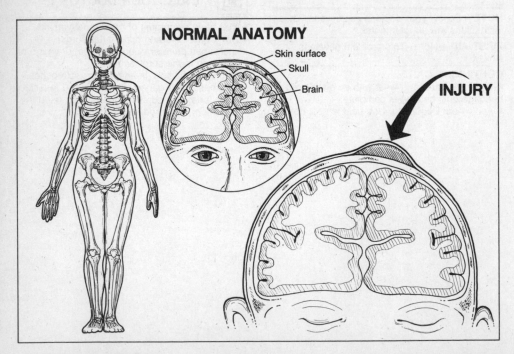

NORMAL ANATOMY

Skin surface
Skull
Brain

INJURY

PROBABLE OUTCOME—Complete recovery is likely with early diagnosis and treatment. Complications can be life-threatening or cause permanent brain damage.

 HOW TO TREAT

NOTE—Follow your doctor's instructions. These instructions are supplemental.

FIRST AID
• Ice helps stop bleeding from any scalp wound. Prepare an ice pack of ice cubes or chips wrapped in plastic or in a container. Place a towel over the injured area to prevent skin damage. Apply ice for 20 minutes, then rest 10 minutes. Repeat applications for 24 to 48 hours after injury.
• Elevate the head above the level of the heart to reduce swelling and prevent accumulation of fluid.

CONTINUING CARE—The extent of injury can be determined only with careful examination and observation. After a doctor's examination, the injured person may be sent home, but a responsible person must stay with the person and watch for serious symptoms. The first 24 hours after injury are critical, although serious aftereffects can appear later. If you are watching the patient, awaken him or her every hour for 24 hours. Report to the doctor immediately if you can't awaken or arouse the person. Report also any of the following:
• Vomiting.
• Inability to move the arms and legs equally well on both sides.
• Temperature above 100F (37.8C).
• Stiff neck.
• Pupils of unequal size or shape.
• Convulsions.
• Noticeable restlessness.
• Severe headache that persists longer than 4 hours after injury.
• Confusion.

MEDICATION—Don't use any medicine—including non-prescription acetaminophen or aspirin—until the extent of injury is certain.

ACTIVITY—Rest in bed until the doctor determines the danger of brain injury is over. Normal activity may then be resumed as symptoms improve.

DIET—Follow a full liquid diet until the danger passes.

REHABILITATION—Depends on the possibility of brain damage. Consult your doctor.

 CALL YOUR DOCTOR IF

You have had a head injury and develop symptoms of a concussion, or you observe the signs and symptoms in someone else.

HEAD INJURY, CEREBRAL CONTUSION

GENERAL INFORMATION

DEFINITION—Bruising of the brain following a blow. Contusions cause bleeding from ruptured small capillaries that allow blood to infiltrate brain tissue.

BODY PARTS INVOLVED
● Brain.
● Skin, subcutaneous tissue, blood vessels (both large vessels and capillaries), periosteum (the outside lining of the skull), muscles of the scalp and connective tissue.

SIGNS & SYMPTOMS—Depends on the extent
of injury. The presence or absence of swelling at the injury site is not related to the seriousness of injury. Signs and symptoms include any or all of the following:
● Drowsiness or confusion.
● Vomiting and nausea.
● Blurred vision.
● Pupils of different size.
● Loss of consciousness—either temporarily or for long periods.
● Amnesia or memory lapses.
● Irritability.
● Headache.
● Bleeding of the scalp, if the skin is broken.

CAUSES—Direct blow to the head, usually from a blunt object.

RISK INCREASES WITH
● Contact sports such as boxing, football or wrestling.
● Auto, motorcycle or bike racing.

HOW TO PREVENT—Wear a protective helmet for any activity at risk for a head injury.

WHAT TO EXPECT

APPROPRIATE HEALTH CARE
● Doctor's diagnosis and care.
● Hospitalization for a serious brain contusion.
● Home care if the initial evaluation doesn't dictate hospitalization.

DIAGNOSTIC MEASURES
● Your own observation of symptoms.
● Physical exam and medical history by a doctor. The total extent of injury may not be apparent for 48 to 72 hours.
● X-rays of the head and neck to assess total injury to soft tissue and to rule out the possibility of a skull fracture.
● CAT scan (see Glossary) of the head.
● Laboratory studies of blood and cerebrospinal fluid.

POSSIBLE COMPLICATIONS
● Permanent brain damage, depending on the extent of injury.
● Excessive cerebral bleeding, causing a clot that puts pressure on the brain.

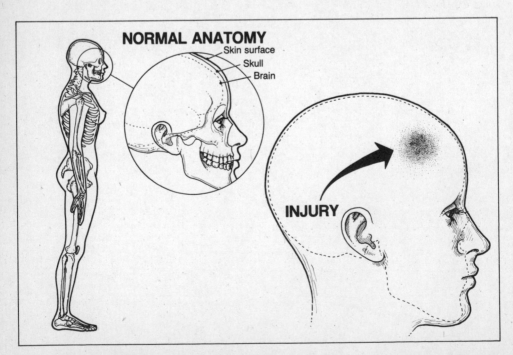

NORMAL ANATOMY
Skin surface
Skull
Brain

INJURY

- Prolonged healing time if vigorous activities are resumed too soon.
- Infection if skin over the contusion site is broken.

PROBABLE OUTCOME—Complete recovery is likely with early diagnosis and treatment. Complications can be life-threatening or cause permanent brain damage.

 # HOW TO TREAT

NOTE—Follow your doctor's instructions. These instructions are supplemental.

FIRST AID
- Ice helps stop internal bleeding. Prepare an ice pack of ice cubes or chips wrapped in plastic or in a container. Place a towel over the injured area to prevent skin damage. Apply ice for 20 minutes, then rest 10 minutes. Repeat applications for 24 to 48 hours after injury.
- Elevate the head above the level of the heart to reduce swelling and prevent accumulation of fluid.

CONTINUING CARE—The extent of injury can be determined only with careful examination and observation. After a doctor's examination, the injured person may be sent home, but a responsible person must stay with the person and watch for serious symptoms. The first 24 hours after injury are critical, although serious aftereffects can appear later. If you are watching the patient, awaken him or her every hour for 24 hours. Report to the doctor immediately if you can't awaken or arouse the person. Report also any of the following:
- Vomiting.
- Inability to move the arms and legs equally well on both sides.
- Temperature above 100F (37.8C).
- Stiff neck.
- Pupils of unequal size or shape.
- Convulsions.
- Noticeable restlessness.
- Severe headache that persists longer than 4 hours after injury.
- Confusion.

MEDICATION—Don't use any medicine—including non-prescription acetaminophen or aspirin—until the extent of injury is certain.

ACTIVITY—Bed rest is necessary until the doctor determines the danger of brain injury is over. Normal activity may then be resumed as symptoms improve.

DIET—A full liquid diet should be followed until the danger passes.

REHABILITATION—Rehabilitation exercises must be individualized. Follow your doctor's or surgeon's directions.

 # CALL YOUR DOCTOR IF

You have had a head injury and develop symptoms of a contusion, or you observe the signs and symptoms in someone else.

HEAD INJURY, EXTRADURAL HEMORRHAGE & HEMATOMA
(Epidural Hemorrhage & Hematoma)

 GENERAL INFORMATION

DEFINITION—Bleeding (hemorrhage) between the skull and the outermost of 3 membranes (meninges) that cover the brain, resulting in a pooling of blood (hematoma) that causes pressure on the brain.

BODY PARTS INVOLVED
- Brain.
- Skull.
- Blood vessels to the brain.
- Meninges.

SIGNS & SYMPTOMS—The following symptoms usually develop within 1 to 96 hours after a head injury:
- Unconsciousness for a short period of time followed by a headache that steadily worsens.
- Drowsiness or unconsciousness.
- Nausea or vomiting.
- Inability to move the arms and legs.
- Change in the size of the eye pupils.

CAUSES—Head injury with skull fracture that tears the middle meningeal artery.

RISK INCREASES WITH
- Contact sports such as boxing, football or hockey.
- Auto, motorcycle or bike racing.
- During surgery, surgical risk increases with smoking and use of drugs, including anticoagulants, muscle relaxants, tranquilizers, sleep inducers, insulin, sedatives, beta-adrenergic blockers, corticosteroids or mind-altering drugs.

HOW TO PREVENT—Wear a protective helmet for any activity at risk for a head injury.

 WHAT TO EXPECT

APPROPRIATE HEALTH CARE
- Doctor's diagnosis.
- Surgery to remove the clot causing pressure on the brain.
- Physical therapy for rehabilitation if there is any residual paralysis or other disability.

DIAGNOSTIC MEASURES
- Your own observation of symptoms.
- Medical history and physical exam by a doctor.
- Laboratory studies of blood and cerebrospinal fluid.
- Hospital diagnostic tests such as X-rays, arteriography, radioactive uptake studies and CAT scan (see Glossary for all).

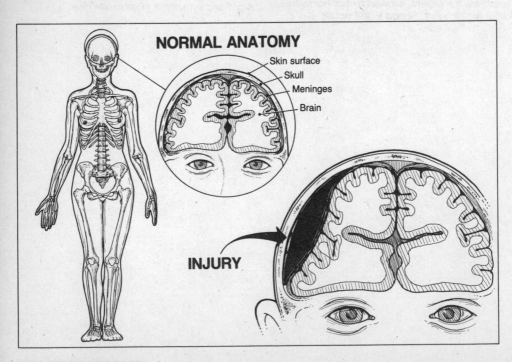

NORMAL ANATOMY

Skin surface
Skull
Meninges
Brain

INJURY

POSSIBLE COMPLICATIONS
• Death or permanent brain damage, including partial or complete paralysis, behavioral and personality changes, and speech problems.
• Convulsions following surgery.

PROBABLE OUTCOME—The degree of recovery depends upon general health, age, severity of the injury, rapidity of the treatment and extensiveness of the bleeding or clot. After the clot is removed, brain tissue that has been compressed usually expands slowly to fill its original space. If speech or muscle control has been damaged, physical therapy or speech therapy may be necessary. The outlook for complete recovery is good with quick diagnosis and prompt surgery.

 ## HOW TO TREAT

NOTE—Follow your doctor's instructions. These instructions are supplemental.

FIRST AID—After any head injury:
• If the victim is wearing headgear with a face guard, cut the face guard off but *don't remove the headgear or move the head or neck for any reason.* Brain injury is frequently associated with neck injury.
• If the victim vomits, support the head and neck completely and carefully while rotating the entire body to the side to prevent aspiration.
• Splint the head and neck and transport the person to the nearest well-equipped emergency facility.
• Elevate the head of the stretcher slightly. Do not use pillows.
• Watch closely for vomiting, convulsions, changes in consciousness, paralysis or impaired breathing. Be ready to render CPR if needed.

CONTINUING CARE—Surgery is the only treatment for an extradural hemorrhage and hematoma. Under local or light general anesthesia, small holes are bored through the skull. The blood clot (which looks like currant jelly) is removed manually or by suction. After surgery, symptoms usually improve rapidly.

MEDICATION—Your doctor may prescribe:
• Corticosteroid drugs to reduce swelling inside the skull.
• Anticonvulsant medication.
• Antibiotics to fight infection.

ACTIVITY—After surgery, stay as active as your strength allows. Work and exercise moderately, and rest often. Once you have had an extradural hemorrhage, don't participate in contact sports.

DIET—During recovery, eat a well-balanced diet that includes extra protein, such as meat, fish, poultry, cheese, milk and eggs. Increase fiber and fluid intake to prevent constipation that may result from decreased activity.

REHABILITATION—Consult your doctor or a physical therapist.

 ## CALL YOUR DOCTOR IF

• You observe signs of an extradural hemorrhage in someone following a head injury. Call immediately. This is an emergency!
• The following occurs after surgery:
Temperature rises to 101F (38.3C) or higher.
Surgical wound becomes red, swollen or tender.
Headache worsens.

HEAD INJURY, INTRACEREBRAL HEMATOMA

GENERAL INFORMATION

DEFINITION—Bleeding (hemorrhage) that causes blood to collect and partially clot (hematoma) inside the brain. The use of CAT scans has shown that this condition occurs more frequently than physicians previously thought.

BODY PARTS INVOLVED
- Brain.
- Blood vessels to the brain.

SIGNS & SYMPTOMS—The following symptoms develop within 1 to 96 hours (occasionally longer) after a head injury:
- Unconsciousness for a short period of time followed by a headache that steadily worsens.
- Drowsiness or unconsciousness.
- Nausea or vomiting.
- Inability to move the arms and legs.
- Change in the size of the eye pupils.

CAUSES—Severe blow to the head.

RISK INCREASES WITH
- Contact sports such as boxing, football or hockey.
- Auto, motorcycle or bike racing.
- During surgery, surgical risk increases with smoking and use of drugs, including anticoagulants, muscle relaxants, tranquilizers, sleep inducers, insulin, sedatives, beta-adrenergic blockers, corticosteroids or mind-altering drugs.

HOW TO PREVENT—Wear a protective helmet for any activity at risk for a head injury.

WHAT TO EXPECT

APPROPRIATE HEALTH CARE
- Doctor's diagnosis.
- Surgery to remove the clot causing pressure on the brain.
- Physical therapy for rehabilitation if there is any residual paralysis or other disability.

DIAGNOSTIC MEASURES
- Your own observation of symptoms.
- Medical history and physical exam by a doctor.
- Laboratory studies of blood and cerebrospinal fluid.
- Hospital diagnostic tests such as X-rays, arteriography, radioactive uptake studies and CAT scan (see Glossary for all).

POSSIBLE COMPLICATIONS
- Death or permanent brain damage, including partial or complete paralysis, behavioral and personality changes and speech problems.
- Convulsions following surgery.

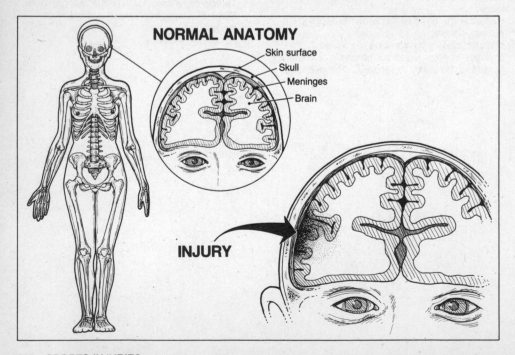

NORMAL ANATOMY

Skin surface
Skull
Meninges
Brain

INJURY

PROBABLE OUTCOME—The degree of recovery depends upon general health, age, severity of the injury, rapidity of the treatment and extensiveness of the bleeding or clot. After the clot is removed, brain tissue that has been compressed usually expands slowly to fill its original space. If speech or muscle control has been damaged, physical therapy or speech therapy may be necessary. The outlook for complete recovery is good with quick diagnosis and prompt surgery.

 ## HOW TO TREAT

NOTE—Follow your doctor's instructions. These instructions are supplemental.

FIRST AID—After any head injury:
● If the victim is wearing headgear with a face guard, cut the face guard off but *don't remove the headgear or move the head or neck for any reason.* Brain injury is frequently associated with neck injury.
● If the victim vomits, support the head and neck completely and carefully while rotating the entire body to the side to prevent aspiration.
● Splint the head and neck and transport the person to the nearest well-equipped emergency facility.
● Elevate the head of the stretcher slightly. Do not use pillows.
● Watch closely for vomiting, convulsions, changes in consciousness, paralysis or impaired breathing. Be ready to render CPR if needed.

CONTINUING CARE—Surgery is the only treatment for an intracerebral hemorrhage and hematoma. Under local or light general anesthesia, small holes are bored through the skull. The blood clot (which looks like currant jelly) is removed manually or by suction. After surgery, symptoms usually improve rapidly.

MEDICATION—Your doctor may prescribe:
● Corticosteroid drugs to reduce swelling inside the skull.
● Anticonvulsant medication.
● Antibiotics to fight infection.

ACTIVITY—After surgery, stay as active as your strength allows. Work and exercise moderately, and rest often. Once you have had an intracerebral hemorrhage, don't participate in contact sports.

DIET—During recovery, eat a well-balanced diet that includes extra protein, such as meat, fish, poultry, cheese, milk and eggs. Increase fiber and fluid intake to prevent constipation that may result from decreased activity.

REHABILITATION—Consult your doctor or a physical therapist.

 ## CALL YOUR DOCTOR IF

● You observe signs of an intracerebral hemorrhage in someone following a head injury. Call immediately. This is an emergency!
● The following occurs after surgery:
   Temperature rises to 101F (38.3C) or higher.
   Surgical wound becomes red, swollen or tender.
   Headache worsens.

HEAD INJURY, SKULL FRACTURE

GENERAL INFORMATION

DEFINITION—Skull fractures may be of two types:
- A closed, or simple, break in the bone without breaking the skin or bone covering (periosteum).
- An open, or compound, break that breaks the skin and periosteum.

BODY PARTS INVOLVED
- Skull.
- Periosteum (fibrous covering of bone).
- Soft tissue adjacent to the skull, including skin and underlying tissue, muscles, nerves and tendons.
- Brain (sometimes), if bone fragments are depressed into the brain.

SIGNS & SYMPTOMS
- Pain and swelling over the skull fracture.
- Bruising over the fracture and around the eyes and nose.
- Profuse bleeding from the scalp if the skin is broken.
- Leakage of clear fluid (cerebrospinal fluid) into the ear or nose.

Additional signs, if brain damage accompanies the skull fracture:
- Drowsiness or confusion.
- Vomiting and nausea.
- Blurred vision.

- Loss of consciousness—either temporarily or for long periods.
- Amnesia or memory lapses.
- Irritability.
- Headache.

CAUSES—Direct blow to the head.

RISK INCREASES WITH
- Contact sports, especially if the head is not protected adequately.
- Sports that involve heavy equipment such as baseball bats or golf clubs.
- Sports such as basketball, gymnastics, diving or cycling, in which falling on the head is possible.
- Poor nutrition, especially calcium deficiency.

HOW TO PREVENT—Wear a protective helmet or other appropriate headgear during athletic activity in which head injury is possible.

WHAT TO EXPECT

APPROPRIATE HEALTH CARE
- Doctor's diagnosis and care.
- Hospitalization (serious skull fractures).
- Home care if hospitalization is not necessary.

DIAGNOSTIC MEASURES
- Your own observation of symptoms.
- Medical history and physical exam by a doctor. Total extent of the injury may not be apparent for 48 to 72 hours following injury.

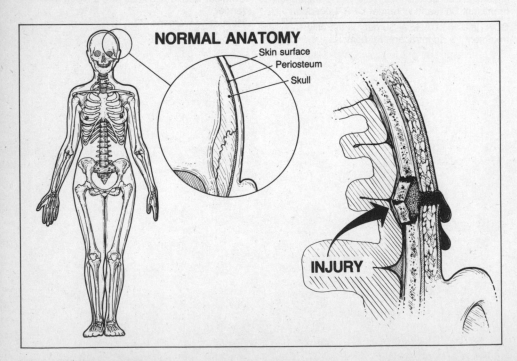

NORMAL ANATOMY

Skin surface
Periosteum
Skull

INJURY

- X-rays of the head and neck to assess total injury to soft tissue.
- CAT scan (see Glossary) of the head.
- Laboratory studies of blood and cerebrospinal fluid.

POSSIBLE COMPLICATIONS
- Hematoma (a collection of blood) that creates pressure on the brain. This can cause permanent brain damage or death, depending on the extent of injury.
- Prolonged healing time if activity is resumed too soon.
- Infection if skin over the skull fracture is broken.

PROBABLE OUTCOME—Most skull fractures without complications heal within 4 to 6 weeks. Prompt medical evaluation and treatment are essential to prevent or treat complications. These can be life-threatening or cause permanent brain damage.

 ## HOW TO TREAT

NOTE—Follow your doctor's instructions. These instructions are supplemental.

FIRST AID—Use instructions for R.I.C.E., the first letters of *rest, ice, compression* and *elevation.* This is critical to minimize bleeding and swelling. See Appendix 1 for details.

CONTINUING CARE—The extent of injury can be determined only with careful examination and observation. After a doctor's examination, the injured person may be sent home—but a responsible person must stay with the person and watch for serious symptoms. The first 24 hours after injury are critical, although serious aftereffects can appear later. If you are watching the patient, awaken him or her every hour for 24 hours. Report to the doctor immediately if you can't awaken or arouse the person. Report also any of the following:
- Vomiting.
- Inability to move arms and legs equally well on both sides.
- Temperature above 100F (37.8C).
- Stiff neck.
- Pupils of unequal size or shape.
- Convulsions.
- Noticeable restlessness.
- Severe headache that persists longer than 4 hours after injury.
- Confusion.

MEDICATION—Don't give *any* medicine—including non-prescription acetaminophen or aspirin—until the extent of injury is certain.

ACTIVITY—The patient should rest in bed until the doctor determines that the danger of complications—especially hematomas—is over. Normal activity may then be resumed as symptoms improve.

DIET—Follow a full liquid diet for 24 to 48 hours until the danger of complications passes.

REHABILITATION—Depends on whether brain damage occurs. Consult your doctor.

 ## CALL YOUR DOCTOR IF

- You have signs and symptoms of a skull fracture after a blow to the head, or you observe signs of a head injury in someone else.
- After returning home, any signs or symptoms appear that are listed under Continuing Care.

HEAD INJURY, SUBDURAL HEMORRHAGE & HEMATOMA

GENERAL INFORMATION

DEFINITION—Bleeding (hemorrhage) that causes blood to collect and clot (hematoma) beneath the membranes (meninges) that cover the brain. There are 2 types of subdural hematomas:
● An acute subdural hematoma occurs soon after a severe head injury. It is the most frequent cause of death from injury in contact sports.
● A chronic subdural hematoma may develop weeks after a head injury. The injury may have been so minor that the patient does not remember it.

BODY PARTS INVOLVED
● Brain.
● Meninges.
● Blood vessels to the brain.
● Skull.

SIGNS & SYMPTOMS
● Recurrent, worsening headaches.
● Fluctuating drowsiness, dizziness, mental changes or confusion.
● Weakness or numbness on one side of the body.
● Vision disturbances.
● Vomiting without nausea.
● Pupils of different size (sometimes).

CAUSES
● Acute: Severe blow to the head that bruises and tears the brain and its blood vessels.
● Chronic: Minor (even forgotten) head injury. Blood in the enclosed space in the brain forms a hematoma that gradually increases with further bleeding.

RISK INCREASES WITH
● Contact sports such as boxing, football or hockey.
● Auto, motorcycle or bike racing.
● During surgery, surgical risk increases with smoking and use of drugs, including anticoagulants, muscle relaxants, tranquilizers, sleep inducers, insulin, sedatives, beta-adrenergic blockers, corticosteroids or mind-altering drugs.

HOW TO PREVENT—Wear a protective helmet for any activity at risk for a head injury.

WHAT TO EXPECT

APPROPRIATE HEALTH CARE
● Doctor's diagnosis.
● Surgery to remove the clot causing pressure on the brain.
● Physical therapy for rehabilitation if there is any residual paralysis or other disability.

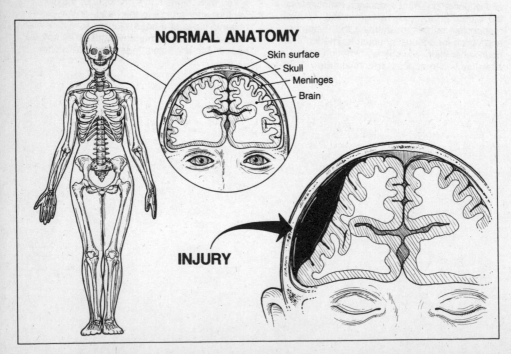

NORMAL ANATOMY

Skin surface
Skull
Meninges
Brain

INJURY

DIAGNOSTIC MEASURES
- Your own observation of symptoms.
- Medical history and physical exam by a doctor.
- Laboratory studies of blood and cerebrospinal fluid.
- Hospital diagnostic tests such as X-rays, arteriography, radioactive uptake studies and CAT scan (see Glossary for all).

POSSIBLE COMPLICATIONS
- Death or permanent brain damage, including partial or complete paralysis, behavioral and personality changes, and speech problems.
- Convulsions following surgery.

PROBABLE OUTCOME—The degree of recovery depends upon general health, age, severity of the injury, rapidity of the treatment and extensiveness of the bleeding or clot. After the clot is removed, brain tissue that has been compressed usually expands slowly to fill its original space. If speech or muscle control has been damaged, physical therapy or speech therapy may be necessary. The outlook for complete recovery is good with quick diagnosis and prompt surgery.

 HOW TO TREAT

NOTE—Follow your doctor's instructions. These instructions are supplemental.

FIRST AID—After any head injury:
- If the victim is wearing headgear with a face guard, cut the face guard off but *don't remove the headgear or move the head or neck for any reason*. Brain injury is frequently associated with neck injury.
- If the victim vomits, support the head and neck completely and carefully while rotating the entire body to the side to prevent aspiration.
- Splint the head and neck and transport the person to the nearest well-equipped emergency facility.

- Elevate the head of the stretcher slightly. Do not use pillows.
- Watch closely for vomiting, convulsions, changes in consciousness, paralysis or impaired breathing. Be ready to render CPR if needed.

CONTINUING CARE—Surgery is the only treatment for a subdural hemorrhage and hematoma. Under local or light general anesthesia, small holes are bored through the skull. The blood clot (which looks like currant jelly) is removed manually or by suction. After surgery, symptoms usually improve rapidly.

MEDICATION—Your doctor may prescribe:
- Corticosteroid drugs to reduce swelling inside the skull.
- Anticonvulsant medication.
- Antibiotics to fight infection.

ACTIVITY—After surgery, stay as active as your strength allows. Work and exercise moderately, and rest often. Once you have had a subdural hemorrhage, don't participate in contact sports.

DIET—During recovery, eat a well-balanced diet that includes extra protein, such as meat, fish, poultry, cheese, milk and eggs. Increase fiber and fluid intake to prevent constipation that may result from decreased activity.

REHABILITATION—Consult your doctor or a physical therapist.

 CALL YOUR DOCTOR IF

- You have had a head injury—even if it seems minor—and you develop any symptoms of a subdural hemorrhage. This is an emergency!
- The following occurs during or after surgery: Temperature rises to 101F (38.3C) or higher. Surgical wound becomes red, swollen or tender.
  Headache worsens.

HIP BURSITIS

GENERAL INFORMATION

DEFINITION—Inflammation of the bursa surrounding either of the big knobs of bone (trochanters) at the top of the femur (thigh bone). Bursitis may vary in degree from mild irritation to an abscess formation that causes excruciating pain.

BODY PARTS INVOLVED
● One of two bursas in the hip joint where the trochanters fit into their socket. A bursa is a soft sac filled with lubricating fluid that facilitates motion in the hip and protects it from injury.
● Soft tissue surrounding the hip joint, including nerves, tendons, ligaments, blood vessels (both large vessels and capillaries), periosteum (the outside lining of bone) and muscles.

SIGNS & SYMPTOMS
● Pain in the hip.
● A "crackling" feeling when moving the hip.
● Tenderness.
● Swelling.
● Redness (sometimes) over the affected bursa.
● A "snapping" noise with stepping or other hip motion.
● Fever if infection is present.
● Limitation of motion in the hip.

CAUSES
● Injury to the hip.
● Acute or chronic infection.
● Arthritis.
● Gout.
● Unknown (frequently).

RISK INCREASES WITH
● Participating in competitive athletics, particularly contact sports.
● Running and bouncing activities.
● Previous history of bursitis in any joint.
● Exposure to cold weather.
● Poor conditioning and inadequate warmup.
● Inadequate protective equipment in contact sports.

HOW TO PREVENT
● Use protective gear such as hip pads for contact sports.
● Warm up adequately before athletic practice or competition.
● Wear warm clothing in cold weather.
● To prevent recurrence, continue to wear extra protection over the hips until healing is complete.

WHAT TO EXPECT

APPROPRIATE HEALTH CARE
● Doctor's diagnosis and treatment.
● Surgery (sometimes), particularly for a frozen hip.

DIAGNOSTIC MEASURES
● Your own observation of symptoms.
● Medical history and physical exam by a doctor.

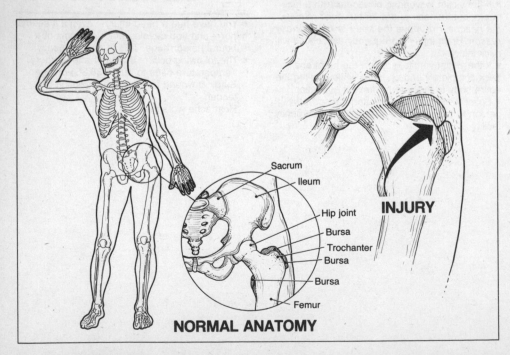

Sacrum
Ileum
Hip joint
Bursa
Trochanter
Bursa
Bursa
Femur

INJURY

NORMAL ANATOMY

- X-rays of the hips.

POSSIBLE COMPLICATIONS
- Frozen hip.
- Permanent limitation of the hip's normal mobility.
- Prolonged healing time if activity is resumed too soon.
- Proneness to repeated flare-ups.
- Unstable or arthritic hip following repeated episodes of bursitis.
- Spontaneous rupture of bursa if severe infection is present.

PROBABLE OUTCOME—Hip bursitis is a common—but not a serious—problem. Painful symptoms usually subside in 3 to 4 weeks with treatment, but they frequently recur.

 HOW TO TREAT

NOTE—Follow your doctor's instructions. These instructions are supplemental.

FIRST AID—None. This problem develops slowly.

CONTINUING CARE
- Use frequent ice massage. Fill a large Styrofoam cup with water and freeze. Tear a small amount of foam from the top so ice protrudes. Massage firmly over the injured area in a circle about the size of a softball. Do this for 15 minutes at a time, 3 or 4 times a day, and before workouts or competition.
- After 72 hours, apply heat instead of ice, if it feels better. Use heat lamps, hot soaks, hot showers, heating pads, or heat liniments or ointments.
- Take whirlpool treatments, if available.
- Use crutches to prevent weight-bearing on the hip joint, if needed. See Appendix 3 (Safe Use of Crutches).
- Elevate the hips above the level of the heart to reduce swelling and prevent accumulation of fluid. Use pillows for propping.
- Gentle massage will frequently provide comfort and decrease swelling.

MEDICATION—Your doctor may prescribe:
- Non-steroidal anti-inflammatory drugs.
- Antibiotics if the bursa is infected.
- Prescription pain relievers for severe pain. Use non-prescription aspirin, acetaminophen or ibuprofen (available under many trade names) for mild pain.
- Injections with a long-lasting local anesthetic mixed with a corticosteroid drug, such as triamcinolone.

ACTIVITY—Rest the inflamed area as much as possible. If you must resume normal activity immediately, use crutches until the pain becomes more bearable. To prevent a frozen hip, begin normal, slow joint movement as soon as possible.

DIET—Eat a well-balanced diet that includes extra protein, such as meat, fish, poultry, cheese, milk and eggs. Increase fiber and fluid intake to prevent constipation that may result from decreased activity. Your doctor may suggest vitamin and mineral supplements to promote healing.

REHABILITATION—See page 457 for rehabilitation exercises.

 CALL YOUR DOCTOR IF

- You have symptoms of hip bursitis.
- Pain increases despite treatment.
- Pain, swelling, tenderness, drainage or bleeding increases in the surgical area.
- You develop signs of infection (headache, muscle aches, dizziness or a general ill feeling and fever).
- New, unexplained symptoms develop. Drugs used in treatment may produce side effects.

HIP DISLOCATION

GENERAL INFORMATION

DEFINITION—A serious hip injury in which adjoining bones in the hip are displaced so they no longer touch each other. Dislocations are frequently accompanied by bone fractures, torn ligaments and torn tendons. Temporary or permanent damage to bone or to the sciatic nerve makes immediate treatment necessary.

BODY PARTS INVOLVED
- Femur (thigh bone) and pelvis.
- Strong ligaments that hold the hip in place.
- Sciatic nerve.
- Soft tissue surrounding the dislocated hip, including periosteum (covering to bone), other nerves, tendons, blood vessels and connective tissue.

SIGNS & SYMPTOMS
- Severe pain in the hip at the time of injury, and when trying to move hip.
- Loss of hip function.
- Visible deformity if the dislocated bones have locked in the dislocated position. The leg may appear shortened and turned in. Bones may spontaneously reposition themselves and leave no deformity, but damage is the same.
- Tenderness over the dislocation.
- Swelling and bruising at the injury site.
- Numbness or paralysis below the dislocation from pressure, pinching or cutting of blood vessels or nerves.

CAUSES
- Direct or indirect blow to a flexed knee and hip.
- End result of a severe hip sprain.
- Congenital abnormality, such as shallow or malformed joint surfaces.

RISK INCREASES WITH
- Contact sports, especially football and hockey.
- Previous hip dislocation or sprain.
- Repeated hip injury of any type.
- Arthritis of any type (rheumatoid, gout).
- Poor muscle conditioning.

HOW TO PREVENT
- Build your overall strength and muscle tone with a long-term conditioning program appropriate for your sport.
- Warm up adequately before physical activity.
- After healing, protect vulnerable joints with special hip pads.
- Consider avoiding contact sports if treatment is unsuccessful in restoring a strong, stable hip.

WHAT TO EXPECT

APPROPRIATE HEALTH CARE
- Doctor's treatment.
- Surgery (sometimes) to restore the joint to its normal position and repair torn ligaments and tendons. Acute or recurring dislocations may require surgical reconstruction or replacement of the joint.

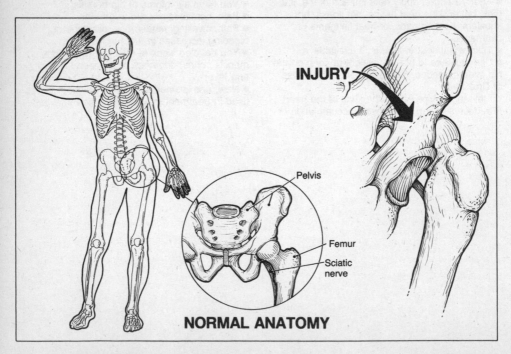

INJURY

Pelvis

Femur

Sciatic nerve

NORMAL ANATOMY

- Self-care during rehabilitation.

DIAGNOSTIC MEASURES
- Your own observation of symptoms.
- Medical history and exam by a doctor.
- X-rays of the hip, pelvis and knee.

POSSIBLE COMPLICATIONS
At the time of injury;
- Shock.
- Pressure on or injury to nearby nerves, ligaments, tendons, muscles, blood vessels and connective tissue.

After treatment or surgery:
- Excessive internal bleeding.
- Impaired blood supply to the dislocated area.
- Death of bone cells due to interruption of the blood supply.
- Infection introduced during surgical treatment.
- Aseptic necrosis (death of tissue without infection) of the head of the femur.
- Prolonged healing if activity is resumed too soon.
- Repeated hip dislocations.
- Unstable or arthritic hip after repeated injury.

PROBABLE OUTCOME—After the dislocation has been corrected, the joint may require immobilization for 4 to 6 weeks in a body cast that encloses the hip. Complete healing of injured ligaments requires a minimum of 6 weeks. Allow at least 3 months of healing before resuming active participation in sports.

 HOW TO TREAT

NOTE—Follow your doctor's instructions. These instructions are supplemental.

FIRST AID
- Keep the person warm with blankets to decrease the possibility of shock.
- Follow instructions for R.I.C.E., the first letters of *rest, ice, compression* and *elevation.* See Appendix 1 for details.
- Support the injured area with pillows during movement or transportation.
- The doctor will manipulate the hip bones to return them to their normal position. Manipulation should be done as soon as possible after injury. Shortly after a hip dislocation, bleeding in the hip area and displacement of body fluids may lead to shock and other major problems. Also, many tissues lose their elasticity and become difficult to return to a normal position within 4 to 6 hours after dislocation.

CONTINUING CARE—At home:
- Apply heat frequently. Use heat lamps, hot soaks, hot showers or heating pads.
- Take whirlpool treatments, if available.
- Massage gently and often to provide comfort and decrease swelling.

MEDICATION—Your doctor may prescribe:
- General anesthesia or muscle relaxants to make joint manipulation possible.
- Acetaminophen to relieve moderate pain.
- Narcotic pain relievers for severe pain.
- Stool softeners to prevent constipation due to decreased activity.
- Antibiotics to fight infection if surgery is required.

ACTIVITY
- Walk only with crutches until after the cast is removed and you can safely bear weight. See Appendix 3 (Safe Use of Crutches).
- Begin weight-bearing and reconditioning of the hip and leg after clearance from your doctor.
- If surgery is necessary, resume normal activities and reconditioning gradually. Don't drive until healing is complete.

DIET
- Drink only water before manipulation or surgery to correct the dislocation. Solid food in your stomach makes vomiting while under general anesthesia more hazardous.
- Eat a well-balanced diet that includes extra protein, such as meat, fish, poultry, cheese, milk and eggs. Increase fiber and fluid intake to prevent constipation that may result from decreased activity.

REHABILITATION
- Begin daily rehabilitation exercises when pain subsides.
- Use ice massage for 10 minutes before and after workouts. Fill a large Styrofoam cup with water and freeze. Tear a small amount of foam from the top so ice protrudes. Massage firmly in a circle over the injured area.
- See page 457 for rehabilitation exercises.

 CALL YOUR DOCTOR IF

- You have symptoms of a hip dislocation. Call immediately if the leg becomes numb, pale, or cold after injury. This is an emergency!
- Any of the following occurs after treatment:
  Swelling above or below the cast.
  Blue or gray skin color beyond the cast, particularly under the toenails.
  Loss of feeling below the hip.
  Nausea or vomiting.
  Constipation.
- Any of the following occur after surgery:
  Increased pain, swelling or drainage in the surgical area.
  Signs of infection (headache, muscle aches, dizziness, or a general ill feeling and fever).
- New, unexplained symptoms develop. Drugs used in treatment may produce side effects.
- Hip dislocations that you can "pop" back into normal position occur repeatedly.

HIP FRACTURE

GENERAL INFORMATION

DEFINITION—A complete or incomplete break in the head of the femur, the major bone in the hip joint.

BODY PARTS INVOLVED
- Femur (the large bone extending from the knee to the hip).
- Acetabulum (hip socket in bony pelvis).
- Hip joint.
- Soft tissue around the fracture site, including muscles, nerves, tendons, ligaments, periosteum (covering to bone), blood vessels and connective tissue.

SIGNS & SYMPTOMS
- Severe pain in the hip.
- Inability to stand.
- Swelling and bruising around the fracture.
- Visible deformity if the fracture is complete and the bone fragments separate enough to distort normal body contours.
- Tenderness to the touch.
- Numbness or coldness in the leg and foot if the blood supply is impaired or nerves are injured.

CAUSES—Direct blow or indirect stress to the hip joint. Indirect stress may be caused by twisting or a violent muscle contraction.

RISK INCREASES WITH
- Adults over 60.
- Contact sports.
- Cycling.
- History of bone or joint disease, especially osteoporosis.
- Obesity.
- Poor nutrition, especially insufficient calcium and protein.
- If surgery is needed, surgical risk increases with smoking and use of drugs, including mind-altering drugs, muscle relaxants, antihypertensives, tranquilizers, sleep inducers, insulin, sedatives, beta-adrenergic blockers or corticosteroids.

HOW TO PREVENT
- Build your strength with a good conditioning program before beginning regular athletic practice or competition. Increased muscle mass helps protect bones and underlying tissue.
- Use appropriate protective equipment, such as hip pads, when competing in contact sports.
- Ensure an adequate calcium intake (1000mg to 1500mg a day) with milk and milk products or calcium supplements.

WHAT TO EXPECT

APPROPRIATE HEALTH CARE
- Doctor's treatment.
- Hospitalization for anesthesia and surgery to set the broken hip fragments, usually by surgically pinning them together.
- Physical therapy and rehabilitation.

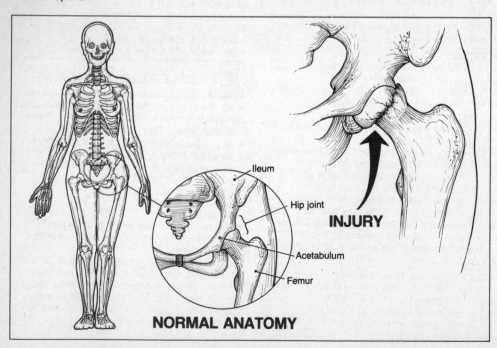

Ileum

Hip joint

Acetabulum

Femur

INJURY

NORMAL ANATOMY

DIAGNOSTIC MEASURES
- Your own observation of symptoms.
- Medical history and exam by a doctor.
- X-rays of the hip, ankle and pelvis.

POSSIBLE COMPLICATIONS
At the time of fracture:
- Shock.
- Pressure on or injury to nearby nerves, ligaments, tendons, blood vessels or connective tissues.

After treatment, including surgery:
- Excessive bleeding.
- Impaired blood supply to the healing bone.
- Avascular necrosis (death of bone cells) due to interruption of the blood supply.
- Problems arising from plaster casts, splints or other immobilizing materials. See Appendix 2 (Care of Casts).
- Shortening or deformity of the fractured bone.
- Poor healing (non-union) of the fracture.
- Arrest of bone growth in young people.
- Infection introduced during surgical treatment.
- Unstable or arthritic hip joint following repeated injury.

PROBABLE OUTCOME—The average healing time for this fracture is 6 to 8 weeks. Healing is considered complete when there is no pain or motion at the fracture site and when X-rays show complete bone union.

HOW TO TREAT

NOTE—Follow your doctor's instructions. These instructions are supplemental.

FIRST AID
- Cut away clothing, if possible, but don't move the injured area to do so.
- Use a padded splint or backboard to immobilize the hip joint before transporting the injured person to an emergency facility.
- Apply ice packs to the injury site to decrease swelling and pain.
- Elevate the foot of the backboard or splint so the pelvis is above the level of the heart. This reduces swelling and fluid accumulation.
- Keep the person warm with blankets to decrease the possibility of shock.
- The doctor will manipulate and set broken bones during surgery. Manipulation should be done as soon as possible after injury. Six or more hours after the fracture, bleeding and displacement of body fluids may lead to shock. Also, many tissues lose elasticity and become difficult to return to a normal position.

CONTINUING CARE
- Immobilization will be necessary. In hip fractures, the fractured bone is usually fixed and held with surgical steel pins or nails. A rigid cast is placed from pelvis to knee.
- Use frequent ice massage after the cast is removed. Fill a large Styrofoam cup with water and freeze. Tear a small amount of foam from the top so ice protrudes. Massage firmly over the injured area in a circle about the size of a softball. Do this for 15 minutes at a time, 3 or 4 times a day.
- Apply heat instead of ice, if it feels better. Use heat lamps, hot soaks, hot showers, heating pads, or heat liniments and ointments.
- Take whirlpool treatments, if available.
- Massage gently and often to provide comfort and decrease swelling.

MEDICATION—Your doctor may prescribe:
- General anesthesia to make joint manipulation possible.
- Narcotic or synthetic narcotic pain relievers for severe pain.
- Stool softeners to prevent constipation due to inactivity.
- Acetaminophen for mild pain.
- Antibiotics to fight infection following surgery.

ACTIVITY
- Begin reconditioning and rehabilitation after clearance from your doctor.
- Resume normal daily activities gradually after treatment.

DIET
- Drink only water before manipulation or surgery to treat the fracture. Solid food in your stomach makes vomiting while under anesthesia more hazardous.
- During recovery, eat a well-balanced diet that includes extra protein, such as meat, fish, poultry, cheese, milk and eggs. Increase fiber and fluid intake to prevent constipation that may result from decreased activity.

REHABILITATION—Begin daily rehabilitation exercises when movement is comfortable. Use ice massage for 10 minutes prior to exercise. See page 457 for rehabilitation exercises.

CALL YOUR DOCTOR IF

- You have signs or symptoms of a hip fracture. Call immediately if you have numbness or loss of feeling below the fracture site. This is an emergency!
- Any of the following occurs after surgery:
  Increased pain, swelling or drainage in the surgical area.
  Signs of infection (headache, muscle aches, dizziness, or a general ill feeling and fever).
  Nausea or vomiting.
  Swelling above or below the cast.
  Blue or gray skin color beyond the cast, especially under the toenails.
  Constipation.

HIP STRAIN

GENERAL INFORMATION

DEFINITION—Injury to the muscles and tendons attached to the trochanter, the large end of the femur (thigh bone) that forms part of the hip joint. Muscles, tendons and bone comprise units. These units stabilize the hip joint and allow its motion. A strain occurs at the weakest part of a unit. Strains are of 3 types:
- Mild (Grade I)—Slightly pulled muscle without tearing of muscle or tendon fibers. There is no loss of strength.
- Moderate (Grade II)—Tearing of fibers in a muscle, tendon or at the attachment to bone. Strength is diminished.
- Severe (Grade III)—Rupture of the muscle-tendon-bone attachment with separation of fibers. Severe strain requires surgical repair. Chronic strains are caused by overuse. Acute strains are caused by direct injury or overstress.

BODY PARTS INVOLVED
- Trochanter of the femur.
- Muscles or tendons that attach to the trochanter.
- Soft tissue surrounding the strain, including nerves, periosteum (covering to bone), blood vessels and lymph vessels.

SIGNS & SYMPTOMS
- Pain when moving, stretching or twisting.
- Muscle spasm in the hip area.
- Swelling around the injury.
- Loss of strength (moderate or severe strain).
- Crepitation ("crackling") feeling and sound when the injured area is pressed with fingers.
- Calcification of muscles or tendons (visible with X-rays).
- Inflammation of the sheath covering a tendon.

CAUSES
- Prolonged overuse of muscle-tendon units in the buttock area or around the hip joint.
- Single violent injury or force applied to the muscle-tendon units in the region of the buttocks and hip joint.

RISK INCREASES WITH
- Contact sports such as football, hockey or soccer.
- Sports that require quick starts, such as running races.
- Any cardiovascular medical problem that results in decreased circulation.
- Medical history of any bleeding disorder.
- Obesity.
- Poor nutrition.
- Previous buttock or hip injury.
- Poor muscle conditioning.

HOW TO PREVENT
- Participate in a strengthening and conditioning program appropriate for your sport.
- Warm up before practice or competition.
- Wear proper protective equipment, such as hip pads for contact sports.

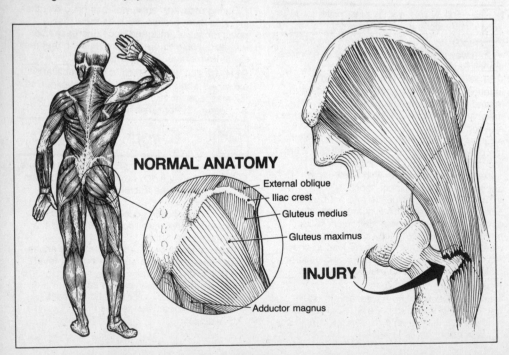

NORMAL ANATOMY

- External oblique
- Iliac crest
- Gluteus medius
- Gluteus maximus
- Adductor magnus

INJURY

WHAT TO EXPECT

APPROPRIATE HEALTH CARE
- Doctor's diagnosis.
- Self-care during rehabilitation.
- Physical therapy (moderate or severe strain).
- Surgery (severe strain).

DIAGNOSTIC MEASURES
- Your own observation of symptoms.
- Medical history and exam by a doctor.
- X-rays of the hip area to rule out fractures.

POSSIBLE COMPLICATIONS
- Prolonged healing time if activity is resumed too soon.
- Proneness to repeated injury.
- Unstable or arthritic hip following repeated injury.
- Inflammation at the attachment to bone (periostitis).
- Prolonged disability (sometimes).

PROBABLE OUTCOME—If this is a first-time injury, proper care and sufficient healing time before resuming activity should prevent permanent disability. Torn ligaments and tendons require as long to heal as fractured bones. Average healing times are:
- Mild strain—2 to 10 days.
- Moderate strain—10 days to 6 weeks.
- Severe strain—6 to 10 weeks.

If this is a repeat injury, complications listed above are more likely to occur.

 # HOW TO TREAT

NOTE—Follow your doctor's instructions. These instructions are supplemental.

FIRST AID—Use instructions for R.I.C.E., the first letters of *rest, ice, compression* and *elevation* (if possible). See Appendix 1 for details.

CONTINUING CARE
- Use ice massage 3 or 4 times a day for 15 minutes at a time. Fill a large Styrofoam cup with water and freeze. Tear a small amount of foam from the top so ice protrudes. Massage firmly over the injured area in a circle about the size of a softball.
- After the first 24 hours, apply heat instead of ice, if it feels better. Use heat lamps, hot soaks, hot showers, heating pads, or heat liniments and ointments.
- Take whirlpool treatments, if available.
- Massage gently and often to provide comfort and decrease swelling.

MEDICATION
- For minor discomfort, you may use:
  Aspirin, acetaminophen or ibuprofen.
  Topical liniments and ointments.
- Your doctor may prescribe:
  Stronger pain relievers.
  Injection of a long-acting local anesthetic to reduce pain.
  Injections of corticosteroids, such as triamcinolone, to reduce inflammation.

ACTIVITY
- For a moderate or severe strain, walk with crutches for at least 72 hours—longer with a cast or splints. See Appendix 3 (Safe Use of Crutches).
- Resume your normal activities gradually.
- Pad the injured area if you participate in contact sports.

DIET—Eat a well-balanced diet that includes extra protein, such as meat, fish, poultry, cheese, milk and eggs. Increase fiber and fluid intake to prevent constipation that may result from decreased activity.

REHABILITATION—Begin daily rehabilitation exercises when pain subsides. See page 457 for rehabilitation exercises.

 # CALL YOUR DOCTOR IF

- You have symptoms of a moderate or severe hip strain, or a mild strain persists longer than 10 days.
- Pain or swelling worsens despite treatment.

HIP SYNOVITIS

GENERAL INFORMATION

DEFINITION—Inflammation of the synovium, the smooth, lubricated lining of the hip joint. The synovium's lubricating fluid allows the hip to move freely and prevents bone surfaces from rubbing against each other. Synovitis is often a complication of an injury, such as a fracture, or of collagen diseases, such as gout or rheumatoid arthritis.

BODY PARTS INVOLVED
- Lining of the hip joint.
- Bones of the hip, including the thigh bone and pelvis.

SIGNS & SYMPTOMS
- Pain in the hip joint with movement.
- Swelling in the hip.
- Tenderness and redness in the hip area, if inflammation is caused from infection or a disease rather than from athletic injury.

CAUSES
- Any direct blow to the hip or other hip injury that damages the synovium of the hip joint. Most hip synovitis can be traced back to an injury, even though the athlete cannot remember the injury.
- Bacterial infection in the hip, usually from gonorrhea or as a complication of an open hip fracture.

- Inflammatory joint disease, such as gout or rheumatoid arthritis.

RISK INCREASES WITH
- Contact sports, such as football or soccer.
- Previous hip injury.
- Vitamin or mineral deficiency, which makes complications following injury more likely.

HOW TO PREVENT
- Engage in a vigorous muscle strengthening and conditioning program prior to beginning regular participation in sports. Overall strength and muscle tone makes injury less likely. Also, warm up adequately before competition or workouts.
- When appropriate, wear hip pads to protect the hip area during participation in contact sports.

WHAT TO EXPECT

APPROPRIATE HEALTH CARE
- Doctor's care.
- Self-care during rehabilitation.
- Physical therapy.

DIAGNOSTIC MEASURES
- Your own observation of symptoms.
- Medical history and physical exam by a doctor.
- X-rays of the hip joint.
- Laboratory examination of any fluid removed.

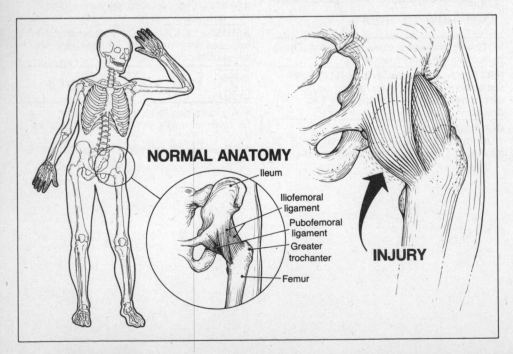

NORMAL ANATOMY

Ileum
Iliofemoral ligament
Pubofemoral ligament
Greater trochanter
Femur

INJURY

POSSIBLE COMPLICATIONS
- Prolonged healing time if activity is resumed too soon.
- Proneness to repeated hip injury.
- Unstable or arthritic hip following repeated bouts of synovitis.
- Chronic synovitis that may prevent athletic participation.

PROBABLE OUTCOME—Hip synovitis can usually be cured completely in 3 to 5 weeks with rest, heat and corticosteroid injections. However, recurrences are common following minor hip injuries.

 HOW TO TREAT

NOTE—Follow your doctor's instructions. These instructions are supplemental.

FIRST AID—None. This condition develops gradually.

CONTINUING CARE
- Follow your doctor's instructions for treatment of any underlying condition.
- Apply heat frequently. Use heat lamps, hot soaks, hot showers, heating pads, or heat liniments and ointments.
- Take whirlpool treatments, if available.
- Massage gently and often to provide comfort and decrease swelling.

MEDICATION
- Your doctor may prescribe:
  Antibiotics if infection is present.
  Non-steroidal anti-inflammatory drugs or antigout medicine.
  Injection of a long-acting local anesthetic mixed with a corticosteroid to help reduce pain and inflammation.
- You may take aspirin or ibuprofen for minor discomfort.

ACTIVITY—Use crutches to prevent weight-bearing until pain subsides. Resume normal activity gradually.

DIET—During recovery, eat a well-balanced diet that includes extra protein, such as meat, fish, poultry, cheese, milk and eggs. Increase fiber and fluid intake to prevent constipation that may result from decreased activity.

REHABILITATION
- Begin daily rehabilitation exercises when pain subsides after clearance from your doctor.
- Use ice massage for 10 minutes before and after exercise. Fill a large Styrofoam cup with water and freeze. Tear a small amount of foam from the top so ice protrudes. Massage firmly over the injured area in a circle about the size of a softball.
- See page 457 for rehabilitation exercises.

 CALL YOUR DOCTOR IF

- Your hip becomes red, hot, tender and painful.
- You develop signs of infection (headache, fever, muscle aches, dizziness or a general ill feeling) after injection of the hip.

JAW DISLOCATION, TEMPORO-MANDIBULAR JOINT

GENERAL INFORMATION

DEFINITION—Injury and displacement of the end of the lower jaw from its normal niche in a small depression at the base of the skull.

BODY PARTS INVOLVED
- Skull.
- Lower jaw (mandible).
- Soft tissue surrounding the dislocation, including nerves, tendons, ligaments, muscles, and blood vessels.

SIGNS & SYMPTOMS
- Inability to close the mouth.
- Excruciating pain in the jaw at the time of injury.
- Visible deformity if dislocated bones lock in the dislocated position. If they spontaneously reposition themselves, no deformity will be apparent, but damage will be the same.
- Tenderness over the dislocation.
- Swelling and bruising around the jaw.
- Numbness or paralysis in muscles of the face, jaw and neck from pressure, pinching or cutting of blood vessels or nerves.

CAUSES
- Direct blow to the jaw.
- Any action that forces the mandible open wider than its normal range on either side. Muscle spasm follows immediately. This can occur with yawning, yelling or taking a very large bite.
- End result of a severe jaw sprain.

RISK INCREASES WITH
- Contact sports such as boxing.
- Previous jaw dislocation or sprain.
- Repeated injury to the temporo-mandibular joint.

HOW TO PREVENT—For participation in contact sports, wear protective equipment, including a mouthpiece and helmet.

? WHAT TO EXPECT

APPROPRIATE HEALTH CARE
- Doctor's treatment. This may include manipulating the joint to reposition the bones.
- Surgery (sometimes) to restore the joint to its normal position. Acute or recurring dislocations may require surgical reconstruction or replacement of the joint.
- Self-care during rehabilitation.

DIAGNOSTIC MEASURES
- Your own observation of symptoms.
- Medical history and exam by a doctor.
- X-rays of the jaw.

POSSIBLE COMPLICATIONS
- Temporary or permanent damage to nearby nerves or major blood vessels, causing numbness and impaired circulation.

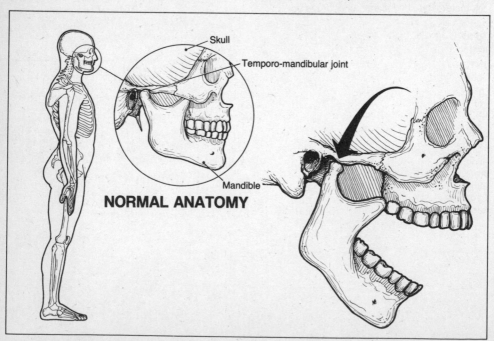

Skull

Temporo-mandibular joint

Mandible

NORMAL ANATOMY

- Shock or loss of consciousness.
- Obstruction of the airway and inhalation of mucus and blood into the lungs, leading to pneumonia. This occurs most often with dislocation and fracture.
- Excessive internal bleeding around the dislocation site.
- Proneness to recurrent jaw dislocations, particularly if a previous dislocation has not healed completely.

PROBABLE OUTCOME—After the dislocation has been corrected, the joint may require immobilization for 2 to 8 weeks with a special device fitted by your doctor or dentist. Complete healing of injured ligaments requires a minimum of 6 weeks.

 ## HOW TO TREAT

NOTE—Follow your doctor's instructions. These instructions are supplemental.

FIRST AID
- Don't panic—try to stay calm. You will not be able to talk. Write messages on paper.
- Don't push or force your mouth or try to make it close. Your mouth cannot close in a normal way until the dislocation is corrected.
- Keep warm with blankets to decrease the possibility of shock.
- Ice helps stop internal bleeding. Prepare an ice pack of ice cubes or chips wrapped in plastic or a container. Place a towel over the injured area to prevent skin damage. Apply ice for 20 minutes, then rest 10 minutes until you obtain medical treatment.
- Go to the nearest dental office or hospital emergency room for help.

CONTINUING CARE
- Continue ice massage 3 or 4 times a day for 15 minutes at a time. Fill a large Styrofoam cup with water and freeze. Tear a small amount of foam from the top so ice protrudes. Massage firmly over the injured area in a circle about the size of a softball.
- After 48 hours, localized heat promotes healing by increasing blood circulation in the injured area. Use hot compresses, heat lamps, heating pads, or heat ointments and liniments.
- If you have recurrent jaw dislocations, you can learn to reposition the jaw. Ask your doctor

or dentist for instructions. Use the following points as reminders:

1. Place your index finger on your back lower teeth (or gums in this area if you have no teeth).
2. At the same time, place both thumbs under the center of your chin.
3. Push the fingers down while simultaneously raising upward with the thumbs. The proper motion is more of a rotating movement than a straight one. It should be gentle—not fast or jerking.
Note: It is probably easier for someone else to perform the relocation than for you to do it.

MEDICATION—Your doctor may prescribe:
- General anesthesia or muscle relaxants to make jaw manipulation easier.
- Acetaminophen or aspirin to relieve moderate pain.
- Narcotic pain relievers for severe pain.

ACTIVITY—No restrictions except those imposed by a mouth appliance. Resume your normal activities gradually over several days. After the dislocation has been corrected, use caution when opening your mouth. Be careful when you yawn, take large bites, yell or scream during excitement, call someone loudly or sing.

DIET—If a mouth appliance is necessary, drink a full liquid diet until the appliance can be removed. If no appliance is necessary, eat a soft diet for a few days until discomfort decreases. Avoid chewy foods that require big bites for a while. Include extra protein, such as meat, fish, poultry, cheese, milk and eggs.

REHABILITATION—Rehabilitation exercises must be individualized. Follow your doctor's or surgeon's directions.

 ## CALL YOUR DOCTOR IF

- You have difficulty moving your jaw after injury.
- Any part of the face becomes numb, pale, or cold after injury. This is an emergency!
- Soft diet causes intestinal upset or constipation.
- Jaw dislocations that you can "pop" back into normal position occur repeatedly.

JAW (MANDIBLE) FRACTURE

GENERAL INFORMATION

DEFINITION—A complete or incomplete break in the lower jaw (the mandible). The temporo-mandibular joints (TMJ) are located just in front of the ears. These joints connect the lower jaw with the skull and are used to open and close the mouth. A fracture usually occurs at the condyle, or head of the mandible.

BODY PARTS INVOLVED
- Lower jawbone (mandible).
- Temporo-mandibular joint.
- Soft tissue surrounding the fracture site, including nerves, muscles, tendons, ligaments and blood vessels.

SIGNS & SYMPTOMS
- Severe pain at the fracture site.
- Swelling of soft tissue surrounding the fracture.
- Blood at the base of the teeth near the fracture site.
- Visible deformity if the fracture is complete and bone fragments separate enough to distort normal facial contours.
- Tenderness to the touch.
- Numbness around the fracture site (sometimes).

CAUSES—Direct blow (usually) or indirect stress to the bone. Indirect stress may be caused by violent muscle contraction.

RISK INCREASES WITH
- Contact sports, especially boxing.
- History of bone or joint disease, especially osteoporosis.
- Poor nutrition, especially calcium deficiency.
- If surgery or anesthesia are needed, surgical risk increases with smoking and use of drugs, including mind-altering drugs, muscle relaxants, antihypertensives, tranquilizers, sleep inducers, insulin, sedatives, beta-adrenergic blockers or corticosteroids.

HOW TO PREVENT—Use appropriate protective equipment, such as a face mask or mouthpiece, when participating in contact sports.

WHAT TO EXPECT

APPROPRIATE HEALTH CARE
- Doctor's or dentist's treatment to manipulate and set the broken bone.
- Hospitalization (sometimes) for anesthesia and surgery to set the fracture and wire the jaw together.
- Self-care during rehabilitation.

DIAGNOSTIC MEASURES
- Your own observation of symptoms.
- Medical history and physical exam by a doctor.
- X-rays of injured areas.

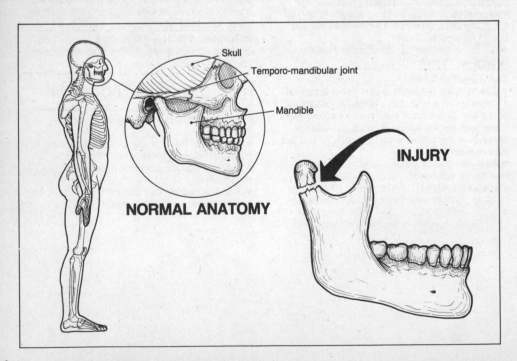

Skull

Temporo-mandibular joint

Mandible

INJURY

NORMAL ANATOMY

POSSIBLE COMPLICATIONS

At the time of injury:
- Shock.
- Pressure on or injury to nearby nerves, ligaments, tendons, muscles, blood vessels or connective tissues.

After treatment or surgery:
- Delayed union or non-union of the fracture (rare).
- Impaired blood supply the fracture site.
- Infection in open fractures (skin broken over fracture site), or at the incision if surgical setting was necessary.
- Proneness to repeated jaw injury.
- Unstable or arthritic jaw following repeated injury.
- Prolonged healing time if activity is resumed too soon.
- Nutritional problems arising because the jaw is wired closed.

PROBABLE OUTCOME—It is impossible to predict exactly how long it will take for any fracture to heal. Variable factors include age, sex, and previous state of health and conditioning. The average healing time for this fracture is 6 to 8 weeks. Healing is considered complete when there is no motion at the fracture site and when X-rays show complete bone union.

 ## HOW TO TREAT

NOTE—Follow your doctor's instructions. These instructions are supplemental.

FIRST AID
- Keep the person warm with blankets to decrease the possibility of shock.
- Use instructions for R.I.C.E., the first letters of *rest, ice, compression* and *elevation*. See Appendix 1 for details.
- The doctor will realign and set the broken bones either with surgery or, if possible, without. Manipulation should be done as soon as possible after injury. Six or more hours after the fracture, bleeding and displacement of body fluids may lead to shock. Also, many tissues lose their elasticity and become difficult to return to a normal position.

CONTINUING CARE
- Immobilization will be necessary. Mandible fractures usually require wiring the jaw together.
- Use an ice pack 3 or 4 times a day. Wrap ice chips or cubes in a plastic bag, and wrap the

bag in a moist towel. Place it over the injured area for 20 minutes at a time.
- After 72 hours, apply heat instead of ice if it feels better. Use heat lamps, hot soaks, hot showers or a heating pad.
- Learn how to "quick-release" your wired teeth for any emergency such as severe coughing or vomiting.

MEDICATION—Your doctor may prescribe:
- General anesthesia, local anesthesia, or muscle relaxants to make bone manipulation and fixation of bone fragments possible.
- Narcotic or synthetic narcotic pain relievers in liquid form for severe pain.
- Stool softeners in liquid form to prevent constipation due to a liquid diet.
- Liquid acetaminophen (available without prescription) for mild pain after initial treatment.

ACTIVITY—Rest quietly for two days, then resume normal activities gradually. Don't exercise to the point that you pant for breath, because breathing may be difficult for a while.

DIET
- Drink only water before manipulation or surgery to treat the fracture. Any food in your stomach makes vomiting while under anesthesia more hazardous.
- During recovery, follow a high-protein liquid diet such as malted milk and eggnog. Add soft foods as you are able. Most people can handle rich soups, ground meat, whipped potatoes and gravy.

REHABILITATION—No special rehabilitation program. Begin using jaw muscles carefully after the fracture heals.

 ## CALL YOUR DOCTOR IF

- You have signs or symptoms of a jaw fracture.
- Any of the following occur after surgery or other treatment:

  Increased pain, swelling or drainage in the surgical area.

  Signs of infection (headache, muscle aches, dizziness, or a general ill feeling and fever).

  Nausea or vomiting.

  Numbness or complete loss of feeling around the jaw.

  Constipation.

JAW (TEMPORO-MANDIBULAR) SPRAIN

GENERAL INFORMATION

DEFINITION—Violent overstretching of one or more ligaments in the temporo-mandibular joint. Sprains involving two or more ligaments cause considerably more disability than single-ligament sprains. When the ligament is overstretched, it becomes tense and gives way at its weakest point, either where it attaches to bone or within the ligament itself. If the ligament pulls loose a fragment of bone, it is called a *sprain-fracture*. There are 3 types of sprains:
- Mild (Grade I)—Tearing of some ligament fibers. There is no loss of function.
- Moderate (Grade II)—Rupture of a portion of the ligament, resulting in some loss of function.
- Severe (Grade III)—Complete rupture of the ligament or complete separation of ligament from bone. There is total loss of function. A severe sprain requires surgical repair.

BODY PARTS INVOLVED
- Ligaments of the temporo-mandibular joint of the jaw.
- Tissue surrounding the sprain, including blood vessels, tendons, bone, periosteum (covering of bone) and muscles.

SIGNS & SYMPTOMS
- Severe pain at the time of injury.
- A feeling of popping or tearing inside the jaw.
- Difficulty opening and closing the mouth.
- Tenderness at the injury site.
- Swelling around the jaw.
- Bruising that appears soon after injury.

CAUSES—Stress that forces the jaw through a wider range of motion than ligaments normally permit.

RISK INCREASES WITH
- Contact sports, especially boxing.
- Previous temporo-mandibular joint injury or disorder.
- Inadequate protection from equipment.

HOW TO PREVENT—Wear protective equipment, such as a face mask and mouthpiece, when appropriate.

WHAT TO EXPECT

APPROPRIATE HEALTH CARE
- Doctor's diagnosis.
- Bandaging or wiring of the jaw (sometimes).
- Biofeedback training (see Glossary) during the healing phase.
- Physical therapy (moderate or severe sprain).
- Surgery (severe sprain).

DIAGNOSTIC MEASURES
- Your own observation of symptoms.
- Medical history and exam by a doctor.
- X-rays of the jaw to rule out fractures or dislocations.

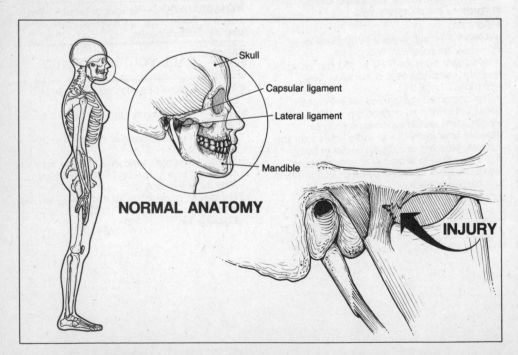

Skull

Capsular ligament

Lateral ligament

Mandible

NORMAL ANATOMY

INJURY

POSSIBLE COMPLICATIONS
- Proneness to repeated jaw injury.
- Inflammation at the ligament attachment to bone (periostitis).

PROBABLE OUTCOME—Jaw sprains usually cause no permanent problems if allowed to heal sufficiently. Ligaments have a poor blood supply, and torn ligaments require as much healing time as fractures. Average healing times are:
- Mild sprains—2 to 6 weeks.
- Moderate sprains—6 to 8 weeks.
- Severe sprains—8 to 10 weeks.

 # HOW TO TREAT

NOTE—Follow your doctor's instructions. These instructions are supplemental.

FIRST AID—Use instructions for R.I.C.E., the first letters of *rest, ice, compression* and *elevation*. See Appendix 1 for details.

CONTINUING CARE
- Continue using an ice pack 3 or 4 times a day. Place ice chips or cubes in a plastic bag. Wrap the bag in a moist towel, and place it over the jaw. Use for 20 minutes at a time.
- After 72 hours, apply heat instead of ice if it feels better. Use heat lamps, hot soaks, hot showers, heating pads, or heat liniments or ointments.
- Massage gently and often to provide comfort and decrease swelling.

MEDICATION
- For minor discomfort, you may use aspirin, acetaminophen or ibuprofen.

- Your doctor may prescribe:
  Stronger pain relievers.
  Injection of a long-acting local anesthetic to reduce pain.
  Injection of a corticosteroid, such as triamcinolone, to reduce inflammation.
  Stool softeners if constipation results from a liquid or soft diet.

ACTIVITY—Resume your normal activities gradually after clearance from your doctor.

DIET—A normal diet may be difficult, especially if the jaw is wired or bandaged. If so, eat soft or liquid foods and increase your protein intake to promote healing.

REHABILITATION—Consult your doctor or oral surgeon for rehabilitation exercises.

 # CALL YOUR DOCTOR IF

- You have symptoms of a moderate or severe temporo-mandibular sprain, or a mild sprain persists longer than 2 weeks.
- Pain, swelling or bruising worsens despite treatment.
- You feel numbness or coldness around the injury.
- Any of the following occur after surgery:
  Increased pain, swelling, redness, drainage or bleeding in the surgical area.
  Signs of infection (headache, muscle aches, dizziness, or a general ill feeling with fever).
- New, unexplained symptoms develop. Drugs used in treatment may produce side effects.

KIDNEY INJURY

GENERAL INFORMATION

DEFINITION—Bruising or tearing of the kidney or ureter. Kidneys filter waste material from the bloodstream and produce urine. Ureters are the tubes that carry urine from the kidneys to the bladder. The most common injury to the kidney is contusion. In contact sports, this may result from a blow from a knee or helmet, with the shock penetrating the flank muscles and reaching the kidney.

BODY PARTS INVOLVED
- Kidney.
- Ureters (tubes that carry urine from the kidney to the bladder).
- Muscles of the abdominal wall.
- Subcutaneous tissue, nerves, blood vessels and connective tissue.
- Urethra (tube that carries urine from the bladder out of the body).

SIGNS & SYMPTOMS
- Pain and tenderness in the flank or back, just below the ribs on the injured side.
- Fever to 101F (38.3C).
- Blood in the urine. There may be enough to make urine look "smoky" or bloody. Lesser bleeding can only be determined by studying urine under the microscope.
- If infection of the injured kidney complicates the injury, sudden onset of:
  Fever and shaking chills.

Burning, frequent urination.
Cloudy urine or blood in the urine.
Aching (sometimes severe) in one or both sides of the lower back.
Abdominal pain.
Marked fatigue.

CAUSES
- A blow or penetrating wound to the kidney, located on the side of the body under the ribs.
- Urinary-tract infection caused by kidney damage that leads to decreased rate of flow of urine. Decreased urinary flow rates allow bacteria to grow and infect the parts of the urinary tract—kidney, ureters, bladder and urethra.

RISK INCREASES WITH
- Contact sports.
- Any underlying abnormality of the kidney or genitourinary tract such as polycystic kidneys.
- Poor muscle conditioning.
- Any bleeding disorder such as hemophilia.

HOW TO PREVENT
- Use adequate protective equipment for contact sports.
- Develop good muscle conditioning in the flank area. Increased muscle mass helps protect underlying organs and other tissues.

WHAT TO EXPECT

APPROPRIATE HEALTH CARE
- Doctor's treatment.

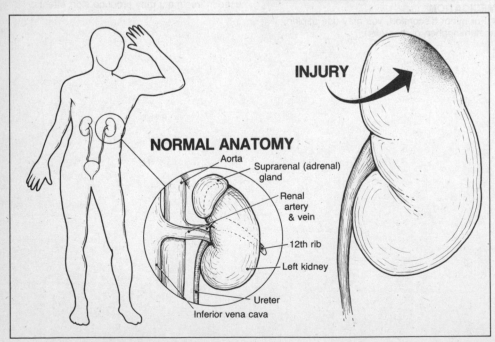

INJURY

NORMAL ANATOMY

Aorta
Suprarenal (adrenal) gland
Renal artery & vein
12th rib
Left kidney
Ureter
Inferior vena cava

- Hospitalization for shock or internal bleeding.
- Surgery to repair the ureter or remove the kidney, if other treatment fails.

DIAGNOSTIC MEASURES
- Your own observation of symptoms.
- Medical history and physical exam by a doctor.
- Laboratory urine studies.
- X-rays of the urinary tract.

POSSIBLE COMPLICATIONS
- Internal bleeding.
- Shock (sweating; faintness; nausea; panting; rapid pulse; pale, cold, moist skin).
- Urine leakage into the abdomen, causing abdominal inflammation or infection.
- Scarring and narrowing of the injured ureter.

PROBABLE OUTCOME—Usually heals with time, bed rest, protection against infection and surgery (sometimes). Surgery to remove an injured kidney (if it does not heal with other measures) is not complicated. After recovery, you can lead a normal life with one kidney, but you must avoid contact sports. Allow about 4 weeks for recovery from surgery.

 ## HOW TO TREAT

NOTE—Follow your doctor's instructions. These instructions are supplemental.

FIRST AID—Use instructions for R.I.C.E., the first letters of *rest, ice, compression* and *elevation*. See Appendix 1 for details.

CONTINUING CARE—No special instructions except those under other headings. If surgery is required, your surgeon will supply postoperative instructions.

MEDICATION—Your doctor may prescribe:
- Pain relievers.
- Antibiotics to treat or protect against infection.

ACTIVITY—You will need bed rest for 1 to 2 weeks after the injury. After recovery, resume normal activities gradually.

DIET
- Drink 6 to 8 glasses of fluid daily.
- Don't drink alcohol.
- During recovery, eat a well-balanced diet that includes extra protein, such as meat, fish, poultry, cheese, milk and eggs. Increase fiber intake to prevent constipation that may result from decreased activity.

REHABILITATION—Rehabilitation exercises must be individualized. Follow your doctor's or surgeon's directions.

 ## CALL YOUR DOCTOR IF

- You have any symptoms of kidney or ureter injury.
- Symptoms recur after treatment, especially blood in the urine.
- You have symptoms of a kidney infection.
- Symptoms and fever persist after 48 hours of antibiotic treatment. Occasionally a different antibiotic is needed.
- Symptoms return (especially if accompanied by fever) after antibiotic treatment.
- New, unexplained symptoms develop. Drugs used in treatment may produce side effects.

KNEE BURSITIS

GENERAL INFORMATION

DEFINITION—Inflammation of a bursa in the knee. Bursitis may vary in degree from mild irritation to an abscess formation that causes excruciating pain. There are many bursas in the knee:
- In front of and behind the kneecap.
- On both sides of the knee.
- Behind the knee (Baker's cyst).
- Just above the knee (popliteal bursa).

BODY PARTS INVOLVED
- Knee bursas—soft sacs in the knee area filled with lubricating fluid that facilitate motion in the knee.
- Soft tissue surrounding the knee, including nerves, tendons, ligaments, blood vessels (both large vessels and capillaries), periosteum (the outside lining of bone) and muscles.

SIGNS & SYMPTOMS
- Pain, especially when moving the knee.
- Tenderness.
- Swelling.
- Redness (sometimes) over the affected bursa.
- Fever if infection is present.
- Limitation of motion in the knee.

CAUSES
- Injury to the knee, especially falling on a bent knee.
- Acute or chronic infection in the knee.
- Arthritis.
- Gout.
- Unknown (frequently).

RISK INCREASES WITH
- Participation in competitive athletics, particularly contact sports such as football.
- Previous history of bursitis in any joint.
- Exposure to cold weather.
- Poor conditioning and inadequate warmup.
- Inadequate protective equipment in contact sports.

HOW TO PREVENT
- Warm up adequately before athletic practice or competition.
- Wear warm clothing in cold weather.
- To prevent recurrence, continue to wear extra knee pads until healing is complete.

WHAT TO EXPECT

APPROPRIATE HEALTH CARE
- Doctor's exam for precise diagnosis and treatment.
- Surgery (sometimes), particularly for a frozen knee.

DIAGNOSTIC MEASURES
- Your own observation of symptoms.
- Medical history and physical exam by a doctor.
- X-rays of the knee.

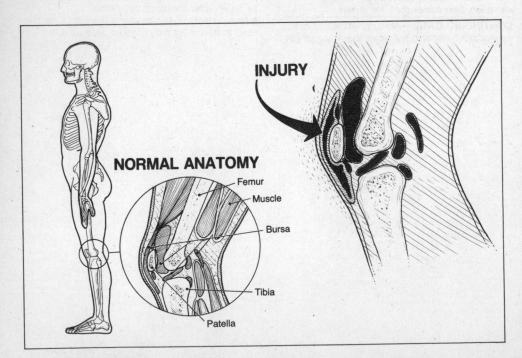

INJURY

NORMAL ANATOMY

Femur

Muscle

Bursa

Tibia

Patella

POSSIBLE COMPLICATIONS
● Frozen knee.
● Permanent limitation of the knee's normal mobility.
● Prolonged healing time if activity or weight-bearing is resumed too soon.
● Proneness to repeated flare-ups.
● Arthritic knee following repeated episodes of bursitis.

PROBABLE OUTCOME—Knee bursitis is commonly a chronic problem. Symptoms may subside with treatment, but recurrent flare-ups are common. If surgery becomes necessary, allow 6 to 8 weeks for healing.

 HOW TO TREAT

NOTE—Follow your doctor's instructions. These instructions are supplemental.

FIRST AID—None. This problem develops slowly.

CONTINUING CARE
● Use frequent ice massage. Fill a large Styrofoam cup with water and freeze. Tear a small amount of foam from the top so ice protrudes. Massage firmly over the injured area in a circle about the size of a softball. Do this for 15 minutes at a time, 3 or 4 times a day, and before workouts or competition.
● After 72 hours, apply heat instead of ice if it feels better. Use heat lamps, hot soaks, hot showers, heating pads, or heat liniments or ointments.
● Take whirlpool treatments, if available.
● Use crutches to prevent weight-bearing on the knee, if needed.
● Whenever possible, elevate the knee above the level of the heart to reduce swelling and prevent accumulation of fluid. Use pillows for propping or elevate the foot of the bed.

● Gentle massage will frequently provide comfort and decrease swelling.

MEDICATION—Your doctor may prescribe:
● Non-steroidal anti-inflammatory drugs.
● Antibiotics if the bursa is infected.
● Prescription pain relievers for severe pain. Use non-prescription aspirin, acetaminophen or ibuprofen (available under many trade names) for mild pain.
● Injection with a long-lasting local anesthetic mixed with a corticosteroid drug, such as triamcinolone.

ACTIVITY—Rest the knee as much as possible. If you must resume normal activity, use crutches until the pain becomes more bearable. To prevent a frozen knee, begin normal, slow knee movement as soon as possible.

DIET—Eat a well-balanced diet that includes extra protein, such as meat, fish, poultry, cheese, milk and eggs. Increase fiber and fluid intake to prevent constipation that may result from decreased activity. Your doctor may suggest vitamin and mineral supplements to promote healing.

REHABILITATION—See page 460 for rehabilitation exercises.

 CALL YOUR DOCTOR IF

● You have symptoms of knee bursitis.
● Pain increases despite treatment.
● Pain, swelling, tenderness, drainage or bleeding increases in the surgical area.
● You develop signs of infection (headache, muscle aches, dizziness or a general ill feeling and fever).
● New, unexplained symptoms develop. Drugs used in treatment may produce side effects.

KNEE-CARTILAGE INJURY
(Meniscus Injury)

 GENERAL INFORMATION

DEFINITION—Damage to cartilage in the knee at the top of the lower leg bone (tibia). Knee-cartilage injuries frequently accompany dislocations of the kneecap or ligament sprains in the knee. This is sometimes a vaguely diagnosed knee injury that resists conservative treatment.

BODY PARTS INVOLVED
- Cartilage at the top of the tibia that normally cushions force to the knee.
- Knee joint.
- Ligaments that lend stability to the knee.
- Soft tissue that includes nerves, synovial membranes, periosteum (covering to bone), blood vessels, lymph vessels and bursae of the knee joint.

SIGNS & SYMPTOMS
- Pain and tenderness in the knee, especially when bearing weight.
- Locking of the knee joint.
- "Giving way" of the knee.
- "Water" on the knee (sometimes).

CAUSES
- Direct blow to the knee.
- Prolonged overuse of an injured knee.
- Twisting or violent muscle contraction.

RISK INCREASES WITH
- Contact sports, especially football.
- Obesity.
- Poor nutrition.
- Previous knee injury.
- Poor muscle conditioning.

HOW TO PREVENT
- Engage in vigorous presport strengthening and conditioning.
- Avoid concrete or asphalt surfaces and other rigid surfaces for continuous conditioning exercises.
- Warm up adequately before practice or competition.
- Tape the knee before practice or competition if you have had a previous knee injury.

 WHAT TO EXPECT

APPROPRIATE HEALTH CARE
- Doctor's care.
- Surgery to remove the damaged meniscus. This is usually done with arthroscopy. Arthroscopy is visual examination of a joint using an arthroscope, a fiber-optic instrument with a lighted tip.
- Self-care during recovery following surgery.
- Physical therapy and rehabilitation after surgery.

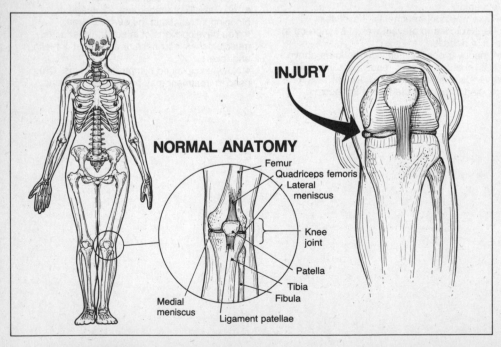

NORMAL ANATOMY

INJURY

Femur
Quadriceps femoris
Lateral meniscus
Knee joint
Patella
Tibia
Fibula
Ligament patellae
Medial meniscus

DIAGNOSTIC MEASURES
- Your own observation of symptoms.
- Medical history and physical exam by a doctor.
- X-rays of the knee to rule out fracture.
- Arthroscopy for knee injuries that have some, but not all, signs of cartilage injury. This instrument Is also used for surgery on the knee.

POSSIBLE COMPLICATIONS
- Prolonged disability, knee instability and pain without surgery.
- Arthritic changes in later years whether surgery was performed or not.
- Proneness to repeated knee injury.
- Postoperative complications, including bleeding into the knee joint, surgical-wound infection and slow healing.

PROBABLE OUTCOME—Surgery is the only definitive treatment for knee-cartilage injuries. With surgery, expect complete healing if no complications occur. Allow 6 weeks for full recovery from surgery.

HOW TO TREAT

NOTE—Follow your doctor's instructions. These instructions are supplemental.

FIRST AID
- Use instructions for R.I.C.E., the first letters of *rest, ice, compression* and *elevation*. See Appendix 1 for details.
- Keep the person warm with blankets to decrease the possibility of shock.
- Cut away clothing, if possible. Don't move the injured knee to remove clothing.
- Use a padded splint or sling to immobilize the knee, hip and ankle before transporting the injured person to the doctor's office or emergency facility.

CONTINUING CARE—During the postoperative phase:
- Walk on crutches until your surgeon instructs otherwise.
- After the cast is removed, use an electric heating pad, heat lamp or a warm compress to relieve incisional pain.
- Take whirlpool treatments, if available.
- Wrap the injured knee with an elasticized bandage between treatments.
- Massage gently and often to provide comfort and decrease swelling.
- On follow-up visits, your surgeon may aspirate fluid that has accumulated in the knee joint.

MEDICATION
- For minor discomfort, you may use non-prescription medicines such as aspirin, acetaminophen or ibuprofen.
- Your doctor may prescribe stronger medicine for pain, if needed.

ACTIVITY—Return gradually to previous level of activity. You may return to full activity when the range of motion and strength in the injured leg is equal to the normal leg.

DIET—During recovery, eat a well-balanced diet that includes extra protein, such as meat, fish, poultry, cheese, milk and eggs. Increase fiber and fluid intake to prevent constipation that may result from decreased activity.

REHABILITATION
- Begin non-weight-bearing rehabilitation exercises the first day after surgery.
- Begin daily rehabilitation exercises when movement is comfortable.
- Use ice massage for 10 minutes before and after exercise. Fill a large Styrofoam cup with water and freeze. Tear a small amount of foam from the top so ice protrudes. Massage firmly over the injured area in a circle about the size of a softball.
- See page 460 for rehabilitation exercises.

CALL YOUR DOCTOR IF

- You have symptoms of a knee-cartilage injury.
- Any of the following occurs after surgery:
  Increased pain, swelling, redness, drainage or bleeding in the surgical area.
  Signs of infection (headache, muscle aches, dizziness or a general ill feeling and fever).
  Nausea or vomiting.

KNEE CONTUSION

GENERAL INFORMATION

DEFINITION—Bruising of the skin and underlying tissues of the knee due to a direct blow. Contusions cause bleeding from ruptured small capillaries that allow blood to infiltrate muscles, tendons or other soft tissue. The knee is highly vulnerable to contusions.

BODY PARTS INVOLVED—Knee, including blood vessels, muscles, tendons, nerves, covering to bone (periosteum) and connective tissue.

SIGNS & SYMPTOMS
● Swelling—either superficial or deep.
● Pain and tenderness over the knee.
● Feeling of firmness when pressure is exerted on the knee.
● Discoloration under the skin, beginning with redness and progressing to the characteristic "black and blue" bruise.
● Restricted knee activity proportional to the extent of injury.
● Break in skin over the contusion (frequent in knee injuries).

CAUSES—Direct blow to the front or side of the knee.

RISK INCREASES WITH
● Contact, running or riding sports, especially if the knees are not adequately protected.
● Medical history of any bleeding disorder such as hemophilia.
● Poor nutrition, including vitamin deficiency.
● Use of anticoagulants or aspirin.

HOW TO PREVENT—Wear protective knee pads during competition or other athletic activity if there is risk of a knee contusion.

WHAT TO EXPECT

APPROPRIATE HEALTH CARE
● Doctor's care unless the injury is quite small.
● Self-care for minor contusions, and for serious contusions during rehabilitation.
● Physical therapy for serious contusions.

DIAGNOSTIC MEASURES
● Your own observation of symptoms.
● Medical history and physical exam by a doctor for all except minor injuries.
● X-rays of the knee to assess total injury to soft tissue and to rule out the possibility of underlying fractures. The total extent of injury may not be apparent for 48 to 72 hours.

POSSIBLE COMPLICATIONS
● Excessive bleeding leading to disability. Infiltrative-type bleeding can sometimes lead to calcification and impaired function of injured muscles, ligaments or tendons.
● Prolonged healing time if usual activities are resumed too soon.

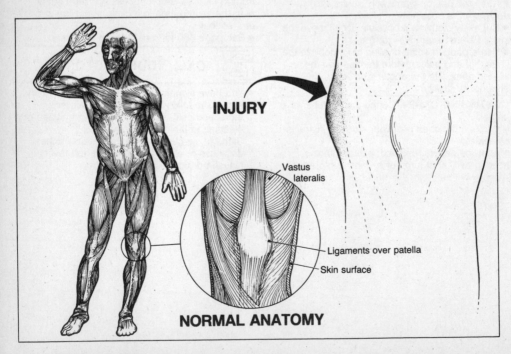

INJURY

Vastus lateralis

Ligaments over patella

Skin surface

NORMAL ANATOMY

• Infection if skin over the contusion is broken.

PROBABLE OUTCOME—Healing time varies from 2 to 6 weeks, depending on the extent of injury.

 ## HOW TO TREAT

NOTE—Follow your doctor's instructions. These instructions are supplemental.

FIRST AID—Use instructions for R.I.C.E., the first letters of *rest, ice, compression* and *elevation*. See Appendix 1 for details.

CONTINUING CARE
• Wrap an elasticized bandage over a felt pad on the knee. Keep the area compressed for about 72 hours.
• Use an ice pack 3 or 4 times a day. Wrap ice chips or cubes in a plastic bag, and wrap the bag in a moist towel. Place it over the injured area for 20 minutes at a time.
• After 72 hours, apply heat instead of ice if it feels better. Use heat lamps, hot soaks, hot showers, heating pads, heat liniments or ointments, or whirlpool treatments.
• Massage gently and often to provide comfort and decrease swelling.

MEDICATION
• For minor discomfort, you may use:
  Acetaminophen or ibuprofen.
  Topical liniments and ointments.

• Your doctor may prescribe stronger medicine for pain.

ACTIVITY—Begin activities slowly and stop exercise as soon as pain begins. Increase activity as healing progresses.

DIET—During recovery, eat a well-balanced diet that includes extra protein, such as meat, fish, poultry, cheese, milk and eggs. Your doctor may prescribe vitamin and mineral supplements to promote healing.

REHABILITATION
• Begin daily rehabilitation exercises when supportive wrapping is no longer needed.
• Use ice massage for 10 minutes before and after workouts. Fill a large Styrofoam cup with water and freeze. Tear a small amount of foam from the top so ice protrudes. Massage firmly over the injured area in a circle about the size of a softball.
• See page 460 for rehabilitation exercises.

 ## CALL YOUR DOCTOR IF

• You have a knee contusion that doesn't improve in 1 or 2 days.
• Skin is broken and signs of infection (drainage, increasing pain, fever, headache, muscle aches, dizziness or a general ill feeling) occur.

KNEE DISLOCATION, TIBIA-FEMUR

GENERAL INFORMATION

DEFINITION—Injury to the knee joint in which the upper and lower leg bones are displaced and no longer touch each other. Knee dislocations often include torn or ruptured ligaments in the knee.

BODY PARTS INVOLVED
- Tibia (large lower leg bone), femur (thigh bone) and patella (kneecap).
- Ligaments of the knee joint.
- Meniscus (cartilage) of the knee joint.
- Soft tissue surrounding the dislocated knee, including periosteum (covering to bone), nerves, tendons, blood vessels and connective tissue.

SIGNS & SYMPTOMS
- Severe knee pain at the time of injury.
- Loss of function of the knee, and severe pain when attempting to move it.
- Visible deformity if the dislocated bones have locked in the dislocated position. Bones may spontaneously reposition themselves and leave no deformity, but damage is the same.
- Tenderness over the dislocation.
- Swelling and bruising around the knee.
- Numbness or paralysis below the dislocation.

CAUSES
- Overextension of the knee.
- Direct blow to the tibia.
- Direct blow to the thigh, driving the knee to either side.

- End result of a severe knee sprain.
- Congenital knee abnormality, such as shallow or malformed joint surfaces.

RISK INCREASES WITH
- Contact sports, especially football or hockey.
- Previous knee sprain or dislocation.
- Repeated knee injury of any sort.
- Poor muscle conditioning.

HOW TO PREVENT
- Build your strength with a conditioning program appropriate for your sport.
- Warm up adequately before physical activity.
- After healing, wear protective equipment such as special knee pads and knee braces during participation in contact sports.

WHAT TO EXPECT

APPROPRIATE HEALTH CARE
- Doctor's treatment.
- Surgery (usually) to restore the knee to its normal position and repair torn ligaments and tendons. Acute or recurring dislocations may require reconstruction or replacement of the joint.

DIAGNOSTIC MEASURES
- Your own observation of symptoms.
- Medical history and exam by a doctor.
- X-rays of the knee, hip and ankle.

POSSIBLE COMPLICATIONS
At the time of injury:
- Shock.

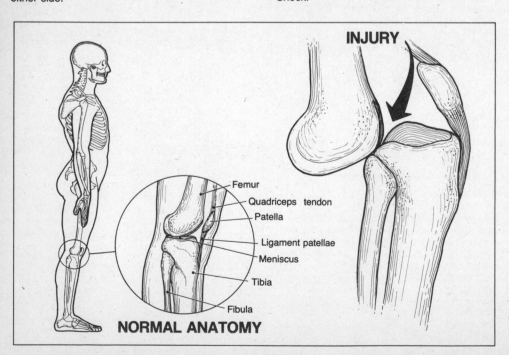

Femur
Quadriceps tendon
Patella
Ligament patellae
Meniscus
Tibia
Fibula

NORMAL ANATOMY

INJURY

- Pressure on or injury to nearby nerves, ligaments, tendons, muscles, blood vessels and connective tissue.

After treatment or surgery:
- Excessive internal bleeding around the knee.
- Impaired blood supply to the knee.
- Death of bone cells from interruption of the blood supply.
- Infection introduced during surgical treatment.
- Recurrent dislocations with progressively less serious provocation.
- Prolonged healing if activity is resumed too soon.
- Unstable or arthritic knee joint following repeated injury.

PROBABLE OUTCOME—After the dislocation has been corrected, the knee may require immobilization with a cast or splint for 6 to 8 weeks. Complete healing of injured ligaments requires a minimum of 6 weeks. Avoid contact sports if all treatments are unsuccessful in restoring a strong, stable knee.

HOW TO TREAT

NOTE—Follow your doctor's instructions. These instructions are supplemental.

FIRST AID
- This is a medical emergency. Get help as soon as possible.
- Follow instructions for R.I.C.E., the first letters of *rest, ice, compression* and *elevation.* See Appendix 1 for details.
- Cut away clothing if possible. Don't move the injured leg to do so.
- Immobilize the knee, hip and ankle joints with padded splints.
- The doctor will repair torn ligaments and tendons and manipulate the dislocated knee to return it to its normal position. Manipulation should be done within 6 hours after injury, or bleeding and displacement of body fluids may lead to shock. Also, many tissues lose elasticity and become difficult to return to a normal position. Manipulation may require spinal or general anesthesia. If blood vessels or nerves have major damage, surgery is mandatory.

CONTINUING CARE—After removal of the cast or splint:
- Use an ice pack 3 or 4 times a day. Place ice chips or cubes in a plastic bag, and wrap the bag in a moist towel. Place it over the injured area for 20 minutes at a time.
- Apply heat instead of ice, if it feels better. Use heat lamps, hot soaks, hot showers, heating pads or whirlpool treatments.
- Wrap the injured knee with an elasticized bandage between treatments.
- Massage gently and often to provide comfort and decrease swelling.

MEDICATION—Your doctor may prescribe:
- General anesthesia, spinal anesthesia or muscle relaxants prior to joint manipulation.
- Acetaminophen to relieve moderate pain.
- Narcotic pain relievers for severe pain.
- Stool softeners to prevent constipation due to decreased activity.
- Antibiotics to fight infection if surgery is necessary.

ACTIVITY
- Walk with crutches while the cast is in place. See Appendix 3 (Safe Use of Crutches). Begin weight-bearing and reconditioning of the knee after clearance from your doctor.
- If surgery is necessary, resume activity gradually. Don't drive until healing is complete.

DIET
- Drink only water before manipulation or surgery to correct the dislocation. Solid food in your stomach makes vomiting while under general anesthesia more hazardous.
- During recovery, eat a well-balanced diet that includes extra protein, such as meat, fish, poultry, cheese, milk and eggs. Increase fiber and fluid intake to prevent constipation that may result from decreased activity.

REHABILITATION
- Begin daily rehabilitation exercises after clearance from your doctor.
- Use ice massage for 10 minutes before and after workouts. Fill a large Styrofoam cup with water and freeze. Tear a small amount of foam from the top so ice protrudes. Massage firmly in a circle over the injured area.
- See page 460 for rehabilitation exercises.

CALL YOUR DOCTOR IF

- You have symptoms of a dislocated knee, even if the knee goes back into position. Call immediately if the leg becomes numb, pale, or cold. This is an emergency!
- Any of the following occur after treatment:
  Nausea or vomiting.
  Swelling above or below the cast.
  Blue or gray skin color below the cast, particularly under the toenails.
  Loss of feeling below the knee.
  Constipation.
- Any of the following occur after surgery:
  Increasing pain, swelling or drainage in the surgical area.
  Signs of infection (headache, muscle aches, dizziness, or a general ill feeling and fever).
- New, unexplained symptoms develop. Drugs used in treatment may produce side effects.
- Knee dislocations that you can "pop" back into normal position occur repeatedly.

KNEE DISLOCATION, TIBIA-FIBULA

GENERAL INFORMATION

DEFINITION—Injury and displacement of the bones of the lower leg so they no longer touch each other. This is less common than dislocation of the kneecap. It often occurs with fracture of the tibia.

BODY PARTS INVOLVED
- Knee joint.
- Lower leg bones (tibia and fibula) where they join the knee joint.
- Soft tissue surrounding the dislocation, including nerves, periosteum (covering of bone), tendons, ligaments, muscles and blood vessels.

SIGNS & SYMPTOMS
- A feeling of the knee "giving way."
- Excruciating pain at the time of injury.
- Locking of the dislocated bones in the abnormal position or spontaneous reposition, leaving no apparent deformity.
- Tenderness over the dislocation.
- Swelling and discoloration of the knee.
- Numbness or paralysis in the lower leg and foot from pressure, pinching or cutting of blood vessels or nerves.

CAUSES
- Direct blow to the knee.
- End result of a severe sprain caused by a twisting injury.
- Powerful muscle contractions related to quick changes of direction while running.

RISK INCREASES WITH
- Contact and running sports.
- Person with a wide pelvis and "knock-knees".
- Previous knee sprains.
- Repeated knee injury.
- Arthritis of any type (rheumatoid, gout).
- Poor muscle conditioning.
- Congenital abnormalities of the knee joint.

HOW TO PREVENT
- Develop your muscle strength and overall conditioning.
- Warm up adequately before physical activity.
- After recovery, protect the knee during contact or running sports by wearing wrapped elastic bandages, tape wraps, knee pads or special support stockings.

WHAT TO EXPECT

APPROPRIATE HEALTH CARE
- Doctor's treatment. This will include manipulation of the knee to reposition the bones.
- Surgery (usually) to restore the knee to normal function.
- Self-care during rehabilitation.

DIAGNOSTIC MEASURES
- Your own observation of symptoms.
- Medical history and exam by a doctor.
- X-rays of the knee joint and adjacent bones.

POSSIBLE COMPLICATIONS
At the time of injury:
- Shock.

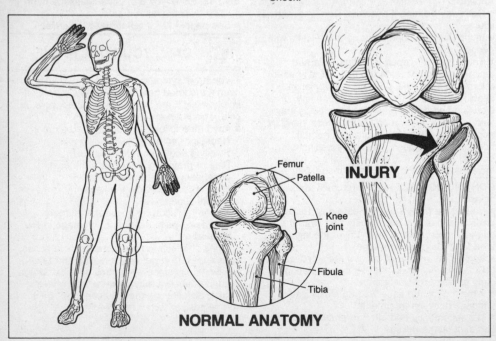

Femur
Patella
Knee joint
Fibula
Tibia

INJURY

NORMAL ANATOMY

- Pressure on or injury to nearby nerves, ligaments, tendons, muscles, blood vessels and connective tissue. This causes numbness, coldness and paleness in the leg or foot.

After treatment or surgery:
- Impaired blood supply to the dislocated area.
- Infection introduced during surgical treatment.
- Excessive internal bleeding around the knee.
- Recurrent dislocations, particularly if the previous dislocation has not healed completely.
- Loss of muscle strength.
- Unstable or arthritic knee following repeated injury.

PROBABLE OUTCOME—After the dislocation has been corrected and the knee has been surgically repaired, the knee may require immobilization in a long leg cast for 3 weeks. Complete healing of injured ligaments requires a minimum of 6 weeks. Avoid contact sports if all treatments are unsuccessful in restoring a strong, stable knee.

HOW TO TREAT

NOTE—Follow your doctor's instructions. These instructions are supplemental.

FIRST AID
- Keep the person warm with blankets to decrease the possibility of shock.
- Cut away clothing if possible. Don't move the injured area to remove clothing.
- Immobilize the knee, hip and ankle joints with padded splints.
- Follow instructions for R.I.C.E., the first letters of *rest, ice, compression* and *elevation.* See Appendix 1 for details.
- The doctor will realign the dislocated bones with surgery or, if possible, without. This should be done as soon as possible after injury. Within 6 hours after the dislocation, bleeding and displacement of body fluids may lead to shock. Also, many tissues lose their elasticity and become difficult to return to a normal position.

CONTINUING CARE—After removal of the cast:
- Use an ice pack 3 or 4 times a day. Wrap ice chips or cubes in a plastic bag, and wrap the bag in a moist towel. Place it over the injured area for 20 minutes at a time.
- You may try heat instead of ice if it feels better. Use heat lamps, hot soaks, hot showers, heating pads, or heat liniments and ointments.
- Take whirlpool treatments, if available.
- Massage gently and often to provide comfort and decrease swelling.

MEDICATION—Your doctor may prescribe:
- General anesthesia or muscle relaxants to make joint manipulation possible.
- Acetaminophen or aspirin to relieve moderate pain.
- Narcotic pain relievers for severe pain.
- Stool softeners to prevent constipation due to decreased activity.
- Antibiotics to fight infection following surgery.

ACTIVITY
- Walk on crutches while the cast is in place.
- Resume usual activities gradually after surgery.
- Begin weight-bearing and reconditioning of the knee after clearance from your doctor.
- Don't drive until healing is complete.

DIET
- Drink only water before manipulation or surgery to correct the dislocation. Solid food in your stomach makes vomiting while under general anesthesia more hazardous.
- During recovery, eat a well-balanced diet that includes extra protein, such as meat, fish, poultry, cheese, milk and eggs. Increase fiber and fluid intake to prevent constipation that may result from decreased activity.

REHABILITATION
- Begin daily rehabilitation exercises after clearance from your doctor.
- Use ice massage for 10 minutes before and after workouts. Fill a large Styrofoam cup with water and freeze. Tear a small amount of foam from the top so ice protrudes. Massage firmly over the injured area in a circle about the size of a softball.
- See page 460 for rehabilitation exercises.

CALL YOUR DOCTOR IF

- You have symptoms of a dislocated knee, even if it repositions itself. Call immediately if the leg becomes numb, pale, or cold. This is an emergency!
- Any of the following occur after treatment or surgery:
  Nausea or vomiting.
  Swelling above or below the cast.
  Blue or gray skin color below the cast, particularly under the toenails.
  Numbness or complete loss of feeling below the knee.
  Increasing pain, swelling or drainage in the surgical area.
  Signs of infection (headache, muscle aches, dizziness, or a general ill feeling and fever).
  Constipation.
- New, unexplained symptoms develop. Drugs used in treatment may produce side effects.
- Knee dislocations that you can "pop" back into normal position occur repeatedly.

KNEE SPRAIN

GENERAL INFORMATION

DEFINITION—Violent overstretching of one or more ligaments in the knee. Sprains involving two or more ligaments cause considerably more disability than single-ligament sprains. When the ligament is overstretched, it becomes tense and gives way at its weakest point, either where it attaches to bone or within the ligament itself. If the ligament pulls loose a fragment of bone, it is called a *sprain-fracture*. There are 3 types of sprains:
- Mild (Grade I)—Tearing of some ligament fibers. There is no loss of function.
- Moderate (Grade II)—Rupture of a portion of the ligament, resulting in some loss of function.
- Severe (Grade III)—Complete rupture of the ligament or complete separation of ligament from bone. There is total loss of function. A severe sprain requires surgical repair.

BODY PARTS INVOLVED
- Any of the many ligaments in the knee.
- Tissue surrounding the sprain, including blood vessels, tendons, bone, periosteum (covering of bone) and muscles.

SIGNS & SYMPTOMS
- Severe pain at the time of injury.
- A feeling of popping or tearing inside the knee.
- Tenderness at the injury site.
- Swelling in the knee.
- Bruising that appears soon after injury.

CAUSES—Stress on a ligament that temporarily forces or pries the knee out of its normal location. Sprains occur frequently in runners, walkers, and those who jump in such sports as basketball, soccer, volleyball, skiing, and distance- or high-jumping. These athletes often accidentally land on the side of the foot.

RISK INCREASES WITH
- Contact, running and jumping sports.
- Previous knee injury.
- Obesity.
- Poor muscle conditioning.
- Inadequate protection from equipment.

HOW TO PREVENT
- Build your strength with a conditioning program appropriate for your sport.
- Warm up before practice or competition.
- Tape vulnerable joints before practice or competition.
- Wear proper protective shoes. A twist or injury to the foot can affect the knee.

WHAT TO EXPECT

APPROPRIATE HEALTH CARE
- Doctor's diagnosis.
- Application of tape, cast or elastic bandage.
- Self-care during rehabilitation.

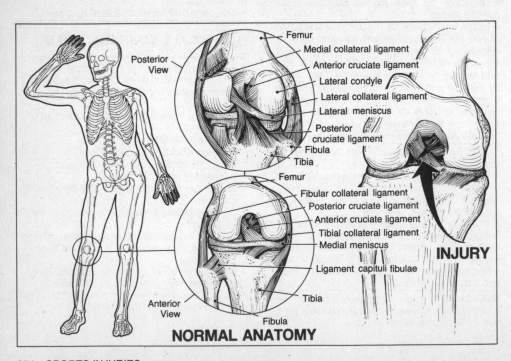

NORMAL ANATOMY

Posterior View

Femur
Medial collateral ligament
Anterior cruciate ligament
Lateral condyle
Lateral collateral ligament
Lateral meniscus
Posterior cruciate ligament
Fibula
Tibia

Femur
Fibular collateral ligament
Posterior cruciate ligament
Anterior cruciate ligament
Tibial collateral ligament
Medial meniscus
Ligament capituli fibulae
Tibia
Fibula

Anterior View

INJURY

- Physical therapy (moderate or severe sprain).
- Surgery (severe sprain).

DIAGNOSTIC MEASURES
- Your own observation of symptoms.
- Medical history and exam by a doctor.
- X-rays of the knee, hip and ankle to rule out fractures.

POSSIBLE COMPLICATIONS
- Prolonged healing time if usual activities are resumed too soon.
- Proneness to repeated injury.
- Inflammation at the ligament attachment to bone (periostitis).
- Prolonged disability (sometimes).
- Unstable or arthritic knee following repeated injury.

PROBABLE OUTCOME—If this is a first-time injury, proper care and sufficient healing time before resuming activity should prevent permanent disability. Ligaments have a poor blood supply, and torn ligaments require as much healing time as fractures. Average healing times are:
- Mild sprains—2 to 6 weeks.
- Moderate sprains—6 to 8 weeks.
- Severe sprains—8 weeks to 10 months.

 HOW TO TREAT

NOTE—Follow your doctor's instructions. These instructions are supplemental.

FIRST AID—Use instructions for R.I.C.E., the first letters of *rest, ice, compression* and *elevation.* See Appendix 1 for details.

CONTINUING CARE—The doctor usually applies a splint from the ankle to the groin to immobilize the sprained knee. If the doctor does not apply a cast, tape or elastic bandage:
- Continue using an ice pack 3 or 4 times a day. Place ice chips or cubes in a plastic bag. Wrap the bag in a moist towel, and place it over the injured knee. Use for 20 minutes at a time.
- Wrap the injured knee with an elasticized bandage.
- After 72 hours, apply heat instead of ice, if it feels better. Use heat lamps, hot soaks, hot showers, heating pads, or heat liniments or ointments.
- Take whirlpool treatments, if available.
- Massage gently and often to provide comfort and decrease swelling.

MEDICATION
- For minor discomfort, you may use:
  Aspirin, acetaminophen or ibuprofen.
  Topical liniments and ointments.
- Your doctor may prescribe:
  Stronger pain relievers.
  Injection of a long-acting local anesthetic to reduce pain.
  Injection of a corticosteroid, such as triamcinolone, to reduce inflammation.
  General anesthetic for surgery or arthroscopy (see Glossary) of the knee joint.

ACTIVITY—Resume your normal activities gradually after clearance from your doctor.

DIET—During recovery, eat a well-balanced diet that includes extra protein, such as meat, fish, poultry, cheese, milk and eggs. Increase fiber and fluid intake to prevent constipation that may result from decreased activity.

REHABILITATION
- Begin daily rehabilitation exercises when the cast or supportive wrapping is no longer necessary.
- Use ice massage for 10 minutes before and after exercise. Fill a large Styrofoam cup with water and freeze. Tear a small amount of foam from the top so ice protrudes. Massage firmly over the injured area in a circle about the size of a softball.
- See page 460 for rehabilitation exercises.

 CALL YOUR DOCTOR IF

- You have symptoms of a moderate or severe knee sprain, or a mild sprain persists longer than 2 weeks.
- Pain, swelling or bruising worsens despite treatment.
- Any of the following occur after casting or splinting:
  Pain, numbness or coldness below the cast or splint.
  Blue, gray or dusky toenails.
- Any of the following occur after surgery:
  Increased pain, swelling, redness, drainage or bleeding in the surgical area.
  Signs of infection (headache, muscle aches, dizziness, or a general ill feeling with fever).
- New, unexplained symptoms develop. Drugs used in treatment may produce side effects.

KNEE STRAIN

GENERAL INFORMATION

DEFINITION—Injury to the muscles or tendons that attach to bones in the knee. Muscles, tendons and bone comprise units. These units stabilize the knee joint and allow its motion. A strain occurs at a unit's weakest part. Strains are of 3 types:
- Mild (Grade I)—Slightly pulled muscle without tearing of muscle or tendon fibers. There is no loss of strength.
- Moderate (Grade II)—Tearing of fibers in a muscle, tendon or at the attachment to bone. Strength is diminished.
- Severe (Grade III)—Rupture of the muscle-tendon-bone attachment with separation of fibers. Severe strain requires surgical repair. Chronic strains are caused by overuse. Acute strains are caused by direct injury or overstress.

BODY PARTS INVOLVED
- Tendons and muscles in the knee region, especially the quadriceps and the hamstrings.
- Bones in the knee area, including the femur, patella, tibia and fibula.
- Soft tissue surrounding the strain, including nerves, periosteum (covering to bone), blood vessels and lymph vessels.

SIGNS & SYMPTOMS
- Pain when moving or stretching the knee.
- Muscle spasm in the knee area.
- Swelling over the injury.
- Loss of strength (moderate or severe strain).
- Crepitation ("crackling") feeling and sound when the injured area is pressed with fingers.
- Calcification of the muscle or tendon (visible with X-rays).
- Inflammation of the tendon sheath.

CAUSES
- Prolonged overuse of muscle-tendon units in the knee.
- Single violent blow or force applied to the knee.

RISK INCREASES WITH
- Contact sports.
- Sports that require quick starts, such as running races.
- Overly "tight" hamstrings or quadriceps muscles or poor muscle conditioning.
- Any cardiovascular medical problem that results in decreased circulation.
- Medical history of any bleeding disorder.
- Obesity.
- Poor nutrition.
- Previous knee injury.

HOW TO PREVENT
- Participate in a stretching, strengthening and conditioning program appropriate for your sport.
- Warm up before practice or competition.
- Tape the knee area before practice or competition.

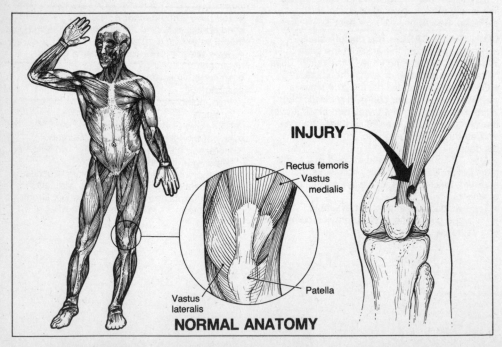

INJURY

Rectus femoris
Vastus medialis
Patella
Vastus lateralis

NORMAL ANATOMY

WHAT TO EXPECT

APPROPRIATE HEALTH CARE
- Doctor's diagnosis.
- Application of tape, plaster splints or casts (sometimes).
- Self-care during rehabilitation.
- Physical therapy (moderate or severe strain).
- Surgery (severe strain).

DIAGNOSTIC MEASURES
- Your own observation of symptoms.
- Medical history and exam by a doctor.
- X-rays of the knee to rule out fractures.

POSSIBLE COMPLICATIONS
- Prolonged healing time if activity is resumed too soon.
- Proneness to repeated injury.
- Unstable or arthritic knee following repeated injury.
- Inflammation at the attachment to bone (periostitis).
- Prolonged disability (sometimes).

PROBABLE OUTCOME—If this is a first-time injury, proper care and sufficient healing time before resuming activity should prevent permanent disability. Torn ligaments and tendons require as long to heal as fractured bones. Average healing times are:
- Mild strain—2 to 10 days.
- Moderate strain—10 days to 6 weeks.
- Severe strain—6 to 10 weeks.
If this is a repeat injury, complications listed above are more likely to occur.

 HOW TO TREAT

NOTE—Follow your doctor's instructions. These instructions are supplemental.

FIRST AID—Use instructions for R.I.C.E., the first letters of *rest, ice, compression* and *elevation.* See Appendix 1 for details.

CONTINUING CARE
- Use ice massage 3 or 4 times a day for 15 minutes at a time. Fill a large Styrofoam cup with water and freeze. Tear a small amount of foam from the top so ice protrudes. Massage firmly over the injured area in a circle about the size of a softball.

- After the first 24 hours, apply heat instead of ice, if it feels better. Use heat lamps, hot soaks, hot showers, heating pads, or heat liniments and ointments.
- Take whirlpool treatments, if available.
- Wrap the injured knee with an elasticized bandage between treatments.
- Massage gently and often to provide comfort and decrease swelling.

MEDICATION
- For minor discomfort, you may use:
  Aspirin, acetaminophen or ibuprofen.
  Topical liniments and ointments.
- Your doctor may prescribe:
  Stronger pain relievers.
  Injection of a long-acting local anesthetic to reduce pain.
  Injections of corticosteroids, such as triamcinolone, to reduce inflammation.

ACTIVITY
- For a moderate or severe strain, walk with crutches for at least 72 hours—longer with a cast or splints. See Appendix 3 (Safe Use of Crutches).
- Do frequent, gentle stretching exercises during the healing phase.
- Resume your normal activities gradually.

DIET—Eat a well-balanced diet that includes extra protein, such as meat, fish, poultry, cheese, milk and eggs. Increase fiber and fluid intake to prevent constipation that may result from decreased activity.

REHABILITATION—Begin daily rehabilitation exercises when supportive wrapping is no longer needed. Use ice massage for 10 minutes prior to exercise. See page 460 for rehabilitation exercises.

 CALL YOUR DOCTOR IF

- You have symptoms of a moderate or severe knee strain, or a mild strain persists longer than 10 days.
- Pain or swelling worsens despite treatment.
- The following occurs with a cast or splints:
  Pain, numbness or coldness below the injury.
  Dusky, blue or gray toenails.

KNEE SYNOVITIS WITH EFFUSION
("Water on the Knee")

 GENERAL INFORMATION

DEFINITION—Inflammation of the synovium, the smooth, lubricated lining of the knee. The synovium's lubricating fluid helps the knee move freely and prevents bone surfaces from rubbing against each other. Inflammation triggers an excess of fluid production and accumulation in the knee. Synovitis with effusion is often a complication of a knee injury or of collagen diseases, such as gout or rheumatoid arthritis.

BODY PARTS INVOLVED
- Synovium of the knee.
- Bones of the knee joint, including the patella (kneecap), femur (thigh bone), and tibia and fibula (lower leg bones).
- Ligaments and soft tissue of the knee joint, including the meniscus (cartilage of the knee).

SIGNS & SYMPTOMS
- Pain in the knee (sometimes).
- Swelling above the kneecap.
- Generalized swelling and redness if the inflammation is caused from infection or joint disease, such as gout, rather than from athletic injury.

CAUSES
- Single injury or repeated injury that damages any part of the knee.
- Bacterial infection (frequently gonorrhea).
- Metabolic disturbance, such as an acute attack of gout or rheumatoid arthritis.

RISK INCREASES WITH
- Participation in contact sports such as football, baseball, soccer or rugby.
- Repeated knee injury.
- Poor muscle strength or conditioning, which makes knee injury more likely.
- Medical history of gout, rheumatoid arthritis, or other inflammatory joint diseases.
- Infection in another joint.
- Vitamin or mineral deficiency, which makes complications following injury more likely.

HOW TO PREVENT
- Engage in a vigorous muscle strengthening and conditioning program prior to beginning regular sports participation. Warm up adequately before workouts or competition.
- Wear protective knee pads during participation in contact sports.

 WHAT TO EXPECT

APPROPRIATE HEALTH CARE
- Doctor's care, including aspiration of fluid from the knee. Because most knee synovitis with effusion is caused by injury to some part of the knee, treating the underlying injury is as important as treating the effusion.

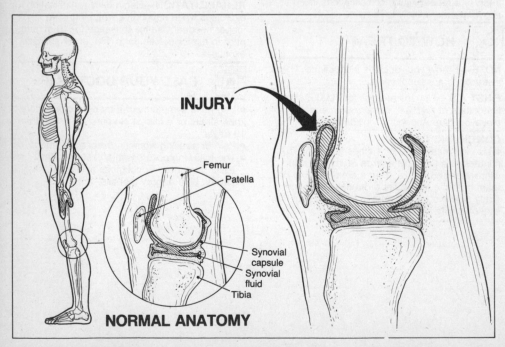

INJURY

Femur
Patella

Synovial capsule
Synovial fluid
Tibia

NORMAL ANATOMY

- Self-care during rehabilitation.
- Physical therapy.

DIAGNOSTIC MEASURES
- Your own observation of symptoms.
- Medical history and physical exam by a doctor.
- X-rays of the knee joint.
- Laboratory examination of fluid removed from the knee.

POSSIBLE COMPLICATIONS
- Prolonged healing time if activity is resumed too soon.
- Proneness to repeated knee injury.
- Unstable or arthritic knee following repeated bouts of synovitis.
- Chronic synovitis that may prevent athletic participation.

PROBABLE OUTCOME—Knee synovitis with effusion can usually be cured completely in 2 to 4 weeks with heat and corticosteroid injections. However, recurrences are common following minor knee injuries.

 HOW TO TREAT

NOTE—Follow your doctor's instructions. These instructions are supplemental.

FIRST AID—None. This condition develops gradually.

CONTINUING CARE
- Follow doctor's instructions for treatment of the underlying condition.
- Use an elastic bandage to compress the knee after fluid has been removed and between physical-therapy sessions.
- Apply heat frequently. Use heat lamps, hot soaks, hot showers, heating pads, or heat liniments and ointments.
- Take whirlpool treatments, if available.

- Massage gently and often to provide comfort and decrease swelling.

MEDICATION
- Your doctor may prescribe:
  Antibiotics if infection is present.
  Non-steroidal anti-inflammatory drugs or antigout medicine.
  Injection of a long-acting local anesthetic mixed with a corticosteroid to help reduce pain and inflammation.
- You may take aspirin or ibuprofen for minor discomfort.

ACTIVITY—Continue your usual activities during treatment if there is no pain, but protect the knee with tape and an elastic bandage during competitive sports. If you do have pain, reduce activities until pain subsides.

DIET—During recovery, eat a well-balanced diet that includes extra protein, such as meat, fish, poultry, cheese, milk and eggs. Increase fiber and fluid intake to prevent constipation that may result from decreased activity.

REHABILITATION
- Begin daily rehabilitation exercises when pain subsides.
- Use ice massage for 10 minutes before and after exercise. Fill a large Styrofoam cup with water and freeze. Tear a small amount of foam from the top so ice protrudes. Massage firmly over the injured area in a circle about the size of a softball.
- See page 460 for rehabilitation exercises.

 CALL YOUR DOCTOR IF

- Your knee becomes red, hot, swollen or painful.
- After aspiration of fluid from the knee, you develop signs of infection (headache, fever, muscle aches, dizziness or a general ill feeling).

KNEECAP (PATELLA) DISLOCATION

GENERAL INFORMATION

DEFINITION—A displacement of the patella (kneecap) so it no longer touches adjoining bones. Adolescents and young adults are most prone to this injury.

BODY PARTS INVOLVED
- Knee joint and patella.
- Femur and tibia, the bones of the lower leg.
- Soft tissue surrounding the dislocation, including nerves, periosteum (covering of bone), tendons, ligaments, muscles and blood vessels.

SIGNS & SYMPTOMS
- A feeling of the knee "giving way."
- Excruciating pain in the knee at the time of injury.
- Loss of function of the knee, and severe pain when attempting to move it.
- Visible deformity if the dislocated bones have locked in the dislocated position. Bones may spontaneously reposition themselves and leave no deformity, but damage is the same.
- Tenderness over the dislocation.
- Swelling and bruising around the knee.
- Numbness or paralysis below the dislocation from pressure, pinching or cutting of blood vessels or nerves.

CAUSES
- Direct blow to the knee.
- End result of a severe knee sprain.

- Powerful muscle contraction.
- "Cutting" moves (movements in which an athlete changes direction suddenly, causing bones in the knee joint to rotate and dislocate the patella).

RISK INCREASES WITH
- Person with a wide pelvis and "knock-knees."
- Contact sports such as football or soccer.
- Running sports.
- Jumping sports such as gymnastics and basketball.
- Previous knee sprains.
- Repeated knee injury of any sort.
- Arthritis of any type (rheumatoid, gout).
- Poor muscle conditioning.
- Congenital abnormalities of the knee joint.

HOW TO PREVENT
- Build your overall strength and muscle tone with a long-term conditioning program appropriate for your sport. Include special exercises for strengthening the knee.
- Warm up adequately before physical activity.
- After injury, protect the knee from reinjury by wearing wrapped elastic bandages, tape wraps, knee pads or special support sleeves.

WHAT TO EXPECT

APPROPRIATE HEALTH CARE
- Doctor's treatment. This will include manipulation of the joint to reposition the bones.

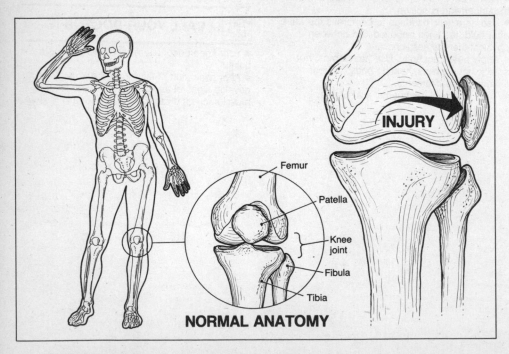

INJURY

Femur

Patella

Knee joint

Fibula

Tibia

NORMAL ANATOMY

● Surgery (usually) to restore normal knee-joint function.

DIAGNOSTIC MEASURES
● Your own observation of symptoms.
● Medical history and exam by a doctor.
● X-rays of the knee joint and adjacent bones.

POSSIBLE COMPLICATIONS
At the time of injury:
● Shock.
● Pressure on or injury to nearby nerves, ligaments, tendons, muscles, blood vessels or connective tissue causing numbness, coldness and paleness in the leg or foot.
● Excessive internal bleeding around the kneecap.
After surgery:
● Impaired blood supply to the dislocated area.
● Infection introduced during surgical treatment.
● Recurrent dislocations, particularly if the previous dislocation has not healed completely.
● Unstable or arthritic knee joint following repeated injury.

PROBABLE OUTCOME—After treatment or surgery to correct the dislocation, the joint may be immobilized with a cast for 6 to 8 weeks. Complete healing of injured ligaments requires a minimum of 6 weeks.

 HOW TO TREAT

NOTE—Follow your doctor's instructions. These instructions are supplemental.

FIRST AID
● Keep the person warm with blankets to decrease the possibility of shock.
● Cut away clothing if possible. Don't move the injured area to remove clothing.
● Immobilize the knee, hip and ankle joints with padded splints.
● Follow instructions for R.I.C.E., the first letters of *rest, ice, compression* and *elevation.* See Appendix 1 for details.
● The doctor will realign the dislocated bones with surgery or, if possible, without. This should be done as soon as possible after injury. Within 6 hours after the dislocation, bleeding and displacement of body fluids may lead to shock. Also, many tissues lose their elasticity and become difficult to return to a normal position.

CONTINUING CARE—After cast removal:
● Use an ice pack 3 or 4 times a day. Wrap ice chips or cubes in a plastic bag, and wrap the bag in a moist towel. Place it over the injured area for 20 minutes at a time.
● You may try heat instead of ice if it feels better. Use heat lamps, hot soaks, hot showers, heating pads, or heat liniments and ointments.
● Take whirlpool treatments, if available.
● Massage gently and often to provide comfort and decrease swelling.

MEDICATION—Your doctor may prescribe:
● General anesthesia or muscle relaxants to make joint manipulation possible.
● Acetaminophen to relieve moderate pain.
● Narcotic pain relievers for severe pain.
● Stool softeners to prevent constipation due to decreased activity.
● Antibiotics to fight infection.

ACTIVITY
● Walk on crutches while the cast is in place.
● Resume usual activities gradually after surgery.
● Begin weight-bearing and reconditioning of the knee after clearance from your doctor.
● Don't drive until healing is complete.

DIET
● Drink only water before manipulation or surgery to correct the dislocation. Solid food in your stomach makes vomiting while under general anesthesia more hazardous.
● During recovery, eat a well-balanced diet that includes extra protein, such as meat, fish, poultry, cheese, milk and eggs. Increase fiber and fluid intake to prevent constipation that may result from decreased activity.

REHABILITATION
● Begin daily rehabilitation exercises when supportive wrapping is no longer needed.
● Use ice massage for 10 minutes before and after workouts. Fill a large Styrofoam cup with water and freeze. Tear a small amount of foam from the top so ice protrudes. Massage firmly in a circle over the injured area.
● See page 460 for rehabilitation exercises.

 CALL YOUR DOCTOR IF

● You have symptoms of a dislocated kneecap. Call immediately if the leg becomes numb, pale, or cold. This is an emergency!
● Any of the following occur after treatment or surgery:
  Swelling above or below the cast.
  Blue or gray skin color below the cast, particularly under the toenails.
  Numbness or complete loss of feeling below the knee.
  Increasing pain, swelling or drainage in the surgical area.
  Signs of infection (headache, muscle aches, dizziness, or a general ill feeling and fever).
  Nausea or vomiting.
  Constipation.
● New, unexplained symptoms develop. Drugs used in treatment may produce side effects.
● Kneecap dislocations that you can "pop" back into normal position occur repeatedly.

KNEECAP (PATELLA) FRACTURE

GENERAL INFORMATION

DEFINITION—A complete or incomplete break in the upper or lower portion of the patella (kneecap). Most fractures of the patella are accompanied by sprain or rupture of ligaments or tendons attached to the patella.

BODY PARTS INVOLVED
- Patella.
- Knee joint.
- Soft tissue surrounding the fracture site, including nerves, tendons, ligaments and blood vessels.

SIGNS & SYMPTOMS
- Severe pain at the fracture site.
- Pain when moving the knee forward or backward.
- Swelling around the fracture.
- Visible deformity if the fracture is complete and bone fragments separate enough to distort normal knee contours.
- "Catching" or locking of the knee.
- Tenderness when pressing the kneecap against underlying bones.
- Numbness and coldness beyond the fracture site if the blood supply is impaired.

CAUSES—Direct blow or indirect stress to the kneecap. Indirect stress may be caused by twisting or violent muscle contraction.

RISK INCREASES WITH
- Contact sports, especially football.
- History of bone or joint disease, especially osteoporosis.
- Obesity.
- Poor nutrition, especially calcium deficiency.
- If surgery or anesthesia is needed, surgical risk increases with smoking and use of drugs, including mind-altering drugs, muscle relaxants, antihypertensives, tranquilizers, sleep inducers, insulin, sedatives, beta-adrenergic blockers or corticosteroids.

HOW TO PREVENT
- Build adequate muscle strength and achieve good conditioning prior to exercise, athletic practice or competition. Increased muscle mass helps protect bones and underlying tissue.
- Use appropriate protective equipment, such as knee pads, when participating in contact sports.

WHAT TO EXPECT

APPROPRIATE HEALTH CARE
- Doctor's treatment to manipulate and set the broken bones.
- Hospitalization (sometimes) for anesthesia and surgery to remove the fractured piece of bone and repair the damage to soft tissue.
- Whirlpool, ultrasound or massage after healing (to displace fluid from the injured joint space).

DIAGNOSTIC MEASURES
- Your own observation of symptoms.

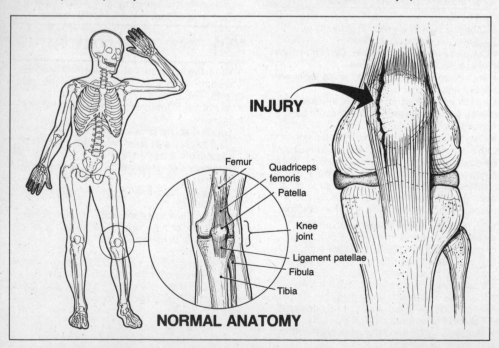

INJURY

Femur
Quadriceps femoris
Patella
Knee joint
Ligament patellae
Fibula
Tibia

NORMAL ANATOMY

- Medical history and exam by a doctor.
- X-rays of the knee joint.

POSSIBLE COMPLICATIONS

At the time of injury:
- Shock.
- Pressure on or injury to nearby nerves, ligaments, tendons, muscles, blood vessels or connective tissues.

After treatment or surgery:
- Delayed union or non-union of the fracture.
- Impaired blood supply to the fracture site.
- Avascular necrosis (death of bone cells) due to interruption of the blood supply.
- Arrest of normal bone growth in children.
- Infection in open fractures (skin broken over fracture site), or at the incision if surgical setting was necessary.
- Proneness to repeated knee problems. After healing, the fracture often leaves a roughened contact surface in the kneecap.
- Unstable or arthritic knee following repeated injury.
- Prolonged healing time if activity is resumed too soon.
- Problems caused by casts. See Appendix 2 (Care of Casts).

PROBABLE OUTCOME—The average healing time for this fracture is 6 to 8 weeks. Healing is considered complete when there is no motion at the fracture site and when X-rays show complete bone union.

 ## HOW TO TREAT

NOTE—Follow your doctor's instructions. These instructions are supplemental.

FIRST AID
- Keep the person warm with blankets to decrease the possibility of shock.
- Cut away clothing, if possible. Don't move the injured knee to remove clothing.
- Use a padded splint to immobilize the hip joint and the ankle joint before transporting the injured person to the doctor's office or emergency facility.
- Follow instructions for R.I.C.E., the first letters of *rest, ice, compression* and *elevation*. See Appendix 1 for details.
- The doctor will realign and set the broken bones with surgery or, if possible, without. Manipulation should be done as soon as possible after injury. Six or more hours after the fracture, bleeding and displacement of body fluids may lead to shock. Also, many tissues lose their elasticity and become difficult to return to a normal position.

CONTINUING CARE
- Immobilization will be necessary. A rigid cast will be used from the upper leg to the ankle.

- After the cast is removed, use frequent ice massage. Fill a large Styrofoam cup with water and freeze. Tear a small amount of foam from the top so ice protrudes. Massage firmly over the injured area in a circle about the size of a softball. Do this for 15 minutes at a time, 3 or 4 times a day, and before workouts or competition.
- Apply heat instead of ice, if it feels better. Use heat lamps, hot soaks, hot showers, heating pads, or heat liniments or ointments.
- Take whirlpool treatments, if available.

MEDICATION—Your doctor may prescribe:
- General anesthesia or local anesthesia for surgery to remove fractured patella fragments.
- Narcotic or synthetic narcotic pain relievers for severe pain.
- Stool softeners to prevent constipation due to inactivity.
- Acetaminophen (available without prescription) for mild pain after initial treatment.

ACTIVITY
- Actively exercise all muscle groups not immobilized. The resulting muscle contractions promote fracture alignment and hasten healing.
- Resume normal activities gradually after treatment. Don't drive until healing is complete.

DIET
- Drink only water before manipulation or surgery to treat the fracture. Solid food in your stomach makes vomiting while under anesthesia more hazardous.
- During recovery, eat a well-balanced diet that includes extra protein, such as meat, fish, poultry, cheese, milk and eggs. Increase fiber and fluid intake to prevent constipation that may result from decreased activity.

REHABILITATION—Begin reconditioning the injured knee after clearance from your doctor. See page 460 for rehabilitation exercises.

 ## CALL YOUR DOCTOR IF

- You have signs or symptoms of a kneecap fracture.
- Any of the following occur after surgery or other treatment:
  Increased pain, swelling or drainage in the surgical area.
  Signs of infection (headache, muscle aches, dizziness, or a general ill feeling and fever).
  Nausea or vomiting.
  Swelling above or below the cast.
  Blue or gray skin color beyond the cast, particularly under the toenails.
  Numbness or complete loss of feeling below the fracture site.
  Constipation.

LEG CONTUSION, LOWER LEG

GENERAL INFORMATION

DEFINITION—Bruising of the skin and underlying tissues of the lower leg due to a direct blow. Contusions cause bleeding from ruptured small capillaries that allow blood to infiltrate muscles, tendons or other soft tissue. The lower leg is particularly susceptible to contusions because it is frequently exposed to direct blows. If the blow is over the tibia (shin bone), it is much more likely to be severe.

BODY PARTS INVOLVED
● Lower-leg tissues, including blood vessels, muscles, tendons, nerves, covering to bone (periosteum) and connective tissue.
● The peroneal nerve where it wraps around the upper portion of the fibula. Injury to the nerve can lead to painful neuritis or temporary paralysis and a dropped foot.

SIGNS & SYMPTOMS
● Swelling—either superficial or deep.
● Pain at the contusion site.
● Feeling of firmness when pressure is exerted on the injury.
● Tenderness.
● Discoloration under the skin, beginning with redness and progressing to the characteristic "black and blue" bruise.
● Restricted leg function proportional to the extent of injury.

● Feeling an "electric shock" followed by temporary muscle paralysis, causing the foot to drop.

CAUSES—Direct blow to the leg, usually from a blunt object.

RISK INCREASES WITH
● Violent contact sports—especially when lower legs are not adequately protected.
● Medical history of any bleeding disorder such as hemophilia.
● Poor nutrition, including vitamin deficiency.
● Use of anticoagulants or aspirin.

HOW TO PREVENT—Wear appropriate protective devices, such as an elastic bandage over felt or sponge rubber, if there is risk of a lower-leg contusion during athletic activity.

WHAT TO EXPECT

APPROPRIATE HEALTH CARE
● Doctor's care unless the contusion is quite small.
● Self-care for minor contusions, and for serious contusions during rehabilitation.
● Physical therapy for serious contusions.

DIAGNOSTIC MEASURES
● Your own observation of symptoms.
● Medical history and physical exam by a doctor for all except minor injuries.

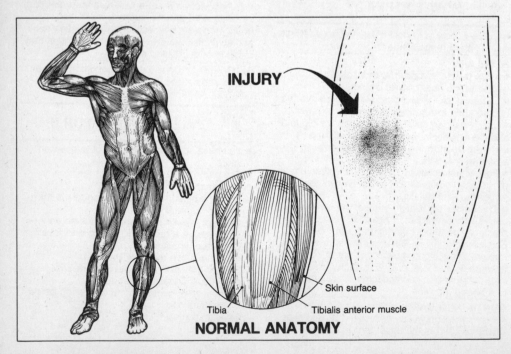

INJURY

Skin surface

Tibia

Tibialis anterior muscle

NORMAL ANATOMY

- X-rays of the lower leg, ankle and knee to assess total injury to soft tissue and to rule out the possibility of underlying fractures. The total extent of injury may not be apparent for 48 to 72 hours.

POSSIBLE COMPLICATIONS
- Excessive bleeding leading to disability. Infiltrative-type bleeding can sometimes lead to calcification and impaired function of the injured muscle.
- Prolonged healing time if usual activities are resumed too soon.
- Infection if skin over the contusion is broken.

PROBABLE OUTCOME—Healing time varies with the extent of injury, but average healing time for a lower-leg contusion is 1 to 2 weeks.

 # HOW TO TREAT

NOTE—Follow your doctor's instructions. These instructions are supplementa1.

FIRST AID—Use instructions for R.I.C.E., the first letters of *rest, ice, compression* and *elevation*. See Appendix 1 for details.

CONTINUING CARE
- Wrap an elasticized bandage over a sponge-rubber donut on the injured area. Keep the area compressed for about 72 hours.
- Continue ice massage. Fill a large Styrofoam cup with water and freeze. Tear a small amount of foam from the top so ice protrudes. Massage gently over the injured area in a circle about the size of a softball. Do this for 15 minutes at a time, 3 or 4 times a day, and before workouts or competition.

- After 72 hours, apply heat instead of ice if it feels better. Use heat lamps, hot soaks, hot showers, heating pads, heat liniments or ointments, or whirlpool treatments.
- Massage gently and often to provide comfort and decrease swelling.

MEDICATION
- For minor discomfort, you may use: Acetaminophen or ibuprofen. Topical liniments and ointments.
- Your doctor may prescribe stronger medicine for pain.

ACTIVITY—Begin activities slowly and stop exercise as soon as pain begins. Increase activity as healing progresses.

DIET—Eat a well-balanced diet that includes extra protein, such as meat, fish, poultry, cheese, milk and eggs. Your doctor may prescribe vitamin and mineral supplements to promote healing.

REHABILITATION—Begin daily rehabilitation exercises when supportive wrapping is no longer needed. See page 462 for rehabilitation exercises.

 # CALL YOUR DOCTOR IF

- You have a lower-leg contusion that doesn't improve in 1 or 2 days.
- Skin is broken and signs of infection (drainage, increasing pain, fever, headache, muscle aches, dizziness or a general ill feeling) occur.
- Signs appear of peroneal-nerve injury (paralysis, dropped foot or loss of sensation in the foot).

LEG EXOSTOSIS

GENERAL INFORMATION

DEFINITION—An overgrowth of bone in the tibia (the larger bone in the lower leg). It extends out from the bone like a spur and is visible on X-rays. An exostosis occurs at the site of repeated injury, usually from direct blows. This benign overgrowth of bone can be mistaken for a bone tumor.

BODY PARTS INVOLVED
- Tibia.
- Knee joint (sometimes).
- Ankle joint (sometimes).
- Soft tissue surrounding the exostosis, including nerves, lymph vessels, blood vessels and periosteum (covering of bone).

SIGNS & SYMPTOMS
- No symptoms for mild cases.
- Pain and tenderness in the lower leg at the site of the exostosis.
- Extreme sensitivity to pressure or even minor injury.
- Change in contour of the tibia, ranging from a slight lump to the appearance of a large calcified spur (1cm or more in length). In the worst cases, the exostosis may break away and feel like a distinct foreign body. An X-ray will show it to be loose in the tissues of the lower leg.

- "Locking" of the lower leg, if a tendon catches on the exostosis during exercise.

CAUSES
- Repeated injury (contusions, sprains or strains) that involve the periosteum—the covering to bone (tibia) in the lower leg.
- Chronic irritation to an already damaged area.

RISK INCREASES WITH
- Participation in contact sports such as football, basketball or soccer.
- History of bone or joint disease, such as osteomyelitis, osteomalacia or osteoporosis.
- Vitamin or mineral deficiency.
- Poor muscle strength or conditioning, which makes injury more likely.
- If surgery or anesthesia are needed, surgical risk increases with smoking, use of mind-altering drugs, muscle relaxants, tranquilizers, sleep inducers, insulin, sedatives, beta-adrenergic blockers or corticosteroids.

HOW TO PREVENT
- Engage in vigorous muscle strengthening and conditioning prior to beginning regular sports participation.
- Warm up adequately before competition or workouts to decrease the risk of injury.
- Allow adequate recovery time for any leg, ankle or knee injury.
- Wear protective equipment, such as shin guards and knee pads, for participation in contact sports.

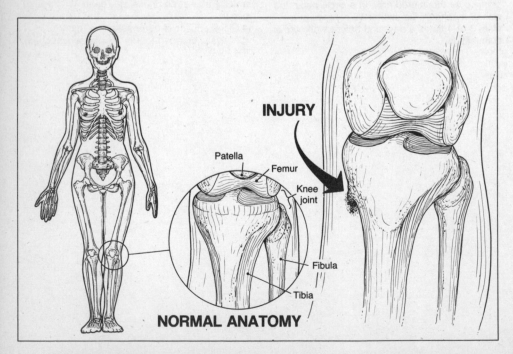

INJURY

Patella

Femur

Knee joint

Fibula

Tibia

NORMAL ANATOMY

- Practice and learn the proper moves and techniques for your sport to decrease the risk of injury.

WHAT TO EXPECT

APPROPRIATE HEALTH CARE
- Doctor's care.
- Surgery (sometimes) to remove the exostosis.
- Self-care during rehabilitation.
- Physical therapy.

DIAGNOSTIC MEASURES
- Your own observation of signs and symptoms.
- Medical history and physical exam by a doctor.
- X-rays of the lower leg, ankle and knee.

POSSIBLE COMPLICATIONS
- Overlooking a mild exostosis that produces no symptoms, despite signs of diminished performance. Athletes and coaches frequently assume that decreased performance is from loss of competitive drive or emotional causes, rather than from the physical disability that actually exists.
- Prolonged healing time if activity is resumed too soon.
- Proneness to repeated injury.
- Unstable or arthritic knee or ankle following repeated injury.
- Pressure on or injury to nearby nerves, ligaments, tendons, blood vessels or connective tissue.
- Impaired blood supply to the injured area.

PROBABLE OUTCOME—Lower-leg exostosis usually causes no disability if it is treated properly. Treatment usually involves resting the injured leg for 2 to 4 weeks, heat treatments, corticosteroid injections and protection against additional injury. In a few cases, surgery is necessary to remove the exostosis.

HOW TO TREAT

NOTE—Follow your doctor's instructions. These instructions are supplemental.

FIRST AID—None. This condition develops gradually.

CONTINUING CARE
- Rest the injured area. Use splints or crutches if needed.
- Apply heat frequently. Use heat lamps, hot soaks, hot showers, heating pads, or heat liniments and ointments.
- Take whirlpool treatments, if available.
- Follow instructions under How to Prevent to avoid a recurrence of the injury.

MEDICATION
- Medicine usually is not necessary for this disorder. For minor pain, you may use non-prescription drugs such as aspirin.
- If surgery is necessary, your doctor may prescribe:
  Non-steroidal anti-inflammatory drugs to help control swelling.
  Stronger pain relievers.
  Antibiotics to fight infection.

ACTIVITY—Decrease activity for 2 to 4 weeks. If surgery is necessary, resume normal activity gradually.

DIET—During recovery, eat a well-balanced diet that includes extra protein, such as meat, fish, poultry, cheese, milk and eggs. Increase fiber and fluid intake to prevent constipation that may result from decreased activity. Your doctor may suggest vitamin and mineral supplements to promote healing.

REHABILITATION
- Begin daily rehabilitation exercises when movement is comfortable.
- Use ice massage for 10 minutes before and 10 minutes after exercise. Fill a large Styrofoam cup with water and freeze. Tear a small amount of foam from the top so ice protrudes. Massage firmly over the injured area in a circle about the size of a softball.
- See pages 460 and 462 for rehabilitation exercises.

CALL YOUR DOCTOR IF

- You have symptoms of lower-leg exostosis.
- Any of the following occur after surgery:
  Increased pain, swelling, redness, drainage, or bleeding in the surgical area.
  Signs of infection (headache, muscle aches, dizziness, or a general ill feeling and fever).
  New, unexplained symptoms. Drugs used in treatment may cause side effects.

LEG FRACTURE, FIBULA

GENERAL INFORMATION

DEFINITION—A complete or incomplete break in the fibula, the smaller of the two bones of the lower leg. Fractures of the fibula are not uncommon, and displacement is seldom severe. They sometimes accompany severe ankle sprains.

BODY PARTS INVOLVED
- Fibula.
- Soft tissue surrounding the fracture site, including nerves, tendons, ligaments and blood vessels.

SIGNS & SYMPTOMS
- Severe pain at the fracture site.
- Swelling of soft tissue surrounding the fracture.
- Visible deformity if the fracture is complete and bone fragments separate enough to distort normal leg contours.
- Tenderness to the touch.
- Numbness or coldness in the foot if the blood supply is impaired.

CAUSES—Direct blow or indirect stress to the bone. Indirect stress may be caused by twisting, turning quickly or violent muscle contraction.

RISK INCREASES WITH
- Contact sports such as football, soccer or hockey.
- History of bone or joint disease, especially osteoporosis.
- Obesity.
- Poor nutrition, especially calcium deficiency.

HOW TO PREVENT—Build adequate muscle strength and achieve good conditioning prior to exercise, athletic practice or competition. Increased muscle mass helps protect bones and underlying tissue.

WHAT TO EXPECT

APPROPRIATE HEALTH CARE
- Doctor's diagnosis. Setting of the fracture is usually not necessary.
- Self-care during rehabilitation.

DIAGNOSTIC MEASURES
- Your own observation of symptoms.
- Medical history and physical exam by a doctor.
- X-rays of injured areas, including the knee and ankle.

POSSIBLE COMPLICATIONS
- Pressure on or injury to nearby nerves, ligaments, tendons, muscles, blood vessels, or connective tissues.
- Delayed union or non-union of the fracture.
- Impaired blood supply to the fracture site.
- Arrest of normal bone growth in children.
- Shortening of the injured bones.
- Prolonged healing time if activity is resumed too soon.
- Proneness to repeated injury.

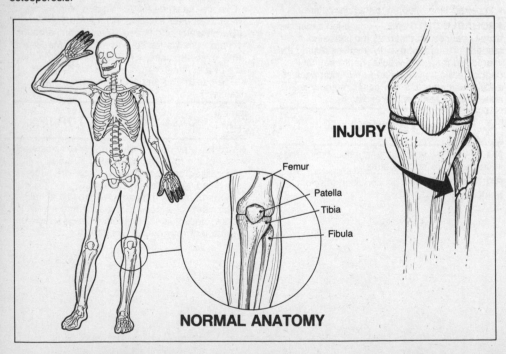

Femur
Patella
Tibia
Fibula

INJURY

NORMAL ANATOMY

PROBABLE OUTCOME—It is impossible to predict exactly how long it will take for any fracture to heal. Variable factors include age, sex and previous state of health and conditioning. The average healing time for this fracture is 4 to 6 weeks. Healing is considered complete when there is no motion at the fracture site and when X-rays show complete bone union.

 HOW TO TREAT

NOTE—Follow your doctor's instructions. These instructions are supplemental.

FIRST AID
- Keep the person warm with blankets to decrease the possibility of shock.
- Cut away clothing, if possible. Don't move the injured area to remove clothing.
- Follow instructions for R.I.C.E., the first letters of *rest, ice, compression* and *elevation*. See Appendix 1 for details.

CONTINUING CARE
- Setting the broken bone for a fibula fracture is usually not necessary. The tibia (the big bone adjacent to the fibula) provides immobilization.
- Fibula fractures usually require only a snug, toe-to-knee cotton elastic bandage. If pain is severe, a walking plaster cast below the knee may be necessary for about 5 weeks.
- After the bandage or cast is removed, use frequent ice massage. Fill a large Styrofoam cup with water and freeze. Tear a small amount of foam from the top so ice protrudes. Massage firmly over the injured area in a circle about the size of a softball. Do this for 15 minutes at a time, 3 or 4 times a day.
- Apply heat instead of ice, if it feels better. Use heat lamps, hot soaks, hot showers, heating pads, or heat liniments and ointments.
- Take whirlpool treatments, if available.

MEDICATION—Your doctor may prescribe:
- Narcotic or synthetic narcotic pain relievers for severe pain.
- Stool softeners to prevent constipation due to inactivity.
- Acetaminophen (available without prescription) for mild pain after initial treatment.

ACTIVITY
- Actively exercise all muscle groups not immobilized. These muscle contractions promote fracture alignment and hasten healing.
- Begin walking and light running when there is no pain or tenderness.
- Resume normal activities gradually after treatment. Don't drive until healing is complete.

DIET—During recovery, eat a well-balanced diet that includes extra protein, such as meat, fish, poultry, cheese, milk and eggs. Increase fiber and fluid intake to prevent constipation that may result from decreased activity.

REHABILITATION
- Begin reconditioning the injured area after clearance from your doctor. Use ice massage for 10 minutes before and after workouts.
- See page 462 for rehabilitation exercises.

 CALL YOUR DOCTOR IF

- You have signs or symptoms of a leg fracture.
- Any of the following occur after surgery or other treatment:
  Signs of infection (headache, muscle aches, dizziness, or a general ill feeling and fever).
  Swelling above or below the bandage or cast.
  Change in skin color to blue or gray beyond the cast, particularly under the toenails.
  Numbness or complete loss of feeling below the fracture site.
  Nausea or vomiting.
  Constipation.

LEG FRACTURE, TIBIA

GENERAL INFORMATION

DEFINITION—A complete or incomplete break in the tibia, one of the two large bones of the leg between the knee and ankle.

BODY PARTS INVOLVED
- Tibia.
- Knee or ankle joints.
- Soft tissue around the fracture site, including nerves, tendons, ligaments and blood vessels.

SIGNS & SYMPTOMS
- Severe leg pain at the time of injury.
- Swelling of soft tissue around the fracture.
- Visible deformity if the fracture is complete and the bone fragments separate enough to distort normal leg contours.
- Tenderness to the touch.
- Numbness and coldness in the leg and foot beyond the fracture site if the blood supply is impaired.

CAUSES
- Direct blow to the leg.
- Weakening of the bone from repeated stress, resulting in a stress fracture that progresses to a complete fracture. This is especially common in joggers, marathon runners and walkers.
- Indirect stress caused by twisting or violent muscle contraction.

RISK INCREASES WITH
- Contact sports.
- History of bone or joint disease.
- Obesity.
- Severe ankle sprain.
- Poor nutrition, especially calcium deficiency.
- If surgery or anesthesia are needed, surgical risk increases with smoking and use of drugs, including mind-altering drugs, muscle relaxants, antihypertensives, tranquilizers, sleep inducers, insulin, sedatives, beta-adrenergic blockers or corticosteroids.

HOW TO PREVENT
- Build your strength with a good conditioning program before beginning regular athletic practice or competition. Increased muscle mass helps protect bones and underlying tissue.
- Use appropriate protective equipment, including good running shoes for running, and shin guards for participation in contact sports.

WHAT TO EXPECT

APPROPRIATE HEALTH CARE
- Doctor's treatment.
- Hospitalization (sometimes) for anesthesia and surgery to set the fracture.
- Whirlpool, ultrasound, or massage after healing (to displace excess fluid from the knee and ankle).

DIAGNOSTIC MEASURES
- Your own observation of symptoms.
- Medical history and exam by a doctor.
- X-rays of the injured area, including the knee joint above and the ankle joint below.

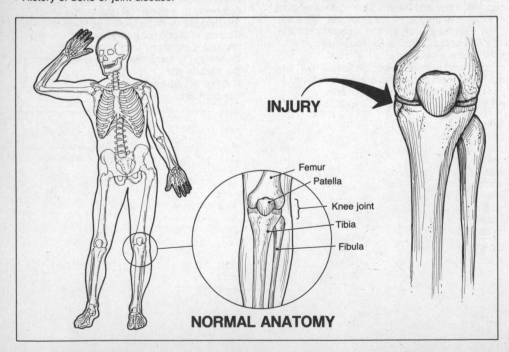

INJURY

Femur
Patella
Knee joint
Tibia
Fibula

NORMAL ANATOMY

POSSIBLE COMPLICATIONS

At the time of injury:
● Shock.
● Pressure on or injury to nearby nerves, ligaments, tendons, muscles, blood vessels or connective tissues.

After treatment or surgery:
● Delayed union or non-union of the fracture.
● Impaired blood supply to the fracture site.
● Avascular necrosis (death of bone cells) due to interruption of the blood supply.
● Shortening of the injured bones.
● Arrest of normal bone growth in children.
● Infection in open fractures (skin broken over fracture site), or at the incision if surgical setting was necessary.
● Unstable or arthritic ankle or knee joint if the fracture is close to either.
● Prolonged healing time if activity is resumed too soon.
● Proneness to repeated leg injury.
● Problems caused by casts. See Appendix 2 (Care of Casts).

PROBABLE OUTCOME—The average healing time for this fracture is 6 to 8 weeks. Healing is considered complete when there is no motion at the fracture site and when X-rays show complete bone union.

HOW TO TREAT

NOTE—Follow your doctor's instructions. These instructions are supplemental.

FIRST AID
● Keep the person warm with blankets to decrease the possibility of shock.
● Cut away clothing, if possible, but don't move the injured leg to do so.
● Follow instructions for R.I.C.E., the first letters of *rest, ice, compression* and *elevation.* See Appendix 1 for details.
● The doctor will set (realign) the broken bones with surgery or, if possible, without. Surgery is seldom performed unless the skin at the injury site is broken. In tibial fractures, the segments are sometimes fixed together with screws or metal plates. Realignment should be done as soon as possible after injury. Six or more hours after the fracture, bleeding and displacement of body fluids may lead to shock. Also, many tissues lose their elasticity and become difficult to return to a normal position.

CONTINUING CARE
● Immobilization will be necessary. A rigid cast is placed around the injured leg to immobilize the knee and ankle.
● After 48 hours, localized heat promotes healing by increasing blood circulation in the injured area. Use a heat lamp or heating pads so heat can penetrate the cast.
● After the cast is removed, use frequent ice massage. Fill a large Styrofoam cup with water and freeze. Tear a small amount of foam from the top so ice protrudes. Massage firmly in a circle over the injured area.

MEDICATION—Your doctor may prescribe:
● General anesthesia, local anesthesia, or muscle relaxants to make bone manipulation and fixation of bone fragments possible.
● Narcotic or synthetic narcotic pain relievers for severe pain.
● Stool softeners to prevent constipation due to inactivity.
● Acetaminophen for mild pain.

ACTIVITY
● Learn to walk with crutches. See Appendix 3 (Safe Use of Crutches).
● Actively exercise all muscle groups not immobilized. These muscle contractions promote fracture alignment and hasten healing.
● Begin reconditioning the injured leg after clearance from your doctor.
● Resume normal activities gradually after treatment. Don't drive until healing is complete.

DIET
● Drink only water before manipulation or surgery to treat the fracture. Solid food in your stomach makes vomiting while under anesthesia more hazardous.
● During recovery, eat a well-balanced diet that includes extra protein, such as meat, fish, poultry, cheese, milk and eggs. Increase fiber and fluid intake to prevent constipation that may result from decreased activity.

REHABILITATION—Begin daily rehabilitation exercises when supportive wrapping is no longer needed. Use ice massage for 10 minutes prior to exercise. See page 462 for rehabilitation exercises.

CALL YOUR DOCTOR IF

● You have signs or symptoms of a tibia fracture.
● Any of the following occurs after surgery or other treatment:
  Increased pain, swelling or drainage in the surgical area.
  Signs of infection (headache, muscle aches, dizziness, or a general ill feeling and fever).
  Swelling above or below the cast.
  Blue or gray skin color beyond the cast, especially under the toenails.
  Loss of feeling below the fracture site.
  Nausea or vomiting.
  Constipation.

LEG HEMATOMA, LOWER LEG

GENERAL INFORMATION

DEFINITION—A collection of pooled blood in a small area of the lower leg. Hematoma in the lower leg can be quite disabling. A large hematoma in the enclosed space over the tibia (the "shin bone") can be a surgical emergency.

BODY PARTS INVOLVED
● Lower leg.
● Soft tissue surrounding the hematoma, including nerves, tendons, ligaments, muscles and blood vessels.

SIGNS & SYMPTOMS
● Swelling over the injury site.
● Fluctuance (feeling of tenseness to the touch, like pushing on an overinflated balloon).
● Tenderness.
● Redness that progresses through several color changes—purple, green-yellow, yellow—before it completely heals.

CAUSES—Direct injury, usually with a blunt object. Bleeding into tissue causes the surrounding tissue to be pushed away.

RISK INCREASES WITH
● Contact sports, especially if the lower leg is not adequately protected.
● Medical history of any bleeding disorder such as hemophilia.

● Poor nutrition, including vitamin deficiency.
● Use of anticoagulants or aspirin.

HOW TO PREVENT—Wear appropriate protective gear and equipment, such as shin pads, during competition or other athletic activity if there is risk of a lower-leg injury.

WHAT TO EXPECT

APPROPRIATE HEALTH CARE
● Doctor's care unless the hematoma is very small.
● Needle aspiration of blood from the hematoma if the hematoma is accessible. At the same time hyaluronidase (an enzyme) can be injected into the hematoma space. Hyaluronidase hastens absorption of blood.
● Self-care for minor hematomas, or for serious hematomas during the rehabilitation phase.
● Physical therapy following serious hematomas.

DIAGNOSTIC MEASURES
● Your own observation of symptoms.
● Physical exam and medical history by a doctor for all except minor injuries.
● X-rays of the injured area to assess total injury to the lower leg and to rule out the possibility of underlying bone fractures. Total extent of the injury may not be apparent for 48 to 72 hours.

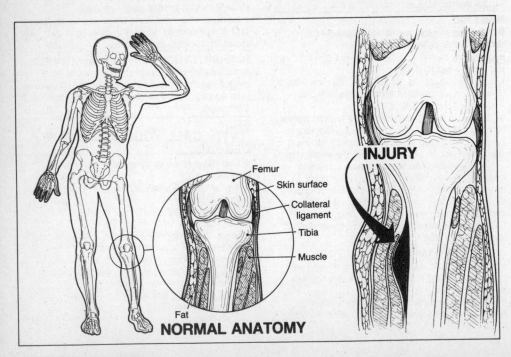

Femur
Skin surface
Collateral ligament
Tibia
Muscle

INJURY

Fat
NORMAL ANATOMY

POSSIBLE COMPLICATIONS
- Permanent damage to muscles and nerves, causing muscle atrophy and a weak foot, if treatment is delayed.
- Infection introduced through a break in the skin at the time of injury or during aspiration of the hematoma by a doctor.
- Prolonged healing time if activity is resumed too soon.
- Calcification of the blood remaining in the hematoma, if the blood is not completely removed or absorbed.

PROBABLE OUTCOME—Average healing time is 2 weeks to 2 months unless blood is removed with aspiration. Healing time is much less with this treatment.

 HOW TO TREAT

NOTE—Follow your doctor's instructions. These instructions are supplemental.

FIRST AID—Use instructions for R.I.C.E., the first letters of *rest, ice, compression* and *elevation.* See Appendix 1 for details.

CONTINUING CARE
- Use an ice pack 3 or 4 times a day. Wrap ice chips or cubes in a plastic bag, and wrap the bag in a moist towel. Place it over the injured area for 20 minutes at a time.
- After 48 hours, localized heat promotes healing by increasing blood circulation in the injured area. Use hot baths, showers, compresses, heat lamps, heating pads, heat ointments and liniments, or whirlpools.
- Don't massage the leg. You may trigger bleeding again.

MEDICATION
- For minor discomfort, you may use: Non-prescription medicines such as acetaminophen or ibuprofen.
  Topical liniments and ointments.
- Your doctor may prescribe stronger medicine for pain, if needed.

ACTIVITY—Begin activities slowly and stop exercise as soon as pain begins. Increase activity as healing progresses. To prevent healing delay, protect the hematoma area against excessive motion soon after injury. Motion breaks down the clot and causes irritation throughout the lower leg, leading to possible scar formation, calcification and restricted movement after healing.

DIET—During recovery, eat a well-balanced diet that includes extra protein, such as meat, fish, poultry, cheese, milk and eggs. Increase fiber and fluid intake to prevent constipation that may result from decreased activity.

REHABILITATION
- Begin daily rehabilitation exercises when supportive wrapping is no longer needed.
- Use gentle ice massage for 10 minutes before and after workouts. Fill a large Styrofoam cup with water and freeze. Tear a small amount of foam from the top so ice protrudes. Massage firmly over the injured area in a circle about the size of a softball.
- See page 462 for rehabilitation exercises.

 CALL YOUR DOCTOR IF

- You have signs or symptoms of a lower-leg hematoma that doesn't begin to improve in 1 or 2 days.
- Skin is broken and signs of infection (drainage, increasing pain, fever, headache, muscle aches, dizziness or a general ill feeling) occur.

LEG SPRAIN

GENERAL INFORMATION

DEFINITION—Violent overstretching of one or more ligaments in the lower leg. Sprains involving two or more ligaments cause considerably more disability than single-ligament sprains. When the ligament is overstretched, it becomes tense and gives way at its weakest point, either where it attaches to bone or within the ligament itself. If the ligament pulls loose a fragment of bone, it is called a *sprain-fracture*. There are 3 types of sprains:
● Mild (Grade I)—Tearing of some ligament fibers. There is no loss of function.
● Moderate (Grade II)—Rupture of a portion of the ligament, resulting in some loss of function.
● Severe (Grade III)—Complete rupture of the ligament or complete separation of ligament from bone. There is total loss of function. A severe sprain requires surgical repair.

BODY PARTS INVOLVED
● Any ligament in the lower leg.
● Tissue surrounding the sprain, including blood vessels, tendons, bone, periosteum (covering of bone) and muscles.

SIGNS & SYMPTOMS
● Severe pain at the time of injury.
● A feeling of popping or tearing inside the lower leg.
● Tenderness at the injury site.
● Swelling in the lower leg.
● Bruising that appears soon after injury.

CAUSES—Stress on a ligament that temporarily forces or pries the tibia and fibula out of their normal location. Sprains occur frequently in runners, walkers, and those who jump in such sports as basketball, soccer, skiing, distance- and high-jumping. These athletes often accidentally land on the side of the foot.

RISK INCREASES WITH
● Contact, running and jumping sports.
● Previous lower-leg injury.
● Obesity.
● Poor muscle conditioning.
● Inadequate protection from equipment.

HOW TO PREVENT
● Build your strength with a conditioning program appropriate for your sport.
● Warm up before practice or competition.
● Tape vulnerable joints before practice or competition.
● Wear proper protective shoes.

WHAT TO EXPECT

APPROPRIATE HEALTH CARE
● Doctor's diagnosis.
● Application of tape, cast or elastic bandage.
● Self-care during rehabilitation.

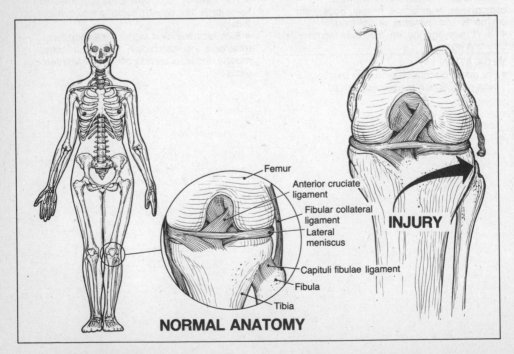

Femur
Anterior cruciate ligament
Fibular collateral ligament
Lateral meniscus
Capituli fibulae ligament
Fibula
Tibia

INJURY

NORMAL ANATOMY

- Physical therapy (moderate or severe sprain).
- Surgery (severe sprain).

DIAGNOSTIC MEASURES
- Your own observation of symptoms.
- Medical history and exam by a doctor.
- X-rays of the lower leg, knee, hip and ankle to rule out fractures.

POSSIBLE COMPLICATIONS
- Prolonged healing time if usual activities are resumed too soon.
- Proneness to repeated injury.
- Inflammation at the ligament attachment to bone (periostitis).
- Prolonged disability (sometimes).

PROBABLE OUTCOME—If this is a first-time injury, proper care and sufficient healing time before resuming activity should prevent permanent disability. Ligaments have a poor blood supply, and torn ligaments require as much healing time as fractures. Average healing times are:
- Mild sprains—2 to 6 weeks.
- Moderate sprains—6 to 8 weeks.
- Severe sprains—8 to 10 weeks.

 HOW TO TREAT

NOTE—Follow your doctor's instructions. These instructions are supplemental.

FIRST AID—Use instructions for R.I.C.E., the first letters of *rest, ice, compression* and *elevation.* See Appendix 1 for details.

CONTINUING CARE—The doctor usually applies a splint from ankle to groin to immobilize the sprained leg. If the doctor does not apply a cast, tape or elastic bandage:
- Use an ice pack 3 or 4 times a day. Put ice chips or cubes in a plastic bag. Wrap the bag in a moist towel, and place it over the injured area. Use for 20 minutes at a time.
- Wrap the injured leg with an elasticized bandage between ice treatments.
- After 72 hours, apply heat instead of ice, if it feels better. Use heat lamps, hot soaks, hot showers, heating pads, or heat liniments and ointments.
- Take whirlpool treatments, if available.
- Massage the leg gently and often to provide comfort and decrease swelling.

MEDICATION
- For minor discomfort, you may use:
  Aspirin, acetaminophen or ibuprofen.
  Topical liniments and ointments.
- Your doctor may prescribe:
  Stronger pain relievers.
  Injection of a long-acting local anesthetic to reduce pain.
  Injection of a corticosteroid, such as triamcinolone, to reduce inflammation.

ACTIVITY—Resume your normal activities gradually after clearance from your doctor.

DIET—During recovery, eat a well-balanced diet that includes extra protein, such as meat, fish, poultry, cheese, milk and eggs. Increase fiber and fluid intake to prevent constipation that may result from decreased activity.

REHABILITATION
- Begin daily rehabilitation exercises when the cast or supportive wrapping is no longer necessary.
- Use ice massage for 10 minutes before and after exercise. Fill a large Styrofoam cup with water and freeze. Tear a small amount of foam from the top so ice protrudes. Massage firmly over the injured area in a circle about the size of a softball.
- See page 462 for rehabilitation exercises.

 CALL YOUR DOCTOR IF

- You have symptoms of a moderate or severe lower-leg sprain, or a mild sprain persists longer than 2 weeks.
- Pain, swelling or bruising worsens despite treatment.
- Any of the following occur after casting or splinting:
  Pain, numbness or coldness below the cast or splint.
  Blue, gray or dusky toenails.
- Any of the following occur after surgery:
  Increased pain, swelling, redness, drainage or bleeding in the surgical area.
  Signs of infection (headache, muscle aches, dizziness, or a general ill feeling with fever).
  New, unexplained symptoms. Drugs used in treatment may produce side effects.

LEG STRAIN, CALF
(Lower-Leg Strain)

GENERAL INFORMATION

DEFINITION—Injury to muscles and tendons in the lower leg (calf). Muscles, tendons and bone comprise units. These units stabilize the knee and allow its motion. A strain occurs at the weakest part of a unit. Strains are of 3 types:
● Mild (Grade I)—Slightly pulled muscle without tearing of muscle or tendon fibers. There is no loss of strength.
● Moderate (Grade II)—Tearing of fibers in a muscle, tendon or at the attachment to bone. Strength is diminished.
● Severe (Grade III)—Rupture of the muscle-tendon-bone attachment with separation of fibers. Severe strain requires surgical repair. Chronic strains are caused by overuse. Acute strains are caused by direct injury or overstress.

BODY PARTS INVOLVED
● Tendons and muscles of the calf and lower leg.
● Leg bones (femur, tibia and fibula).
● Soft tissue surrounding the strain, including nerves, periosteum (covering to bone), blood vessels and lymph vessels.

SIGNS & SYMPTOMS
● Pain when moving or stretching the foot or ankle.
● Muscle spasm in the calf.
● Muscle spasm in the calf.
● Swelling over the injury.
● Loss of strength (moderate or severe strain).
● Crepitation ("crackling") feeling and sound when the injured area is pressed with fingers.
● Calcification of the muscle or the tendon (visible with X-rays).
● Inflammation of tendon sheath.

CAUSES
● Prolonged overuse of muscle-tendon units in the calf.
● Single violent injury or force applied to the calf.

RISK INCREASES WITH
● Contact sports such as football, soccer or hockey.
● Sports that require quick starts, such as running races.
● Any cardiovascular medical problem that results in decreased circulation.
● Medical history of any bleeding disorder.
● Obesity.
● Poor nutrition.
● Previous lower-leg injury.
● Poor muscle conditioning.

HOW TO PREVENT
● Participate in a strengthening and conditioning program appropriate for your sport.
● Warm up before practice or competition.

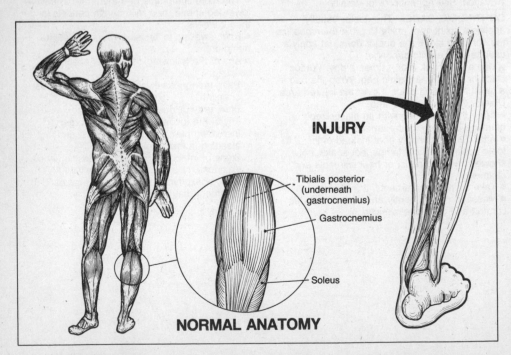

INJURY

Tibialis posterior (underneath gastrocnemius)

Gastrocnemius

Soleus

NORMAL ANATOMY

WHAT TO EXPECT

APPROPRIATE HEALTH CARE
- Doctor's care.
- Self-care during rehabilitation.
- Physical therapy (for moderate and severe strains).
- Surgery (severe strain).

DIAGNOSTIC MEASURES
- Your own observation of symptoms.
- Medical history and exam by a doctor.
- X-rays of the leg, ankle, knee and foot to rule out fractures.

POSSIBLE COMPLICATIONS
- Prolonged healing time if activity is resumed too soon.
- Proneness to repeated injury.
- Unstable or arthritic knee following repeated injury.
- Inflammation at the attachment to bone (periostitis).
- Prolonged disability (sometimes).

PROBABLE OUTCOME—If this is a first-time injury, proper care and sufficient healing time before resuming activity should prevent permanent disability. Torn ligaments and tendons require as long to heal as fractured bones. Average healing times are:
- Mild strain—2 to 10 days.
- Moderate strain—10 days to 6 weeks.
- Severe strain—6 to 10 weeks.
If this is a repeat injury, complications listed above are more likely to occur.

 HOW TO TREAT

NOTE—Follow your doctor's instructions. These instructions are supplemental.

FIRST AID—Use instructions for R.I.C.E., the first letters of *rest, ice, compression* and *elevation*. See Appendix 1 for details.

CONTINUING CARE—If a cast or splints are necessary, keep toes free and exercise them frequently. If a cast or splints are not necessary:
- Use ice massage 3 or 4 times a day for 15 minutes at a time. Fill a large Styrofoam cup with water and freeze. Tear a small amount of foam from the top so ice protrudes. Massage

firmly over the injured area in a circle about the size of a softball.
- Apply heat instead of ice, if it feels better. Use heat lamps, hot soaks, hot showers, heating pads, or heat liniments and ointments.
- Take whirlpool treatments, if available.
- Wrap the injured leg with an elasticized bandage between treatments.
- Massage gently and often to provide comfort and decrease swelling.
- Elevate the heels of your shoes to relax the calf. Use 1/2 of a heel pad in each shoe.

MEDICATION
- For minor discomfort, you may use:
  Aspirin, acetaminophen or ibuprofen.
  Topical liniments and ointments.
- Your doctor may prescribe:
  Stronger pain relievers.
  Injection of a long-acting local anesthetic to reduce pain (rare).
  Injections of a corticosteroid, such as triamcinolone, to reduce inflammation (rare).

ACTIVITY
- For a moderate or severe strain, walk with crutches for at least 72 hours—longer with a cast or splints. See Appendix 3 (Safe Use of Crutches).
- Resume your normal activities gradually as pain subsides.

DIET—Eat a well-balanced diet that includes extra protein, such as meat, fish, poultry, cheese, milk and eggs. Increase fiber and fluid intake to prevent constipation that may result from decreased activity.

REHABILITATION—Begin daily rehabilitation exercises when supportive wrapping is no longer needed. Use ice massage for 10 minutes prior to exercise. See page 462 for rehabilitation exercises.

 CALL YOUR DOCTOR IF

- You have symptoms of a moderate or severe calf strain, or a mild strain persists longer than 10 days.
- Pain or swelling worsens despite treatment.
- The following occurs with a cast or splints:
  Pain, numbness or coldness below the injury.
  Dusky, blue or gray toenails.

LEG STRESS-FRACTURE, FIBULA
(Fatigue Fracture of the Fibula)

 GENERAL INFORMATION

DEFINITION—A hairline fracture of the fibula that develops after repeated stress, such as prolonged standing, marching, running, jogging or walking.

BODY PARTS INVOLVED
- Fibula (smaller bone in the lower leg).
- Soft tissue around the fracture site, including muscles, joints, nerves, tendons, ligaments, periosteum (covering to bone), blood vessels and connective tissue.

SIGNS & SYMPTOMS
- Pain at the fracture site that lessens or disappears when the load is taken off the legs.
- Tenderness to the touch.
- Warmth over the site of the fractured fibula.

CAUSES—Fatigue of the fibula bone caused by repeated overload.

RISK INCREASES WITH
- Walking, running, jogging or standing for long periods.
- History of bone or joint disease, especially osteoporosis.
- Obesity.
- Poor nutrition, especially calcium deficiency.

HOW TO PREVENT
- Heed early warnings of an impending fracture, such as leg pain during or after extended standing, walking or running. Reduce activities before a fracture occurs.
- Ensure an adequate calcium intake (1000mg to 1500mg a day) with milk and milk products or calcium supplements.

 WHAT TO EXPECT

APPROPRIATE HEALTH CARE
- Doctor's diagnosis and care.
- Self-care during rehabilitation.

DIAGNOSTIC MEASURES
- Your own observation of symptoms.
- Medical history and physical exam by a doctor.
- X-rays of the lower leg. X-rays are often normal for 10 to 24 days after symptoms begin before changes appear.
- Radioactive technetium 99 scan (see Glossary), if symptoms are typical but X-rays are negative.

POSSIBLE COMPLICATIONS
- Complete fibula fracture with possible dislocation of broken fragments, if overuse of the leg continues after symptoms begin.

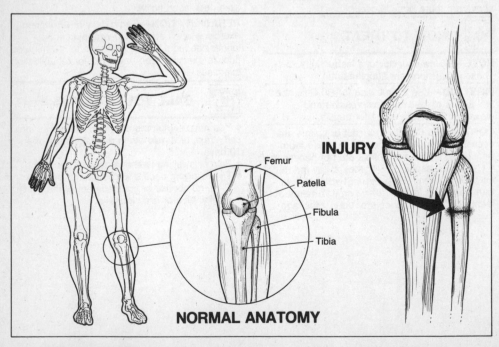

Femur
Patella
Fibula
Tibia

INJURY

NORMAL ANATOMY

- Pressure on or injury to nearby nerves, ligaments, tendons, blood vessels or connective tissues.
- Unstable or arthritic knee or ankle joint following repeated injury.

PROBABLE OUTCOME—It is impossible to predict exactly how long it will take for any fracture to heal. Variable factors include age, sex and previous state of health and conditioning. The average healing time for this fracture is 6 to 8 weeks with adequate treatment. Healing is considered complete when there is no pain at the fracture site and when X-rays show complete bone union.

 HOW TO TREAT

NOTE—Follow your doctor's instructions. These instructions are supplemental.

FIRST AID—None. This injury develops gradually.

CONTINUING CARE
- This fracture does not require setting (realignment) because the fractured bone is not displaced.
- Use frequent ice massage. Fill a large Styrofoam cup with water and freeze. Tear a small amount of foam from the top so ice protrudes. Massage firmly over the injured area in a circle about the size of a softball. Do this for 15 minutes at a time, 3 or 4 times a day, and before workouts or competition.
- Apply heat instead of ice if it feels better. Use heat lamps, hot soaks, hot showers, heating pads, or heat liniments and ointments.
- Take whirlpool treatments, if available.
- Massage gently and often to provide comfort and decrease swelling.

MEDICATION—Your doctor may prescribe:
- Narcotic or synthetic narcotic pain relievers for severe pain.
- Stool softeners to prevent constipation due to inactivity.
- Acetaminophen or ibuprofen (available without prescription) for mild pain after initial treatment.

ACTIVITY
- Don't bear weight on the injured leg. Learn to walk with crutches (see Appendix 3, Safe Use of Crutches) and prop your leg up whenever possible. Immobilization in a cast is not usually necessary.
- Begin reconditioning and rehabilitation after clearance from your doctor.
- Resume normal daily activities gradually after treatment.

DIET—During recovery, eat a well-balanced diet that includes extra protein, such as meat, fish, poultry, cheese, milk and eggs. Increase fiber and fluid intake to prevent constipation that may result from decreased activity.

REHABILITATION—Begin daily rehabilitation exercises when movement is comfortable. Use ice massage for 10 minutes prior to exercise. See page 462 for rehabilitation exercises.

 CALL YOUR DOCTOR IF

- You have symptoms of a fibula stress-fracture.
- After diagnosis, pain worsens despite treatment.

LEG STRESS-FRACTURE, TIBIA
(Fatigue Fracture of the Tibia)

GENERAL INFORMATION

DEFINITION—A hairline fracture of the tibia that develops after repeated stress, such as prolonged standing, marching, running, jogging or walking.

BODY PARTS INVOLVED
- Tibia (large bone in the lower leg).
- Soft tissue around the fracture site, including muscles, joints, nerves, tendons, ligaments, periosteum (covering to bone), blood vessels and connective tissue.

SIGNS & SYMPTOMS
- Pain at the fracture site that lessens or disappears when the load is taken off the legs.
- Tenderness to the touch.
- Warmth over the site of the fractured tibia.

CAUSES—Fatigue of the tibia bone caused by repeated overload.

RISK INCREASES WITH
- Walking, running, jogging or standing for long periods.
- History of bone or joint disease, especially osteoporosis.
- Obesity.
- Poor nutrition, especially calcium deficiency.

HOW TO PREVENT
- Heed early warnings of an impending fracture, such as leg pain during or after extended standing, walking or running. Reduce activities before a fracture occurs.
- Ensure an adequate calcium intake (1000mg to 1500mg a day) with milk and milk products or calcium supplements.

WHAT TO EXPECT

APPROPRIATE HEALTH CARE
- Doctor's diagnosis and care.
- Self-care during rehabilitation.

DIAGNOSTIC MEASURES
- Your own observation of symptoms.
- Medical history and physical exam by a doctor.
- X-rays of the lower leg. X-rays are often normal for 10 to 24 days after symptoms begin before bone changes appear.
- Radioactive technetium 99 scan (see Glossary), if symptoms are typical but X-rays are negative.

POSSIBLE COMPLICATIONS
- Complete fracture with possible dislocation of broken bone fragments if overuse of leg continues after symptoms begin.
- Pressure on or injury to nearby nerves, ligaments, tendons, blood vessels or connective tissues.

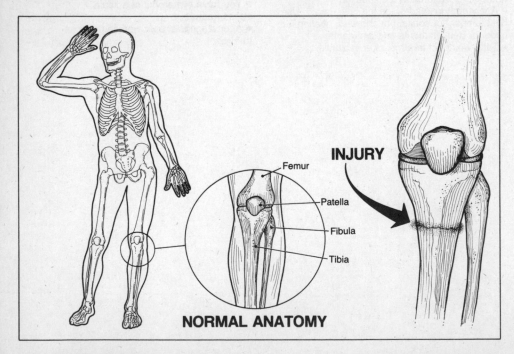

Femur
Patella
Fibula
Tibia

INJURY

NORMAL ANATOMY

- Problems arising from plaster casts, splints or other immobilizing materials. See Appendix 2 (Care of Casts).
- Unstable or arthritic knee or ankle joint following repeated injury.

PROBABLE OUTCOME—It is impossible to predict exactly how long it will take for any fracture to heal. Variable factors include age, sex and previous state of health and conditioning. The average healing time for this fracture is 6 to 8 weeks with adequate rest and treatment. Healing is considered complete when there is no pain at the fracture site and when X-rays show complete bone union.

 ## HOW TO TREAT

NOTE—Follow your doctor's instructions. These instructions are supplemental.

FIRST AID—None. This injury develops gradually.

CONTINUING CARE
- This fracture does not require setting (realignment) because the fractured bone is not displaced.
- Immobilization is sometimes required. If so, a rigid walking cast is placed around the lower leg.
- After cast removal, use frequent ice massage. Fill a large Styrofoam cup with water and freeze. Tear a small amount of foam from the top so ice protrudes. Massage firmly over the injured area in a circle about the size of a baseball. Do this for 15 minutes at a time, 3 or 4 times a day, and before workouts or competition.
- Apply heat instead of ice, if it feels better. Use heat lamps, hot soaks, hot showers, heating pads, and heat liniments or ointments.
- Take whirlpool treatments, if available.
- Massage gently and often to provide comfort and decrease swelling.

MEDICATION—Your doctor may prescribe:
- Narcotic or synthetic narcotic pain relievers for severe pain.
- Stool softeners to prevent constipation due to inactivity.
- Acetaminophen or ibuprofen (available without prescription) for mild pain after initial treatment.

ACTIVITY
- Don't bear weight on the injured leg. Learn to walk with crutches, and prop your leg up whenever possible. See Appendix 3 (Safe Use of Crutches).
- Begin reconditioning and rehabilitation after clearance from your doctor.
- Resume normal daily activities gradually as symptoms disappear.

DIET—During recovery, eat a well-balanced diet that includes extra protein, such as meat, fish, poultry, cheese, milk and eggs. Increase fiber and fluid intake to prevent constipation that may result from decreased activity.

REHABILITATION—Begin daily rehabilitation exercises when movement is comfortable. Use ice massage for 10 minutes prior to exercise. See page 462 for rehabilitation exercises.

 ## CALL YOUR DOCTOR IF

- You have symptoms of a tibia stress-fracture.
- Toes become dark, blue, cold or numb while the cast is on.

LIVER INJURY

GENERAL INFORMATION

DEFINITION—Laceration, contusion or rupture of the liver. A severe liver injury is an emergency!

BODY PARTS INVOLVED
- Liver.
- Muscles of the abdominal wall.
- Peritoneum (membranous covering to the intestines).
- Ribs (sometimes) if fractured at the same time the liver is injured.

SIGNS & SYMPTOMS
- Vomiting.
- Pain in the abdomen.
- Abdominal tenderness.
- Pain in the right shoulder or right side of the neck.
- Rapid heart rate.
- Low blood pressure.
- Signs of shock: pale, moist and sweaty skin; anxiety with a feeling of impending doom; shortness of breath and rapid breathing; disorientation; and confusion.

CAUSES—Direct blow to the liver, located in the upper abdomen or right side of the chest.

RISK INCREASES WITH
- Contact sports.
- Recent injury to the right side of the abdomen or flank (side or back between ribs and hip).
- Rib fracture.
- Any bleeding disorder such as hemophilia.
- Any illness that causes enlargement of the liver.
- If surgery is necessary, surgical risk increases with smoking, use of mind-altering drugs, muscle relaxants, tranquilizers, sleep inducers, insulin, sedatives, beta-adrenergic blockers or corticosteroids.

HOW TO PREVENT—Avoid causes and risk factors when possible.

WHAT TO EXPECT

APPROPRIATE HEALTH CARE
- Doctor's treatment.
- Hospitalization for intravenous fluids or transfusions to treat shock.
- Surgery under general anesthesia to clamp off bleeding blood vessels and repair the injured liver.

DIAGNOSTIC MEASURES
Before surgery:
- Blood and urine studies;
- X-rays of the abdomen and chest.
After surgery:
- Examination of all removed tissue.
- Additional blood studies.

POSSIBLE COMPLICATIONS
At the time of injury:
- Rapid deterioration due to internal bleeding, possibly leading to death.

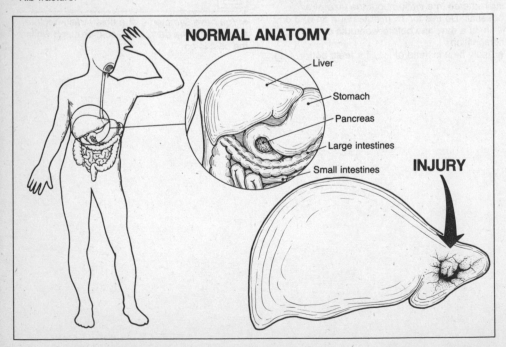

NORMAL ANATOMY

Liver

Stomach

Pancreas

Large intestines

Small intestines

INJURY

After surgery:
- Excessive bleeding.
- Infection.
- Incisional hernia.
- Lung collapse.
- Inflammation of the pancreas.
- Deep-vein blood clots.
- Pneumonia.

PROBABLE OUTCOME—Expect complete healing if no complications occur. Allow about 4 weeks for recovery from surgery.

 ## HOW TO TREAT

NOTE—Follow your doctor's instructions. These instructions are supplemental.

FIRST AID
- Cover the victim with a blanket to combat shock.
- Carry the injured person to the nearest emergency facility.
- Don't give the person water or food. If surgery is necessary, food or water in the stomach makes vomiting while under general anesthesia more dangerous.
- Don't give the person pain relievers. They may mask symptoms and hinder diagnosis.

CONTINUING CARE—No specific instructions except those under other headings. If surgery is required, your surgeon will supply postoperative instructions.

MEDICATION
- Your doctor may prescribe:
  Pain relievers. Don't take prescription pain medication longer than 4 to 7 days. Use only as much as you need.
  Antibiotics to fight infection.
  Stool softeners to prevent constipation.
  Pneumonia vaccinations.
- You may use non-prescription drugs such as acetaminophen for minor pain.

ACTIVITY—Return to work, play and normal activity as soon as possible. This reduces postoperative depression, which is common. Avoid vigorous exercise for 6 weeks after surgery.

DIET—No food or water before surgery. Following surgery, a clear liquid diet will be necessary until the gastrointestinal tract functions again. During recovery, follow a well-balanced diet that includes extra protein, such as meat, fish, poultry, cheese, milk and eggs. Increase fiber and fluid intake to prevent constipation that may result from decreased activity.

REHABILITATION—Rehabilitation exercises must be individualized. Follow your doctor's or surgeon's directions.

 ## CALL YOUR DOCTOR IF

- You receive an abdominal injury and the symptoms last longer than a few minutes, or symptoms diminish and recur within hours or days. This may be an emergency!
- Any of the following occur after surgery:
  You develop signs of infection (headache, muscle aches, dizziness or a general ill feeling and fever).
  Pain, swelling, redness, drainage or bleeding increases in the surgical area.
  New, unexplained symptoms develop. Drugs used in treatment may produce side effects.
- Symptoms return after recovery.

NECK (CERVICAL SPINE) DISLOCATION

 GENERAL INFORMATION

DEFINITION—A displacement of spinal vertebrae in the neck so that adjoining bones no longer touch each other. *Subluxation* is a minor dislocation. Joint surfaces still touch, but not in normal relation to each other. Neck subluxation followed by spontaneous reposition occurs frequently in athletes. A neck dislocation is a serious injury that can lead to spinal-cord damage and paralysis of all four extremities, and sometimes leads to death.

BODY PARTS INVOLVED
● Vertebrae of the spine in the cervical (neck) region.
● Ligaments that hold the vertebrae in proper alignment.
● Cartilage between the vertebrae that cushions the bones.
● Spinal-cord and nerve roots (sometimes).

SIGNS & SYMPTOMS
● Excruciating pain at the time of injury.
● Loss of function in the neck and severe pain when attempting to move it.
● Visible deformity if the dislocated bones have locked in the dislocated position. Bones may spontaneously reposition themselves and leave no deformity, but damage is the same.
● Tenderness over the dislocation.
● Swelling and bruising in the neck.
● Numbness or paralysis below the neck

dislocation site from pressure, pinching or cutting of blood vessels or nerves.

CAUSES
● Forceful flexing, extension or rotation of the neck.
● Direct blow or violent force on the neck or head.
● End result of a severe neck sprain.

RISK INCREASES WITH
● Contact and collision sports such as football, hockey or basketball.
● Gymnastics or diving.
● Previous neck dislocation or sprain.
● Repeated neck injury of any sort.
● Arthritis of any type (rheumatoid, gout).
● Poor muscle conditioning.

HOW TO PREVENT
● Build your overall muscle tone with a conditioning program appropriate for your sport.
● Warm up adequately before physical activity.
● After healing, wear protective devices (such as a soft or rigid neck collar) to decrease the likelihood of reinjury during participation in any sports. Avoid all contact or collision sports.

? WHAT TO EXPECT

APPROPRIATE HEALTH CARE
● Doctor's treatment.
● Surgery (sometimes) to restore the cervical vertebrae and torn ligaments to normal position

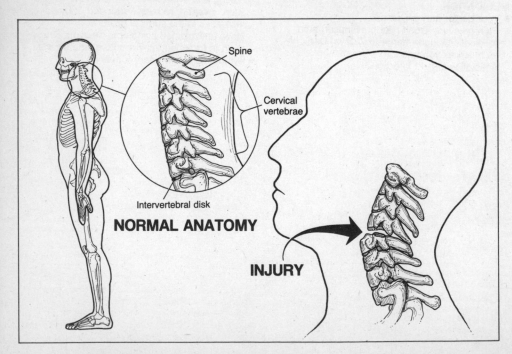

Spine

Cervical vertebrae

Intervertebral disk

NORMAL ANATOMY

INJURY

and repair torn ligaments and tendons.
- Self-care during rehabilitation.

DIAGNOSTIC MEASURES
- Your own observation of symptoms.
- Medical history and exam by a doctor.
- X-rays of the neck and skull.

POSSIBLE COMPLICATIONS
At time of injury:
- Shock.
- Serious injury to neck cartilage, the spinal cord and roots of spinal nerves as they emerge from between vertebrae to serve other parts of the body. Neck dislocation can lead to paralysis from the neck down.
- Pressure on or damage to other nearby smaller nerves, tendons, muscles, blood vessels and connective tissue.

After treatment or surgery:
- Excessive internal bleeding in the neck area.
- Impaired blood supply to the dislocated area.
- Death of bone cells due to interruption of the blood supply.
- Infection introduced during surgical treatment.
- Prolonged healing if activity is resumed too soon.
- Unstable or arthritic neck joint following repeated injury.

PROBABLE OUTCOME—After the dislocation has been corrected, the neck may require immobilization with a soft or rigid collar for 8 weeks or more. Complete healing of injured ligaments requires a minimum of 6 weeks.

 HOW TO TREAT

NOTE—Follow your doctor's instructions. These instructions are supplemental.

FIRST AID
- *Don't move anyone with a neck injury* except on sturdy boards and with the neck immobilized. Don't remove the victim's headgear.
- Transport the victim immediately to an emergency facility.
- Ice helps stop internal bleeding. Prepare an ice pack of ice cubes or chips wrapped in plastic or a container. Place a towel over the injured area to prevent skin damage. Apply ice for 20 minutes, then rest 10 minutes until medical help is available. Compress the area with a loose-fitting elastic wrap to hold ice in place. Don't wrap too tightly. This can cause further damage.
- The doctor will manipulate the dislocated bones or apply traction for 12 to 24 hours to return bones to their normal position. Manipulation should be done as soon as possible after injury. Six or more hours after dislocation, bleeding and displacement of body fluids may lead to compression of the spinal cord—a surgical emergency. Also, many

tissues lose their elasticity and become difficult to return to a normal functional position.

CONTINUING CARE—At home:
- Apply heat frequently. Use heat lamps, hot soaks, hot showers or heating pads.
- Take whirlpool treatments, if available.
- Massage gently and often to provide comfort and decrease swelling.

MEDICATION—Your doctor may prescribe:
- General anesthesia or muscle relaxants prior to joint manipulation or application of traction.
- Acetaminophen, aspirin or non-steroidal anti-inflammatory drugs for mild pain.
- Narcotic pain relievers for severe pain.
- Stool softeners to prevent constipation due to decreased activity.
- Antibiotics to fight infection, if surgery is necessary.

ACTIVITY
- Begin reconditioning the neck after clearance from your doctor.
- If surgery is necessary, resume usual activities gradually after surgery. Don't drive until healing is complete.

DIET
- Drink only water before manipulation or surgery to correct the dislocation. Solid food in your stomach makes vomiting while under general anesthesia more hazardous.
- During recovery, eat a well-balanced diet that includes extra protein, such as meat, fish, poultry, cheese, milk and eggs. Increase fiber and fluid intake to prevent constipation that may result from decreased activity.

REHABILITATION—Begin daily rehabilitation exercises after clearance from your doctor. See page 464 for rehabilitation exercises.

 CALL YOUR DOCTOR IF

- You have any neck injury—especially if any part of your body becomes numb, pale, or cold after injury. This is an emergency!
- Any of the following occur after treatment:
  Loss of feeling below the dislocation site.
  Blue or gray skin color, particularly under the fingernails or toenails.
  Swelling above or below the neck collar.
  Nausea or vomiting.
  Constipation.
- Any of the following occur after surgery:
  Increased pain, swelling or drainage in the surgical area.
  Signs of infection (headache, muscle aches, dizziness, or a general ill feeling and fever).
- New, unexplained symptoms develop. Drugs used in treatment may produce side effects.
- Neck dislocations that you can "pop" back into normal position occur repeatedly.

NECK (CERVICAL SPINE) FRACTURE

GENERAL INFORMATION

DEFINITION—A complete or incomplete break in a bone in the neck (cervical spine). Injuries to this region of the spine are frequently a combination of sprain, dislocation and fracture. The most serious can injure the spinal cord, leading to paralysis or death.

BODY PARTS INVOLVED
- Bones in the neck (cervical spine).
- Joints in the cervical spine.
- Spinal cord (sometimes).
- Soft tissue surrounding the fracture site, including muscles, nerves, tendons, ligaments, periosteum (covering to bone), blood vessels and connective tissue.

SIGNS & SYMPTOMS
- Severe pain in the neck at the fracture site.
- Swelling of soft tissue around the fracture.
- Tenderness to touch.
- Numbness below the fracture site (sometimes).

CAUSES—Direct blow or indirect stress to the neck. Indirect stress may be caused by twisting.

RISK INCREASES WITH
- Diving.
- Gymnastics (tumbling or trampoline activities).
- Contact sports, particularly football.
- History of bone or joint disease, especially osteoporosis.
- Obesity.
- Poor nutrition, especially insufficient calcium.
- If surgery or anesthesia is necessary, surgical risk increases with smoking and use of drugs, including mind-altering drugs, muscle relaxants, antihypertensives, tranquilizers, sleep inducers, insulin, sedatives, beta-adrenergic blockers or corticosteroids.

HOW TO PREVENT
- Build your strength with a good conditioning program before beginning regular athletic practice or competition. Increased muscle mass provides additional protection to your bones.
- Use a "spotter" (helper) when attempting difficult moves in gymnastics or similar activities.
- Use appropriate protective equipment, such as padded collars and shoulder pads, when competing in contact sports.
- Ensure an adequate calcium intake (1000mg to 1500mg a day) with milk and milk products or calcium supplements.

WHAT TO EXPECT

APPROPRIATE HEALTH CARE
- Doctor's treatment.
- Hospitalization for traction to the skull so the fracture can heal properly.
- Whirlpool, ultrasound or massage to displace excess fluid from the injured joint space.

DIAGNOSTIC MEASURES
- Your own observation of symptoms.
- Medical history and exam by a doctor.

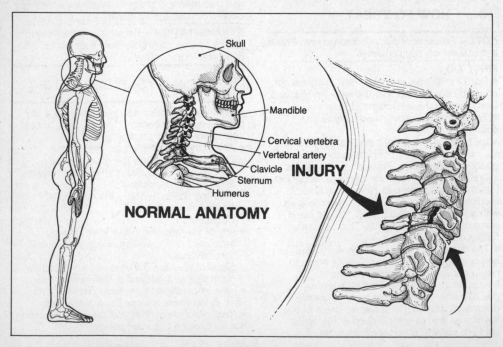

Skull

Mandible

Cervical vertebra

Vertebral artery

Clavicle

Sternum

Humerus

INJURY

NORMAL ANATOMY

- X-rays of the skull and neck.

POSSIBLE COMPLICATIONS
At the time of injury:
- Shock.
- Pressure or injury to the spinal cord and nearby nerves, ligaments, tendons, muscles, blood vessels or connective tissues.

After treatment:
- Paralysis—temporary or permanent, partial or complete—below the neck.
- Delayed union or non-union of the fracture.
- Impaired blood supply to the fracture site.
- Avascular necrosis (death of bone cells) due to interruption of the blood supply.
- Infection in open fractures (skin broken over the fracture site), or at the incision if surgical setting was necessary.
- Prolonged healing time if activity is resumed too soon.
- Proneness to repeated neck injury.
- Unstable or arthritic neck joint following repeated injury.

PROBABLE OUTCOME—The average healing time for this fracture is 6 to 12 weeks in traction, followed by 2 months in a neck brace. Healing is complete when there is no pain or motion at the fracture site and when X-rays show complete bone union.

 ## HOW TO TREAT

NOTE—Follow your doctor's instructions. These instructions are supplemental.

FIRST AID
- Keep the person warm with blankets to decrease the possibility of shock.
- *Don't move the injured area.* Don't try to remove a helmet or other headgear.
- Use a stretcher or spineboard with sandbags or a cervical collar to immobilize the neck while transporting the injured person to an emergency facility. Do this only if you are trained in emergency medical assistance or if no help is available.
- The doctor will apply traction to manipulate the broken bones slowly back to their original position. Traction lines up and holds the broken neck bones as close to their normal position as possible. Manipulation should be done as soon as possible after injury. Six or more hours after the fracture, bleeding and loss of body fluids may lead to shock. Also, many tissues lose their elasticity and become difficult to return to a normal position.
- Immobilization will be necessary. The best method must be determined by your doctor based on your age, sex and the possibility of spinal-cord injury.

CONTINUING CARE—Treatment after manipulation and healing:
- Take whirlpool treatments, if available.
- Massage *gently* and often to provide comfort and decrease swelling.

MEDICATION—Your doctor may prescribe:
- Narcotic or synthetic narcotic pain relievers for severe pain.
- Special corticosteroids, such as dexamethasone, to reduce swelling and minimize spinal-cord damage.
- Stool softeners to prevent constipation due to inactivity.
- Acetaminophen for mild pain.
- Antibiotics to fight infection if skin is broken or surgery is needed.

ACTIVITY
- Actively exercise all muscle groups not immobilized. These muscle contractions promote fracture alignment and hasten healing.
- Resume normal daily activities gradually after treatment.

DIET
- Drink only water before manipulation or surgery to treat the fracture. Solid food in your stomach makes vomiting while under anesthesia more hazardous.
- During recovery, eat a well-balanced diet that includes extra protein, such as meat, fish, poultry, cheese, milk and eggs. Increase fiber and fluid intake to prevent constipation that may result from decreased activity.

REHABILITATION
- Begin reconditioning and rehabilitation after clearance from your doctor.
- Use ice massage for 10 minutes before and after workouts. Fill a large Styrofoam cup with water and freeze. Tear a small amount of foam from the top so ice protrudes. Massage firmly over the injured area in a circle about the size of a softball.
- See page 464 for rehabilitation exercises.

 ## CALL YOUR DOCTOR IF

- You have any serious neck injury.
- You develop signs of infection (headache, muscle aches, dizziness, or a general ill feeling and fever) while in traction.
- You experience muscle weakness, numbness or complete loss of feeling below the fracture site.
- You experience nausea, vomiting or constipation.

NECK SPRAIN

GENERAL INFORMATION

DEFINITION—Violent overstretching of one or more ligaments in the cervical (neck) region of the vertebral column. Sprains involving two or more ligaments cause considerably more disability than single-ligament sprains. When the ligament is overstretched, it becomes tense and gives way at its weakest point, either where it attaches to bone or within the ligament itself. If the ligament pulls loose a fragment of bone, it is called a *sprain-fracture*. There are 3 types of sprains:
- Mild (Grade I)—Tearing of some ligament fibers. There is no loss of function.
- Moderate (Grade II)—Rupture of a portion of the ligament, resulting in some loss of function.
- Severe (Grade III)—Complete rupture of the ligament or complete separation of ligament from bone. There is total loss of function. A severe sprain requires surgical repair.

BODY PARTS INVOLVED
- Any ligament in the neck.
- Tissue surrounding the sprain, including blood vessels, tendons, bone, periosteum (covering of bone) and muscles.

SIGNS & SYMPTOMS
- Severe pain at the time of injury.
- A feeling of popping or tearing inside the neck.

- Muscle spasm with soreness and stiffness in the neck.
- Tenderness at the injury site.
- Swelling in the neck.
- Bruising that appears soon after injury.

CAUSES—Stress on a ligament that temporarily forces the joints in the neck out of their normal location. Neck sprains occur frequently in contact sports and auto accidents.

RISK INCREASES WITH
- Contact sports, especially football and wrestling.
- Diving or gymnastics.
- Auto racing.
- Previous neck injury.
- Obesity.
- Poor muscle conditioning.
- Inadequate protection from equipment.

HOW TO PREVENT
- Build your strength with a conditioning program appropriate for your sport.
- Warm up before practice or competition.
- Wear protective equipment, such as padded soft collars, for participation in contact sports.

WHAT TO EXPECT

APPROPRIATE HEALTH CARE
- Doctor's diagnosis.
- Traction (sometimes).

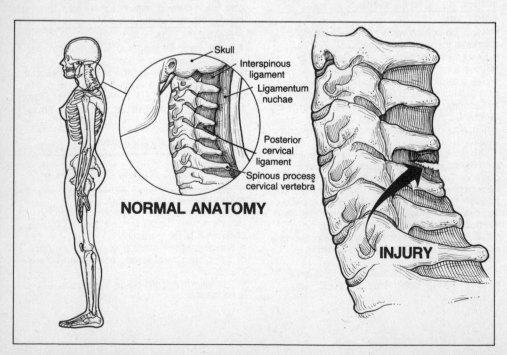

Skull
Interspinous ligament
Ligamentum nuchae
Posterior cervical ligament
Spinous process cervical vertebra

NORMAL ANATOMY

INJURY

- Self-care during rehabilitation.
- Physical therapy (moderate or severe sprain).
- Surgery (severe sprain).

DIAGNOSTIC MEASURES
- Your own observation of symptoms.
- Medical history and exam by a doctor.
- X-rays of the neck to rule out fractures.

POSSIBLE COMPLICATIONS
- Prolonged healing time if usual activities are resumed too soon.
- Proneness to repeated injury.
- Inflammation at the ligament attachment to bone (periostitis).
- Prolonged disability (sometimes).

PROBABLE OUTCOME—If this is a first-time injury, proper care and sufficient healing time before resuming activity should prevent permanent disability. Ligaments have a poor blood supply, and torn ligaments require as much healing time as fractures. Average healing times are:
- Mild sprains—2 to 6 weeks.
- Moderate sprains—6 to 8 weeks.
- Severe sprains—8 to 10 weeks.

HOW TO TREAT

NOTE—Follow your doctor's instructions. These instructions are supplemental.

FIRST AID—Use instructions for R.I.C.E., the first letters of *rest, ice, compression* and *elevation*. See Appendix 1 for details.

CONTINUING CARE
- Your doctor may suggest an adjustable cervical brace, a plastic cervical collar or a cloth collar to immobilize the neck while it heals.
- Continue using an ice pack 3 or 4 times a day. Wrap ice chips or cubes in a plastic bag. Wrap the bag in a moist towel, and place it over the injured area. Use for 20 minutes at a time.
- After 72 hours, apply heat instead of ice, if it feels better. Use heat lamps, hot soaks, hot showers, heating pads, or heat liniments or ointments.
- Take whirlpool treatments, if available.
- Massage gently and often to provide comfort and decrease swelling.

- Cervical traction devices that can be rented or purchased may provide pain relief. Follow your doctor's or manufacturer's instructions.

MEDICATION
- For minor discomfort, you may use:
  Aspirin, acetaminophen or ibuprofen.
  Topical liniments and ointments.
- Your doctor may prescribe:
  Stronger pain relievers.
  Injection of a long-acting local anesthetic to reduce pain.
  Injection of a corticosteroid, such as triamcinolone, to reduce inflammation.

ACTIVITY—Resume your normal activities gradually after clearance from your doctor.

DIET—During recovery, eat a well-balanced diet that includes extra protein, such as meat, fish, poultry, cheese, milk and eggs. Increase fiber and fluid intake to prevent constipation that may result from decreased activity.

REHABILITATION
- Begin daily rehabilitation exercises when the supportive collar is no longer necessary.
- Use ice massage for 10 minutes before and after exercise. Fill a large Styrofoam cup with water and freeze. Tear a small amount of foam from the top so ice protrudes. Massage firmly over the injured area in a circle about the size of a softball.
- See page 464 for rehabilitation exercises.

CALL YOUR DOCTOR IF

- You have symptoms of a moderate or severe neck sprain, or a mild sprain persists longer than 2 weeks.
- Pain, swelling or bruising worsens despite treatment.
- Numbness or weakness occurs in muscles of the face, shoulder, arm or hand.
- Any of the following occur after surgery:
  Increased pain, swelling, redness, drainage or bleeding in the surgical area.
  Signs of infection (headache, muscle aches, dizziness, or a general ill feeling with fever).
  New, unexplained symptoms. Drugs used in treatment may produce side effects.

NECK STRAIN

GENERAL INFORMATION

DEFINITION—Injury to the muscles or tendons that attach to the vertebral column in the neck, to the skull and to the shoulder. Muscles, tendons and bones comprise units. These units stabilize the neck and head and allow their motion. A strain occurs at a unit's weakest part. Strains are of 3 types:
● Mild (Grade I)—Slightly pulled muscle without tearing of muscle or tendon fibers. There is no loss of strength.
● Moderate (Grade II)—Tearing of fibers in a muscle, tendon or at the attachment to bone. Strength is diminished.
● Severe (Grade III)—Rupture of the muscle-tendon-bone attachment with separation of fibers. Severe strain requires surgical repair. Chronic strains are caused by overuse. Acute strains are caused by direct injury or overstress.

BODY PARTS INVOLVED
● Tendons and muscles with multiple attachments to bones in the neck, skull and shoulder.
● Bones in the neck, shoulder and skull.
● Soft tissue surrounding the strain, including nerves, periosteum (covering to bone), blood vessels and lymph vessels.

SIGNS & SYMPTOMS
● Pain when moving or stretching the neck.
● Muscle spasm in the neck.
● Swelling in the neck area.
● Loss of strength (moderate or severe strain).
● Crepitation ("crackling") feeling and sound when the injured area is pressed with fingers.
● Calcification (visible with X-ray) of the injured muscle or tendon.

CAUSES
● Prolonged overuse of muscle-tendon units in the neck.
● Single violent injury or force applied to the muscle-tendon units in the neck.

RISK INCREASES WITH
● Contact sports, especially wrestling and football.
● Any cardiovascular medical problem that results in decreased circulation.
● Medical history of any bleeding disorder.
● Obesity.
● Poor nutrition.
● Previous neck strain.
● Poor muscle conditioning.

HOW TO PREVENT
● Participate in a strengthening and conditioning program appropriate for your sport.
● Warm up before practice or competition.
● Wear proper protective equipment, such as fabric neck rolls.

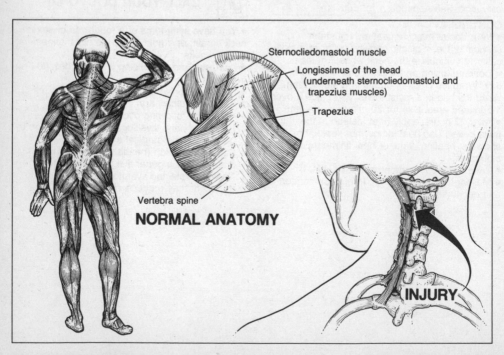

Sternocliedomastoid muscle
Longissimus of the head (underneath sternocliedomastoid and trapezius muscles)
Trapezius
Vertebra spine
NORMAL ANATOMY
INJURY

WHAT TO EXPECT

APPROPRIATE HEALTH CARE
- Doctor's diagnosis.
- Self-care during rehabilitation.
- Physical therapy (moderate or severe strain).
- Surgery (severe strain).

DIAGNOSTIC MEASURES
- Your own observation of symptoms.
- Medical history and exam by a doctor.
- X-rays of the neck to rule out fractures.

POSSIBLE COMPLICATIONS
- Prolonged healing time if activity is resumed too soon.
- Proneness to repeated injury.
- Unstable or arthritic neck joints following repeated injury.
- Inflammation at the attachment to bone (periostitis).
- Prolonged disability (sometimes).

PROBABLE OUTCOME—If this is a first-time injury, proper care and sufficient healing time before resuming activity should prevent permanent disability. Torn ligaments and tendons require as long to heal as fractured bones. Average healing times are:
- Mild strain—2 to 10 days.
- Moderate strain—10 days to 6 weeks.
- Severe strain—6 to 10 weeks.

If this is a repeat injury, complications listed above are more likely to occur.

 ## HOW TO TREAT

NOTE—Follow your doctor's instructions. These instructions are supplemental.

FIRST AID—Use instructions for R.I.C.E., the first letters of *rest, ice, compression* and *elevation.* See Appendix 1 for details.

CONTINUING CARE
- Rest in bed with traction on the neck if your doctor advises you to do so.
- Use ice massage 3 or 4 times a day for 15 minutes at a time. Fill a large Styrofoam cup with water and freeze. Tear a small amount of foam from the top so ice protrudes. Massage firmly over the injured area in a circle about the size of a softball.
- After the first 24 hours, apply heat instead of ice, if it feels better. Use heat lamps, hot soaks, hot showers, heating pads, or heat liniments and ointments.
- Use a support collar to reduce movement and support the neck during healing.
- Massage gently and often to comfort and decrease swelling.

MEDICATION
- For minor discomfort, you may use:
  Aspirin, acetaminophen or ibuprofen.
  Topical liniments and ointments.
- Your doctor may prescribe:
  Stronger pain relievers.
  Muscle relaxants.
  Tranquilizers.
  Injection of a long-acting local anesthetic to reduce pain (rare).
  Injection of a corticosteroid, such as triamcinolone, to reduce inflammation (rare).

ACTIVITY—Resume your normal activities gradually after pain subsides.

DIET—Eat a well-balanced diet that includes extra protein, such as meat, fish, poultry, cheese, milk and eggs. Increase fiber and fluid intake to prevent constipation that may result from decreased activity.

REHABILITATION—Begin daily rehabilitation exercises when support collar is no longer needed. Use ice massage for 10 minutes prior to exercise. See page 464 for rehabilitation exercises.

 ## CALL YOUR DOCTOR IF

- You have symptoms of a moderate or severe neck strain, or a mild strain persists longer than 5 days.
- Pain or swelling worsens despite treatment.
- Symptoms of neck strain recur after treatment.

NOSE INJURY

GENERAL INFORMATION

DEFINITION—Nose injuries include:
- Fractures of the nasal bones.
- Dislocations of nasal bones and cartilage.
- Contusions of the nose.
- Nosebleed.

BODY PARTS INVOLVED
- Nasal bones and cartilage.
- Skin.
- Sinuses and eustachian tubes (indirectly, sometimes).
- Soft tissue surrounding the injury: eyes, periosteum (covering to bone), nerves, blood vessels, mucous membrane lining the inside of the nose, connective tissue.

SIGNS & SYMPTOMS
- Pain or tenderness in the nose.
- Swollen, bruised nose.
- Inability to breathe through the nose.
- Crooked or misshapen nose (sometimes).
- Brisk bleeding or blood oozing from the nostril. If the nosebleed is close to the nostril, the blood is bright red. If the nosebleed is deeper in the nose, the blood may be bright or dark.
- Lightheadedness from blood loss.
- Rapid heartbeat, shortness of breath and pallor (with significant blood loss only).

CAUSES—Direct blow to the nose.

RISK INCREASES WITH
- Contact sports, particularly boxing and wrestling. The nose is fairly well protected by a faceguard in football.
- Previous nose injury.
- Blood disorders, including leukemia and hemophilia.
- Use of certain drugs, such as anticoagulants, aspirin, or prolonged use of nosedrops.
- Exposure to irritating chemicals.
- High altitude or dry climate.

HOW TO PREVENT—Protect your nose from injury whenever possible. Wear protective headgear for contact sports or when riding motorcycles or bicycles. Wear auto seat belts.

WHAT TO EXPECT

APPROPRIATE HEALTH CARE
- Self-care (see Continuing Care).
- Doctor's treatment or emergency room treatment if self-care is unsuccessful.
- Surgery (for severe bleeding only) to tie off the artery feeding the bleeding area.
- Surgery, if the nose is crooked or breathing is impaired.

DIAGNOSTIC MEASURES
- Your own observation of symptoms.
- Medical history and physical exam by a doctor.
- Laboratory blood tests if bleeding is heavy.
- X-rays of the nose.

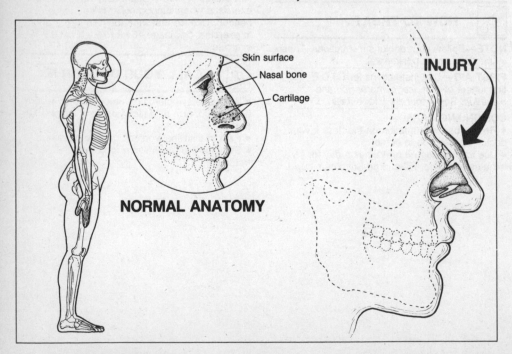

Skin surface
Nasal bone
Cartilage

NORMAL ANATOMY

INJURY

POSSIBLE COMPLICATIONS
- Infection of the nose and sinuses.
- Shock from loss of blood (rare).
- Bleeding severe enough to require a transfusion.
- Permanent breathing difficulty.
- Permanent change in appearance.

PROBABLE OUTCOME
- Minor fractures and contusions with no deformity usually heal in 4 weeks.
- Major fractures can be repaired with surgery. If surgery is necessary, it should be done within 2 weeks or not until 6 months after injury.
- Most bleeding can be controlled with home treatment. Severe bleeding requires hospitalization.

 # HOW TO TREAT

NOTE—Follow your doctor's instructions. These instructions are supplemental.

FIRST AID
- Apply ice packs to the nose immediately after injury to minimize swelling and decrease bleeding.
- If the nose is deformed or if the nosebleed is heavy or cannot be stopped, obtain emergency medical treatment. Gauze packing may be inserted to absorb blood, stop dripping and exert pressure on ruptured blood vessels. Continued bleeding may require cauterization (see Glossary).

CONTINUING CARE
- If surgery is required to set a broken nose or insert a nasal pack, your surgeon will give you postoperative instructions.

For a nosebleed without fracture:
- Sit up with your head bent forward.
- Clamp your nose closed with your fingers for 5 uninterrupted minutes. During this time, breathe through your mouth.
- If bleeding stops and recurs, repeat—but pinch your nose firmly on both sides for 8 to 10 minutes. Holding your nose tightly closed allows the blood to clot and seal the damaged blood vessels.
- You may apply cold compresses at the same time.
- Don't blow your nose for 12 hours after bleeding stops to avoid dislodging the blood clot.
- Don't swallow blood. It may upset your stomach or make you gag, causing you to inhale blood.
- Don't talk (also to avoid gagging).

MEDICATION
- For minor discomfort, you may use non-prescription drugs such as acetaminophen. Aspirin should not be used because it makes bleeding more likely.
- Your doctor may prescribe:
  Stronger pain relievers, if needed.
  Antibiotics if infection develops.
  Drugs to treat any underlying serious disorder.

ACTIVITY—Resume your normal activities as soon as bleeding stops or other symptoms improve.

DIET—After surgery, eat a well-balanced diet that includes extra protein, such as meat, fish, poultry, cheese, milk and eggs. Increase fiber and fluid intake to prevent constipation that may result from decreased activity. Otherwise, no special diet.

REHABILITATION—Rehabilitation exercises must be individualized. Follow your doctor's or surgeon's directions.

 # CALL YOUR DOCTOR IF

- You have a nosebleed that won't stop with self-care described above.
- After the nosebleed, you become nauseous or vomit.
- After the nose has been packed, your temperature rises to 101F (38.3C) or higher.

PELVIS STRAIN, HIP-TRUNK

GENERAL INFORMATION

DEFINITION—Injury to the muscles or tendons in the region of the hip and trunk where these parts attach to the upper pelvis. Tendons, muscles and bones comprise units. These units stabilize the pelvis and allow its motion. A strain occurs at the weakest part of a unit. Strains are of 3 types:
- Mild (Grade I)—Slightly pulled muscle without tearing of muscle or tendon fibers. There is no loss of strength.
- Moderate (Grade II)—Tearing of fibers in a muscle, tendon or at the attachment to bone. Strength is diminished.
- Severe (Grade III)—Rupture of the muscle-tendon-bone attachment with separation of fibers. Severe strain requires surgical repair. Chronic strains are caused by overuse. Acute strains are caused by direct injury or overstress.

BODY PARTS INVOLVED
- Muscles and tendons of the trunk and hip.
- Iliac-crest bone.
- Soft tissue surrounding the strain, including nerves, periosteum (covering to bone), blood vessels and lymph vessels.

SIGNS & SYMPTOMS
- Pain when moving or stretching the leg or trunk.
- Muscle spasm at the injury site.
- Swelling at the injury site.
- Weakened trunk and thigh muscles (moderate or severe strain).
- Crepitation ("crackling") feeling and sound when the injured area is pressed with fingers.
- Calcification of the muscle or tendon (visible with X-rays).
- Inflammation of the tendon sheath.

CAUSES
- Prolonged overuse of muscle-tendon units in the region of the iliac crest.
- Single violent injury or force applied to the muscle-tendon units in the upper pelvic area.

RISK INCREASES WITH
- Contact sports such as football, soccer or hockey.
- Sports that require quick starts, such as running races.
- Any cardiovascular medical problem that results in decreased circulation.
- Medical history of any bleeding disorder.
- Obesity.
- Poor nutrition.
- Previous pelvic injury.
- Poor muscle conditioning.

HOW TO PREVENT
- Participate in a strengthening and conditioning program appropriate for your sport.
- Warm up before practice or competition.
- Wear proper protective equipment for contact sports.

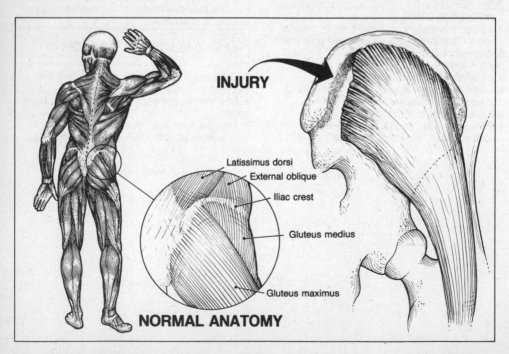

INJURY

Latissimus dorsi
External oblique
Iliac crest
Gluteus medius
Gluteus maximus

NORMAL ANATOMY

WHAT TO EXPECT

APPROPRIATE HEALTH CARE
- Doctor's diagnosis.
- Self-care during rehabilitation.
- Physical therapy (moderate or severe strain).
- Surgery (severe strain).

DIAGNOSTIC MEASURES
- Your own observation of symptoms.
- Medical history and exam by a doctor.
- X-rays of the hip, thigh and pelvis to rule out fractures.

POSSIBLE COMPLICATIONS
- Prolonged healing time if activity is resumed too soon.
- Proneness to repeated injury.
- Inflammation at the attachment to bone (periostitis).
- Prolonged disability (sometimes).

PROBABLE OUTCOME—If this is a first-time injury, proper care and sufficient healing time before resuming activity should prevent permanent disability. Torn ligaments and tendons require as long to heal as fractured bones do. Average healing times are:
- Mild strain—2 to 10 days.
- Moderate strain—10 days to 6 weeks.
- Severe strain—6 to 10 weeks.

If this is a repeat injury, complications listed above are more likely to occur.

 HOW TO TREAT

NOTE—Follow your doctor's instructions. These instructions are supplemental.

FIRST AID—Use instructions for R.I.C.E., the first letters of *rest, ice, compression* and *elevation* (if possible). See Appendix 1 for details.

CONTINUING CARE
- Use ice massage 3 or 4 times a day for 15 minutes at a time. Fill a large Styrofoam cup with water and freeze. Tear a small amount of foam from the top so ice protrudes. Massage firmly over the injured area in a circle about the size of a softball.
- After the first 24 hours, apply heat instead of ice, if it feels better. Use heat lamps, hot soaks, hot showers, heating pads, or heat liniments and ointments.
- Take whirlpool treatments, if available.
- Massage gently and often to provide comfort and decrease swelling.

MEDICATION
- For minor discomfort, you may use:
  Aspirin, acetaminophen or ibuprofen.
  Topical liniments and ointments.
- Your doctor may prescribe:
  Stronger pain relievers.
  Injection of a long-acting local anesthetic to reduce pain.
  Injections of corticosteroids, such as triamcinolone, to reduce inflammation.

ACTIVITY
- For a moderate or severe strain, walk with crutches for at least 72 hours. See Appendix 3 (Safe Use of Crutches).
- Resume your normal activities gradually.

DIET—Eat a well-balanced diet that includes extra protein, such as meat, fish, poultry, cheese, milk and eggs. Increase fiber and fluid intake to prevent constipation that may result from decreased activity.

REHABILITATION—Begin daily rehabilitation exercises when pain subsides. Use ice massage for 10 minutes prior to exercise. See page 457 for rehabilitation exercises.

 CALL YOUR DOCTOR IF

- You have symptoms of a moderate or severe hip-trunk pelvic strain, or a mild strain persists longer than 10 days.
- Pain or swelling worsens despite treatment.

PELVIS STRAIN, ISCHIUM

GENERAL INFORMATION

DEFINITION—Injury to the muscles or tendons of the lower pelvis (ischium), or injury at places where muscles attach to pelvic bones. Tendons, muscles and bones comprise units. These units stabilize the pelvis and allow its motion. A strain occurs at the weakest part of a unit. Strains are of 3 types:
- Mild (Grade I)—Slightly pulled muscle without tearing of muscle or tendon fibers. There is no loss of strength.
- Moderate (Grade II)—Tearing of fibers in a muscle, tendon or at the attachment to bone. Strength is diminished.
- Severe (Grade III)—Rupture of the muscle-tendon-bone attachment with separation of fibers. Severe strain requires surgical repair. Chronic strains are caused by overuse. Acute strains are caused by direct injury or overstress.

BODY PARTS INVOLVED
- Tendons and muscles of the lower pelvic region, including thigh, abdominal and back muscles.
- Bones of the pelvis, thigh and lower spine.
- Soft tissue surrounding the strain, including nerves, periosteum (covering to bone), blood vessels and lymph vessels.

SIGNS & SYMPTOMS
- Pain when moving or stretching the thigh.
- Spasm in muscles that attach to the pelvis.
- Swelling in the lower pelvic area.
- Loss of strength (moderate or severe strain).
- Crepitation ("crackling") feeling and sound when the injured area is pressed with fingers.
- Calcification of the muscle or tendon (visible with X-rays).
- Inflammation of the tendon sheath.

CAUSES
- Prolonged overuse of muscle-tendon units in the pelvis.
- Single violent injury or force applied to the muscle-tendon units in the lower pelvis. Strains of pelvic muscles are common in sports in which the hip is bent and the knee is straight, as with a hurdler's leading leg. Forceful straight leg-raising exercises also lead to pelvic strain.

RISK INCREASES WITH
- Hurdling, high-jumping, vaulting or long jumping.
- Sports that require quick starts.
- Contact sports.
- Any cardiovascular medical problem that results in decreased circulation.
- Medical history of any bleeding disorder.
- Obesity.
- Poor nutrition.
- Previous pelvic injury.
- Poor muscle conditioning.

HOW TO PREVENT
- Participate in a strengthening and conditioning program appropriate for your sport.
- Warm up before practice or competition.

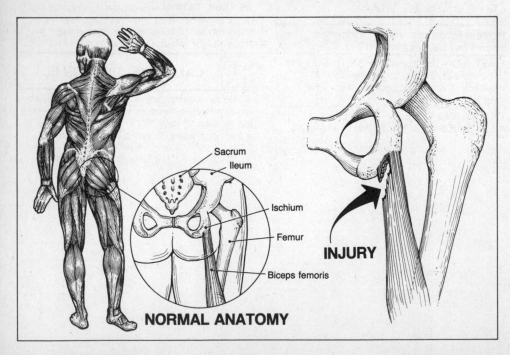

Sacrum
Ileum
Ischium
Femur
Biceps femoris

NORMAL ANATOMY

INJURY

? WHAT TO EXPECT

APPROPRIATE HEALTH CARE
- Doctor's diagnosis.
- Self-care during rehabilitation.
- Physical therapy (moderate or severe strain).
- Surgery (severe strain).

DIAGNOSTIC MEASURES
- Your own observation of symptoms.
- Medical history and exam by a doctor.
- X-rays of pelvic bones to rule out fractures.

POSSIBLE COMPLICATIONS
- Prolonged healing time if activity is resumed too soon.
- Proneness to repeated injury.
- Unstable or arthritic hip and lower back following repeated injury.
- Inflammation at the attachment to bone (periostitis).
- Prolonged disability (sometimes).

PROBABLE OUTCOME—If this is a first-time injury, proper care and sufficient healing time before resuming activity should prevent permanent disability. Torn ligaments and tendons require as long to heal as fractured bones do. Average healing times are:
- Mild strain—2 to 10 days.
- Moderate strain—10 days to 6 weeks.
- Severe strain—6 to 10 weeks.

If this is a repeat injury, complications listed above are more likely to occur.

✎ HOW TO TREAT

NOTE—Follow your doctor's instructions. These instructions are supplemental.

FIRST AID—Use instructions for R.I.C.E., the first letters of *rest, ice, compression* and *elevation* (if possible). See Appendix 1 for details.

CONTINUING CARE
- Use ice massage 3 or 4 times a day for 15 minutes at a time. Fill a large Styrofoam cup with water and freeze. Tear a small amount of foam from the top so ice protrudes. Massage firmly over the injured area in a circle about the size of a softball.
- After the first 24 hours, apply heat instead of ice, if it feels better. Use heat lamps, hot soaks, hot showers, heating pads, or heat liniments and ointments.
- Take whirlpool treatments, if available.
- Wrap the injured pelvic muscles loosely with an elasticized bandage or wear a corset between treatments.
- Massage gently and often to provide comfort and decrease swelling.

MEDICATION
- For minor discomfort, you may use:
  Aspirin, acetaminophen or ibuprofen.
  Topical liniments and ointments.
- Your doctor may prescribe:
  Stronger pain relievers.
  Injection of a long-acting local anesthetic to reduce pain (rare).
  Injections of a corticosteroid, such as triamcinolone, to reduce inflammation (rare).

ACTIVITY
- For a moderate or severe strain, walk with crutches for at least 72 hours. See Appendix 3 (Safe Use of Crutches).
- Resume your normal activities gradually.

DIET—Eat a well-balanced diet that includes extra protein, such as meat, fish, poultry, cheese, milk and eggs. Increase fiber and fluid intake to prevent constipation that may result from decreased activity.

REHABILITATION—Begin daily rehabilitation exercises when supportive wrapping is no longer needed. Use ice massage for 10 minutes prior to exercise. See page 457 for rehabilitation exercises.

☎ CALL YOUR DOCTOR IF

- You have symptoms of a moderate or severe lower pelvic strain, or a mild strain persists longer than 10 days.
- Pain or swelling worsens despite treatment.

PERINEUM CONTUSION

GENERAL INFORMATION

DEFINITION—A direct blow to the floor of the pelvis and associated structures including the genitals, causing bruising of skin and underlying tissues. Contusions cause bleeding from ruptured small capillaries that allow blood to infiltrate muscles, tendons, nerves or other soft tissue.

BODY PARTS INVOLVED
- The perineum.
- Vaginal lips, mons pubis (pubic mound), vagina, anus, penis, scrotum, testicles.
- Skin, subcutaneous tissue, tendons, ligaments, blood vessels (both large vessels and capillaries), periosteum (the outside lining of bone), muscles and connective tissue.

SIGNS & SYMPTOMS
- Swelling in the perineal area—either superficial or deep.
- Pain in the perineum.
- Feeling of firmness when pressure is exerted from outside.
- Tenderness.
- Discoloration under the skin beginning with redness and progressing to the characteristic "black and blue" discoloration.

CAUSES
- Direct blow to the perineum, usually by a blunt object or because of a fall.

- Damage to tiny blood vessels causing bleeding that infiltrates into muscle and other surrounding tissue.

RISK INCREASES WITH
- Ice skating.
- Gymnastics.
- Cycling.
- Horseback riding.
- Medical history of any bleeding disorder such as hemophilia.
- Poor nutrition.
- Inadequate protection of exposed areas during sports.
- Obesity.

HOW TO PREVENT—Usually cannot be prevented.

WHAT TO EXPECT

APPROPRIATE HEALTH CARE
- Doctor's care unless the injury is quite small.
- Self-care for minor contusions.

DIAGNOSTIC MEASURES
- Your own observation of symptoms.
- Physical exam and medical history by a doctor for all except minor injuries. The total extent of injury may not be apparent for 48 to 72 hours.
- X-rays of the pelvis to assess total injury to perineal soft tissue and to rule out the possibility of underlying fracture.

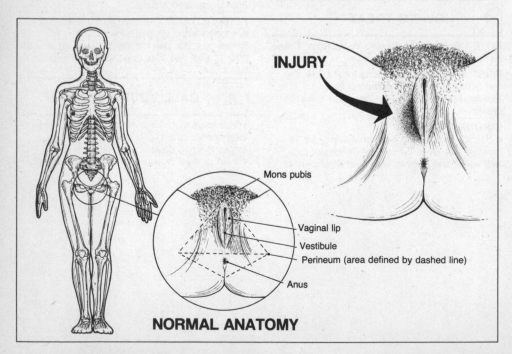

INJURY

Mons pubis

Vaginal lip

Vestibule

Perineum (area defined by dashed line)

Anus

NORMAL ANATOMY

POSSIBLE COMPLICATIONS
- Excessive bleeding leading to disability. Infiltrative type bleeding can (rarely) lead to calcification and impaired function of injured muscle.
- Prolonged healing time if usual activities are resumed too soon.
- Infection if skin over the injury site was broken.
- Scarring and narrowing of the birth canal in women.

PROBABLE OUTCOME—Healing is usually complete in 1 to 4 weeks, depending on the extent of injury.

 HOW TO TREAT

NOTE—Follow your doctor's instructions. These instructions are supplemental.

FIRST AID—Use instructions for R.I.C.E., the first letters of *rest, ice, compression* and *elevation* (if possible). See Appendix 1 for details.

CONTINUING CARE
- Use an ice pack 3 or 4 times a day. Wrap ice chips or cubes in a plastic bag, and wrap the bag in a moist towel. Place it over the injured area for 20 minutes at a time.
- After 72 hours, apply heat instead of ice, if it feels better. Use heat lamps, hot soaks, hot showers, heating pads, or heat liniments or ointments.
- Take whirlpool treatments, if available.
- Protect the injured area with pads between treatments.

MEDICATIONS
- For minor discomfort, you may use non-prescription medicines such as acetaminophen or ibuprofen (available under many different brand names). Do not use aspirin for injuries involving bleeding.
- Your doctor may prescribe stronger medicine for pain, if needed.

ACTIVITY
- Begin activities slowly and stop exercise as soon as pain begins. Increase activity as healing progresses.
- Delay sexual activity until healing is complete.

DIET—Eat a well-balanced diet that includes extra protein, such as meat, fish, poultry, cheese, milk and eggs. Increase fiber and fluid intake to prevent constipation that may result from decreased activity.

REHABILITATION—None.

 CALL YOUR DOCTOR IF

- The injured perineum doesn't improve within a day or two.
- Signs of infection (drainage from skin, headache, muscle aches, dizziness, fever or a general ill feeling) occur if skin was broken.
- You have discomfort with sexual intercourse after healing.

RIB DISLOCATION

GENERAL INFORMATION

DEFINITION—Injury and displacement of a rib where it joins the sternum (breastbone) or spinal column. *Dislocation* means the rib and adjoining bones no longer touch each other. *Subluxation* is a minor dislocation in which the joint surfaces still touch, but not in normal relation to each other.

BODY PARTS INVOLVED
- Rib and sternum or spinal column.
- Ligaments attaching ribs to the sternum or spinal column.
- Soft tissue surrounding the dislocation or subluxation site, including periosteum (covering to bone), nerves, tendons, blood vessels and connective tissue.

SIGNS & SYMPTOMS
- Excruciating pain at the time of injury.
- Loss of function of the injured rib, causing breathing difficulty.
- Severe pain when moving.
- Visible deformity (lump) if the dislocated bones have locked in the dislocated position. Bones may spontaneously reposition themselves and leave no deformity, but damage is the same.
- Tenderness over the dislocation.
- Swelling and bruising over the rib.
- Pain when taking a deep breath, coughing or laughing.

- Numbness or paralysis of other ribs below the dislocation or subluxation from pressure, pinching or cutting of blood vessels or nerves.

CAUSES
- Direct blow to the ribs.
- End result of a severe rib sprain.

RISK INCREASES WITH
- Contact sports, especially football, boxing, wrestling, basketball or hockey.
- Previous rib dislocation or sprain.
- Repeated chest injury.
- Arthritis of any type (rheumatoid, gout).
- Poor muscle conditioning.

HOW TO PREVENT
- Build your overall strength and muscle tone with a long-term conditioning program appropriate for your sport.
- Warm up adequately before physical activity.
- After healing, wear protective devices, such as wrapped elastic bandages or a special rib vest, to prevent reinjury during participation in contact sports.
- Consider avoiding contact sports if treatment is unsuccessful in restoring strong, normal rib connections.

WHAT TO EXPECT

APPROPRIATE HEALTH CARE
- Doctor's treatment.
- Surgery (rare) to restore the rib to its normal

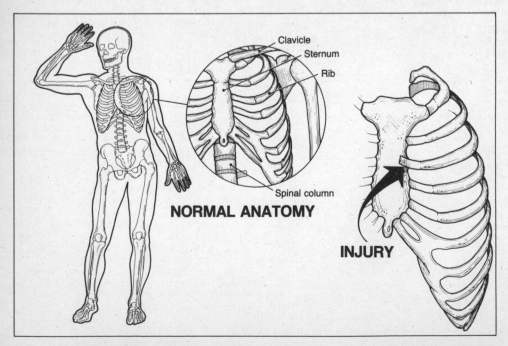

Clavicle
Sternum
Rib
Spinal column

NORMAL ANATOMY

INJURY

position and repair torn ligaments and tendons.

DIAGNOSTIC MEASURES
- Your own observation of symptoms.
- Medical history and exam by a doctor.
- X-rays of the chest and spine.

POSSIBLE COMPLICATIONS
At the time of injury:
- Shock.
- Pressure or damage to nearby nerves, ligaments, tendons, muscles, blood vessels or connective tissue.
- Injury to the underlying lung.
After treatment or surgery:
- Excessive internal bleeding.
- Impaired blood supply to the dislocated area.
- Death of bone cells due to interruption of the blood supply.
- Infection introduced during surgical treatment.
- Continuing dislocations, often with progressively less provocation.
- Prolonged healing if activity is resumed too soon.
- Unstable or arthritic rib joints following repeated injury.

PROBABLE OUTCOME—After the dislocation has been corrected, the chest may require padding and gentle compression with an elasticized bandage. Injured ligaments require a minimum of 6 weeks to heal.

 HOW TO TREAT

NOTE—Follow your doctor's instructions. These instructions are supplemental.

FIRST AID
- Use instructions for R.I.C.E., the first letters of *rest, ice, compression* and *elevation.* See Appendix 1 for details.
- The doctor may manipulate the dislocated rib to return it to its normal position. Manipulation should be done within 6 hours, if possible. After that time, internal bleeding and displacement of body fluids may lead to shock. Also, many tissues lose their elasticity and become difficult to return to a normal position.

CONTINUING CARE—At home:
- Use an ice pack 3 or 4 times a day. Wrap ice chips or cubes in a plastic bag, and wrap the bag in a moist towel. Place it over the injured area for 20 minutes at a time.
- After 48 hours, apply heat instead of ice if it feels better. Use heat lamps, hot soaks, hot showers, heating pads, or heat liniments and ointments.
- Take whirlpool treatments, if available.
- Wrap the injured chest with an elasticized bandage between treatments.

- Massage gently and often to provide comfort and decrease swelling.

MEDICATION—Your doctor may prescribe:
- General anesthesia or muscle relaxants to make joint manipulation possible.
- Acetaminophen to relieve moderate pain.
- Narcotic pain relievers for severe pain.
- Stool softeners after manipulation to prevent constipation due to decreased activity.
- Antibiotics to fight infection if surgery is necessary.

ACTIVITY
- Begin reconditioning the chest area after clearance from your doctor.
- If surgery is necessary, resume normal activities and reconditioning gradually after surgery. Don't drive until healing is complete.

DIET
- Drink only water before manipulation or surgery to correct the dislocation. Solid food in your stomach makes vomiting while under general anesthesia more hazardous.
- During recovery, eat a well-balanced diet that includes extra protein, such as meat, fish, poultry, cheese, milk and eggs. Increase fiber and fluid intake to prevent constipation that may result from decreased activity.
- Your doctor may suggest vitamin and mineral supplements to promote healing.

REHABILITATION
- Begin daily rehabilitation exercises when supportive wrapping is no longer needed.
- Use ice massage for 10 minutes before and after workouts. Fill a large Styrofoam cup with water and freeze. Tear a small amount of foam from the top so ice protrudes. Massage firmly in a circle over the injured area.
- See page 451 for rehabilitation exercises.

 CALL YOUR DOCTOR IF

- Any of the following occur after chest injury: The skin of the chest wall becomes numb, pale or cold.
  You experience nausea or vomiting.
  You feel very short of breath or have an extreme air hunger.
- Any of the following occur after surgery: Increasing pain, swelling or drainage in the surgical area.
  Numbness or loss of feeling below the dislocation site.
  Signs of infection (headache, muscle aches, dizziness, or a general ill feeling and fever).
- New, unexplained symptoms develop. Drugs used in treatment may produce side effects.
- Rib dislocations that you can "pop" back into normal position occur repeatedly.

RIB FRACTURE

GENERAL INFORMATION

DEFINITION—A complete or incomplete fracture of any of the 12 ribs on either side. Most rib fractures are accompanied by sprain or rupture of muscles, tendons or ligaments between the ribs (intercostal structures). Rib fractures are relatively common injuries in athletes, particularly those who compete in contact sports.

BODY PARTS INVOLVED
- Any one or several of the 12 ribs.
- Soft tissue surrounding the fracture site, including nerves, tendons, ligaments, cartilage and blood vessels.

SIGNS & SYMPTOMS
- Severe pain at the fracture site.
- Tenderness to the touch.
- A feeling that the "wind has been knocked out" (sometimes).
- Abdominal pain if the fractured ribs are below the diaphragm (the 11th and 12th ribs).
- Severe chest pain when coughing, sneezing or breathing deeply.
- A feeling of small air pockets under the skin of the chest or neck if the lung has been injured and leaked air.
- Swelling and bruising over the fracture site.

CAUSES
- Direct blow to the chest from a blunt object, such as an arm or elbow.
- Compression of the chest, as when a player falls on his side with a ball or helmet between him and the ground, or when a player is crushed in a pileup.

RISK INCREASES WITH
- Contact sports, especially football, hockey, boxing, wrestling or rugby.
- History of bone or joint disease.
- Poor nutrition, especially calcium deficiency.
- If surgery is needed to remove air or blood from the chest, surgical risk increases with smoking and use of drugs, including mind-altering drugs, muscle relaxants, antihypertensives, tranquilizers, sleep inducers, insulin, sedatives, beta-adrenergic blockers or corticosteroids.

HOW TO PREVENT—No specific preventive measures. The chance of reinjury can be minimized by using a chest support or binder that has a rigid pad in it to prevent a direct blow to the injured area.

WHAT TO EXPECT

APPROPRIATE HEALTH CARE
- Doctor's diagnosis.

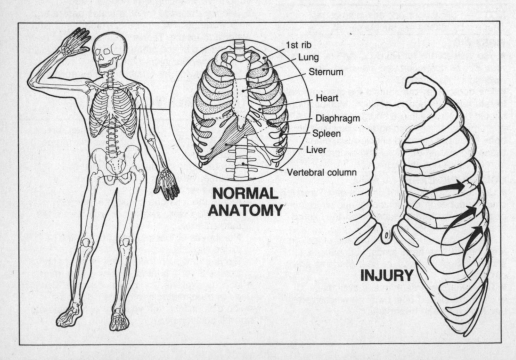

NORMAL ANATOMY

1st rib
Lung
Sternum
Heart
Diaphragm
Spleen
Liver
Vertebral column

INJURY

• Application of a wide elastic wrap or chest binder to decrease movement of the chest muscles and reduce pain with breathing. The binder should be applied around the lower chest beneath the breasts, even if the rib fracture is in the upper chest.
• Hospitalization if symptoms of injury to the lung, spleen or liver appear. Blood or air in the chest may need to be removed if the lung is punctured from the raw edge of a fractured rib. A lacerated liver may need to be surgically repaired. A ruptured spleen frequently requires surgical removal.

DIAGNOSTIC MEASURES
• Your own observation of symptoms.
• Medical history and exam by a doctor.
• X-rays of the ribs and vertebral column. Early X-rays may not show fractures if they are not dislocated, but repeat X-rays taken 4 or more days later usually reveal them. The early treatment for an uncomplicated rib fracture is the same as for bruised ribs, so a delay in diagnosis does not hinder treatment.

POSSIBLE COMPLICATIONS
• Rupture of the lung with bleeding or escape of air into the chest wall or under the skin in the neck.
• Injury to the liver if the right 11th or 12th ribs are fractured and have jagged edges.
• Injury or rupture of the spleen if the 11th and 12th ribs on the left are fractured and have jagged edges.
• Prolonged pain and slow healing.

PROBABLE OUTCOME—If this is a first-time chest injury and there are no complications of internal injury, proper care and sufficient healing time before resuming contact sports should prevent later complications. Healing is usually complete in 4 to 6 weeks.

 ## HOW TO TREAT

NOTE—Follow your doctor's instructions. These instructions are supplemental.

FIRST AID—With uncomplicated rib fractures, no first aid is necessary. If injury to the lung, liver or spleen is suspected, transport the player to the nearest emergency facility.

CONTINUING CARE
• Use the binder or wrap as long as needed for pain and support—usually 4 to 6 weeks.
• Use an ice pack 3 or 4 times a day. Place chips in a plastic bag. Wrap the bag in a moist towel and place over the injured area. Use for 20 minutes at a time.
• After 2 or 3 days, if heat is more soothing than ice, use heat lamps, hot soaks, hot showers or heating pads.

MEDICATION
• For minor discomfort, you may use:
  Aspirin, acetaminophen or ibuprofen.
  Topical liniments and ointments.
• Your doctor may prescribe:
  Stronger pain relievers.
  Injection of long-acting local anesthesia into the fracture site to reduce pain and allow normal breathing (sometimes).

ACTIVITY—Resume your normal activities gradually after clearance from your doctor.

DIET—During recovery, eat a well-balanced diet that includes extra protein, such as meat, fish, poultry, cheese, milk and eggs. Increase fiber and fluid intake to prevent constipation that may result from decreased activity.

REHABILITATION—None. Continue exercising uninjured parts during recovery.

 ## CALL YOUR DOCTOR IF

• You have symptoms of a fractured rib.
• Any of the following occur after diagnosis:
  Shortness of breath.
  Uncontrollable chest pain.
  Sudden or severe abdominal pain.
  Nausea or vomiting.
  Swelling of the abdomen.
  New unexplained symptoms. Drugs used in treatment may produce side effects.

RIB SPRAIN
(Osteo-Chondral Sprain; Costral-Chondral Sprain; Costral-Vertebral Sprain)

GENERAL INFORMATION

DEFINITION—Violent overstretching of one or more ligaments where ribs attach to the vertebral column in the back or the breastbone (sternum) in the front. Sprains involving two or more ligaments cause considerably more disability than single-ligament sprains. When the ligament is overstretched, it becomes tense and gives way at its weakest point, either where it attaches to bone or within the ligament itself. If the ligament pulls loose a fragment of bone, it is called a *sprain-fracture*. There are 3 types of sprains:
- Mild (Grade I)—Tearing of some ligament fibers. There is no loss of function.
- Moderate (Grade II)—Rupture of a portion of the ligament, resulting in some loss of function.
- Severe (Grade III)—Complete rupture of the ligament or complete separation of ligament from bone. There is total loss of function. A severe sprain requires surgical repair.

BODY PARTS INVOLVED
- Ligaments attaching ribs to the vertebral column or to cartilage of the breastbone.
- Tissue surrounding the sprain, including blood vessels, tendons, bone, periosteum (covering of bone) and muscles.

SIGNS & SYMPTOMS
- Severe pain at the time of injury.
- A feeling of popping or tearing at the injury site.
- Swelling and tenderness over the injury.
- Bruising that appears soon after injury.
- Pain when rotating the body, coughing, sneezing or breathing deeply.

CAUSES—Stress on a ligament, temporarily forcing or prying ligaments attached to ribs out of their normal location.

RISK INCREASES WITH
- Contact sports.
- Gymnastics.
- Skiing.
- Crewing.
- Previous back or chest injury.
- Obesity.
- Poor muscle conditioning.
- Inadequate protection from equipment, especially shoulder pads.

HOW TO PREVENT
- Build your strength with a conditioning program appropriate for your sport.
- Warm up before practice or competition.
- Wear protective equipment appropriate for your sport.

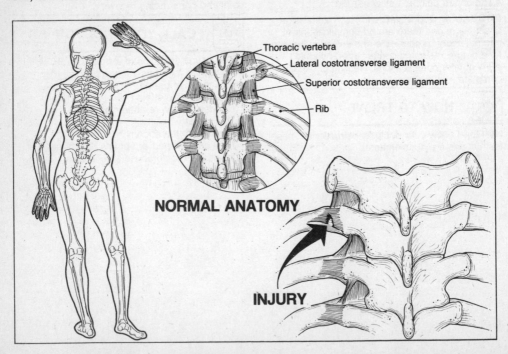

Thoracic vertebra
Lateral costotransverse ligament
Superior costotransverse ligament
Rib

NORMAL ANATOMY

INJURY

WHAT TO EXPECT

APPROPRIATE HEALTH CARE
- Doctor's diagnosis.
- Application of an elastic bandage or rib belt.
- Self-care during rehabilitation.
- Physical therapy (moderate or severe sprain).
- Surgery (severe sprain).

DIAGNOSTIC MEASURES
- Your own observation of symptoms.
- Medical history and exam by a doctor.
- X-rays of the ribs and injury site to rule out fractures.

POSSIBLE COMPLICATIONS
- Prolonged healing time if usual activities are resumed too soon.
- Proneness to repeated injury.
- Inflammation at the ligament attachment to bone (periostitis).
- Prolonged disability (sometimes).
- Unstable or arthritic rib attachment to the sternum or vertebra following repeated injury.

PROBABLE OUTCOME—If this is a first-time injury, proper care and sufficient healing time before resuming activity should prevent permanent disability. Ligaments have a poor blood supply, and torn ligaments require as much healing time as fractures. Average healing times are:
- Mild sprains—2 to 6 weeks.
- Moderate sprains—6 to 8 weeks.
- Severe sprains—8 to 10 weeks.

HOW TO TREAT

NOTE—Follow your doctor's instructions. These instructions are supplemental.

FIRST AID—Use instructions for R.I.C.E., the first letters of *rest, ice, compression* and *elevation*. See Appendix 1 for details.

CONTINUING CARE
- If your doctor fits you with an elastic wrap, rib belt or rib binder, continue to use it for pain and support—usually 4 to 6 weeks.
- Use an ice pack 3 or 4 times a day. Wrap ice chips or cubes in a plastic bag. Wrap the bag in a moist towel, and place it over the injured area. Use for 20 minutes at a time.

- After 72 hours, apply heat instead of ice if it feels better. Use heat lamps, hot soaks, hot showers, heating pads, or heat liniments or ointments.
- Take whirlpool treatments, if available.
- Massage gently and often to provide comfort and decrease swelling.

MEDICATION
- For minor discomfort, you may use:
  Aspirin, acetaminophen or ibuprofen.
  Topical liniments and ointments.
- Your doctor may prescribe:
  Stronger pain relievers.
  Injection of a long-acting local anesthetic to reduce pain.
  Injection of a corticosteroid such as triamcinolone to reduce inflammation.

ACTIVITY—Resume your normal activities gradually after clearance from your doctor.

DIET—During recovery, eat a well-balanced diet that includes extra protein, such as meat, fish, poultry, cheese, milk and eggs. Increase fiber and fluid intake to prevent constipation that may result from decreased activity.

REHABILITATION
- Begin daily rehabilitation exercises when supportive wrapping is no longer necessary.
- Use ice massage for 10 minutes before and after exercise. Fill a large Styrofoam cup with water and freeze. Tear a small amount of foam from the top so ice protrudes. Massage firmly over the injured area in a circle about the size of a softball.
- See pages 451 and 465 for rehabilitation exercises.

CALL YOUR DOCTOR IF

- You have symptoms of a moderate or severe rib sprain, or a mild sprain persists longer than 2 weeks.
- Pain, swelling or bruising worsens despite treatment.
- Any of the following occur after surgery:
  Increased pain, swelling, redness, drainage or bleeding in the surgical area.
  Signs of infection (headache, muscle aches, dizziness, or a general ill feeling with fever).
- New, unexplained symptoms develop. Drugs used in treatment may produce side effects.

RIB STRAIN

GENERAL INFORMATION

DEFINITION—Injury to any of the muscles or tendons that attach to the ribs. A muscle, tendon and rib comprise a unit. The units stabilize the chest, breastbone and upper spine and allow their motion. A strain occurs at the weakest part of a unit. Strains are of 3 types:
- Mild (Grade I)—Slightly pulled muscle without tearing of muscle or tendon fibers. There is no loss of strength.
- Moderate (Grade II)—Tearing of fibers in a muscle, tendon or at the attachment to a rib. Strength is diminished.
- Severe (Grade III)—Rupture of the muscle-tendon-rib attachment with separation of fibers. Severe strain requires surgical repair. Chronic strains are caused by overuse. Acute strains are caused by direct injury or overstress.

BODY PARTS INVOLVED
- Tendons and muscles of the chest, back and abdomen that attach to any of the ribs.
- Ribs.
- Soft tissue surrounding the strain, including nerves, periosteum (covering to bone), blood vessels and lymph vessels.

SIGNS & SYMPTOMS
- Pain with motion, breathing or stretching.
- Muscle spasm.
- Tenderness to the touch.
- Swelling.
- Crepitation ("crackling") feeling and sound when the injured area is pressed with fingers.
- Calcification of the muscle or tendon (visible with X-rays).
- Loss of strength (moderate or severe strain).

CAUSES
- Prolonged overuse of muscle-tendon units that attach to the ribs.
- Single violent injury or force applied to the muscle-tendon units in the chest.

RISK INCREASES WITH
- Contact sports such as wrestling.
- Weight-lifting.
- Any cardiovascular medical problem that results in decreased circulation.
- Medical history of any bleeding disorder.
- Obesity.
- Poor nutrition.
- Previous rib injury.
- Poor muscle conditioning.

HOW TO PREVENT
- Participate in a strengthening and conditioning program appropriate for your sport.
- Warm up before practice or competition.
- To prevent a recurrence, tape the rib area before practice or competition.

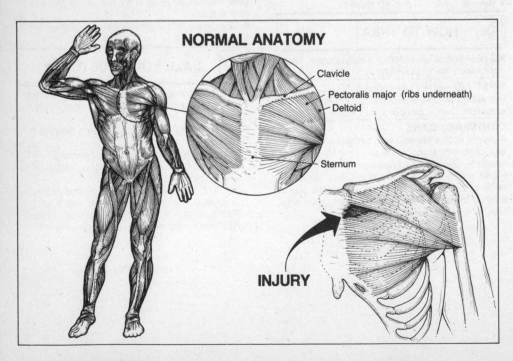

NORMAL ANATOMY

Clavicle

Pectoralis major (ribs underneath)

Deltoid

Sternum

INJURY

WHAT TO EXPECT

APPROPRIATE HEALTH CARE
- Doctor's diagnosis.
- Application of tape or elastic wrap (sometimes).
- Self-care during rehabilitation.
- Physical therapy (moderate or severe strain).
- Surgery (rare).

DIAGNOSTIC MEASURES
- Your own observation of symptoms.
- Medical history and exam by a doctor.
- X-rays of the chest to rule out fractures.

POSSIBLE COMPLICATIONS
- Prolonged healing time if activity is resumed too soon.
- Proneness to repeated injury.
- Inflammation at the attachment to the rib (periostitis).

PROBABLE OUTCOME—Most rib strains are more painful than disabling. If this is a first-time injury, proper care and sufficient healing time before resuming activity should prevent permanent disability. Average healing times are:
- Mild strain—2 to 10 days.
- Moderate strain—10 days to 6 weeks.
- Severe strain—6 to 10 weeks.

If this is a repeat injury, complications listed above are more likely to occur.

HOW TO TREAT

NOTE—Follow your doctor's instructions. These instructions are supplemental.

FIRST AID—Follow instructions for R.I.C.E., the first letters of *rest, ice, compression* and *elevation* (if possible). See Appendix 1 for details.

CONTINUING CARE
- Continue ice massage 3 or 4 times a day for 15 minutes at a time. Fill a large Styrofoam cup with water and freeze. Tear a small amount of foam from the top so ice protrudes. Massage firmly over the injured area in a circle about the size of a softball.
- After the first 24 hours, apply heat instead of ice, if it feels better. Use heat lamps, hot soaks, hot showers, heating pads, or heat liniments and ointments.
- Take whirlpool treatments, if available.
- Wrap the injured chest cage with an elasticized bandage or rib belt between treatments.
- Massage gently and often to provide comfort and decrease swelling.

MEDICATION
- For minor discomfort, you may use:
  Aspirin, acetaminophen or ibuprofen.
  Topical liniments and ointments.
- Your doctor may prescribe:
  Stronger pain relievers.
  Injection of a long-acting local anesthetic to reduce pain (rare).
  Injection of corticosteroids, such as triamcinolone, to reduce inflammation (rare).

ACTIVITY—Resume your normal activities gradually after treatment.

DIET—Eat a well-balanced diet that includes extra protein, such as meat, fish, poultry, cheese, milk and eggs. Increase fiber and fluid intake to prevent constipation that may result from decreased activity.

REHABILITATION—Begin daily rehabilitation exercises when supportive wrapping is no longer needed. Use ice massage for 10 minutes prior to exercise. See page 451 for rehabilitation exercises.

CALL YOUR DOCTOR IF

- You have symptoms of a moderate or severe rib strain, or a mild strain persists longer than 10 days.
- Pain or swelling worsens despite treatment.

SHOULDER BURSITIS, GLENO-HUMERAL

GENERAL INFORMATION

DEFINITION—Inflammation of one of the bursas in the shoulder. Bursitis may vary in degree from mild irritation to an abscess formation that causes excruciating pain.

BODY PARTS INVOLVED
- Gleno-humeral joint or other shoulder joint.
- Bursa (soft sacs filled with lubricating fluid that facilitate motion in the shoulder).
- Soft tissue surrounding the shoulder, including nerves, tendons, ligaments, blood vessels (both large vessels and capillaries), periosteum (the outside lining of bone) and muscles.

SIGNS & SYMPTOMS
- Shoulder pain, especially when moving the shoulder.
- Tenderness.
- Swelling.
- Redness (sometimes) over the affected bursa.
- Fever if infection is present.
- Limitation of shoulder motion.

CAUSES
- Injury to the shoulder.
- Acute or chronic infection.
- Arthritis.
- Gout.
- Unknown (frequently).

RISK INCREASES WITH
- Participation in competitive athletics, particularly contact sports such as football or soccer.
- Previous history of bursitis in any joint.
- Previous shoulder injury involving muscles of the "rotator cuff" (see Glossary).
- Exposure to cold weather.
- Poor conditioning and inadequate warmup.
- Inadequate protective equipment in contact sports.

HOW TO PREVENT
- Use protective gear for contact sports.
- Warm up adequately before athletic practice or competition.
- Wear warm clothing in cold weather.
- To prevent recurrence, continue to wear extra protection over the shoulder until healing is complete.

WHAT TO EXPECT

APPROPRIATE HEALTH CARE
- Doctor's diagnosis and treatment.
- Surgery (sometimes), particularly for a frozen shoulder.

DIAGNOSTIC MEASURES
- Your own observation of symptoms.
- Medical history and physical exam by a doctor.
- X-rays of the shoulder.

POSSIBLE COMPLICATIONS
- Frozen shoulder.

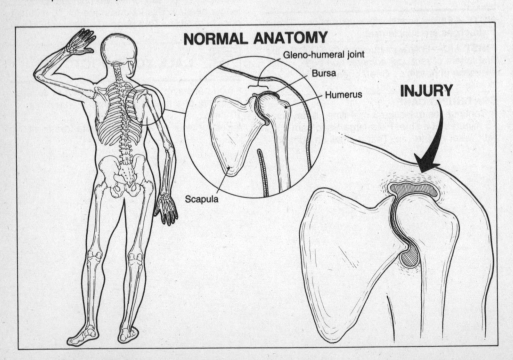

NORMAL ANATOMY

Gleno-humeral joint

Bursa

Humerus

Scapula

INJURY

- Permanent limitation of the shoulder's normal mobility.
- Prolonged healing time if activity is resumed too soon.
- Proneness to repeated flare-ups.
- Unstable or arthritic shoulder following repeated episodes of bursitis.
- Spontaneous rupture of bursa if severe infection is present.

PROBABLE OUTCOME—Mild, acute shoulder bursitis is a common—but not serious—problem. Symptoms usually subside in 7 to 14 days with treatment. Chronic or recurrent bursitis, resulting from undertreatment of the acute form, can lead to a frozen shoulder and years of discomfort.

 ## HOW TO TREAT

NOTE—Follow your doctor's instructions. These instructions are supplemental.

FIRST AID—None. This problem develops slowly.

CONTINUING CARE

- Use ice massage. Fill a large Styrofoam cup with water and freeze. Tear a small amount of foam from the top so ice protrudes. Massage firmly over the injured area in a circle about the size of a softball. Do this for 15 minutes at a time, 3 or 4 times a day, and before workouts or competition.
- Apply heat instead of ice, if it feels better. Use heat lamps, hot soaks, hot showers, heating pads, or heat liniments or ointments. Sometimes heat makes pain worse. If so, discontinue and use ice only.
- Use a sling to support the shoulder joint, if needed.
- Elevate the shoulder above the level of the heart to reduce swelling and prevent accumulation of fluid. Use pillows for propping.
- Gentle massage will frequently provide comfort and decrease swelling.

MEDICATION—Your doctor may prescribe:
- Non-steroidal anti-inflammatory drugs.
- Prescription pain relievers for severe pain. Use non-prescription aspirin, acetaminophen or ibuprofen (available under many trade names) for mild pain.
- Your doctor may inject the inflamed bursa with a long-lasting local anesthetic mixed with a corticosteroid drug, such as triamcinolone.

ACTIVITY—Rest the inflamed area as much as possible. If you must resume normal activity immediately, wear a sling until the pain becomes more bearable. To prevent a frozen shoulder, begin normal, slow joint movement as soon as possible.

DIET—Eat a well-balanced diet that includes extra protein, such as meat, fish, poultry, cheese, milk and eggs. Increase fiber and fluid intake to prevent constipation that may result from decreased activity. Your doctor may suggest vitamin and mineral supplements to promote healing.

REHABILITATION—See page 465 for rehabilitation exercises.

 ## CALL YOUR DOCTOR IF

- You have symptoms of shoulder bursitls.
- Pain increases despite treatment.
- Pain, swelling, tenderness, drainage or bleeding increases in the surgical area.
- You develop signs of infection (headache, muscle aches, dizziness or a general ill feeling and fever).
- New, unexplained symptoms develop. Drugs used in treatment may produce side effects.

SHOULDER BURSITIS, SUBACROMIAL
(Subdeltoid Bursitis)

 GENERAL INFORMATION

DEFINITION—Inflammation of the subdeltoid bursa, one of the important bursas of the shoulder. Bursitis may vary in degree from mild irritation to an abscess formation that causes excruciating pain.

BODY PARTS INVOLVED
● Subacromial bursa (a soft sac filled with lubricating fluid that facilitates motion in the shoulder).
● Soft tissue surrounding the shoulder, including nerves, tendons, ligaments, blood vessels (both large vessels and capillaries), periosteum (the outside lining of bone) and muscles.

SIGNS & SYMPTOMS
● Pain in the shoulder area.
● Tenderness.
● Swelling.
● Redness (sometimes) over the affected bursa.
● Fever if infection is present.
● Limitation of motion in the shoulder.

CAUSES
● Injury to the shoulder.
● Acute or chronic infection.
● Arthritis.
● Gout.
● Unknown (frequently).

RISK INCREASES WITH
● Participation in competitive athletics, particularly contact sports such as football.
● Previous history of bursitis in any joint.
● Previous shoulder injury involving the "rotator cuff" (see Glossary).
● Exposure to cold weather.
● Poor conditioning and inadequate warmup.
● Inadequate protective equipment in contact sports.

HOW TO PREVENT
● Use protective gear for contact sports.
● Warm up adequately before athletic practice or competition.
● Wear warm clothing in cold weather.
● To prevent recurrence, continue to wear extra protection over the shoulder until healing is complete.

 WHAT TO EXPECT

APPROPRIATE HEALTH CARE
● Doctor's diagnosis and treatment.
● Surgery (sometimes) in worst cases, particularly for a frozen shoulder.

DIAGNOSTIC MEASURES
● Your own observation of symptoms.
● Medical history and physical exam by a doctor.

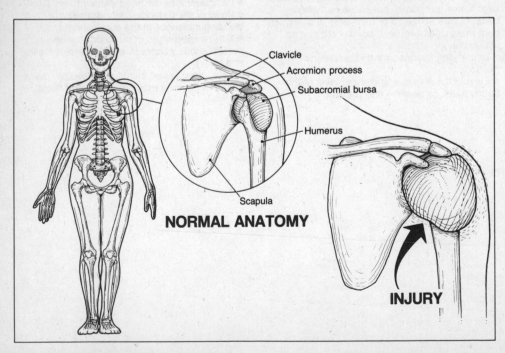

Clavicle
Acromion process
Subacromial bursa
Humerus
Scapula

NORMAL ANATOMY

INJURY

• X-rays of the shoulder.

POSSIBLE COMPLICATIONS
• Frozen shoulder, with temporary or permanent limitation of the shoulder's normal mobility.
• Prolonged healing time if activity is resumed too soon.
• Proneness to repeated flare-ups.
• Unstable or arthritic shoulder following repeated episodes of bursitis.
• Spontaneous rupture of bursa if severe infection is present.

PROBABLE OUTCOME—Mild, subdeltoid bursitis is a common—but not a serious—problem. Symptoms usually subside in 7 to 14 days with treatment. Chronic bursitis in any bursa of the shoulder can cause recurrent flare-ups.

 ## HOW TO TREAT

NOTE—Follow your doctor's instructions. These instructions are supplemental.

FIRST AID—None. This problem develops slowly.

CONTINUING CARE
• Use ice massage. Fill a large Styrofoam cup with water and freeze. Tear a small amount of foam from the top so ice protrudes. Massage firmly over the injured area in a circle about the size of a softball. Do this for 15 minutes at a time, 3 or 4 times a day, and before workouts or competition.
• Apply heat instead of ice, if it feels better. Use heat lamps, hot soaks, hot showers, heating pads, or heat liniments or ointments. Sometimes heat makes pain worse. If so, discontinue and use ice only.
• Use a sling to support the shoulder joint, if needed.
• Elevate the shoulder above the level of the heart to reduce swelling and prevent accumulation of fluid. Use pillows for propping.
• Gentle massage will frequently provide comfort and decrease swelling.

MEDICATION—Your doctor may prescribe:
• Non-steroidal anti-inflammatory drugs.
• Prescription pain relievers for severe pain. Use non-prescription aspirin, acetaminophen or ibuprofen (available under many trade names) for mild pain.
• Injections into the inflamed bursa of a long-lasting local anesthetic mixed with a corticosteroid drug, such as triamcinolone.

ACTIVITY—Rest the inflamed area as much as possible. If you must resume normal activity immediately, wear a sling until the pain becomes more bearable. To prevent a frozen shoulder, begin normal, slow joint movement as soon as possible.

DIET—Eat a well-balanced diet that includes extra protein, such as meat, fish, poultry, cheese, milk and eggs. Increase fiber and fluid intake to prevent constipation that may result from decreased activity. Your doctor may suggest vitamin and mineral supplements to promote healing.

REHABILITATION—See page 465 for rehabilitation exercises.

 ## CALL YOUR DOCTOR IF

• You have symptoms of shoulder bursitis.
• Pain increases despite treatment.
• Pain, swelling, tenderness, drainage or bleeding increases in the surgical area.
• You develop signs of infection (headache, muscle aches, dizziness or a general ill feeling and fever).
• New, unexplained symptoms develop. Drugs used in treatment may produce side effects.

SHOULDER CONTUSION

GENERAL INFORMATION

DEFINITION—Bruising of the skin and underlying tissue of the shoulder due to a direct blow. Contusions cause bleeding from ruptured small capillaries that allow blood to infiltrate muscles, tendons or other soft tissue.

BODY PARTS INVOLVED
- Shoulder, particularly the part over the acromium, the outer front end of the shoulder.
- Blood vessels, muscles, tendons, nerves, covering to bone (periosteum) and connective tissue.
- Injury to the axillary nerve, the most serious possible injury resulting from shoulder contusion and sometimes requiring surgery for repair.

SIGNS & SYMPTOMS
- Local swelling—either superficial or deep.
- Pain at the site of injury.
- Numbness and decreased function of the arm and hand if the axillary nerve was seriously damaged.
- Feeling of firmness when pressure is exerted on the shoulder.
- Tenderness.
- Discoloration under the skin, beginning with redness and progressing to the characteristic "black and blue" bruise.
- Restricted activity of the shoulder directly proportional to the extent of injury.

CAUSES—Direct blow to the shoulder, usually from a blunt object.

RISK INCREASES WITH
- Contact sports, especially football, soccer, hockey, baseball or basketball.
- Medical history of any bleeding disorder such as hemophilia.
- Poor nutrition, including vitamin deficiency.
- Inadequate protection of exposed areas during contact sports.
- Use of anticoagulants or aspirin.

HOW TO PREVENT—Wear appropriate protective gear and equipment, such as shoulder pads, during competition or other athletic activity if there is risk of a shoulder contusion.

WHAT TO EXPECT

APPROPRIATE HEALTH CARE
- Doctor's care unless the contusion is quite small.
- Self-care for minor contusions and during rehabilitation following serious contusions.
- Physical therapy for serious contusions.
- Possible surgery if the axillary nerve is damaged severely.

DIAGNOSTIC MEASURES
- Your own observation of symptoms.
- Medical history and physical exam by a

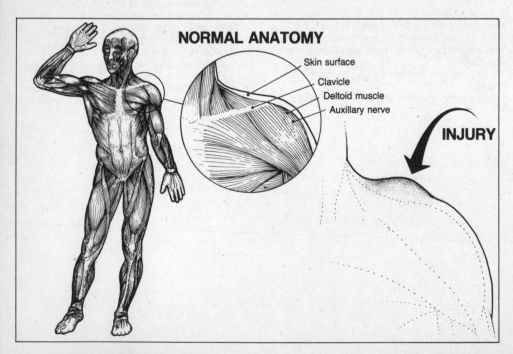

NORMAL ANATOMY

Skin surface
Clavicle
Deltoid muscle
Auxillary nerve

INJURY

doctor, with particular attention to the possibility of axillary-nerve damage for all except minor injuries.
- X-rays of the shoulder to assess total injury to soft tissue and to rule out the possibility of underlying fracture. The total extent of injury may not be apparent for 48 to 72 hours.

POSSIBLE COMPLICATIONS
- Excessive bleeding leading to disability. Infiltrative-type bleeding can sometimes lead to calcification and impaired function of the injured muscle.
- Prolonged healing time if usual activities are resumed too soon.
- Infection if skin over the contusion is broken.
- Unstable or arthritic shoulder joint following repeated injury.

PROBABLE OUTCOME—Healing time varies from 2 to 6 weeks, depending on the site and extent of injury.

 HOW TO TREAT

NOTE—Follow your doctor's instructions. These instructions are supplemental.

FIRST AID—Use instructions for R.I.C.E., the first letters of *rest, ice, compression* and *elevation*. See Appendix 1 for details.

CONTINUING CARE
- Wrap an elasticized bandage over a felt pad on the injured area. Keep the area compressed for about 72 hours.
- Use an ice pack 3 or 4 times a day. Wrap ice chips or cubes in a plastic bag, and wrap the bag in a moist towel. Place it over the injured area for 20 minutes at a time.
- After 72 hours, apply heat instead of ice if it feels better. Use heat lamps, hot soaks, hot showers, heating pads, heat liniments or ointments, or whirlpool treatments.
- Massage gently and often to provide comfort and decrease swelling.

MEDICATION
- For minor discomfort, you may use:
  Acetaminophen or ibuprofen.
  Topical liniments and ointments.
- Your doctor may prescribe stronger medicine for pain.

ACTIVITY—Begin activities slowly and stop exercise as soon as pain begins. Increase activity as healing progresses.

DIET—Eat a well-balanced diet that includes extra protein, such as meat, fish, poultry, cheese, milk and eggs. Your doctor may prescribe vitamin and mineral supplements to promote healing.

REHABILITATION
- Begin daily rehabilitation exercises when a sling is no longer needed.
- Use ice massage for 10 minutes before and after workouts. Fill a large Styrofoam cup with water and freeze. Tear a small amount of foam from the top so ice protrudes. Massage firmly over the injured area in a circle about the size of a softball.
- See page 465 for rehabilitation exercises.

 CALL YOUR DOCTOR IF

- You have a contusion that doesn't improve in 1 or 2 days.
- Skin is broken and signs of infection (drainage, increasing pain, fever, headache, muscle aches, dizziness or a general ill feeling) occur.
- Numbness or tingling in the arm begins. These may be signs of axillary-nerve damage.

SHOULDER DISLOCATION

GENERAL INFORMATION

DEFINITION—Displacement of the humerus (upper-arm bone) from its socket in the shoulder joint. A forward displacement of the humerus is the most common type of shoulder dislocation.

BODY PARTS INVOLVED
- Shoulder joint.
- Humerus.
- Soft tissue surrounding the dislocation, including nerves, tendons, ligaments, muscles, and blood vessels. Injury to nerves in the axilla (armpit) is quite common.

SIGNS & SYMPTOMS
- Excruciating pain at the time of injury.
- Loss of function of the dislocated shoulder joint and severe pain when attempting to move it.
- Visible deformity if dislocated bones lock in the dislocated position. If they spontaneously reposition themselves, no deformity will be visible, but damage will be the same.
- Tenderness over the dislocation.
- Swelling and bruising at the injury site.
- Numbness or paralysis in the arm from pressure, pinching or cutting of blood vessels or nerves.

CAUSES
- Direct upward blow to the shoulder or backward force on an extended arm.
- End result of a severe shoulder sprain.

- Congenital abnormality, including shallow or malformed joint surfaces.
- Powerful muscle twisting or a violent muscle contraction. Some people can willfully produce a recurrent dislocation.

RISK INCREASES WITH
- Contact sports, especially football, wrestling or basketball.
- Any activity that involves forceful throwing, lifting, hitting or twisting.
- Shoulder fracture (25% occurrence).
- Previous shoulder dislocation or sprain.
- Repeated shoulder injury of any sort.
- Arthritis of any type (rheumatoid, gout).
- Poor muscle conditioning.

HOW TO PREVENT
- Build your overall strength and muscle tone with a long-term conditioning program appropriate for your sport.
- Warm up adequately before physical activity.
- For participation in contact sports, protect shoulders with special equipment such as shoulder pads. After recovery, strapping or elastic wraps may protect against reinjury.

? WHAT TO EXPECT

APPROPRIATE HEALTH CARE
- Doctor's treatment. This will include manipulation of the joint to reposition the bones.
- Surgery (sometimes) to restore the joint to its normal position. Acute or recurring dislocations

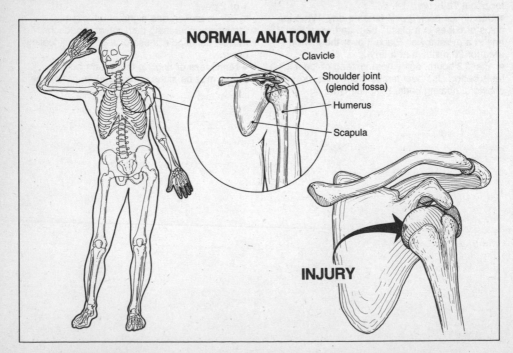

NORMAL ANATOMY

Clavicle

Shoulder joint (glenoid fossa)

Humerus

Scapula

INJURY

may require surgical reconstruction or replacement of the joint.
- Self-care during rehabilitation.

DIAGNOSTIC MEASURES
- Your own observation of symptoms.
- Medical history and exam by a doctor.
- X-rays of the shoulder joint and adjacent bones.

POSSIBLE COMPLICATIONS
- Temporary or permanent damage to nearby nerves or major blood vessels, causing numbness, coldness and paleness.
- Excessive internal bleeding.
- Shock or loss of consciousness.
- Recurrent dislocations, particularly if the previous dislocation is not healed completely. Most recurrent dislocations are anterior dislocations caused by repeated injury or congenital abnormalities of the gleno-humeral joint.

PROBABLE OUTCOME—After the shoulder dislocation has been corrected, it may require immobilization with a cast or sling for 2 to 8 weeks. Complete healing of injured ligaments requires a minimum of 6 weeks. If customary treatment does not prevent a recurrence, then athletic activities should be modified until surgery can be done to cure the problem. Surgery should be followed by rehabilitation to prevent reinjury.

 ## HOW TO TREAT

NOTE—Follow your doctor's instructions. These instructions are supplemental.

FIRST AID
- Keep the person warm with blankets to decrease the possibility of shock.
- Cut away clothing if possible, but don't move the injured area to remove clothing. Untrained persons should not attempt to reposition a dislocated shoulder.
- Immobilize the neck, dislocated shoulder, and elbow with padded splints or a sling.
- Follow instructions for R.I.C.E., the first letters of *rest, ice, compression* and *elevation*. See Appendix 1 for details.
- The doctor will manipulate the dislocated bones to return them to their normal position. Manipulation should be done within 6 hours, if possible. After that time, internal bleeding and displacement of body fluids may lead to shock. Also, many tissues lose their elasticity and become difficult to return to a normal position. Relocating a dislocated shoulder frequently requires general anesthesia.

CONTINUING CARE—At home:
- Use an ice pack 3 or 4 times a day. Wrap ice chips or cubes in a plastic bag, and wrap the

bag in a moist towel. Place it over the injured area for 20 minutes at a time.
- After 48 hours, localized heat promotes healing by increasing blood circulation in the injured area. Use hot baths, showers, compresses, heat lamps, heating pads, heat ointments or liniments, or whirlpools.
- Exercise all muscle groups not immobilized in a cast or sling. Muscle contractions promote alignment and hasten healing.
- Massage gently and often to provide comfort and decrease swelling.

MEDICATION—Your doctor may prescribe:
- General anesthesia or muscle relaxants to make joint manipulation possible.
- Acetaminophen to relieve moderate pain.
- Narcotic pain relievers for severe pain.
- Antibiotics to fight infection if surgery is necessary.

ACTIVITY—Resume your normal activities gradually after treatment. Don't drive until healing is complete.

DIET
- Drink only water before manipulation or surgery to correct the dislocation. Solid food in your stomach makes vomiting while under general anesthesia more hazardous.
- During recovery, eat a well-balanced diet that includes extra protein, such as meat, fish, poultry, cheese, milk and eggs. Increase fiber and fluid intake to prevent constipation that may result from decreased activity.

REHABILITATION
- Begin daily rehabilitation exercises when a supportive sling is no longer needed.
- Use ice massage for 10 minutes before and after workouts. Fill a large Styrofoam cup with water and freeze. Tear a small amount of foam from the top so ice protrudes. Massage firmly in a circle over the injured area.
- See page 465 for rehabilitation exercises. Review them with your doctor.

 ## CALL YOUR DOCTOR IF

- You have difficulty moving your shoulder after dislocation.
- Your arm becomes numb, pale, or cold after a dislocation. This is an emergency!
- Any of the following occur after surgery:
  Increased pain, swelling or drainage in the surgical area.
  Signs of infection (headache, muscle aches, dizziness, or a general ill feeling and fever).
  Constipation.
  New, unexplained symptoms. Drugs used in treatment may produce side effects.
- Dislocations occur repeatedly that you can "pop" back into normal position.

SHOULDER SPRAIN, ACROMIO-CLAVICULAR

 GENERAL INFORMATION

DEFINITION—Violent overstretching of the acromio-clavicular ligaments in the shoulder where it meets the collarbone (clavicle). Sprains involving two or more ligaments cause considerably more disability than single-ligament sprains. When the ligament is overstretched, it becomes tense and gives way at its weakest point, either where it attaches to bone or within the ligament itself. If the ligament pulls loose a fragment of bone, it is called a *sprain-fracture*. There are 3 types of sprains:
● Mild (Grade I)—Tearing of some ligament fibers. There is no loss of function.
● Moderate (Grade II)—Rupture of a portion of the ligament, resulting in some loss of function.
● Severe (Grade III)—Complete rupture of the ligament or complete separation of ligament from bone. There is total loss of function. A severe sprain requires surgical repair.

BODY PARTS INVOLVED
● Acromio-clavicular ligaments of the shoulder and collarbone.
● Tissue surrounding the sprain, including blood vessels, tendons, bone, periosteum (covering of bone) and muscles.

SIGNS & SYMPTOMS
● Severe pain at the time of injury.
● A feeling of popping or tearing inside the shoulder.
● Tenderness at the injury site.
● Swelling in the collarbone and shoulder.
● Bruising that appears soon after injury.

CAUSES
● Downward stress on the shoulder that temporarily forces the shoulder bones away from the collarbone.
● Falling on an outstretched hand or on the point of the elbow.

RISK INCREASES WITH
● Contact sports.
● Throwing sports.
● Racket sports.
● Previous shoulder sprain or dislocation.
● Obesity.
● Poor muscle conditioning.
● Inadequate protection from equipment.

HOW TO PREVENT
● Build your strength with a conditioning program appropriate for your sport.
● Warm up before practice or competition.
● Wear protective equipment appropriate for your sport.
● To prevent reinjury, tape vulnerable joints before practice or competition.

 WHAT TO EXPECT

APPROPRIATE HEALTH CARE
● Doctor's diagnosis.

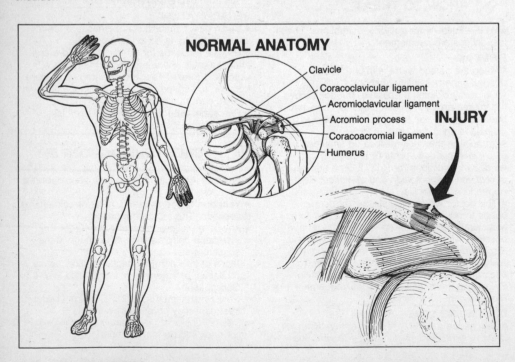

NORMAL ANATOMY

Clavicle
Coracoclavicular ligament
Acromioclavicular ligament
Acromion process
Coracoacromial ligament
Humerus

INJURY

- Application of a cast, sling, tape or elastic bandage.
- Self-care during rehabilitation.
- Physical therapy (moderate or severe sprain).
- Surgery (severe sprain).

DIAGNOSTIC MEASURES
- Your own observation of symptoms.
- Medical history and exam by a doctor.
- X-rays of the shoulder, elbow and collarbone to rule out fractures.

POSSIBLE COMPLICATIONS
- Prolonged healing time if usual activities are resumed too soon.
- Proneness to repeated injury.
- Inflammation at the ligament attachment to bone (periostitis).
- Prolonged disability (sometimes).
- Unstable or arthritic shoulder following repeated injury.

PROBABLE OUTCOME—If this is a first-time injury, proper care and sufficient healing time before resuming activity should prevent permanent disability. Ligaments have a poor blood supply, and torn ligaments require as much healing time as fractures. Average healing times are:
- Mild sprains—2 to 6 weeks.
- Moderate sprains—6 to 8 weeks.
- Severe sprains—8 to 10 weeks.

 ## HOW TO TREAT

NOTE—Follow your doctor's instructions. These instructions are supplemental.

FIRST AID—Use instructions for R.I.C.E., the first letters of *rest, ice, compression* and *elevation*. See Appendix 1 for details.

CONTINUING CARE—If the doctor does not apply a cast, sling, tape or elastic bandage:
- Continue using an ice pack 3 or 4 times a day. Place ice chips or cubes in a plastic bag. Wrap the bag in a moist towel, and place it over the injured area. Use for 20 minutes at a time.
- Wrap the injured shoulder with an elasticized bandage between treatments.
- After 72 hours, apply heat instead of ice, if it feels better. Use heat lamps, hot soaks, hot showers, heating pads, or heat liniments or ointments.
- Take whirlpool treatments, if available.

- Massage the shoulder and collarbone gently and often to provide comfort and decrease swelling.

MEDICATION
- For minor discomfort, you may use: Aspirin, acetaminophen or ibuprofen. Topical liniments and ointments.
- Your doctor may prescribe: Stronger pain relievers. Injection of a long-acting local anesthetic to reduce pain. Injection of a corticosteroid, such as triamcinolone, to reduce inflammation.

ACTIVITY—Resume your normal activities gradually after clearance from your doctor.

DIET—During recovery, eat a well-balanced diet that includes extra protein, such as meat, fish, poultry, cheese, milk and eggs. Increase fiber and fluid intake to prevent constipation that may result from decreased activity.

REHABILITATION
- Begin daily rehabilitation exercises when the cast or supportive wrapping is no longer necessary.
- Use ice massage for 10 minutes before and after exercise. Fill a large Styrofoam cup with water and freeze. Tear a small amount of foam from the top so ice protrudes. Massage firmly over the injured area in a circle about the size of a softball.
- See page 465 for rehabilitation exercises.

 ## CALL YOUR DOCTOR IF

- You have symptoms of a moderate or severe shoulder sprain, or a mild sprain persists longer than 2 weeks.
- Pain, swelling or bruising worsens despite treatment.
- You experience pain, numbness or coldness in the arm.
- Blue, gray or dusky color appears in the fingernails.
- Any of the following occur after surgery: Increased pain, swelling, redness, drainage or bleeding in the surgical area. Signs of infection (headache, muscle aches, dizziness, or a general ill feeling with fever).
- New, unexplained symptoms develop. Drugs used in treatment may produce side effects.

SHOULDER SPRAIN, GLENO-HUMERAL

GENERAL INFORMATION

DEFINITION—Violent overstretching of one or more ligaments in the gleno-humeral joint of the shoulder. Sprains involving two or more ligaments cause considerably more disability than single-ligament sprains. When the ligament is overstretched, it becomes tense and gives way at its weakest point, either where it attaches to bone or within the ligament itself. If the ligament pulls loose a fragment of bone, it is called a *sprain-fracture*. There are 3 types of sprains:
● Mild (Grade I)—Tearing of some ligament fibers. There is no loss of function.
● Moderate (Grade II)—Rupture of a portion of the ligament, resulting in some loss of function.
● Severe (Grade III)—Complete rupture of the ligament or complete separation of ligament from bone. There is total loss of function. A severe sprain requires surgical repair.

BODY PARTS INVOLVED
● Ligaments of the gleno-humeral joint of the shoulder.
● Tissue surrounding the sprain, including blood vessels, tendons, bone, periosteum (covering of bone) and muscles.

SIGNS & SYMPTOMS
● Severe pain at the time of injury.
● A feeling of popping or tearing inside the shoulder.
● Tenderness at the injury site.
● Swelling in the shoulder.
● Bruising that appears soon after injury.

CAUSES—Backward and upward stress that temporarily forces or pries the ligaments and bones of the shoulder joint out of their normal location.

RISK INCREASES WITH
● Contact sports such as boxing or wrestling.
● "Throwing" sports such as baseball, football and track events.
● Skiing.
● Previous shoulder injury.
● Obesity.
● Poor muscle conditioning.
● Inadequate protection from equipment.

HOW TO PREVENT
● Build your strength with a conditioning program appropriate for your sport.
● Warm up before practice or competition.
● Tape vulnerable joints before practice or competition.
● Wear protective equipment such as shoulder pads.

WHAT TO EXPECT

APPROPRIATE HEALTH CARE
● Doctor's diagnosis.
● Application of a cast, sling, tape or elastic bandage.

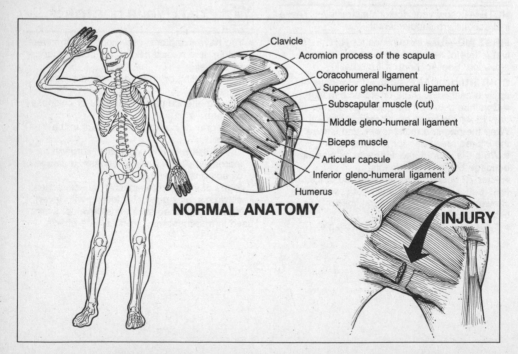

Clavicle
Acromion process of the scapula
Coracohumeral ligament
Superior gleno-humeral ligament
Subscapular muscle (cut)
Middle gleno-humeral ligament
Biceps muscle
Articular capsule
Inferior gleno-humeral ligament
Humerus

NORMAL ANATOMY

INJURY

- Self-care during rehabilitation.
- Physical therapy (moderate or severe sprain).
- Surgery (severe sprain).

DIAGNOSTIC MEASURES
- Your own observation of symptoms.
- Medical history and exam by a doctor.
- X-rays of the shoulder joint to rule out fractures.

POSSIBLE COMPLICATIONS
- Prolonged healing time if usual activities are resumed too soon.
- Proneness to repeated injury.
- Inflammation at the ligament attachment to bone (periostitis).
- Prolonged disability (sometimes).
- Unstable or arthritic shoulder following repeated injury.

PROBABLE OUTCOME—If this is a first-time injury, proper care and sufficient healing time before resuming activity should prevent permanent disability. Ligaments have a poor blood supply, and torn ligaments require as much healing time as fractures. Average healing times are:
- Mild sprains—2 to 6 weeks.
- Moderate sprains—6 to 8 weeks.
- Severe sprains—8 to 10 weeks.

 # HOW TO TREAT

NOTE—Follow your doctor's instructions. These instructions are supplemental.

FIRST AID—Use instructions for R.I.C.E., the first letters of *rest, ice, compression* and *elevation*. See Appendix 1 for details.

CONTINUING CARE—If the doctor does not apply a cast, sling, tape or elastic bandage:
- Continue using an ice pack 3 or 4 times a day. Place ice chips or cubes in a plastic bag. Wrap the bag in a moist towel, and place it over the injured area. Use for 20 minutes at a time.
- Wrap the injured shoulder with an elasticized bandage between ice treatments.
- After 72 hours, apply heat instead of ice, if it feels better. Use heat lamps, hot soaks, hot showers, heating pads, or heat liniments or ointments.
- Take whirlpool treatments, if available.

- Massage the shoulder gently and often to provide comfort and decrease swelling.

MEDICATION
- For minor discomfort, you may use:
  Aspirin, acetaminophen or ibuprofen.
  Topical liniments and ointments.
- Your doctor may prescribe:
  Stronger pain relievers.
  Injection of a long-acting local anesthetic to reduce pain.
  Injection of a corticosteroid, such as triamcinolone, to reduce inflammation.

ACTIVITY—Resume your normal activities gradually after clearance from your doctor.

DIET—During recovery, eat a well-balanced diet that includes extra protein, such as meat, fish, poultry, cheese, milk and eggs. Increase fiber and fluid intake to prevent constipation that may result from decreased activity.

REHABILITATION
- Begin daily rehabilitation exercises when the cast or supportive wrapping is no longer necessary.
- Use ice massage for 10 minutes before and after exercise. Fill a large Styrofoam cup with water and freeze. Tear a small amount of foam from the top so ice protrudes. Massage firmly over the injured area in a circle about the size of a softball.
- See page 465 for rehabilitation exercises.

 # CALL YOUR DOCTOR IF

- You have symptoms of a moderate or severe shoulder sprain, or a mild sprain persists longer than 2 weeks.
- Pain, swelling or bruising worsens despite treatment.
- You experience pain, numbness or coldness in the arm or hand.
- Blue, gray or dusky color appears in the fingernails.
- Any of the following occur after surgery:
  Increased pain, swelling, redness, drainage or bleeding in the surgical area.
  Signs of infection (headache, muscle aches, dizziness, or a general ill feeling with fever).
- New, unexplained symptoms develop. Drugs used in treatment may produce side effects.

SHOULDER STRAIN

GENERAL INFORMATION

DEFINITION—Injury to muscles or tendons that attach to bones in the shoulder. Muscles, tendons and bones comprise units. These units stabilize the shoulder and allows its motion. A strain occurs at a unit's weakest part. Strains are of 3 types:
● Mild (Grade I)—Slightly pulled muscle without tearing of muscle or tendon fibers. There is no loss of strength.
● Moderate (Grade II)—Tearing of fibers in a muscle, tendon or at the attachment to bone. Strength is diminished.
● Severe (Grade III)—Rupture of the muscle-tendon-bone attachment with separation of fibers. Severe strain requires surgical repair. Chronic strains are caused by overuse. Acute strains are caused by direct injury or overstress.

BODY PARTS INVOLVED
● Muscles and tendons that attach to bones in the shoulder.
● Bones in the shoulder area, including the humerus, scapula and clavicle.
● Soft tissue surrounding the strain, including nerves, periosteum (covering to bone), blood vessels and lymph vessels.

SIGNS & SYMPTOMS
● Pain when moving or stretching the shoulder.
● Muscle spasm in the shoulder.
● Swelling over the injury.
● Loss of strength (moderate or severe strain).
● Crepitation ("crackling") feeling and sound when the injured area is pressed with fingers.
● Calcification of the shoulder muscle or tendon (visible with X-rays).
● Inflammation of the tendon sheath.

CAUSES
● Prolonged overuse of muscle-tendon units in the shoulder.
● Single violent blow or force applied to the shoulder.

RISK INCREASES WITH
● Contact sports such as boxing, wrestling or rugby.
● "Throwing" sports, such as baseball, football, basketball or tennis.
● Any cardiovascular medical problem that results in decreased circulation.
● Medical history of any bleeding disorder.
● Obesity.
● Poor nutrition.
● Previous shoulder injury.
● Poor muscle conditioning.

HOW TO PREVENT
● Participate in a strengthening and conditioning program appropriate for your sport.
● Warm up before practice or competition.
● Wear protective equipment, such as shoulder pads, for contact sports.

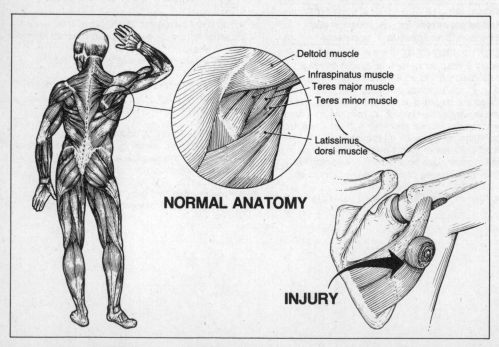

Deltoid muscle
Infraspinatus muscle
Teres major muscle
Teres minor muscle
Latissimus dorsi muscle

NORMAL ANATOMY

INJURY

- Avoid overuse. For example, rest between games if you are a pitcher or quarterback.
- To prevent a recurrence, tape the shoulder area before practice or competition.

 ## WHAT TO EXPECT

APPROPRIATE HEALTH CARE
- Doctor's diagnosis.
- Self-care during rehabilitation.
- Physical therapy (moderate or severe strain).
- Surgery (severe strain).

DIAGNOSTIC MEASURES
- Your own observation of symptoms.
- Medical history and exam by a doctor.
- X-rays of injured areas to rule out fractures.

POSSIBLE COMPLICATIONS
- Prolonged healing time if activity is resumed too soon.
- Proneness to repeated injury.
- Unstable or arthritic shoulder following repeated injury.
- Inflammation at the attachment to bone (periostitis).
- Prolonged disability (sometimes).

PROBABLE OUTCOME—If this is a first-time injury, proper care and sufficient healing time before resuming activity should prevent permanent disability. Torn ligaments and tendons require as long to heal as fractured bones do. Average healing times are:
- Mild strain—2 to 10 days.
- Moderate strain—10 days to 6 weeks.
- Severe strain—6 to 10 weeks.
If this is a repeat injury, complications listed above are more likely to occur.

 ## HOW TO TREAT

NOTE—Follow your doctor's instructions. These instructions are supplemental.

FIRST AID—Use instructions for R.I.C.E., the first letters of *rest, ice, compression* and *elevation*. See Appendix 1 for details.

CONTINUING CARE
- Use ice massage 3 or 4 times a day for 15 minutes at a time. Fill a large Styrofoam cup with water and freeze. Tear a small amount of foam from the top so ice protrudes. Massage firmly over the injured area in a circle about the size of a softball.
- After the first 24 hours, apply heat instead of ice, if it feels better. Use heat lamps, hot soaks, hot showers, heating pads, or heat liniments or ointments.
- Take whirlpool treatments, if available.
- Wrap the injured shoulder with an elasticized bandage between treatments.
- Massage gently and often to provide comfort and decrease swelling.

MEDICATION
- For minor discomfort, you may use:
  Aspirin, acetaminophen or ibuprofen.
  Topical liniments and ointments.
- Your doctor may prescribe:
  Stronger pain relievers.
  Injection of a long-acting local anesthetic to reduce pain.
  Injections of corticosteroids, such as triamcinolone, to reduce inflammation.

ACTIVITY
- For a moderate or severe strain, use a sling for at least 72 hours.
- Resume your normal activities gradually.

DIET—Eat a well-balanced diet that includes extra protein, such as meat, fish, poultry, cheese, milk and eggs. Increase fiber and fluid intake to prevent constipation that may result from decreased activity.

REHABILITATION—Begin daily rehabilitation exercises when supportive wrapping is no longer needed. Use ice massage for 10 minutes prior to exercise. See page 465 for rehabilitation exercises.

 ## CALL YOUR DOCTOR IF

- You have symptoms of a moderate or severe shoulder strain, or a mild strain persists longer than 10 days.
- Pain or swelling worsens despite treatment.

SHOULDER TENDINITIS & TENOSYNOVITIS

 GENERAL INFORMATION

DEFINITION—Inflammation of a tendon (tendinitis) or the lining of a tendon sheath (tenosynovitis) in the shoulder. The lining secretes a fluid that lubricates the tendon. When the lining or the sheath becomes inflamed, the tendon cannot glide smoothly in its covering.

BODY PARTS INVOLVED
- Tendons of the shoulder muscles. These muscles include the teres minor, infraspinatus, suprapinatus, subscapularis, deltoid and biceps. These muscles and tendons allow movement of the shoulder and hold the head of the humerus snugly against the glenoid cavity to stabilize the shoulder joint.
- Lining of the tendon sheaths (tough, fibrous tissue covering the tendons).
- Soft tissue in the surrounding area, including blood vessels, nerves, ligaments, periosteum (covering to bone) and connective tissue.

SIGNS & SYMPTOMS
- Constant pain or pain with motion of the shoulder.
- Limited motion of the shoulder.
- Crepitation (a "crackling" sound when the tendon moves or is touched).

- Redness and tenderness over the injured tendon.

CAUSES
- Strain from unusual use or overuse of the shoulder.
- Direct blow or injury to muscles and tendons in the shoulder. Tenosynovitis becomes more likely with repeated injury.
- Infection introduced through broken skin at the time of injury or through a surgical incision after injury.

RISK INCREASES WITH
- Contact sports, especially football and basketball.
- "Throwing" sports such as baseball.
- Swimming or water polo.
- If surgery is needed, surgical risk increases with smoking, poor nutrition, alcoholism or drug abuse, and recent or chronic illness.

HOW TO PREVENT
- Engage in a vigorous program of physical conditioning before beginning regular sports participation.
- Warm up adequately before practice or competition.
- Wear protective gear such as shoulder pads, if they are appropriate for your sport.
- Learn proper moves and techniques for your sport.

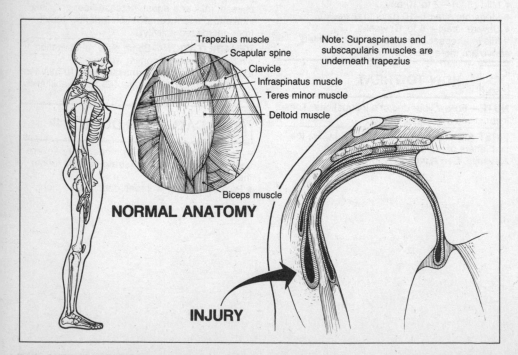

Trapezius muscle
Scapular spine
Clavicle
Infraspinatus muscle
Teres minor muscle
Deltoid muscle

Note: Supraspinatus and subscapularis muscles are underneath trapezius

Biceps muscle

NORMAL ANATOMY

INJURY

WHAT TO EXPECT

APPROPRIATE HEALTH CARE
- Doctor's examination and diagnosis.
- Surgery (sometimes) to enlarge the tunnel of the tendon covering and restore a smooth gliding motion. The surgical procedure under general anesthesia is performed in an outpatient surgical facility or hospital operating room.

DIAGNOSTIC MEASURES
- Your own observations of symptoms and signs.
- Medical history and physical examination by your doctor.
- X-rays of the shoulder and arm to rule out other abnormalities.
- Laboratory studies:
  Blood and urine studies before surgery.
  Tissue examination after surgery.

POSSIBLE COMPLICATIONS
- Prolonged healing time if activity is resumed too soon.
- Proneness to repeated shoulder injury.
- Adhesive tenosynovitis: The tendon and its covering become bound together. Loss of motion may be complete or partial. Surgery is necessary to remove the covering or transfer the tendon to a new area.
- Constrictive tenosynovitis: The walls of the covering thicken and narrow the opening, preventing the tendon from sliding through. Surgery is necessary to cut away part of the covering.

PROBABLE OUTCOME—Tendinitis and tenosynovitis are usually curable in about 6 weeks with heat treatments, corticosteroid injections and rest of the inflamed area. Recovery is usually quicker if the inflammation is caused by a direct blow rather than by a strain or sprain.

HOW TO TREAT

NOTE—Follow your doctor's instructions. These instructions are supplemental.

FIRST AID—None. This problem develops slowly.

CONTINUING CARE
- Use a sling to rest the shoulder.
- Apply heat frequently. Use heat lamps, hot soaks, hot showers, heating pads, or heat liniments and ointments.
- Take whirlpool treatments, if available.

MEDICATION—You may use non-prescription drugs such as acetaminophen for minor pain. Your doctor may prescribe:
- Stronger pain relievers. Don't take prescription pain medication longer than 4 to 7 days. Use only as much as you need.
- Injection of the tendon covering with a combination of a long-acting local anesthetic and a non-absorbable corticosteroid such as triamcinolone.

ACTIVITY—Resume normal activities gradually.

DIET—During recovery, eat a well-balanced diet that includes extra protein, such as meat, fish, poultry, cheese, milk and eggs. Your doctor may suggest vitamin and mineral supplements to promote healing.

REHABILITATION
- Begin daily rehabilitation exercises when you can raise or work your hand overhead without pain, and supportive wrapping is no longer needed.
- Use ice massage for 10 minutes before and after exercise. Fill a large Styrofoam cup with water and freeze. Tear a small amount of foam from the top so ice protrudes. Massage firmly over the injured area in a circle about the size of a baseball.
- See page 465 for rehabilitation exercises.

CALL YOUR DOCTOR IF

- You have symptoms of shoulder tendinitis or tenosynovitis.
- Any of the following occur after surgery:
  Increased pain, swelling, redness, drainage or bleeding in the surgical area.
  Signs of infection (headache, muscle aches, dizziness, or a general ill feeling and fever).
  New, unexplained symptoms. Drugs used in treatment may produce side effects.

SHOULDER-BLADE (SCAPULA) BURSITIS

GENERAL INFORMATION

DEFINITION—Inflammation of any of the bursas of the scapula (shoulder blade or wingbone). Bursitis may vary in degree from mild irritation to an abscess formation that causes excruciating pain. There are several bursas around the body of the scapula. Scapula bursitis develops most frequently in the bursa between the body of the scapula and muscles of the chest wall.

BODY PARTS INVOLVED
● Scapula bursas (soft sacs filled with lubricating fluid that facilitate motion in the scapula area).
● Soft tissue surrounding the scapula, including nerves, tendons, ligaments, large blood vessels, capillaries, periosteum (the outside lining of bone) and muscles.

SIGNS & SYMPTOMS
● Pain around or under the scapula.
● Tenderness.
● Swelling.
● Redness (sometimes) over the affected bursa.
● Fever if infection is present.
● Limitation of motion in the scapula area, including the shoulder.

CAUSES
● Injury to the scapula.
● Acute or chronic infection.
● Arthritis.
● Gout.
● Unknown (frequently).

RISK INCREASES WITH
● Participation in competitive athletics, particularly contact sports such as football.
● Previous history of bursitis in any joint.
● Exposure to cold weather.
● Poor conditioning and inadequate warmup.
● Inadequate protective equipment in contact sports.

HOW TO PREVENT
● Use protective gear for contact sports.
● Warm up adequately before athletic practice or competition.
● Wear warm clothing in cold weather.
● To prevent recurrence, continue to wear extra protection over the scapula until healing is complete.

WHAT TO EXPECT

APPROPRIATE HEALTH CARE
● Doctor's diagnosis and treatment.
● Surgery (sometimes), particularly for a frozen joint.

DIAGNOSTIC MEASURES
● Your own observation of symptoms.
● Medical history and physical exam by a doctor.
● X-rays of the shoulder and scapula.

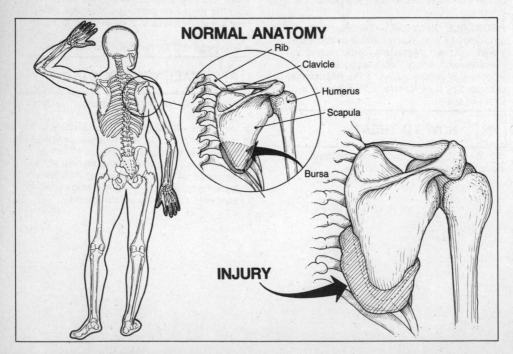

NORMAL ANATOMY

Rib
Clavicle
Humerus
Scapula
Bursa

INJURY

POSSIBLE COMPLICATIONS
• Frozen scapula, with temporary or permanent limitation of the normal mobility of both scapula and shoulder.
• Prolonged healing time if activity is resumed too soon.
• Proneness to repeated flare-ups.
• Unstable or arthritic scapula following repeated episodes of bursitis.
• Spontaneous rupture of bursa if severe infection is present.

PROBABLE OUTCOME—Scapula bursitis is a common problem. Symptoms usually subside in 7 to 14 days with treatment. Chronic bursitis may require 6 to 8 months to heal.

 ## HOW TO TREAT

NOTE—Follow your doctor's instructions. These instructions are supplemental.

FIRST AID—None. This problem develops slowly.

CONTINUING CARE
• Use ice massage. Fill a large Styrofoam cup with water and freeze. Tear a small amount of foam from the top so ice protrudes. Massage firmly over the injured area in a circle about the size of a softball. Do this for 15 minutes at a time, 3 or 4 times a day, and before workouts or competition.
• After 72 hours of ice treatment, apply heat if it feels better. Use heat lamps, hot soaks, hot showers, heating pads, or heat liniments or ointments.
• Use a sling to support the shoulder and scapula, if needed.
• Elevate the inflamed scapula and shoulder above the level of the heart to reduce swelling and prevent accumulation of fluid. Use pillows for propping.

• Gentle massage will frequently provide comfort and decrease swelling.

MEDICATION—Your doctor may prescribe:
• Non-steroidal anti-inflammatory drugs.
• Prescription pain relievers for severe pain. Use non-prescription aspirin, acetaminophen or ibuprofen (available under many trade names) for mild pain.
• Injections into the inflamed bursa of a long-lasting local anesthetic mixed with a corticosteroid drug, such as triamcinolone.

ACTIVITY—Rest the inflamed area as much as possible. If you must resume normal activity immediately, use a sling to immobilize the shoulder and scapula and help reduce pain. To prevent a frozen shoulder, begin normal, slow joint movement as soon as possible.

DIET—Eat a well-balanced diet that includes extra protein, such as meat, fish, poultry, cheese, milk and eggs. Increase fiber and fluid intake to prevent constipation that may result from decreased activity. Your doctor may suggest vitamin and mineral supplements to promote healing.

REHABILITATION—See page 465 for rehabilitation exercises.

 ## CALL YOUR DOCTOR IF

• You have symptoms of scapula bursitis.
• Pain increases despite treatment.
• Pain, swelling, tenderness, drainage or bleeding increases in the surgical area.
• You develop signs of infection (headache, muscle aches, dizziness or a general ill feeling and fever).
• New, unexplained symptoms develop. Drugs used in treatment may produce side effects.

SHOULDER-BLADE (SCAPULA) CONTUSION

GENERAL INFORMATION

DEFINITION—Bruising of skin and underlying tissues caused by a direct blow to the scapula (shoulder blade or wingbone). Contusions cause bleeding from ruptured small capillaries that allow blood to infiltrate muscles, tendons, or other soft tissue.

BODY PARTS INVOLVED—Tissues surrounding the scapula, including blood vessels, tendons, nerves, covering to the bone (periosteum) and connective tissue between the scapula and the skin.

SIGNS & SYMPTOMS
- Local swelling—either superficial or deep.
- Pain and tenderness over the injury.
- Feeling of firmness when pressure is exerted on the injured area.
- Discoloration under the skin, beginning with redness and progressing to the characteristic "black and blue" bruise.
- Restricted shoulder-blade motion proportional to the extent of injury.

CAUSES—Direct blow to the skin, usually from a blunt object.

RISK INCREASES WITH
- Contact sports, especially when the shoulder area is not adequately protected.
- Medical history of any bleeding disorder such as hemophilia.
- Poor nutrition, including vitamin deficiency.
- Use of anticoagulants or aspirin.

HOW TO PREVENT—Wear appropriate protective gear and equipment , such as shoulder pads, during competition or other athletic activity if there is risk of a scapula contusion.

WHAT TO EXPECT

APPROPRIATE HEALTH CARE
- Doctor's care unless the contusion is quite small.
- Self-care for minor contusions, and for serious contusions during the rehabilitation phase.
- Physical therapy following serious contusions.

DIAGNOSTIC MEASURES
- Your own observation of symptoms.
- Medical history and physical exam by a doctor for all except minor injuries.
- X-rays of the clavicle, shoulder and scapula to assess total injury to soft tissue and to rule out the possibility of underlying fractures. The total extent of injury may not be apparent for 48 to 72 hours.

POSSIBLE COMPLICATIONS
- Excessive bleeding leading to disability. Infiltrative-type bleeding can (rarely) lead to calcification and impaired function of injured muscle.

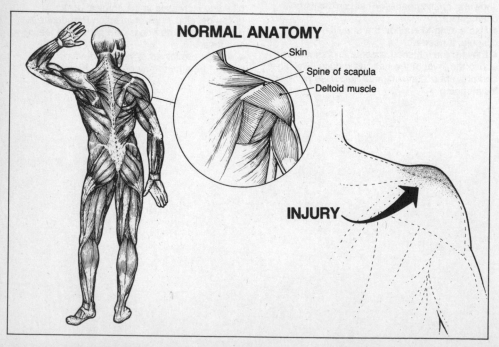

NORMAL ANATOMY

Skin

Spine of scapula

Deltoid muscle

INJURY

- Prolonged healing time if usual activities are resumed too soon.
- Infection if skin is broken over the contusion.

PROBABLE OUTCOME—Healing time varies with the extent of injury, but all but the most serious contusions should heal in 6 to 10 days.

 # HOW TO TREAT

NOTE—Follow your doctor's instructions. These instructions are supplemental.

FIRST AID—Use instructions for R.I.C.E., the first letters of *rest, ice, compression* and *elevation*. See Appendix 1 for details.

CONTINUING CARE
- Use an ice pack 3 or 4 times a day. Wrap ice chips or cubes in a plastic bag, and wrap the bag in a moist towel. Place it over the injured area for 20 minutes at a time.
- After 72 hours, apply heat instead of ice if it feels better. Use heat lamps, hot soaks, hot showers, heating pads, heat liniments or ointments, or whirlpool treatments.
- Massage gently and often to provide comfort and decrease swelling.

MEDICATION
- For minor discomfort, you may use:
  Acetaminophen or ibuprofen.
  Topical liniments and ointments.
- Your doctor may prescribe stronger medicine for pain.

ACTIVITY—Begin activities slowly and stop exercise as soon as pain begins. Increase activity as healing progresses.

DIET—During recovery, eat a well-balanced diet that includes extra protein, such as meat, fish, poultry, cheese, milk and eggs. Your doctor may prescribe vitamin and mineral supplements to promote healing.

REHABILITATION
- Begin daily rehabilitation exercises when pain subsides.
- Use ice massage for 10 minutes before and after workouts. Fill a large Styrofoam cup with water and freeze. Tear a small amount of foam from the top so ice protrudes. Massage firmly over the injured area in a circle about the size of a softball.
- See page 465 for rehabilitation exercises.

 # CALL YOUR DOCTOR IF

- You have a contusion that doesn't improve in 1 or 2 days.
- Skin is broken and signs of infection (drainage, increasing pain, fever, headache, muscle aches, dizziness or a general ill feeling) occur.

SHOULDER-BLADE (SCAPULA) FRACTURE, ACROMION

GENERAL INFORMATION

DEFINITION—A complete or incomplete break of the acromion (the part of the shoulder blade that projects over the shoulder joint and forms the highest point of the shoulder).

BODY PARTS INVOLVED
- Acromion.
- Shoulder joint.
- Soft tissue around the fracture site, including nerves, tendons, ligaments and blood vessels.
- Ribs. Broken ribs frequently accompany any scapula fracture.

SIGNS & SYMPTOMS
- Severe pain at the fracture site.
- Swelling of soft tissue around the fracture.
- Visible deformity if the fracture is complete and bone fragments separate enough to distort normal body contours.
- Tenderness to the touch.
- Numbness and coldness in the arm if the blood supply is impaired.

CAUSES
- Direct injury caused by an upward blow occurring at the same time as a shoulder dislocation. This can result in a major injury requiring surgery for repair.
- Indirect stress caused by twisting or by a violent muscle contraction.

RISK INCREASES WITH
- Contact sports such as football, soccer and hockey.
- History of bone or joint disease.
- Obesity.
- Poor nutrition, especially calcium deficiency.
- If surgery or anesthesia are needed, surgical risk increases with smoking and use of drugs, including mind-altering drugs, muscle relaxants, antihypertensives, tranquilizers, sleep inducers, insulin, sedatives, beta-adrenergic blockers or corticosteroids.

HOW TO PREVENT
- Build your strength with a good conditioning program before beginning regular athletic practice or competition. Increased muscle mass helps protect bones and underlying tissue.
- Use appropriate protective equipment, such as shoulder pads for contact sports.

WHAT TO EXPECT

APPROPRIATE HEALTH CARE
- Doctor's treatment to manipulate and set the broken bones.
- Hospitalization (sometimes) for anesthesia and surgery to set the fracture.
- Self-care during rehabilitation.
- Whirlpool, ultrasound or massage (to displace excess fluid from the injured joint space).

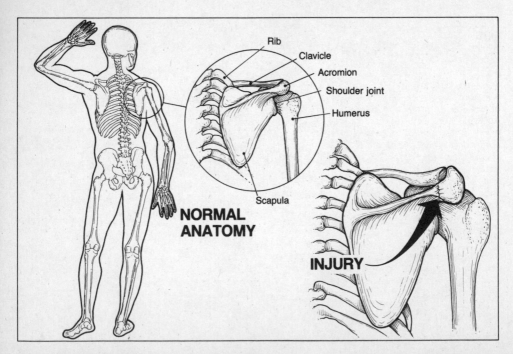

Rib
Clavicle
Acromion
Shoulder joint
Humerus
Scapula

NORMAL ANATOMY

INJURY

DIAGNOSTIC MEASURES
- Your own observation of symptoms.
- Medical history and physical exam by a doctor.
- X-rays of injured areas.

POSSIBLE COMPLICATIONS
At the time of injury:
- Shock.
- Pressure on or injury to nearby nerves, ligaments, tendons, muscles, blood vessels or connective tissues.

After treatment or surgery:
- Delayed union or non-union of the fracture.
- Impaired blood supply to the fracture site.
- Arrest of normal bone growth in children.
- Infection in open fractures (skin broken over fracture site), or at the incision if surgical setting was necessary.
- Shortening of the injured bones.
- Unstable or arthritic joint following repeated injury.
- Prolonged healing time if activity is resumed too soon.
- Proneness to repeated injury.

PROBABLE OUTCOME—The average healing time for this fracture is 6 to 8 weeks. Healing is considered complete when there is no motion at the fracture site and when X-rays show complete bone union.

 ## HOW TO TREAT

NOTE—Follow your doctor's instructions. These instructions are supplemental.

FIRST AID
- Keep the person warm with blankets to decrease the possibility of shock.
- Cut away clothing, if possible, but don't move the injured area to do so.
- Follow instructions for R.I.C.E., the first letters of *rest, ice, compression* and *elevation*. See Appendix 1 for details.
- The doctor will set the broken bones with surgery or, if possible, without. Manipulation should be done as soon as possible after injury. Six or more hours after the fracture, bleeding and displacement of body fluids may lead to shock. Also, many tissues lose their elasticity and become difficult to return to a normal position.

CONTINUING CARE
- Immobilization will be necessary. A firm compression bandage plus suspension of the arm in a sling usually supplies satisfactory support and immobilization. Casts are rarely used for this injury.
- Use frequent ice massage. Fill a large Styrofoam cup with water and freeze. Tear a small amount of foam from the top so ice protrudes. Massage firmly over the injured area in a circle about the size of a baseball. Do this for 15 minutes at a time, 3 or 4 times a day, and before workouts or competition.
- After 48 hours, localized heat promotes healing by increasing blood circulation in the injured area. Use hot baths, showers, compresses, heat lamps, heating pads, heat ointments, or liniments and whirlpools.

MEDICATION—Your doctor may prescribe:
- General anesthesia, local anesthesia, or muscle relaxants to make bone manipulation and fixation of bone fragments possible.
- Narcotic or synthetic narcotic pain relievers for severe pain.
- Stool softeners to prevent constipation due to inactivity.
- Acetaminophen (available without prescription) for mild pain after initial treatment.

ACTIVITY
- Actively exercise all muscle groups not immobilized. These muscle contractions promote fracture alignment and hasten healing.
- Resume normal activities gradually after treatment. Don't drive until healing is complete.
- Begin reconditioning the injured area after clearance from your doctor.

DIET—During recovery, eat a well-balanced diet that includes extra protein, such as meat, fish, poultry, cheese, milk and eggs. Increase fiber and fluid intake to prevent constipation that may result from decreased activity.

REHABILITATION—Begin daily rehabilitation exercises when movement is comfortable. Use ice massage for 10 minutes prior to exercise. See page 465 for rehabilitation exercises.

 ## CALL YOUR DOCTOR IF

- You have signs or symptoms of a shoulder-blade injury.
- Any of the following occurs after surgery or treatment:
  Pain, swelling or drainage increases in the surgical area.
  You develop signs of infection (headache, muscle aches, dizziness, or a general ill feeling and fever).
  You experience nausea or vomiting.
  You notice swelling above or below the bandage.
  Color of skin changes beyond the bandage to blue or gray, particularly under the fingernails.
  You have numbness or complete loss of feeling below the fracture site.
  You become constipated.

SHOULDER-BLADE (SCAPULA) FRACTURE, CORACOID PROCESS

GENERAL INFORMATION

DEFINITION—A complete or incomplete break in the coracoid process of the scapula (shoulder blade).

BODY PARTS INVOLVED
- Scapula.
- Shoulder joint.
- Soft tissue around the fracture site, including nerves, tendons, ligaments and blood vessels.

SIGNS & SYMPTOMS
- Severe pain at the fracture site.
- Swelling of soft tissue around the fracture.
- Tenderness to the touch.

CAUSES—Direct blow or indirect stress to the bone. Indirect stress may be caused by twisting or violent muscle contraction.

RISK INCREASES WITH
- Contact sports such as football, soccer or hockey.
- History of bone or joint disease, especially osteoporosis.
- Poor nutrition, especially calcium deficiency.

HOW TO PREVENT
- Build your strength with a good conditioning program before beginning regular athletic practice or competition. Increased muscle mass helps protect bones and underlying tissue.
- Use appropriate protective equipment.

WHAT TO EXPECT

APPROPRIATE HEALTH CARE
- Doctor's diagnosis.
- Self-care during rehabilitation.

DIAGNOSTIC MEASURES
- Your own observation of symptoms.
- Medical history and physical exam by a doctor.
- X-rays of injured areas.

POSSIBLE COMPLICATIONS
At the time of injury:
- Shock.
- Pressure on or injury to nearby nerves, ligaments, tendons, muscles, blood vessels or connective tissues.

After treatment or surgery:
- Delayed union or non-union of the fracture.
- Impaired blood supply to the fracture site.
- Arrest of normal bone growth in children.
- Infection in open fractures (skin broken over fracture site), or at the incision if surgical setting was necessary.
- Shortening of the injured bones.
- Unstable or arthritic joint following repeated injury.
- Prolonged healing time if activity is resumed too soon.

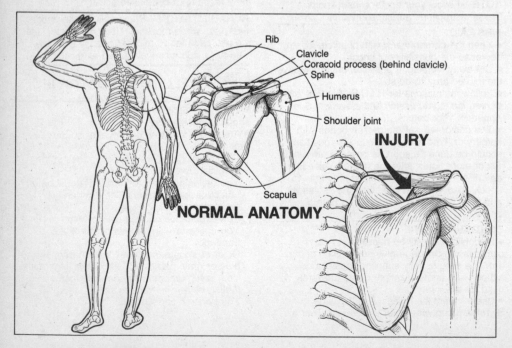

Rib
Clavicle
Coracoid process (behind clavicle)
Spine
Humerus
Shoulder joint
Scapula

NORMAL ANATOMY

INJURY

• Proneness to repeated injury.

PROBABLE OUTCOME—It is impossible to predict exactly how long it will take for any fracture to heal. Variable factors include age, sex, and previous state of health and conditioning. The average healing time for this fracture is 6 to 8 weeks. Healing is complete when there is no motion at the fracture site and when X-rays show complete bone union.

HOW TO TREAT

NOTE—Follow your doctor's instructions. These instructions are supplemental.

FIRST AID
• Keep the person warm with blankets to decrease the possibility of shock.
• Cut away clothing, if possible. Don't move the injured area to do so.
• Follow instructions for R.I.C.E., the first letters of *rest, ice, compression* and *elevation*. See Appendix 1 for details.

CONTINUING CARE
• If bone fragments are displaced, the doctor will set the broken bones with surgery or, if possible, without. The bones should be set as soon as possible after injury. Six or more hours after the fracture, bleeding and displacement of body fluids may lead to shock. Also, many tissues lose their elasticity and become difficult to return to a normal position.
• If bone fragments are not displaced, these fractures require only simple treatment and heal relatively quickly. The strong muscles that attach to and surround the scapula usually prevent the displacement of the fractured parts.
• Immobilization with a compression bandage and sling will be necessary for 14 days.
• After 48 hours, localized heat promotes healing by increasing blood circulation in the injured area. Use hot baths, showers, compresses, heat lamps, heating pads, and heat ointments or liniments.
After immobilization:
• Use ice massage. Fill a large Styrofoam cup with water and freeze. Tear a small amount of foam from the top so ice protrudes. Massage firmly over the injured area in a circle about the size of a baseball. Do this for 15 minutes at a time, 3 or 4 times a day, and before workouts or competition.

MEDICATION—Your doctor may prescribe:
• Narcotic or synthetic narcotic pain relievers for severe pain.
• Stool softeners to prevent constipation due to inactivity.
• Acetaminophen (available without prescription) for mild pain after initial treatment.

ACTIVITY
• Actively exercise all muscle groups not immobilized. These muscle contractions promote fracture alignment and hasten healing.
• Resume normal activities gradually after treatment.
• Begin reconditioning the injured area after clearance from your doctor.
• Resume driving only after healing is complete.

DIET—During recovery, eat a well-balanced diet that includes extra protein, such as meat, fish, poultry, cheese, milk and eggs. Increase fiber and fluid intake to prevent constipation that may result from decreased activity.

REHABILITATION—Begin shoulder exercises (see page 465) 10 to 14 days after injury. Use ice massage for 10 minutes prior to exercise.

CALL YOUR DOCTOR IF

• You have signs or symptoms of a shoulder-blade fracture.
• Any of the following occurs after surgery or treatment:
   Pain, swelling or drainage increases in the surgical area.
   You develop signs of infection (headache, muscle aches, dizziness, or a general ill feeling and fever).
   You experience nausea or vomiting.
   You notice swelling above or below the compression bandage.
   You have numbness or complete loss of feeling below the fracture site.
   Pain continues for more than 6 weeks.
   You become constipated.

SHOULDER-BLADE (SCAPULA) FRACTURE, GLENOID FOSSA

GENERAL INFORMATION

DEFINITION—A complete or incomplete break in the glenoid fossa of the scapula (wingbone). The glenoid fossa functions as a receptacle—like a socket—for the upper end of the humerus (the large bone between the elbow and shoulder). The glenoid fossa, along with bones, tendons, joint capsules and other soft tissue, forms the shoulder.

BODY PARTS INVOLVED
- Glenoid fossa of the scapula.
- Shoulder joint.
- Soft tissue around the fracture site, including nerves, tendons, ligaments, joint membranes and capsules, and blood vessels.

SIGNS & SYMPTOMS
- Severe pain at the fracture site.
- Swelling of soft tissue around the fracture.
- Visible deformity if the fracture is complete and the bone fragments separate enough to distort normal body contours.
- Tenderness to the touch.
- Numbness in the arm and hand (sometimes).
- Cold arm and hand if the blood supply is impaired.

CAUSES
- Direct injury: A direct blow to the side of the shoulder produces a star-shaped minor fracture of the glenoid fossa.
- Indirect injury: Falling on a bent elbow can fracture the glenoid fossa.

RISK INCREASES WITH
- Participation in contact sports such as football, soccer or hockey.
- History or bone or joint disease, especially osteoporosis.
- Obesity.
- Poor nutrition, especially calcium deficiency.
- If surgery or anesthesia is needed, surgical risk increases with smoking and use of drugs, including mind-altering drugs, muscle relaxants, antihypertensives, tranquilizers, sleep inducers, insulin, sedatives, beta-adrenergic blockers or corticosteroids.

HOW TO PREVENT
- Build your strength with a good conditioning program before beginning regular athletic practice or competition. Increased muscle mass helps protect bones and underlying tissue.
- Try to avoid falling on a bent elbow.
- Use appropriate protective equipment, such as shoulder pads for contact sports.

WHAT TO EXPECT

APPROPRIATE HEALTH CARE
- Doctor's treatment to manipulate and set the broken bones.
- Hospitalization for anesthesia and surgery to set bones for all except minimal fractures

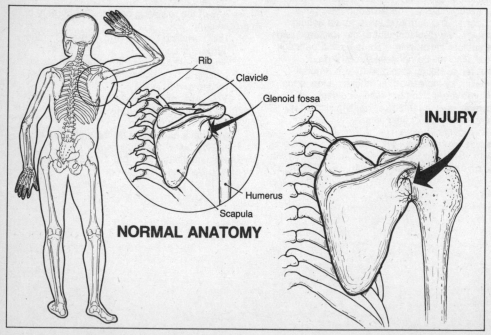

NORMAL ANATOMY

Rib
Clavicle
Glenoid fossa
Humerus
Scapula

INJURY

without displacement.
- Self-care during rehabilitation.
- Ultrasound or massage (to displace excess fluid from the injured joint space).

DIAGNOSTIC MEASURES
- Your own observation of symptoms.
- Medical history and physical exam by a doctor.
- X-rays of injured areas.

POSSIBLE COMPLICATIONS
At the time of injury:
- Shock.
- Pressure on or injury to nearby nerves, ligaments, tendons, muscles, blood vessels or connective tissues.
After treatment or surgery:
- Delayed union or non-union of the fracture.
- Impaired blood supply to the fracture site.
- Arrest of normal bone growth in children.
- Infection in open fractures (skin broken over fracture site), or at the incision if surgical setting was necessary.
- Shortening of the injured bones.
- Unstable or arthritic joint following repeated injury.
- Prolonged healing time if activity is resumed too soon.
- Proneness to repeated injury.

PROBABLE OUTCOME—It is impossible to predict exactly how long it will take for any fracture to heal. Variable factors include age, sex, and previous state of health and conditioning. The average healing time for this fracture is 8 to 10 weeks. Healing is complete when there is no motion at the fracture site and when X-rays show complete bone union.

HOW TO TREAT

NOTE—Follow your doctor's instructions. These instructions are supplemental.

FIRST AID
- Keep the person warm with blankets to decrease the possibility of shock.
- Cut away clothing, if possible, but don't move the injured area to do so.
- Follow instructions for R.I.C.E., the first letters of *rest, ice, compression* and *elevation*. See Appendix 1 for details.
- The doctor will set the broken bones with surgery or, if possible, without. This should be done as soon as possible after injury. Six or more hours after the fracture, bleeding and displacement of body fluids may lead to shock. Also, many tissues lose their elasticity and become difficult to return to a normal position. Most injuries to the glenoid fossa require surgical treatment.

CONTINUING CARE
- Immobilization will be necessary. A triangular sling for 3 to 4 weeks is usually sufficient.
- Use frequent ice massage. Fill a large Styrofoam cup with water and freeze. Tear a small amount of foam from the top so ice protrudes. Massage firmly over the injured area in a circle about the size of a baseball. Do this for 15 minutes at a time, 3 or 4 times a day, and before workouts or competition.
- After 48 hours, localized heat promotes healing by increasing blood circulation in the injured area. Use hot baths, showers, compresses, heat lamps, heating pads, and heat ointments or liniments.

MEDICATION—Your doctor may prescribe:
- General anesthesia, local anesthesia, or muscle relaxants to make bone manipulation possible.
- Narcotic or synthetic narcotic pain relievers for severe pain.
- Stool softeners to prevent constipation due to inactivity.
- Acetaminophen (available without prescription) for mild pain after initial treatment.

ACTIVITY
- Actively exercise all muscle groups not immobilized. These muscle contractions promote fracture alignment and hasten healing.
- Resume normal activities gradually after treatment. Don't drive until healing is complete.
- Begin reconditioning the injured area after clearance from your doctor.

DIET—During recovery, eat a well-balanced diet that includes extra protein, such as meat, fish, poultry, cheese, milk and eggs. Increase fiber and fluid intake to prevent constipation that may result from decreased activity.

REHABILITATION—Start shoulder exercises 2 weeks after injury. Use ice massage for 10 minutes prior to exercise. See page 465 for rehabilitation exercises.

CALL YOUR DOCTOR IF

- You have signs or symptoms of a shoulder-blade fracture.
- Any of the following occurs after surgery or other treatment:
    Increased pain, swelling or drainage in the surgical area.
    Signs of infection (headache, muscle aches, dizziness, or a general ill feeling and fever).
    Nausea or vomiting.
    Change in skin color beyond the fracture to blue or gray, particularly under the fingernails.
    Numbness or complete loss of feeling below the fracture site.
    Constipation.

SHOULDER-BLADE (SCAPULA) FRACTURE, NECK

GENERAL INFORMATION

DEFINITION—A complete or incomplete break in the neck of the scapula (shoulder blade). This injury results in marked displacement of the broken bone.

BODY PARTS INVOLVED
- Scapula.
- Shoulder joint.
- Soft tissue around the fracture site, including nerves, tendons, ligaments, joint membranes and blood vessels.

SIGNS & SYMPTOMS
- Severe pain at the fracture site.
- Swelling of soft tissue around the fracture.
- Visible deformity if the fracture is complete and bone fragments separate enough to distort normal body contours.
- Tenderness to the touch.
- Numbness in the arm and hand (sometimes).
- Cold arm and hand if the blood supply is impaired.

CAUSES—Direct blow or indirect stress on the bone. Indirect stress may be caused by twisting or violent muscle contraction.

RISK INCREASES WITH
- Contact sports such as football.
- History of bone or joint disease, especially osteoporosis.
- Poor nutrition, especially calcium deficiency.
- Obesity.
- If surgery or anesthesia are needed, surgical risk increases with smoking and use of drugs, including mind-altering drugs, muscle relaxants, antihypertensives, tranquilizers, sleep inducers, insulin, sedatives, beta-adrenergic blockers or corticosteroids.

HOW TO PREVENT
- Build your strength with a good conditioning program before beginning regular athletic practice or competition. Increased muscle mass helps protect bones and underlying tissue.
- Use appropriate protective equipment, such as shoulder pads for contact sports.

WHAT TO EXPECT

APPROPRIATE HEALTH CARE
- Doctor's treatment to manipulate and set the broken bones.
- Hospitalization (sometimes) for anesthesia and surgery to set the fracture.
- Hospitalized for traction (sometimes).
- Self-care during rehabilitation.
- Ultrasound or massage after healing (to displace excess fluid from the injured joint space).

DIAGNOSTIC MEASURES
- Your own observation of symptoms.
- Medical history and exam by a doctor.

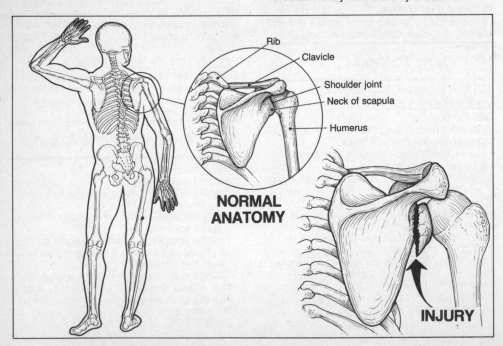

Rib
Clavicle
Shoulder joint
Neck of scapula
Humerus

NORMAL ANATOMY

INJURY

- X-rays of injured areas.

POSSIBLE COMPLICATIONS

At the time of injury:
- Shock.
- Pressure on or injury to nearby nerves, ligaments, tendons, muscles, blood vessels or connective tissues.

After treatment or surgery:
- Delayed union or non-union of the fracture.
- Impaired blood supply to the fracture site.
- Arrest of normal bone growth in children.
- Infection in open fractures (skin broken over fracture site), or at the incision if surgical setting was necessary.
- Shortening of the injured bones.
- Unstable or arthritic joint following repeated injury.
- Prolonged healing time if activity is resumed too soon.
- Proneness to repeated injury.
- Problems caused by casts. See Appendix 2 (Care of Casts).

PROBABLE OUTCOME—It is impossible to predict exactly how long it will take for any fracture to heal. Variable factors include age, sex, and previous state of health and conditioning. The average healing time for this fracture is 6 to 8 weeks. Healing is complete when there is no motion at the fracture site and when X-rays show complete bone union.

 HOW TO TREAT

NOTE—Follow your doctor's instructions. These instructions are supplemental.

FIRST AID
- Keep the person warm with blankets to decrease the possibility of shock.
- Cut away clothing, if possible, but don't move the injured area to do so.
- Use instructions for R.I.C.E., the first letters of *rest, ice, compression* and *elevation*. See Appendix 1 for details.

CONTINUING CARE
- The doctor will set the broken bones with surgery or, if possible, without. Manipulation should be done as soon as possible after injury. Six or more hours after the fracture, bleeding and displacement of body fluids may lead to shock. Also, many tissues lose their elasticity and become difficult to return to a normal position.
- Immobilization will be necessary. A rigid cast placed around the injured area is the most common technique. Skeletal traction is sometimes necessary.
- After traction or surgery, use a triangular sling for 2 weeks and begin progressive shoulder exercises on a regular schedule (5 to 10

minutes every waking hour).
- After immobilization, use frequent ice massage. Fill a large Styrofoam cup with water and freeze. Tear a small amount of foam from the top so ice protrudes. Massage firmly over the injured area in a circle about the size of a baseball. Do this for 15 minutes at a time, 3 or 4 times a day, and before workouts or competition.
- Apply heat instead of ice, if it feels better. Use heat lamps, hot soaks, hot showers, heating pads, or heat liniments or ointments.

MEDICATION—Your doctor may prescribe:
- General anesthesia, local anesthesia, or muscle relaxants to make bone manipulation and fixation of bone fragments possible.
- Narcotic or synthetic narcotic pain relievers for severe pain.
- Stool softeners to prevent constipation due to inactivity.
- Acetaminophen (available without prescription) for mild pain after initial treatment.

ACTIVITY
- Actively exercise all muscle groups not immobilized. These muscle contractions promote fracture alignment and hasten healing.
- Resume normal activities gradually after treatment. Don't drive until healing is complete.
- Begin reconditioning the injured area after clearance from your doctor.

DIET—During recovery, eat a well-balanced diet that includes extra protein, such as meat, fish, poultry, cheese, milk and eggs. Increase fiber and fluid intake to prevent constipation that may result from decreased activity.

REHABILITATION—Begin daily rehabilitation exercises when movement is comfortable. Use ice massage for 10 minutes prior to exercise. See page 465 for rehabilitation exercises.

 CALL YOUR DOCTOR IF

- You have signs or symptoms of a shoulder-blade fracture.
- Any of the following occurs after surgery or treatment:
    Pain, swelling or drainage increases in the surgical area.
    You develop signs of infection (headache, muscle aches, dizziness, or a general ill feeling and fever).
    You experience nausea or vomiting.
    You notice swelling above or below the cast.
    Color of skin changes beyond the cast to blue or gray, particularly under the fingernails.
    You have numbness or complete loss of feeling below the fracture site.
    You become constipated.

SHOULDER-BLADE (SCAPULA) STRAIN

GENERAL INFORMATION

DEFINITION—Injury to muscles or tendons that attach to bone in the area of the scapula (shoulder blade). Muscles, tendons and bone comprise units. Units stabilize the shoulder and allows its motion. A strain occurs at a unit's weakest part. Strains are of 3 types:
● Mild (Grade I)—Slightly pulled muscle without tearing of muscle or tendon fibers. There is no loss of strength.
● Moderate (Grade II)—Tearing of fibers in a muscle, tendon or at the attachment to bone. Strength is diminished.
● Severe (Grade III)—Rupture of the muscle-tendon-bone attachment with separation of fibers. Severe strain requires surgical repair. Chronic strains are caused by overuse. Acute strains are caused by direct injury or overstress.

BODY PARTS INVOLVED
● Tendons and muscles that attach the shoulder blade to the arm and chest wall.
● Shoulder blade, collarbone (clavicle), upper armbone (humerus) or spinal column.
● Soft tissue surrounding the strain, including nerves, periosteum (covering to bone), blood vessels and lymph vessels.

SIGNS & SYMPTOMS
● Pain when moving or stretching muscles of the shoulder blade.

● Muscle spasm in the shoulder-blade area.
● Swelling in the shoulder-blade area.
● Loss of strength (moderate or severe strain).
● Crepitation ("crackling") feeling and sound when the injured area is pressed with fingers.
● Calcification of the muscle or its tendon (visible with X-ray).
● Inflammation of sheath covering the tendon.

CAUSES
● Prolonged overuse of muscle-tendon units of the shoulder blade.
● Single violent injury or force applied to the muscle-tendon unit of the shoulder blade.

RISK INCREASES WITH
● Any "throwing" sport or exercise, such as baseball, basketball, tennis, shotput or javelin.
● Contact sports.
● Any cardiovascular medical problem that results in decreased circulation.
● Medical history of any bleeding disorder.
● Obesity.
● Poor nutrition.
● Previous shoulder or shoulder-blade injury.
● Poor muscle conditioning.

HOW TO PREVENT
● Participate in a strengthening and conditioning program appropriate for your sport.
● Warm up before practice or competition.
● Wear proper protective equipment, such as shoulder pads, for contact sports.

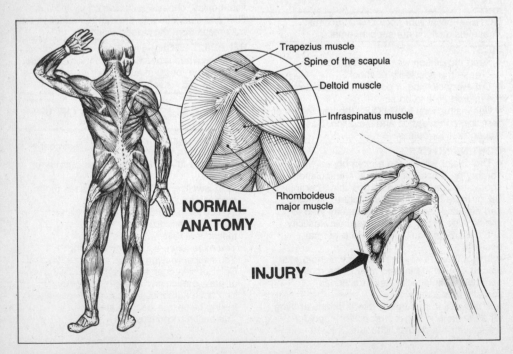

Trapezius muscle
Spine of the scapula
Deltoid muscle
Infraspinatus muscle
Rhomboideus major muscle

NORMAL ANATOMY

INJURY

WHAT TO EXPECT

APPROPRIATE HEALTH CARE
- Doctor's diagnosis.
- Self-care during rehabilitation.
- Physical therapy (moderate or severe strain).
- Surgery (rare).

DIAGNOSTIC MEASURES
- Your own observation of symptoms.
- Medical history and exam by a doctor.
- X rays of the chest and shoulder to rule out fractures.

POSSIBLE COMPLICATIONS
- Prolonged healing time if activity is resumed too soon.
- Proneness to repeated injury.
- Unstable or arthritic shoulder and spine following repeated injury.
- Inflammation at the attachment to bone (periostitis).
- Prolonged disability (sometimes).

PROBABLE OUTCOME—If this is a first-time injury, proper care and sufficient healing time before resuming activity should prevent permanent disability. Torn ligaments and tendons require as long to heal as fractured bones do. Average healing times are:
- Mild strain—2 to 10 days.
- Moderate strain—10 days to 6 weeks.
- Severe strain—6 to 10 weeks.
If this is a repeat injury, complications listed above are more likely to occur.

 ## HOW TO TREAT

NOTE—Follow your doctor's instructions. These instructions are supplemental.

FIRST AID—Use instructions for R.I.C.E., the first letters of *rest, ice, compression* and *elevation*. See Appendix 1 for details.

CONTINUING CARE
- Use ice massage 3 or 4 times a day for 15 minutes at a time. Fill a large Styrofoam cup with water and freeze. Tear a small amount of foam from the top so ice protrudes. Massage firmly over the injured area in a circle about the size of a softball.
- After the first 24 hours, apply heat instead of ice, if it feels better. Use heat lamps, hot soaks, hot showers, heating pads, or heat liniments and ointments.
- Take whirlpool treatments, if available.
- Wrap the injured chest and shoulder blade with an elasticized bandage between treatments.
- Massage gently and often to provide comfort and decrease swelling.

MEDICATION
- For minor discomfort, you may use:
  Aspirin, acetaminophen or ibuprofen.
  Topical liniments and ointments.
- Your doctor may prescribe:
  Stronger pain relievers.
  Injection of a long-acting local anesthetic to reduce pain.
  Injections of corticosteroids, such as triamcinolone, to reduce inflammation.

ACTIVITY
- For a moderate or severe strain, use a sling for at least 72 hours—longer if it lessens discomfort.
- Resume your normal activities gradually.

DIET—Eat a well-balanced diet that includes extra protein, such as meat, fish, poultry, cheese, milk and eggs. Increase fiber and fluid intake to prevent constipation that may result from decreased activity.

REHABILITATION—Begin daily rehabilitation exercises when supportive wrapping is no longer needed. See page 465 for rehabilitation exercises.

 ## CALL YOUR DOCTOR IF

- You have symptoms of a moderate or severe shoulder-blade strain, or a mild strain persists longer than 10 days.
- Pain or swelling worsens despite treatment.

SKIN ABRASION

GENERAL INFORMATION

DEFINITION—Scraped skin or mucous membrane. An abrasion is usually a minor injury, but it can be serious if it covers a large area or if foreign materials become imbedded in it.

BODY PARTS INVOLVED—Skin or mucous membranes. The most common sites are usually over bone or other firm tissue.

SIGNS & SYMPTOMS
- Skin that looks scraped or irritated.
- Bleeding at the abrasion site.
- Immediate pain that lasts a short time.
- Crusting over of the abraded area in 3 to 5 days.

CAUSES
- Falling on a hard, rough or jagged surface.
- Rough fabric, seams in clothing, ill-fitting shoes, or other parts of athletic equipment such as helmets and shoulder pads that constantly irritate the skin.

RISK INCREASES WITH
- Athletic activity on rough terrain, such as bicycling, or playing football or baseball (sliding).
- Skin that is not properly covered or protected, especially when playing on rough terrain.

HOW TO PREVENT
- Wear protective clothing, including long sleeves, high socks, knee and elbow pads, and special clothing designed for your sport.
- Wear good-quality, well-fitting footgear to help avoid falls and to prevent foot abrasion.
- Choose athletic clothing wisely to avoid irritating fabric and poorly placed seams. A combination of cotton and synthetic may be the most comfortable. Seams on the inside of the thigh of shorts can be particularly irritating, and should be checked for roughness before purchase.
- Avoid poor-quality playing fields.

WHAT TO EXPECT

APPROPRIATE HEALTH CARE
- Self-care for minor, non-infected wounds.
- Doctor's care for extensive contaminated abrasions.

DIAGNOSTIC MEASURES
- Your own observation of symptoms.
- Medical history and exam by a doctor.
- X-rays of underlying tissue (sometimes) to rule out other injuries.

POSSIBLE COMPLICATIONS
- Infection.
- "Tattooing", if imbedded, dark-colored foreign material is not carefully removed.

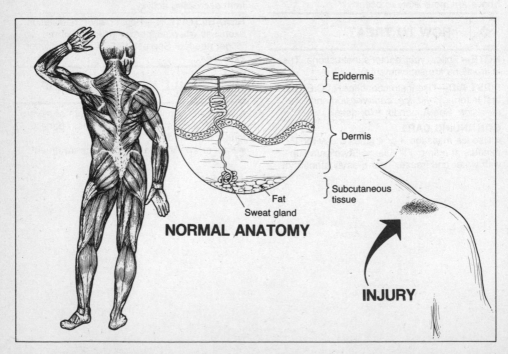

Epidermis

Dermis

Subcutaneous tissue

Fat

Sweat gland

NORMAL ANATOMY

INJURY

• Scarring, if deeper layers of skin are affected (rare).

PROBABLE OUTCOME—The wound will heal in 3 to 10 days, depending on its location.

 ## HOW TO TREAT

NOTE—Follow your doctor's Instructions. These instructions are supplemental.

FIRST AID
• For a scrape, wash the abraded area with plain soap and warm water as soon as possible. Scrub with a soft brush if possible. Soap acts as a solvent for imbedded dirt.
• For an irritation, protect the area against further abrasion. Use gauze or moleskin.

CONTINUING CARE
• If foreign material is imbedded too deeply or the wound is too painful to cleanse thoroughly, seek medical help.
• Cleanse lightly each day. If crusting or oozing occurs, soak in warm water with a little dishwashing or laundry detergent.
• Between soakings, apply non-prescription antibiotic ointment.
• Cover lightly with a bandage during the day, but leave the wound open to air at night.
• If infection occurs, use warm soaks more frequently. Keep the injured area elevated above the level of the heart, when possible.

MEDICATION
• Apply non-prescription antibiotic ointment to prevent infection.
• Spray with tincture of benzoin to reduce pain, if necessary.
• Don't use strong antiseptics such as iodine, Merthiolate, mercurochrome or alcohol. They will further irritate the skin.
• For minor discomfort, use aspirin, acetaminophen or Ibuprofen.
• Your doctor may prescribe antibiotics if the abrasion becomes infected.

ACTIVITY—Resume normal activities as healing progresses, but don't overuse the abraded area until it heals. Protect it against repeat injury.

DIET—No special diet.

REHABILITATION—None.

 ## CALL YOUR DOCTOR IF

• You cannot clean all debris from an abrasion.
• Signs of infection begin (fever, headache, or tenderness, increased oozing, redness, swelling and pain at the injury site).
• New, unexplained symptoms develop. Drugs used in treatment may produce side effects.

SKIN LACERATION

GENERAL INFORMATION

DEFINITION—A skin cut that has sharp or ragged edges. Athletic injuries are usually a combination of a contusion and a laceration, producing a bruised, jagged, irregular cut.

BODY PARTS INVOLVED—Any part of the body.

SIGNS & SYMPTOMS
● Cut of any type in the skin. Athletic injuries frequently produce lacerations at such a steep angle that they create flaps of skin.
● Pain at the lacerated site.
● Bleeding. This is especially heavy in lacerations of the scalp and forehead.
● Swelling, redness and tenderness around the laceration (sometimes).

CAUSES—Direct blow with a sharp or blunt object (boxer's glove, shoe, spike, cleat or sharp edge of another player's equipment).

RISK INCREASES WITH
● Contact sports.
● Auto, motorcycle or bicycle racing.
● Uneven terrain for a playing field.

HOW TO PREVENT
● Wear protective padding and equipment appropriate for your sport.
● Avoid playing on rough terrain when possible.
● Use seat belts in automobiles.

WHAT TO EXPECT

APPROPRIATE HEALTH CARE
● Doctor's treatment, which may include cleaning and evening jagged edges as well as suturing (stitching) a laceration.
● Self-care after treatment.

DIAGNOSTIC MEASURES
● Your own observation of symptoms.
● Medical history and physical exam by a doctor.
● X-rays of bones adjacent to the laceration to rule out fractures.

POSSIBLE COMPLICATIONS
● Fluid collection under the sutures.
● Allergy to local anesthetics.
● Wound infection due to bacterial contamination of the laceration. If infection complicates healing, fever, pain and edema (collection of fluid) around the incision will occur. The edema may cause the sutures to become tighter and break.
● Scarring and disfigurement (sometimes).

PROBABLE OUTCOME—Lacerations usually heal in 2 weeks if they are sutured properly and do not become infected. Sutures are usually removed in about 10 days. Sutures for facial lacerations may be removed sooner. You will experience discomfort as the wound swells in the 6 to 20 hours after injury.

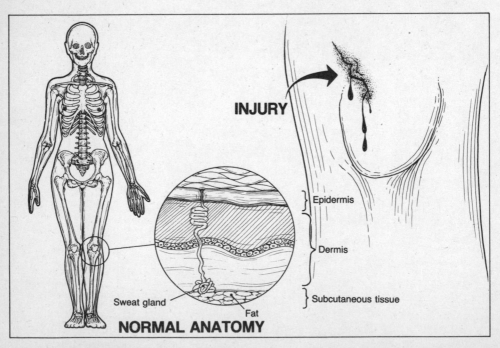

INJURY

Epidermis

Dermis

Subcutaneous tissue

Sweat gland

Fat

NORMAL ANATOMY

HOW TO TREAT

NOTE—Follow your doctor's instructions. These instructions are supplemental.

FIRST AID
For brisk bleeding:
- Cover the injured area with a cloth or your bare hands, if no cloth is available.
- Apply strong pressure directly to the laceration for 10 minutes while awaiting an ambulance or transportation to an emergency room.
- If direct pressure doesn't control brisk bleeding and bleeding is from an arm or leg, use a *light* tourniquet. Make a tourniquet from a length of cloth or similar material. Wrap and tie the tourniquet around the extremity, above the wound. Place a stick or other rigid object between the cloth and the extremity. Twist the rigid object several times until the pressure is tight and bleeding stops. Note how long the tourniquet is in place so emergency medical personnel will know. Don't leave the tourniquet on longer than 20 minutes.

For wound care without brisk bleeding:
- Clean the wound carefully with soap and water.
- The wound will be cleaned again and sutured in the doctor's office or an emergency medical facility, usually under local anesthesia.

CONTINUING CARE
- Keep the wound covered with a bandage and moderate compression for 2 days to help prevent fluid collection under the sutures.
- If the bandage gets wet, replace it and apply non-prescription antibiotic ointment.
- If bleeding occurs after suturing, control it by applying firm pressure to the wound with a facial tissue or clean cloth. Hold the pressure for 10 minutes.
- Prevent tetanus by getting a booster dose of tetanus toxoid or human antitetanic serum.
- Protect a laceration with extra padding during contact sports until it heals.

MEDICATION
- For minor discomfort, you may use non-prescription drugs such as acetaminophen. Don't use aspirin. It makes bleeding more likely.
- Your doctor may prescribe:
  Antibiotics to fight infection.
  Stronger pain medicine if needed.

ACTIVITY—Resume your normal activities gradually after treatment.

DIET—During recovery from serious lacerations, eat a well-balanced diet that includes extra protein, such as meat, fish, poultry, cheese, milk and eggs. Increase fiber and fluid intake to prevent constipation that may result from decreased activity.

REHABILITATION—None.

 ## CALL YOUR DOCTOR IF

- You have a lacerated wound.
- You develop signs of a wound infection (fever, headache, or increasing pain, redness and fluid with pus at the laceration site).
- A healed laceration leaves a scar and you would like to consider cosmetic surgery.

SKIN PUNCTURE WOUND

GENERAL INFORMATION

DEFINITION—Wound produced by any object that penetrates the skin to the soft tissue, bones or joint below.

BODY PARTS INVOLVED—Any part of the body.

SIGNS & SYMPTOMS—Hole in the skin with a puckered and discolored edge. The hole may appear smaller than the object that caused it, due to partial re-expansion of the damaged tissues.

CAUSES—Any foreign body that penetrates the skin and underlying tissue (cleats, javelin, splinters, glass).

RISK INCREASES WITH
- Contact sports.
- Athletic activities on rough terrain.

HOW TO PREVENT—Avoid rough terrain for athletic activities.

WHAT TO EXPECT

APPROPRIATE HEALTH CARE—Doctor's treatment to clean the wound and sometimes to explore it surgically to determine the extent of damage.

DIAGNOSTIC MEASURES
- Your own observation of symptoms.
- Medical history and physical exam by a doctor.
- X-rays of the underlying area to rule out fractures and joint damage.

POSSIBLE COMPLICATIONS
- Fluid collection under a closed penetrating wound.
- Wound infection.

PROBABLE OUTCOME—With treatment, a puncture wound usually heals without complications.

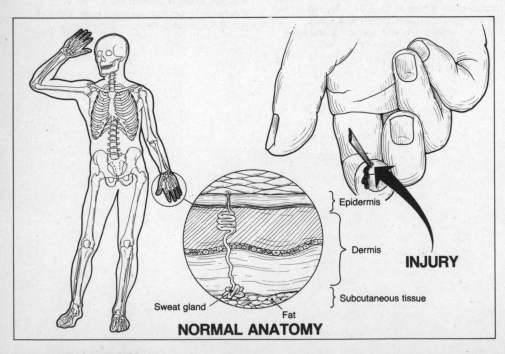

Epidermis

Dermis

INJURY

Subcutaneous tissue

Sweat gland

Fat

NORMAL ANATOMY

HOW TO TREAT

NOTE—Follow your doctor's instructions. These instructions are supplemental.

FIRST AID
● Remove any foreign material (splinter, glass or others) if you can.
● Clean the area with warm water and soap.

CONTINUING CARE
● Extensive or deep penetrating wounds may need to be enlarged and explored surgically under antiseptic conditions.
● If bleeding occurs, control it by applying firm pressure to the wound with a cloth.
● Use warm immersion soaks (see Glossary) to relieve pain and swelling.
● Rest the injured part until it heals.
● Wear a snug elastic bandage over the injured area if you can. This will decrease fluid collection under the wound and minimize further bleeding.
● Get a tetanus toxoid booster.

MEDICATION
● For minor discomfort, you may use non-prescription drugs such as acetaminophen.
● Your doctor may prescribe antibiotics to fight infection.

ACTIVITY—Resume normal activity slowly after clearance by your doctor.

DIET—For a serious puncture wound, eat a well-balanced diet that includes extra protein, such as meat, fish, poultry, cheese, milk and eggs.

REHABILITATION—None.

 CALL YOUR DOCTOR IF

● You receive a puncture wound and have not had a tetanus booster in 10 years.
● You develop signs of a wound infection (fever, headache, or increasing pain, redness and fluid with pus at the puncture site).

SPINE FRACTURE, LOWER THORACIC & LUMBAR REGION

 GENERAL INFORMATION

DEFINITION—A complete or incomplete break in a bone in the lower thoracic or the lumbar spine. The lowest part of the thoracic spine and the first two bones of the lumbar spine are the most common sites for fractures in this region. This is due to the change in the spine's curvature and the lack of rib-cage support.

BODY PARTS INVOLVED
- Bones of the lower thoracic and lumbar spine.
- Joints between segments of the spine.
- Soft tissue around the fracture site, including muscles, nerves, tendons, ligaments, periosteum (covering to bone), blood vessels and connective tissue.

SIGNS & SYMPTOMS
- Severe pain in the spine.
- Swelling and bruising around the fracture.
- Visible deformity if the fracture is complete and the bone fragments separate enough to distort normal back contours.
- Tenderness to the touch.
- Paralysis of legs and muscles in the pelvis, if the spinal cord is injured.

CAUSES—Direct blow or indirect stress to the bone. Indirect stress can be excessive spinal flexing, extension, rotation or bending. Common situations that cause this fracture include:
- A hard fall in which the person lands on the heels.
- Sitting down hard, especially for an older person with osteoporosis.
- A heavy load falling on a bent back, such as someone jumping on a swimmer's back.

RISK INCREASES WITH
- Sledding or toboggan riding.
- "Horseplay" around swimming pools and diving boards.
- Contact sports.
- History of bone or joint disease, especially osteoporosis.
- Obesity.
- Poor nutrition, especially calcium deficiency.
- If surgery or anesthesia are needed, surgical risk increases with smoking and use of drugs, including mind-altering drugs, muscle relaxants, antihypertensives, tranquilizers, sleep inducers, insulin, sedatives, beta-adrenergic blockers or corticosteroids.

HOW TO PREVENT
- Build your strength with a good conditioning program before beginning regular athletic practice or competition. Increased muscle mass helps protect bones and underlying tissue.
- Ensure an adequate calcium intake (1000mg to 1500mg a day) with milk and milk products or calcium supplements.

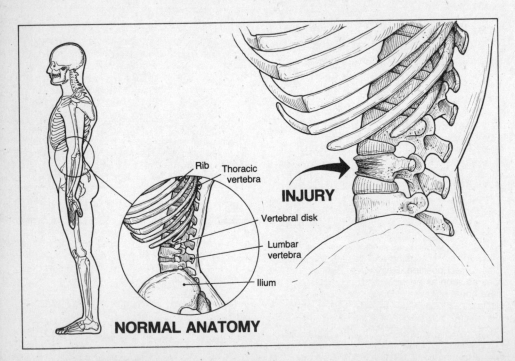

Rib   Thoracic vertebra

INJURY

Vertebral disk

Lumbar vertebra

Ilium

NORMAL ANATOMY

WHAT TO EXPECT

APPROPRIATE HEALTH CARE
- Traction.
- Surgery (sometimes) to set and immobilize the fracture.
- Long rehabilitation program and physical therapy, if the spinal cord is damaged.

DIAGNOSTIC MEASURES
- Your own observation of symptoms.
- Medical history and exam by a doctor.
- X-rays of the spine.

POSSIBLE COMPLICATIONS
At the time of fracture:
- Shock.
- Pressure on or injury to the spinal cord, nearby nerves, ligaments, tendons, blood vessels or connective tissues.

After treatment or surgery:
- Excessive bleeding.
- Impaired blood supply to the healing bone.
- Avascular necrosis (death of bone cells) due to interruption of blood supply.
- Arrest of bone growth in young people.
- Infection introduced during surgical treatment.
- Unstable or arthritic joint after repeated injury.
- Paralysis (sometimes).

PROBABLE OUTCOME—The average healing time for this fracture is 6 to 12 weeks. Healing is considered complete when there is no pain or motion at the fracture site and when X-rays show complete bone union.

 HOW TO TREAT

NOTE—Follow your doctor's instructions. These instructions are supplemental.

FIRST AID
- Cut away clothing, if possible, but don't move the injured area to do so.
- Use a spineboard to immobilize the back while transporting the injured person to an emergency facility.
- Elevate the injured part above the level of the heart to reduce swelling and prevent accumulation of excess fluid. To do so, elevate the foot of the spineboard or the bed.
- Keep the patient warm with blankets to decrease the possibility of shock.
- Treatment consists of surgically or non-surgically realigning and holding the spine in its correct position. Realignment should be done as soon as possible after injury. Six or more hours after the fracture, bleeding and displacement of body fluids may lead to shock. Also, many tissues lose their elasticity and become difficult to return to a normal position.

CONTINUING CARE
- Immobilization will be necessary. This may mean immobilization of the patient with bed rest in a rehabilitation facility, or immobilization of the fractured bones with internal wires or screws. A cast is rarely used.
- After treatment, use ice massage if possible. Fill a large Styrofoam cup with water and freeze. Tear a small amount of foam from the top so ice protrudes. Massage firmly over the injured area in a circle about the size of a softball. Do this for 15 minutes at a time, 3 or 4 times a day.
- After 72 hours, you may apply heat instead of ice if it feels better. Use heat lamps, hot soaks, hot showers or heating pads.
- Take whirlpool treatments, if available.
- Massage gently and often to provide comfort and decrease swelling.

MEDICATION—Your doctor may prescribe:
- General anesthesia, local anesthesia or muscle relaxants to make bone manipulation possible.
- Narcotic or synthetic narcotic pain relievers for severe pain.
- Stool softeners to prevent constipation due to inactivity.
- Acetaminophen (available without prescription) for mild pain after initial treatment.
- Antibiotics to fight infection if the skin is broken or surgery is needed.

ACTIVITY—Begin reconditioning and rehabilitation after clearance from your doctor. Resume normal daily activities gradually after treatment.

DIET
- Drink only water before manipulation or surgery to treat the fracture. Solid food in your stomach makes vomiting while under anesthesia more hazardous.
- During recovery, eat a well-balanced diet that includes extra protein, such as meat, fish, poultry, cheese, milk and eggs. Increase fiber and fluid intake to prevent constipation.

REHABILITATION—Begin daily rehabilitation exercises when movement is comfortable. Use ice massage for 10 minutes prior to exercise. See pages 448 and 451 for rehabilitation exercises.

 CALL YOUR DOCTOR IF

- You have signs or symptoms of a spine fracture.
- Any of the following occurs after treatment or surgery:
  Numbness, complete loss of feeling or paralysis below the fracture site.
  Increased pain, swelling or drainage in the surgical area.
  Signs of infection (headache, muscle aches, dizziness, or a general ill feeling and fever).
  Nausea or vomiting.
  Constipation.

SPINE FRACTURE, SACRUM

GENERAL INFORMATION

DEFINITION—A complete or incomplete break in the sacrum. This is a serious injury because it frequently damages important nerves that supply the rectum, bladder and genitals. Signs of this nerve damage may not appear for several days after injury.

BODY PARTS INVOLVED
● Sacrum.
● Lumbo-sacral and sacroiliac joints.
● Soft tissue around the fracture site, including muscles, nerves, tendons, ligaments, periosteum (covering to bone), blood vessels and connective tissue.

SIGNS & SYMPTOMS
● Severe pain in the lower spine.
● Swelling and bruising of soft tissue around the fracture.
● Visible deformity if the fracture is complete and the bone fragments separate enough to distort normal body contours.
● Tenderness to the touch.
● Numbness beyond the fracture site (sometimes).

CAUSES
● Direct blow to the lower back.
● Indirect stress caused by twisting or other injury to the low back.

RISK INCREASES WITH
● Skating.
● Contact sports.
● History of bone or joint disease, especially osteoporosis.
● Obesity.
● Poor nutrition, especially calcium deficiency.
● If surgery or anesthesia are needed, surgical risk increases with smoking and use of drugs, including mind-altering drugs, muscle relaxants, antihypertensives, tranquilizers, sleep inducers, insulin, sedatives, beta-adrenergic blockers or cortisone.

HOW TO PREVENT
● Build your strength with a good conditioning program before beginning regular athletic practice or competition. Increased muscle mass helps protect bones and underlying tissue.
● Use appropriate protective equipment, such as sacral or "tailbone" pads, when participating in contact sports.
● Ensure an adequate calcium intake (1000mg to 1500mg a day) with milk and milk products or calcium supplements.

WHAT TO EXPECT

APPROPRIATE HEALTH CARE
● Doctor's treatment to manipulate the broken bones or to prescribe bed rest and support with a sacral corset.

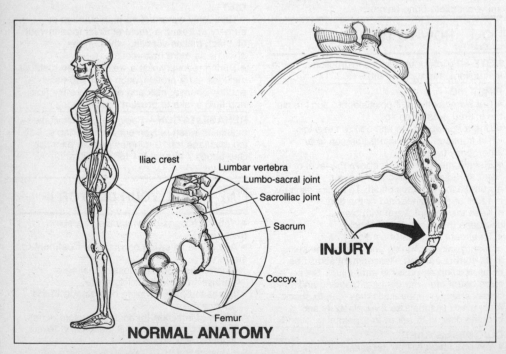

Iliac crest
Lumbar vertebra
Lumbo-sacral joint
Sacroiliac joint
Sacrum
Coccyx
Femur

INJURY

NORMAL ANATOMY

- Surgery (sometimes) to set the fracture if the fractured ends are displaced, or to relieve pressure if there is evidence of nerve damage.

DIAGNOSTIC MEASURES
- Your own observation of symptoms.
- Medical history and exam by a doctor.
- X-rays of the lower back region, including the pelvis and hips.

POSSIBLE COMPLICATIONS
At the time of fracture:
- Shock.
- Pressure on or injury to nearby nerves, ligaments, tendons, blood vessels or connective tissues.
- Injury to the rectum.
After treatment or surgery:
- Excessive bleeding.
- Impaired blood supply to the healing bone.
- Interference with bladder, rectal and sexual functions caused by postoperative swelling and pressure on nerves and blood vessels.
- Avascular necrosis (death of bone cells) due to interruption of the blood supply.
- Infection introduced during surgical treatment.
- Unstable or arthritic spinal joint following repeated injury.

PROBABLE OUTCOME—The average healing time for this fracture is 6 to 12 weeks. Healing is considered complete when there is no pain at the fracture site and when X-rays show complete bone union.

HOW TO TREAT

NOTE—Follow your doctor's instructions. These instructions are supplemental.

FIRST AID
- Use a spineboard to immobilize the back while transporting the injured person to an emergency facility.
- Keep the person warm with blankets to decrease the possibility of shock.
- The doctor may manipulate the broken bones in surgery to return them to their normal position. Manipulation should be done as soon as possible after injury, particularly if there is evidence of injury to major nerves in the lower-back region. Six or more hours after the fracture, bleeding and displacement of body fluids may lead to shock. Also, many tissues lose their elasticity and become difficult to return to a normal position.

CONTINUING CARE
- Immobilization will be necessary. Non-displaced sacrum fractures usually require a corset. Displaced fractures may require more complicated immobilization techniques such as traction.
- After treatment, use ice massage if possible. Fill a large Styrofoam cup with water and freeze.

Tear a small amount of foam from the top so ice protrudes. Massage firmly over the injured area in a circle about the size of a softball. Do this for 15 minutes at a time, 3 or 4 times a day.
- Apply heat instead of ice if it feels better. Use heat lamps, hot soaks, hot showers, heating pads or whirlpool treatments.
- Massage gently and often to provide comfort and decrease swelling.

MEDICATION—Your doctor may prescribe:
- General anesthesia, local anesthesia or muscle relaxants before joint manipulation.
- Narcotic or synthetic narcotic pain relievers for severe pain.
- Acetaminophen for mild pain.
- Stool softeners to prevent constipation due to inactivity.
- Antibiotics to fight infection if skin is broken or surgery is needed.

ACTIVITY
- Bed rest will be necessary for 2 to 6 weeks. You will need to wear a corset for support once you begin activity.
- During recovery, actively exercise all muscle groups not immobilized. These muscle contractions promote fracture alignment and hasten healing.
- Begin reconditioning and rehabilitation after clearance from your doctor.
- Resume normal daily activities gradually.

DIET
- Drink only water before manipulation or surgery to treat the fracture. Solid food in your stomach makes vomiting while under anesthesia more hazardous.
- During recovery, eat a well-balanced diet that includes extra protein, such as meat, fish, poultry, cheese, milk and eggs. Increase fiber and fluid intake to prevent constipation that may result from decreased activity.

REHABILITATION—Begin daily rehabilitation exercises when movement is comfortable. Use ice massage for 10 minutes prior to exercise. See page 448 for rehabilitation exercises.

CALL YOUR DOCTOR IF

- You have signs and symptoms of a sacrum fracture, or observe these signs in someone else.
- Any of the following occur after treatment or surgery:
  Loss of feeling below the fracture site.
  Increased pain, swelling or drainage in the surgical area.
  Signs of infection (headache, muscle aches, dizziness, or a general ill feeling and fever).
  Nausea or vomiting.
  Impaired bladder, rectal or sexual function.

SPINE FRACTURE, TAILBONE (COCCYX)

GENERAL INFORMATION

DEFINITION—A complete or incomplete break in the coccyx (tailbone).

BODY PARTS INVOLVED
- Coccyx (lower tip of the spine).
- Joints connecting the coccyx to the sacrum.
- Soft tissue around the fracture site, including muscles, nerves, tendons, ligaments, periosteum (covering to bone), blood vessels and connective tissue.

SIGNS & SYMPTOMS
- Pain at the fracture site.
- Swelling and bruising of soft tissue around the fracture.
- Tenderness to the touch.

CAUSES
- Falling into a sitting position on the tailbone.
- Direct blow or kick to the tailbone.

RISK INCREASES WITH
- Skating.
- Contact sports.
- History of bone or joint disease, especially osteoporosis.
- Obesity.
- Poor nutrition, especially calcium deficiency.
- If surgery or anesthesia are needed, surgical risk increases with smoking and use of drugs, including mind-altering drugs, muscle relaxants, antihypertensives, tranquilizers, sleep inducers, insulin, sedatives, beta-adrenergic blockers or corticosteroids.

HOW TO PREVENT
- Use appropriate protective equipment, such as sacral or "tailbone" pads, during participation in contact sports.
- Ensure an adequate calcium intake (1000mg to 1500mg a day) with milk and milk products or calcium supplements.

WHAT TO EXPECT

APPROPRIATE HEALTH CARE
- Doctor's treatment to manipulate the broken coccyx.
- Hospitalization (sometimes) for anesthesia and surgery to remove the fractured coccyx.
- Physical therapy and rehabilitation exercises.
- Self-care during rehabilitation.

DIAGNOSTIC MEASURES
- Your own observation of symptoms.
- Medical history and exam by a doctor.
- X-rays of injured areas, including all of the lower back, pelvis and hips.

POSSIBLE COMPLICATIONS
At the time of fracture:
- Shock.
- Pressure on or injury to nearby nerves, ligaments, tendons, blood vessels or connective tissues.

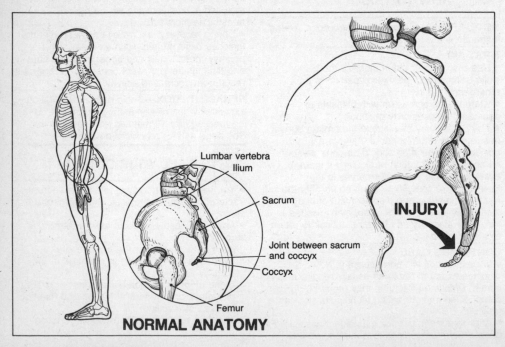

Lumbar vertebra
Ilium
Sacrum
Joint between sacrum and coccyx
Coccyx
Femur

NORMAL ANATOMY

INJURY

After treatment or surgery:
- Excessive bleeding.
- Impaired blood supply to the healing bone.
- Infection introduced during surgical treatment.
- Unstable or arthritic tailbone joint following repeated injury.
- Continuing pain long after injury.
- Avascular necrosis (death of bone cells) due to interruption of the blood supply.

PROBABLE OUTCOME—The average healing time for this fracture is 6 to 8 weeks. Healing is considered complete when there is no motion at the fracture site and when X-rays show complete bone union.

HOW TO TREAT

NOTE—Follow your doctor's instructions. These instructions are supplemental.

FIRST AID
- Cut away clothing, if possible, but don't move the injured area to do so.
- Apply ice packs to the injured site to decrease swelling and pain.
- Elevate the injured part above the level of the heart to reduce swelling and prevent accumulation of excess fluid. Use pillows to prop the lower part of the body or elevate the foot of the bed.
- Keep the injured person warm. Cover with blankets to decrease the possibility of shock.
- The doctor will manipulate the broken coccyx into normal position in a "closed" procedure (without surgery) or will remove the coccyx surgically. Manipulation should be done as soon as possible after injury. Six or more hours after the fracture, bleeding around the injury and displacement of body fluids may lead to shock. Also, many tissues lose their elasticity and become difficult to return to a normal position.

CONTINUING CARE—Treatment after manipulation or surgical removal:
- Use frequent ice massage. Fill a large Styrofoam cup with water and freeze. Tear a small amount of foam from the top so ice protrudes. Massage firmly over the tailbone area in a circle about the size of a softball. Do this for 15 minutes at a time, 3 or 4 times a day.

- Apply heat instead of ice, if it feels better. Use heat lamps, hot soaks, hot howers, heating pads, or heat liniments or ointments.
- Take whirlpool treatments, if available.
- Massage gently and often to provide comfort and decrease swelling.

MEDICATION—Your doctor may prescribe:
- General, spinal or local anesthesia during surgery to remove the fractured coccyx.
- Narcotic or synthetic narcotic pain relievers for severe pain, and acetaminophen for mild pain.
- Stool softeners to prevent constipation due to inactivity.
- Antibiotics to fight infection if skin is broken or surgery is needed.

ACTIVITY—Begin reconditioning and rehabilitation after clearance from your doctor. Resume normal daily activities gradually after treatment.

DIET
- Drink only water before manipulation or surgery to treat the fracture. Solid food in your stomach makes vomiting while under anesthesia more hazardous.
- During recovery, eat a well-balanced diet that includes extra protein, such as meat, fish, poultry, cheese, milk and eggs. Increase fiber and fluid intake to prevent constipation that may result from decreased activity.

REHABILITATION—Begin daily rehabilitation exercises when movement is comfortable. Use ice massage for 10 minutes prior to exercise. See pages 448 and 457 for rehabilitation exercises.

CALL YOUR DOCTOR IF

- You have signs or symptoms of a fractured tailbone after a hard fall or injury.
- Any of the following occur after surgery:
  Increased pain, swelling or drainage in the surgical area.
  Signs of infection (headache, muscle aches, dizziness, or a general ill feeling and fever).
  Numbness or complete loss of feeling below the fracture site.
  Nausea or vomiting
  Constipation.

SPINE STRESS-FRACTURE, NECK OR BACK

GENERAL INFORMATION

DEFINITION—A hairline fracture of the spine in the neck or back (cervical, thoracic or lumbar spine) that develops after repeated stress. A stress fracture is sometimes called a *fatigue* fracture. X-ray changes may not appear clearly for several weeks after pain begins. The X-ray appearance may be similar to a bone tumor.

BODY PARTS INVOLVED
- Any segment of the spinal column in the neck or back.
- Any joint connecting segments of the spinal column.
- Soft tissue surrounding the fracture site, including muscles, nerves, tendons, ligaments, periosteum (covering to bone), blood vessels and connective tissue.

SIGNS & SYMPTOMS
- Severe pain in the neck or back following injury.
- Swelling and bruising of soft tissue around the fracture.
- Tenderness to the touch.
- Warmth over the fracture site.
- Numbness beyond the fracture site (sometimes).

CAUSES—Direct or indirect stress to the bone. Indirect stress may be caused by twisting or violent muscle contraction.

RISK INCREASES WITH
- Contact sports such as football, wrestling, boxing or soccer.
- History of bone or joint disease, especially osteoporosis.
- Obesity.
- Poor nutrition, especially insufficient calcium and protein.
- If surgery or anesthesia are needed, surgical risk increases with smoking and use of drugs, including mind-altering drugs, muscle relaxants, antihypertensives, tranquilizers, sleep inducers, insulin, sedatives, beta-adrenergic blockers or corticosteroids.

HOW TO PREVENT
- Build your strength with a good conditioning program before beginning regular athletic practice or competition. Increased muscle mass helps protect bones and underlying tissue.
- Ensure an adequate calcium intake (1000mg to 1500mg a day) with milk and milk products or calcium supplements.

? WHAT TO EXPECT

APPROPRIATE HEALTH CARE
- Doctor's diagnosis and care.
- Physical therapy and rehabilitation.
- Self-care during rehabilitation.

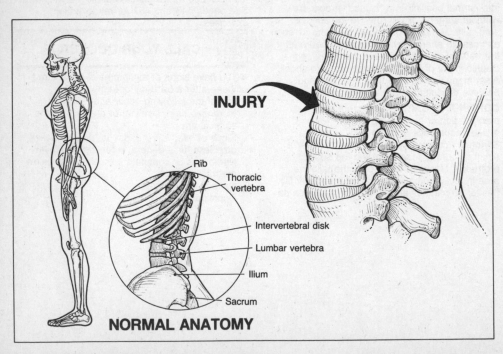

INJURY

Rib

Thoracic vertebra

Intervertebral disk

Lumbar vertebra

Ilium

Sacrum

NORMAL ANATOMY

DIAGNOSTIC MEASURES
- Your own observation of symptoms.
- Medical history and physical exam by a doctor.
- X-rays of the neck and back.

POSSIBLE COMPLICATIONS
- Pressure on or injury to nearby nerves, ligaments, tendons, blood vessels or connective tissues.
- Complete fracture and spinal-cord damage from continued activity after symptoms begin.
- Problems arising from plaster casts, splints or other immobilizing materials. See Appendix 2 (Care of Casts).
- Arrest of bone growth in young people.
- Unstable or arthritic joint following repeated injury.

PROBABLE OUTCOME—It is impossible to predict exactly how long a fracture will take to heal. Variable factors include age, sex, previous health and general conditioning. The average healing time for this fracture is 6 to 8 weeks. Healing is considered complete when there is no pain at the fracture site and when X-rays show complete bone union.

 ## HOW TO TREAT

NOTE—Follow your doctor's instructions. These instructions are supplemental.

FIRST AID—None. This fracture develops gradually and does not require setting. The fractured bone is not displaced.

CONTINUING CARE
- Immobilization will be necessary, usually with a cast or corset.
- After cast removal, use frequent ice massage. Fill a large Styrofoam cup with water and freeze. Tear a small amount of foam from the top so

ice protrudes. Massage firmly over the injured area in a circle about the size of a softball. Do this for 15 minutes at a time, 3 or 4 times a day.
- Apply heat instead of ice, if it feels better. Use heat lamps, hot soaks, hot showers, heating pads, or heat liniments and ointments.
- Take whirlpool treatments, if available.
- Massage gently and often to provide comfort and decrease swelling.

MEDICATION—Your doctor may prescribe:
- Narcotic or synthetic narcotic pain relievers for severe pain.
- Stool softeners to prevent constipation due to inactivity.
- Acetaminophen (available without prescription) for mild pain after initial treatment.

ACTIVITY
- Actively exercise all muscle groups not immobilized. These muscle contractions promote fracture alignment and hasten healing.
- Resume normal daily activities gradually after treatment.
- Begin reconditioning and rehabilitation after clearance from your doctor.

DIET—During recovery, eat a well-balanced diet that includes extra protein, such as meat, fish, poultry, cheese, milk and eggs. Increase fiber and fluid intake to prevent constipation that may result from decreased activity.

REHABILITATION—Begin daily rehabilitation exercises when movement is allowed. Use ice massage for 10 minutes prior to exercise. See pages 448, 451 or 464 for rehabilitation exercises, depending on the area of injury.

 ## CALL YOUR DOCTOR IF

You have symptoms of a spinal stress-fracture, especially unexplained persistent numbness or pain in the neck or back.

SPLEEN RUPTURE

GENERAL INFORMATION

DEFINITION—Injury to the spleen, causing it to rupture. Bleeding of a ruptured spleen can be fatal. The spleen is vulnerable to injury, particularly if it is enlarged due to any underlying disorder (infectious mononucleosis is the most common). Spleen injuries are infrequent in athletes but, when they do occur, they can be disastrous.

BODY PARTS INVOLVED
● Spleen.
● Muscles of the abdominal wall.
● Peritoneum (membranous covering to the intestines).
● Ribs (sometimes) if fractured at the same time the spleen is injured.

SIGNS & SYMPTOMS
● Recent injury to the abdomen or flank.
● Rib fracture on the left side.
● Vomiting.
● Abdominal pain and tenderness.
● Pain in the left shoulder or left side of the neck.
● Rapid heart rate.
● Low blood pressure.
● Other signs of shock: pale, moist and sweaty skin; anxiety with feelings of impending doom; shortness of breath and rapid breathing; disorientation and confusion.

CAUSES—Direct injury to the left upper abdomen or left side of the chest.

RISK INCREASES WITH
● Contact sports.
● Bleeding disorders such as hemophilia.
● Infectious mononucleosis or any other illness that causes spleen enlargement.
● If surgery is necessary, surgical risk increases with smoking, use of mind-altering drugs, muscle relaxants, tranquilizers, sleep inducers, insulin, sedatives, beta-adrenergic blockers or corticosteroids.

HOW TO PREVENT—Avoid causes and risk factors when possible. Don't return to athletic activities until a spleen enlarged by disease has returned to normal.

WHAT TO EXPECT

APPROPRIATE HEALTH CARE
● Doctor's exam. When abdominal symptoms follow a blow to the abdomen, it is imperative that a diagnosis be established as soon as possible. Injury to any organ in the abdomen (spleen, liver, intestines, kidney, bladder, pancreas) causes an acute surgical emergency.
● Hospitalization for intravenous fluids or transfusions to treat shock.
● Surgery under general anesthesia to remove the ruptured spleen.

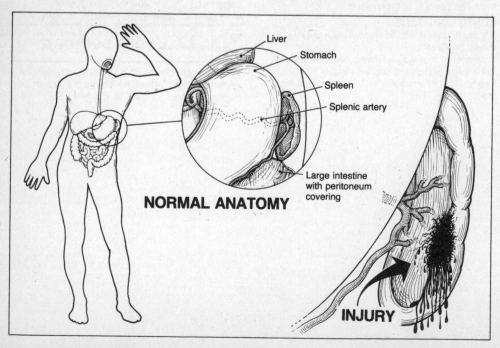

Liver
Stomach
Spleen
Splenic artery
Large intestine with peritoneum covering

NORMAL ANATOMY

INJURY

DIAGNOSTIC MEASURES

Before surgery:
- Blood and urine studies.
- X-rays of the abdomen and chest.

After surgery:
- Examination of all removed tissue.
- Additional blood studies.

POSSIBLE COMPLICATIONS

At the time of injury:
- Rapid deterioration due to internal bleeding, possibly leading to death.

Following surgery:
- Excessive bleeding.
- Infection.
- Incisional hernia.
- Lung collapse.
- Inflammation of the pancreas.
- Deep-vein blood clots.
- Pneumonia.

PROBABLE OUTCOME—Expect complete healing if no complications occur. Allow about 4 weeks for recovery from surgery.

 HOW TO TREAT

NOTE—Follow your doctor's instructions. These instructions are supplemental.

FIRST AID—Cover the victim with a blanket to combat shock, and take to the nearest emergency facility. Do not give water, food or pain relievers.

CONTINUING CARE—No specific instructions except those under other headings. If surgery is required, your surgeon will supply postoperative instructions.

MEDICATION
- Do not give pain relievers at the time of injury. They may mask symptoms.
- After surgery, your doctor may prescribe:
  Pain relievers. Don't take prescription pain medication longer than 4 to 7 days. Use only as much as you need.
  Antibiotics to fight infection.
  Pneumonia vaccinations.
  Stool softeners to prevent constipation.
  Non-prescription drugs such as acetaminophen for minor pain.

ACTIVITY
- Return to work, play and normal activity as soon as possible. This reduces postoperative depression, which is common.
- Avoid vigorous exercise for 6 weeks after surgery.
- Resume driving 4 weeks after returning home.

DIET
- No food or water before surgery.
- Drink a clear liquid diet until the gastrointestinal tract functions again. Then eat a well-balanced diet that includes extra protein, such as meat, fish, poultry, cheese, milk and eggs. Increase fiber and fluid intake to prevent constipation that may result from decreased activity.

REHABILITATION—Rehabilitation exercises must be individualized. Follow your doctor's or surgeon's directions.

 CALL YOUR DOCTOR IF

- You receive any abdominal injury and the symptoms last longer than a few minutes, worsen, or recur within hours or days. This may be an emergency!
- Any of the following occur after surgery:
  You develop signs of infection (headache, muscle aches, dizziness or a general ill feeling and fever).
  Pain, swelling, redness, drainage or bleeding increases in the surgical area.
  New, unexplained symptoms develop. Drugs used in treatment may produce side effects.

THIGH-BONE (FEMUR) FRACTURE

GENERAL INFORMATION

DEFINITION—A complete or incomplete break in the shaft of the femur (the large bone extending from the hip to the knee). This is a serious injury, but unusual in sports—the ankle, lower leg or knee will usually give way before the shaft of the femur does.

BODY PARTS INVOLVED
● Femur (usually in the middle of the bone).
● Soft tissue around the fracture site, including muscles, nerves, tendons, ligaments, periosteum (covering to bone), blood vessels and connective tissue.

SIGNS & SYMPTOMS
● Severe pain in the midthigh at the time of injury.
● Swelling and bruising around the fracture.
● Visible deformity if the fracture is complete and the bone fragments separate enough to distort normal leg contours.
● Tenderness to the touch.
● Numbness and coldness in the leg and foot beyond the fracture site if the blood supply is impaired.

CAUSES
● Direct blow to the thigh.
● Indirect stress caused by twisting or violent muscle contraction.

RISK INCREASES WITH
● Contact sports.
● Field and track events.
● History of bone or joint disease, especially osteoporosis.
● Obesity.
● Poor nutrition, especially calcium deficiency.
● If surgery or anesthesia are needed, surgical risk increases with smoking and use of drugs, including mind-altering drugs, muscle relaxants, antihypertensives, tranquilizers, sleep inducers, insulin, sedatives, beta-adrenergic blockers or corticosteroids.

HOW TO PREVENT
● Build your strength with a good conditioning program before beginning regular athletic practice or competition. Increased muscle mass helps protect bones and underlying tissue.
● Ensure an adequate calcium intake (1000mg to 1500mg a day) with milk and milk products or calcium supplements.
● Use appropriate protective equipment, such as thigh pads, for participation in contact sports.

WHAT TO EXPECT

APPROPRIATE HEALTH CARE
● Doctor's care.
● Surgery to set the broken femur.
● Traction (sometimes) for 6 to 8 weeks in a hospital, extended-care facility or at home.
● Immobilization with a cast (sometimes).
● Physical therapy and rehabilitation.

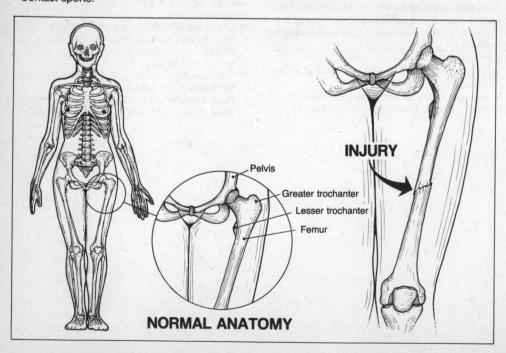

INJURY

Pelvis
Greater trochanter
Lesser trochanter
Femur

NORMAL ANATOMY

DIAGNOSTIC MEASURES
- Your own observation of symptoms.
- Medical history and exam by a doctor.
- X-rays of the ankle, knee, femur and pelvis.

POSSIBLE COMPLICATIONS
At the time of fracture:
- Shock.
- Pressure on or injury to nearby nerves, ligaments, tendons, blood vessels or connective tissue.

After treatment or surgery:
- Excessive bleeding.
- Poor healing (non-union) of the fracture.
- Impaired blood supply to the healing bone.
- Avascular necrosis (death of bone cells) due to interruption of the blood supply.
- Shortening or deformity of the fractured femur.
- Arrest of normal bone growth in children.
- Infection introduced during surgery.
- Problems caused by plaster casts. See Appendix 2 (Care of Casts).

PROBABLE OUTCOME—The average healing time for this fracture is 6 to 8 weeks. Healing is considered complete when there is no pain or motion at the fracture site, and when X-rays show complete bone union.

 # HOW TO TREAT

NOTE—Follow your doctor's instructions. These instructions are supplemental.

FIRST AID
- Keep the person warm with blankets to decrease the possibility of shock.
- Cut away clothing, if possible, but don't move the injured leg to do so.
- Follow instructions for R.I.C.E., the first letters of *rest, ice, compression* and *elevation.* See Appendix 1 for details.
- Use a padded splint or backboard to immobilize the hip and leg before transporting the injured person to an emergency facility.
- The doctor will set (realign) the broken bones with surgery or, if possible, without. Realignment should be done as soon as possible after injury. Six or more hours after the fracture, bleeding and displacement of body fluids may lead to shock. Also, many tissues lose their elasticity and become difficult to return to a normal position.

CONTINUING CARE
- Immobilization will be necessary, either with traction or with a rigid hip-to-knee cast following surgery to pin bone fragments together.
- After 48 hours, localized heat promotes healing by increasing blood circulation in the injured area. Use a heat lamp or heating pad so heat can penetrate the cast.
- When the cast is removed, take whirlpool treatments, if available.

MEDICATION—Your doctor may prescribe:
- General anesthesia to make joint manipulation possible.
- Narcotic or synthetic narcotic pain relievers for severe pain.
- Stool softeners to prevent constipation due to inactivity.
- Acetaminophen for mild pain.
- Antibiotics to fight infection if necessary.

ACTIVITY
- Exercise the uninjured leg and arms vigorously during recuperation. These muscle contractions promote fracture alignment and hasten healing.
- Resume normal daily activities gradually after treatment. Don't drive until healing is complete.

DIET
- Drink only water before manipulation or surgery to treat the fracture. Solid food in your stomach makes vomiting while under anesthesia more hazardous.
- During recovery, eat a well-balanced diet that includes extra protein, such as meat, fish, poultry, cheese, milk and eggs. Increase fiber and fluid intake to prevent constipation that may result from decreased activity.

REHABILITATION
- Begin daily rehabilitation exercises after clearance from your doctor when movement is comfortable.
- Use ice massage for 10 minutes before and after exercise. Fill a large Styrofoam cup with water and freeze. Tear a small amount of foam from the top so ice protrudes. Massage firmly in a circle over the injured area.
- See pages 457, 460 and 471 for rehabilitation exercises.

 # CALL YOUR DOCTOR IF

- You have signs or symptoms of a femur fracture. Call immediately if you have numbness or complete loss of feeling below the fracture site. This is an emergency!
- Any of the following occur after surgery or other treatment:
  Increased pain, swelling or drainage in the surgical area.
  Signs of infection (headache, muscle aches, dizziness, or a general ill feeling and fever).
  Swelling above or below the cast.
  Blue or gray skin color beyond the cast, especially under the toenails.
  Nausea or vomiting.
  Constipation.

THIGH CONTUSION

GENERAL INFORMATION

DEFINITION—Bruising of skin and underlying tissues of the thigh (between knee and hip) due to a direct blow. Contusions cause bleeding from ruptured small capillaries that allow blood to infiltrate muscles, tendons or other soft tissue. The thigh is well-suited to absorb direct blows, but contusions do occur here.

BODY PARTS INVOLVED—The thigh, including blood vessels, muscles, tendons, nerves, covering to bone (periosteum) and connective tissue.

SIGNS & SYMPTOMS
- Swelling of the thigh—either superficial or deep.
- Pain and tenderness in the thigh.
- Feeling of firmness when pressure is exerted at the injury site.
- Discoloration under the skin, beginning with redness and progressing to the characteristic "black and blue" bruise.
- Restricted activity of the injured leg proportional to the extent of injury.

CAUSES—Direct blow to the thigh, usually from a blunt object (frequently the edge of a thigh pad in football pants.)

RISK INCREASES WITH
- Violent contact sports, especially football.

- Medical history of any bleeding disorder such as hemophilia.
- Poor nutrition, including vitamin deficiency.
- Inadequate protection of exposed areas during contact sports.
- Use of anticoagulants or aspirin.

HOW TO PREVENT—Wear appropriate protective gear and equipment, such as thigh pads, during competition or other athletic activity if there is risk of a thigh contusion. Keep thigh pads strapped in position.

WHAT TO EXPECT

APPROPRIATE HEALTH CARE
- Doctor's care unless the contusion is quite small.
- Self-care for minor contusions and for serious contusions during the rehabilitation phase.
- Physical therapy following serious contusions.

DIAGNOSTIC MEASURES
- Your own observation of symptoms.
- Medical history and physical exam by a doctor for all except minor injuries.
- X-rays of the thigh, knee and hip to assess total injury to soft tissue and to rule out the possibility of underlying fractures. The total extent of injury may not be apparent for 48 to 72 hours.

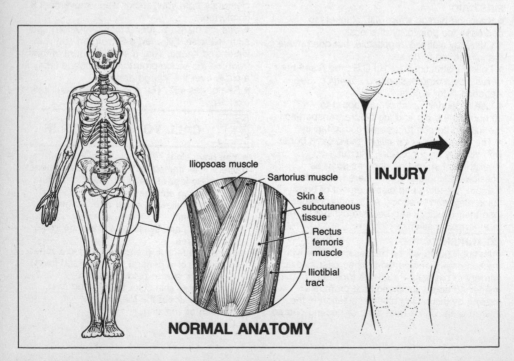

Iliopsoas muscle
Sartorius muscle
Skin & subcutaneous tissue
Rectus femoris muscle
Iliotibial tract

INJURY

NORMAL ANATOMY

POSSIBLE COMPLICATIONS

- Excessive bleeding leading to disability. Infiltrative type bleeding can often lead to calcification and impaired function of injured muscle.
- Prolonged healing time if usual activities are resumed too soon.
- Infection if skin over the contusion is broken.

PROBABLE OUTCOME—Healing time varies with the extent of injury, but average healing time for a thigh contusion is 1 to 2 weeks.

 ## HOW TO TREAT

NOTE—Follow your doctor's instructions. These instructions are supplemental.

FIRST AID—Use instructions for R.I.C.E., the first letters of *rest, ice, compression* and *elevation.* See Appendix 1 for details.

CONTINUING CARE

- Wrap an elasticized bandage over a felt pad on the injured area. Keep the area compressed for about 72 hours.
- Use ice massage. Fill a large Styrofoam cup with water and freeze. Tear a small amount of foam from the top so ice protrudes. Massage gently over the injured area in a circle about the size of a softball. Do this for 15 minutes at a time, 3 or 4 times a day, and before workouts or competition.
- Massage gently and often to provide comfort and decrease swelling.

MEDICATION

- For minor discomfort, you may use:
  Acetaminophen or ibuprofen.
  Topical liniments and ointments.
- Your doctor may prescribe stronger medicine for pain.

ACTIVITY—Begin activities slowly and stop exercise as soon as pain begins. Increase activity as healing progresses.

DIET—Eat a well-balanced diet that includes extra protein, such as meat, fish, poultry, cheese, milk and eggs. Your doctor may prescribe vitamin and mineral supplements to promote healing.

REHABILITATION—Begin daily rehabilitation exercises when supportive wrapping is no longer needed. See pages 457, 460 and 471 for rehabilitation exercises.

 ## CALL YOUR DOCTOR IF

- You have a thigh contusion that doesn't improve in 1 or 2 days.
- Skin is broken and signs of infection (drainage, increasing pain, fever, headache, muscle aches, dizziness or a general ill feeling) occur.

THIGH HEMATOMA

GENERAL INFORMATION

DEFINITION—A collection of pooled blood in the thigh within a relatively constricted area. Thigh hematomas probably accompany all serious contusions of the thigh, but they are difficult to diagnose because of the large muscle mass in the thigh.

BODY PARTS INVOLVED—Thigh, including soft tissue (nerves, tendons, ligaments, muscles and blood vessels) surrounding the hematoma.

SIGNS & SYMPTOMS
- Swelling at the injury site.
- Fluctuance (feeling of tenseness to touch, like pushing on an overinflated balloon).
- Tenderness.
- Redness that progresses through several color changes—purple, green-yellow, yellow—before it completely heals.

CAUSES—Direct injury, usually with a blunt object. Bleeding into tissues causes the surrounding tissue to be pushed away.

RISK INCREASES WITH
- Contact sports, especially if the thigh is not adequately protected.
- Medical history of any bleeding disorder such as hemophilia.
- Poor nutrition, including vitamin deficiency.
- Use of anticoagulants or aspirin.

HOW TO PREVENT—Wear appropriate protective gear and equipment, such as thigh pads, during competition or other athletic activity if there is a risk of a thigh injury.

WHAT TO EXPECT

APPROPRIATE HEALTH CARE
- Doctor's care unless the hematoma is very small.
- Needle aspiration of blood from the hematoma if the hematoma is accessible. At the same time, hyaluronidase (an enzyme) can be injected into the hematoma space. Hyaluronidase hastens absorption of blood.
- Self-care for minor hematomas, or for serious hematomas during the rehabilitation phase.
- Physical therapy following serious hematomas.

DIAGNOSTIC MEASURES
- Your own observation of symptoms.
- Physical exam and medical history by a doctor for all except minor injuries.
- X-rays of the injured area to assess total injury and to rule out the possibility of an underlying bone fracture. Total extent of the injury may not be apparent for 48 to 72 hours following injury.

POSSIBLE COMPLICATIONS
- Infection introduced either through a break in

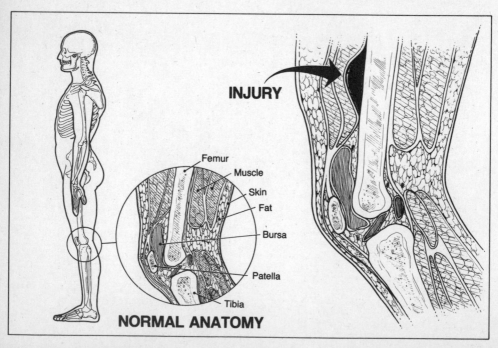

INJURY

Femur
Muscle
Skin
Fat
Bursa
Patella
Tibia

NORMAL ANATOMY

the skin at the time of injury or during aspiration of the hematoma.
- Prolonged healing time if activity is resumed too soon.
- Calcification of the blood remaining in the hematoma if blood is not completely removed or absorbed.

PROBABLE OUTCOME—Average healing time is 2 weeks to 2 months unless blood is removed with aspiration. Healing time is much less with this treatment.

 HOW TO TREAT

NOTE—Follow your doctor's instructions. These instructions are supplemental.

FIRST AID—Use instructions for R.I.C.E., the first letters of *rest, ice, compression* and *elevation*. See Appendix 1 for details.

CONTINUING CARE
- Continue ice massage 3 or 4 times a day for 15 minutes at a time. Fill a large Styrofoam cup with water and freeze. Tear a small amount of foam from the top so ice protrudes. Massage firmly over the injured area in a circle about the size of a softball.
- Don't massage the thigh. You may trigger bleeding again.

MEDICATION
- For minor discomfort, you may use:
  Non-prescription medicines such as acetaminophen or ibuprofen.

Topical liniments and ointments.
- Your doctor may prescribe stronger medicine for pain, if needed.

ACTIVITY—Begin activities slowly and stop exercise as soon as pain begins. Increase activity as healing progresses. To prevent a delay in healing, protect the hematoma area against excessive motion soon after injury. Motion breaks down the clot and causes irritation throughout the thigh, leading to possible scar formation, calcification and restricted movement after healing.

DIET—During recovery, eat a well-balanced diet that includes extra protein, such as meat, fish, poultry, cheese, milk and eggs. Increase fiber and fluid intake to prevent constipation that may result from decreased activity.

REHABILITATION—Begin daily rehabilitation exercises when supportive wrapping is no longer needed. Use gentle ice massage for 10 minutes prior to exercise. See pages 457, 460 and 471 for rehabilitation exercises.

 CALL YOUR DOCTOR IF

- You have signs or symptoms of a thigh hematoma that doesn't begin to improve in 1 or 2 days.
- Skin is broken and signs of infection (drainage, increasing pain, fever, headache, muscle aches, dizziness or a general ill feeling) occur.

THIGH INJURY, HAMSTRING

GENERAL INFORMATION

DEFINITION—An injury to a hamstring tendon. The hamstrings connect the muscles of the thigh to the back and side of the knee. These tendons can be felt behind the knee on either side. They feel like tough rope. Hamstring tendons, muscles and bone comprise units that stabilize the knee and allow its motion. The injury, usually a strain, occurs at the weakest part of a unit. Hamstring strains are of 3 types:
- Mild (Grade I)—Slightly pulled muscle without tearing of muscle or tendon fibers. There is no loss of strength.
- Moderate (Grade II)—Tearing of fibers of the muscle, tendon or at the attachment to bone. Strength is diminished.
- Severe (Grade III)—Rupture of the muscle-tendon-bone attachment with separation of fibers. Severe strain requires surgical repair. Chronic strains are caused by overuse. Acute strains are caused by direct injury or overstress.

BODY PARTS INVOLVED
- Hamstring tendons and associated muscles.
- Bones in the pelvis and knee joints.
- Soft tissue surrounding the injury, including nerves, periosteum (covering to bone), blood vessels and lymph vessels.

SIGNS & SYMPTOMS
- Pain when moving or stretching the leg.
- Muscle spasm of the injured muscles.
- Swelling over the injury.
- Weakened leg (moderate or severe strain).
- Crepitation ("crackling") feeling and sound when the injured area is pressed with fingers.
- Calcification of the hamstring tendon or muscles (visible with X-rays).
- Inflammation of the sheath covering the hamstring tendon.

CAUSES
- Prolonged overuse of muscle-tendon units in the leg.
- Single violent injury or force applied to the muscle-tendon unit in the leg.

RISK INCREASES WITH
- Contact sports.
- Running, jumping and quick-start sports.
- Any cardiovascular medical problem that results in decreased circulation.
- Medical history of any bleeding disorder.
- Obesity.
- Poor nutrition.
- Previous pelvic or knee injury.
- Poor muscle conditioning.

HOW TO PREVENT
- Build your strength with a long-term conditioning program.
- Warm up adequately before practice or competition.
- Use proper protective equipment, such as knee pads and thigh pads, during participation in contact sports.

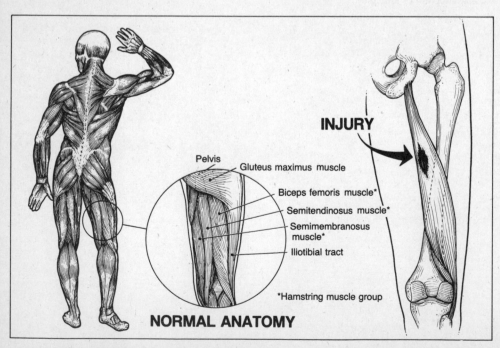

Pelvis
Gluteus maximus muscle
Biceps femoris muscle*
Semitendinosus muscle*
Semimembranosus muscle*
Iliotibial tract

INJURY

*Hamstring muscle group

NORMAL ANATOMY

WHAT TO EXPECT

APPROPRIATE HEALTH CARE
- Doctor's care.
- Application of tape, plaster splints or a cast (sometimes) if a muscle ruptures or the muscle-tendon-bone attachment loosens.
- Self-care during rehabilitation.
- Physical therapy (moderate and severe injury).
- Surgery (severe injury).

DIAGNOSTIC MEASURES
- Your own observation of symptoms.
- Medical history and exam by a doctor.
- X-rays of the pelvis, femur and knee to rule out fractures.

POSSIBLE COMPLICATIONS
- Prolonged healing time if activity is resumed too soon.
- Proneness to repeated injury.
- Unstable or arthritic knee following repeated injury.
- Inflammation at the attachment to bone (periostitis).
- Prolonged disability (sometimes).

PROBABLE OUTCOME—If this is a first-time injury, proper care and sufficient healing time before resuming activity should prevent permanent disability. Torn ligaments and tendons require as long to heal as fractured bones. Average healing times are:
- Mild strain—2 to 10 days.
- Moderate strain—10 days to 6 weeks.
- Severe strain—6 to 10 weeks.

If this is a repeat injury, complications listed above are more likely to occur.

 ## HOW TO TREAT

NOTE—Follow your doctor's instructions. These instructions are supplemental.

FIRST AID—Use instructions for R.I.C.E., the first letters of *rest, ice, compression* and *elevation*. See Appendix 1 for details.

CONTINUING CARE
- Continue using an ice pack 3 or 4 times a day. Place ice chips or cubes in a plastic bag. Wrap the bag in a moist towel, and place it over the injured area. Use for 20 minutes at a time.

- After 24 hours, apply heat instead of ice if it feels better. Use heat lamps, hot soaks, hot showers, heating pads, or heat liniments and ointments.
- Take whirlpool treatments, if available.
- Wrap the injured leg with an elasticized bandage between ice or heat treatments.
- Massage gently and often to provide comfort and decrease swelling.

MEDICATION
- For minor discomfort, you may use:
  Non-prescription medicines such as aspirin, acetaminophen or ibuprofen.
  Topical liniments and ointments.
- Your doctor may prescribe:
  Stronger medicine for pain, if needed.
  Injection of a long-acting local anesthetic to reduce pain.
  Injection of a corticosteroid, such as triamcinolone, to reduce inflammation.

ACTIVITY
- For a moderate or severe injury, use crutches for at least 72 hours.
- Resume your normal activities gradually.

DIET—During recovery, eat a well-balanced diet that includes extra protein, such as meat, fish, poultry, cheese, milk and eggs. Increase fiber and fluid intake to prevent constipation that may result from decreased activity.

REHABILITATION
- Begin daily rehabilitation exercises when supportive wrapping is no longer needed.
- Use ice massage for 10 minutes before and after exercise. Fill a large Styrofoam cup with water and freeze. Tear a small amount of foam from the top so ice protrudes. Massage firmly over the injured area in a circle about the size of a softball.
- See pages 457, 460 and 471 for rehabilitation exercises.

 ## CALL YOUR DOCTOR IF

- You have symptoms of a moderate or severe hamstring injury, or a mild injury persists longer than 10 days.
- Pain or swelling worsens despite treatment.
- Either of the following occurs with a cast or splints:
  Pain, numbness or coldness below the injury.
  Dusky, blue or gray toenails.

THIGH STRAIN

GENERAL INFORMATION

DEFINITION—Injury to the muscles or tendons of the thigh. Muscles, tendons and bones comprise units. These units stabilize the thigh and allow its motion. A strain occurs at the weakest part of a unit. Strains are of 3 types:
● Mild (Grade I)—Slightly pulled muscle without tearing of muscle or tendon fibers. There is no loss of strength.
● Moderate (Grade II)—Tearing of fibers in a muscle, tendon or at the attachment to bone. Strength is diminished.
● Severe (Grade III)—Rupture of the muscle-tendon-bone attachment with separation of fibers. Severe strain requires surgical repair. Chronic strains are caused by overuse. Acute strains are caused by direct injury or overstress.

BODY PARTS INVOLVED
● Any tendons or muscles of the thigh.
● Bones of the thigh area, including the femur, pelvis, knee, tibia and fibula.
● Soft tissue surrounding the strain, including nerves, periosteum (covering to bone), blood vessels and lymph vessels.

SIGNS & SYMPTOMS
● Pain when moving or stretching the hip or knee.
● Muscle spasm of the injured muscle.
● Swelling over the injury.

● Weakened thigh muscles (moderate or severe strain).
● Crepitation ("crackling") feeling and sound when the injured area is pressed with fingers.
● Calcification of the muscle or tendon (visible with X-rays).
● Inflammation of sheath covering a tendon in the thigh.

CAUSES
● Prolonged overuse of muscle-tendon units in the thigh.
● Single episode of stressful overactivity, in which muscles are under maximum stress and additional tension is applied when the knee is sharply flexed.
● Single violent blow or force applied to the thigh.

RISK INCREASES WITH
● Contact sports.
● Sports that require quick starts, such as running races, football and basketball.
● Any cardiovascular medical problem that results in decreased circulation.
● Medical history of any bleeding disorder.
● Obesity.
● Poor nutrition.
● Previous thigh injury.
● Poor muscle conditioning.

HOW TO PREVENT
● Participate in a strengthening and conditioning program appropriate for your sport.

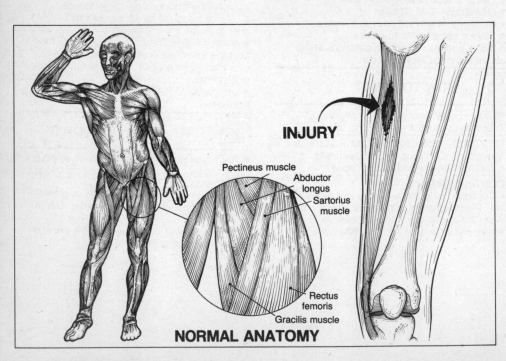

INJURY

Pectineus muscle
Abductor longus
Sartorius muscle
Rectus femoris
Gracilis muscle

NORMAL ANATOMY

- Warm up (include stretching exercises) before practice or competition.

 ## WHAT TO EXPECT

APPROPRIATE HEALTH CARE
- Doctor's diagnosis.
- Application of tape, plaster splints or casts If the muscle ruptures or muscle-tendon-bone attachment loosens.
- Self-care during rehabilitation.
- Physical therapy (moderate or severe strain).
- Surgery (severe strain).

DIAGNOSTIC MEASURES
- Your own observation of symptoms.
- Medical history and exam by a doctor.
- X-rays of the thigh area to rule out fractures.

POSSIBLE COMPLICATIONS
- Prolonged healing time if activity is resumed too soon.
- Proneness to repeated injury.
- Unstable or arthritic knee or hip following repeated injury.
- Inflammation at the attachment to bone (periostitis).
- Prolonged disability (sometimes).

PROBABLE OUTCOME—If this is a first-time injury, proper care and sufficient healing time before resuming activity should prevent permanent disability. Torn ligaments and tendons require as long to heal as fractured bones do. Average healing times are:
- Mild strain—2 to 10 days.
- Moderate strain—10 days to 6 weeks.
- Severe strain—6 to 10 weeks.
If this is a repeat injury, complications listed above are more likely to occur.

 ## HOW TO TREAT

NOTE—Follow your doctor's instructions. These instructions are supplemental.

FIRST AID—Use instructions for R.I.C.E., the first letters of *rest, ice, compression* and *elevation*. See Appendix 1 for details.

CONTINUING CARE
- Use ice massage 3 or 4 times a day for 15 minutes at a time. Fill a large Styrofoam cup with water and freeze. Tear a small amount of foam from the top so ice protrudes. Massage firmly over the injured area in a circle about the size of a softball.
- After the first 24 hours, apply heat instead of ice, if it feels better. Use heat lamps, hot soaks, hot showers, heating pads, or heat liniments and ointments.
- Take whirlpool treatments, if available.
- Wrap the injured thigh with an elasticized bandage between treatments.
- Massage gently and often to provide comfort and decrease swelling.

MEDICATION
- For minor discomfort, you may use:
  Aspirin, acetaminophen or ibuprofen.
  Topical liniments and ointments.
- Your doctor may prescribe:
  Stronger pain relievers.
  Injection of a long-acting local anesthetic to reduce pain.
  Injections of corticosteroids, such as triamcinolone, to reduce inflammation.

ACTIVITY
- For a moderate or severe strain, walk with crutches for at least 72 hours—longer with a cast or splints. See Appendix 3 (Safe Use of Crutches).
- Resume normal activities gradually.

DIET—During recovery, eat a well-balanced diet that includes extra protein, such as meat, fish, poultry, cheese, milk and eggs. Increase fiber and fluid intake to prevent constipation that may result from decreased activity.

REHABILITATION—Begin daily rehabilitation exercises when supportive wrapping is no longer needed. Use ice massage for 10 minutes prior to exercise. See page 471 for rehabilitation exercises.

 ## CALL YOUR DOCTOR IF

- You have symptoms of a moderate or severe thigh strain, or a mild strain persists longer than 10 days.
- Pain or swelling worsens despite treatment.
- The following occurs with a cast or splints:
  Pain, numbness or coldness below the injury.
  Dusky, blue or gray toenails.

THIGH STRAIN, QUADRICEPS

GENERAL INFORMATION

DEFINITION—Injury to the quadriceps femoris muscle or its tendons. The quadriceps femoris is a large muscle at the front of the thigh. The muscle, tendon and attached bone comprise a unit. The unit stabilizes the thigh and allows its motion. A strain occurs at the weakest part of a unit. Strains are of 3 types:
- Mild (Grade I)—Slightly pulled muscle without tearing of muscle or tendon fibers. There is no loss of strength.
- Moderate (Grade II)—Tearing of fibers in the muscle, tendon or at the attachment to bone. Strength is diminished.
- Severe (Grade III)—Rupture of the muscle-tendon-bone attachment with separation of fibers. Severe strain requires surgical repair. Chronic strains are caused by overuse. Acute strains are caused by direct injury or overstress.

BODY PARTS INVOLVED
- Quadriceps femoris muscle or its various tendons.
- Femur (thigh bone), patella (kneecap) or tibia (large lower-leg bone).
- Soft tissue surrounding the strain, including nerves, periosteum (covering to bone), blood vessels and lymph vessels.

SIGNS & SYMPTOMS
- Pain when moving, stretching or flexing the thigh.
- Muscle spasm of the quadriceps femoris.
- Swelling around the injury.
- Loss of strength (moderate or severe strain).
- Crepitation ("crackling") feeling and sound when the injured area is pressed with fingers.
- Calcification of the muscle or tendon (visible with X-rays).
- Inflammation of the tendon sheath.

CAUSES
- Prolonged overuse of muscle-tendon units in the thigh or knee.
- Single violent blow or force applied to the knee or the quadriceps area of the thigh.

RISK INCREASES WITH
- Sports that require quick starts, such as running races and other track events.
- Contact sports.
- Any cardiovascular medical problem that results in decreased circulation.
- Medical history of any bleeding disorder.
- Obesity.
- Poor nutrition.
- Previous thigh, hip or knee injury.
- Poor muscle conditioning.

HOW TO PREVENT
- Participate in a strengthening and conditioning program appropriate for your sport.
- Warm up before practice or competition.
- Wear proper protective equipment, such as thigh pads, for contact sports.

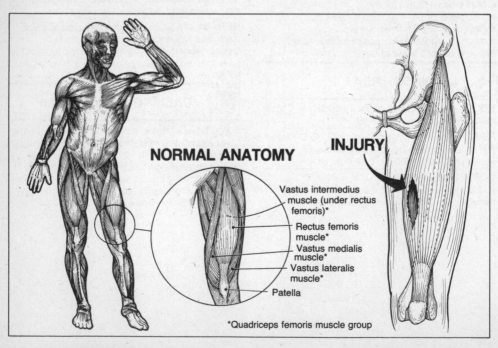

NORMAL ANATOMY

INJURY

Vastus intermedius muscle (under rectus femoris)*

Rectus femoris muscle*

Vastus medialis muscle*

Vastus lateralis muscle*

Patella

*Quadriceps femoris muscle group

WHAT TO EXPECT

APPROPRIATE HEALTH CARE
- Doctor's diagnosis.
- Self-care during rehabilitation.
- Physical therapy (moderate or severe strain).
- Surgery (severe strain).

DIAGNOSTIC MEASURES
- Your own observation of symptoms.
- Medical history and exam by a doctor.
- X-rays of the hip, thigh and knee to rule out fractures.

POSSIBLE COMPLICATIONS
- Prolonged healing time if activity is resumed too soon.
- Proneness to repeated injury.
- Unstable or arthritic knee following repeated injury.
- Inflammation at the attachment to bone (periostitis).
- Prolonged disability (sometimes).

PROBABLE OUTCOME—If this is a first-time injury, proper care and sufficient healing time before resuming activity should prevent permanent disability. Torn ligaments and tendons require as long to heal as fractured bones. Average healing times are:
- Mild strain—2 to 10 days.
- Moderate strain—10 days to 6 weeks.
- Severe strain—6 to 10 weeks.
If this is a repeat injury, complications listed above are more likely to occur.

 HOW TO TREAT

NOTE—Follow your doctor's instructions. These instructions are supplemental.

FIRST AID—Use instructions for R.I.C.E., the first letters of *rest, ice, compression* and *elevation*. See Appendix 1 for details.

CONTINUING CARE
- Use ice massage 3 or 4 times a day for 15 minutes at a time. Fill a large Styrofoam cup with water and freeze. Tear a small amount of foam from the top so ice protrudes. Massage firmly over the injured area in a circle about the size of a softball.
- After the first 24 hours, apply heat instead of ice, if it feels better. Use heat lamps, hot soaks, hot showers, heating pads, or heat liniments and ointments.
- Take whirlpool treatments, if available.
- Wrap the injured quadriceps muscle loosely with an elasticized bandage between treatments.
- Massage gently and often to provide comfort and decrease swelling.

MEDICATION
- For minor discomfort, you may use:
  Aspirin, acetaminophen or ibuprofen.
  Topical liniments and ointments.
- Your doctor may prescribe:
  Stronger pain relievers.
  Injection of a long-acting local anesthetic to reduce pain.
  Injections of corticosteroids, such as triamcinolone, to reduce inflammation.

ACTIVITY
- For a moderate or severe strain, walk with crutches for at least 72 hours. See Appendix 3 (Safe Use of Crutches).
- Resume your normal activities gradually.

DIET—Eat a well-balanced diet that includes extra protein, such as meat, fish, poultry, cheese, milk and eggs. Increase fiber and fluid intake to prevent constipation that may result from decreased activity.

REHABILITATION—Begin daily rehabilitation exercises when supportive wrapping is no longer needed. See page 471 for rehabilitation exercises.

 CALL YOUR DOCTOR IF

- You have symptoms of a moderate or severe quadriceps strain, or a mild strain persists longer than 10 days.
- Pain or swelling worsens despite treatment.

THUMB FRACTURE

GENERAL INFORMATION

DEFINITION—A complete or incomplete break in the metacarpal bone of the thumb.

BODY PARTS INVOLVED
- Metacarpal bone of the thumb.
- Joint between the two longer bones of the thumb, and joint between the lowest bone of the thumb and the wrist.
- Soft tissue around the fracture site, including nerves, tendons, ligaments and blood vessels.

SIGNS & SYMPTOMS
- Severe thumb pain at the fracture site.
- Swelling of soft tissue around the fracture.
- Visible deformity if the fracture is complete and the bone fragments separate enough to distort the thumb.
- Tenderness to the touch.
- Numbness or coldness in the thumb, if the blood supply is impaired.

CAUSES
- Direct stress, frequently caused by hitting with the fist or by catching the thumb on an object.
- Indirect stress that may be caused by twisting or violent muscle contraction.

RISK INCREASES WITH
- Contact sports such as hockey.
- Skiing.
- History of bone or joint disease, especially osteoporosis.

- Poor nutrition, especially calcium deficiency.
- If surgery or anesthesia is needed, surgical risk increases with smoking and use of drugs, including mind-altering drugs, muscle relaxants, antihypertensives, tranquilizers, sleep inducers, insulin, sedatives, beta-adrenergic blockers or corticosteroids.

HOW TO PREVENT
- Develop strength in your hands.
- Use appropriate taping, padding or protective equipment for the hand and thumb.

WHAT TO EXPECT

APPROPRIATE HEALTH CARE
- Doctor's treatment to manipulate the broken bones.
- Hospitalization (sometimes) for anesthesia and surgery to set the fracture.
- Self-care during rehabilitation.

DIAGNOSTIC MEASURES
- Your own observation of symptoms.
- Medical history and exam by a doctor.
- X-rays of the hand.

POSSIBLE COMPLICATIONS
At the time of injury:
- Shock.
- Pressure on or injury to nearby nerves, ligaments, tendons, muscles, blood vessels or connective tissues.

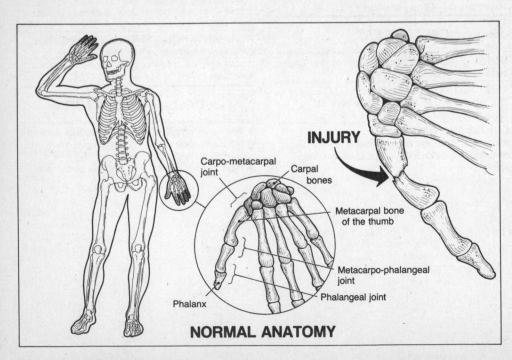

Carpo-metacarpal joint

Carpal bones

Metacarpal bone of the thumb

Metacarpo-phalangeal joint

Phalangeal joint

Phalanx

INJURY

NORMAL ANATOMY

After surgery or treatment:
- Delayed union or non-union of the fracture.
- Impaired blood supply to the fracture site.
- Avascular necrosis (death of bone cells) due to interruption of the blood supply.
- Infection in open fractures (skin broken over fracture site), or at the incision if surgical setting was necessary.
- Shortening of the injured bones.
- Unstable or arthritic thumb following repeated injury.
- Prolonged healing time if activity is resumed too soon.
- Proneness to repeated thumb injury.
- Problems caused by casts. See Appendix 2 (Care of Casts).

PROBABLE OUTCOME—The average healing time for this fracture is 6 to 8 weeks. Healing is complete when there is no motion at the fracture site and when X-rays show complete bone union.

 ## HOW TO TREAT

NOTE—Follow your doctor's instructions. These instructions are supplemental.

FIRST AID
- Use a padded splint or sling to immobilize the hand and wrist before taking the injured person to the doctor's office or emergency facility.
- Keep the person warm with blankets to decrease the possibility of shock.
- Follow instructions for R.I.C.E., the first letters of *rest, ice, compression* and *elevation*. See Appendix 1 for details.
- The doctor will set the broken bones with surgery or, if possible, without. This manipulation should be done as soon as possible after injury. Six or more hours after the fracture, bleeding and displacement of body fluids may lead to shock. Also, many tissues lose their elasticity and become difficult to return to a normal position.
- Shaft fractures of the metacarpal can sometimes be realigned without surgery, but the broken bones must be fixed in place with a wire across the base of the metacarpal bone. This wire passes through the bone fragment into one of the bones of the hand.

CONTINUING CARE
- Immobilization will be necessary. A rigid cast is used to immobilize the thumb and wrist. This cast can usually be removed in 3 weeks.
- After 48 hours, localized heat promotes

healing by increasing blood circulation in the injured area. Use a heat lamp or heating pad so heat can penetrate the cast.
- After the cast is removed, use frequent ice massage. Fill a large Styrofoam cup with water and freeze. Tear a small amount of foam from the top so ice protrudes. Massage firmly over the injured area.

MEDICATION—Your doctor may prescribe:
- General anesthesia, local anesthesia, or muscle relaxants to make bone manipulation and fixation of bone fragments possible.
- Narcotic or synthetic narcotic pain relievers for severe pain.
- Acetaminophen (available without prescription) for mild pain after initial treatment.

ACTIVITY
- Actively exercise all muscle groups not immobilized. These muscle contractions promote fracture alignment and hasten healing.
- Begin reconditioning the thumb and hand after clearance from your doctor.
- Resume normal activities gradually after treatment. Don't drive until healing is complete.

DIET
- Drink only water before manipulation or surgery to treat the fracture. Solid food in your stomach makes vomiting while under anesthesia more hazardous.
- During recovery, eat a well-balanced diet that includes extra protein, such as meat, fish, poultry, cheese, milk and eggs.

REHABILITATION—Begin daily rehabilitation exercises when movement is comfortable. Use ice massage for 10 minutes prior to exercise. See page 474 for rehabilitation exercises.

 ## CALL YOUR DOCTOR IF

- You have signs or symptoms of a thumb fracture.
- Any of the following occurs after surgery or other treatment:
  Increased pain, swelling or drainage in the surgical area.
  Signs of infection (headache, muscle aches, dizziness, or a general ill feeling and fever).
  Swelling above or below the cast.
  Blue or gray skin color under the fingernails or the thumb.
  Numbness or complete loss of feeling anywhere in the hand.
  Nausea or vomiting.

THUMB SPRAIN

GENERAL INFORMATION

DEFINITION—Violent overstretching of one or more ligaments in the joint of the thumb. Sprains involving two or more ligaments cause considerably more disability than single-ligament sprains. When the ligament is overstretched, it becomes tense and gives way at its weakest point, either where it attaches to bone or within the ligament itself. If the ligament pulls loose a fragment of bone, it is called a *sprain-fracture*. There are 3 types of sprains:
● Mild (Grade I)—Tearing of some ligament fibers. There is no loss of function.
● Moderate (Grade II)—Rupture of a portion of the ligament, resulting in some loss of function.
● Severe (Grade III)—Complete rupture of the ligament or complete separation of ligament from bone. There is total loss of function. A severe sprain requires surgical repair.

BODY PARTS INVOLVED
● Ligaments that hold the metacarpo-phalangeal joint of the thumb together.
● Tissue surrounding the sprain, including blood vessels, tendons, bone, periosteum (covering of bone) and muscles.

SIGNS & SYMPTOMS
● Severe pain at the time of injury.
● A feeling of popping or tearing inside the thumb.
● Tenderness at the injury site.
● Swelling and redness in the injured thumb.
● Bruising that appears soon after injury.

CAUSES—Stress on a ligament that temporarily forces or pries the thumb out of its normal location. Thumb sprains occur frequently in baseball players, particularly catchers, but they may occur in other exercise or sports activities.

RISK INCREASES WITH
● Contact sports, especially "catching" sports such as baseball, football or basketball.
● Skiing.
● Previous thumb injury.
● Poor muscle conditioning.

HOW TO PREVENT—Tape vulnerable joints before practice or competition to prevent reinjury. Immobilization after healing can be provided by a slip-on protector devised by a brace-maker.

❓ WHAT TO EXPECT

APPROPRIATE HEALTH CARE
● Doctor's diagnosis.
● Application of a cast, tape or elastic bandage.
● Self-care during rehabilitation.
● Physical therapy (moderate or severe sprain).
● Surgery (severe sprain).

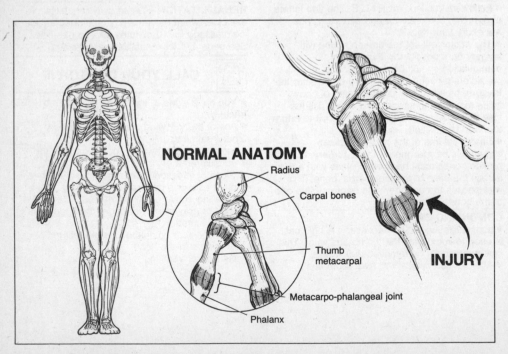

NORMAL ANATOMY

Radius

Carpal bones

Thumb metacarpal

Metacarpo-phalangeal joint

Phalanx

INJURY

DIAGNOSTIC MEASURES
- Your own observation of symptoms.
- Medical history and exam by a doctor.
- X-rays of the thumb, hand and wrist to rule out fractures.

POSSIBLE COMPLICATIONS
- Prolonged healing time if usual activities are resumed too soon.
- Proneness to repeated injury.
- Inflammation at the ligament attachment to bone (periostitis).
- Prolonged disability (sometimes).
- Unstable or arthritic thumb following repeated injury.

PROBABLE OUTCOME—If this is a first-time injury, proper care and sufficient healing time before resuming activity should prevent permanent disability. Ligaments have a poor blood supply, and torn ligaments require as much healing time as fractures. Average healing times are:
- Mild sprains—2 to 6 weeks.
- Moderate sprains—6 to 8 weeks.
- Severe sprains—8 to 10 weeks.

HOW TO TREAT

NOTE—Follow your doctor's instructions. These instructions are supplemental.

FIRST AID—Use instructions for R.I.C.E., the first letters of *rest, ice, compression* and *elevation*. See Appendix 1 for details.

CONTINUING CARE—If the doctor does not apply a cast, tape or elastic bandage:
- Continue using an ice pack 3 or 4 times a day. Place ice chips or cubes in a plastic bag. Wrap the bag in a moist towel, and place it over the injured thumb. Use for 20 minutes at a time.
- After 72 hours, apply heat instead of ice, if it feels better. Use heat lamps, hot soaks, hot showers, heating pads, or heat liniments or ointments.
- Take whirlpool treatments, if available.
- Massage gently and often to provide comfort and decrease swelling.

MEDICATION
- For minor discomfort, you may use:
  Aspirin, acetaminophen or ibuprofen.
  Topical liniments and ointments.
- Your doctor may prescribe:
  Stronger pain relievers.
  Injection of a long-acting local anesthetic to reduce pain.
  Injection of a corticosteroid, such as triamcinolone, to reduce inflammation.

ACTIVITY—Resume your normal activities gradually after clearance from your doctor.

DIET—During recovery, eat a well-balanced diet that includes extra protein, such as meat, fish, poultry, cheese, milk and eggs.

REHABILITATION
- Begin daily rehabilitation exercises when the cast or supportive wrapping is no longer necessary.
- Use ice massage for 10 minutes before and after exercise. Fill a large Styrofoam cup with water and freeze. Tear a small amount of foam from the top so ice protrudes. Massage firmly over the injured area.
- See page 474 for rehabilitation exercises.

CALL YOUR DOCTOR IF

- You have symptoms of a moderate or severe thumb sprain, or a mild sprain persists longer than 2 weeks.
- Pain, swelling or bruising worsens despite treatment.
- Any of the following occur after casting or splinting:
  Pain, numbness or coldness in the tip of the thumb.
  Blue, gray or dusky thumbnail.
- Any of the following occur after surgery:
  Increased pain, swelling, redness, drainage or bleeding in the surgical area.
  Signs of infection (headache, muscle aches, dizziness, or a general ill feeling with fever).
- New, unexplained symptoms develop. Drugs used in treatment may produce side effects.

TOE DISLOCATION

GENERAL INFORMATION

DEFINITION—Injury to any toe joint so that adjoining bones are displaced from their normal position and no longer touch each other. Fractures and ligament sprains frequently accompany this dislocation. Toe dislocations are a common problem for athletes.

BODY PARTS INVOLVED
- Bones of the toes.
- Ligaments that hold toe bones in place.
- Soft tissue surrounding the dislocation site, including periosteum (covering to bone), nerves, tendons, blood vessels and connective tissue.

SIGNS & SYMPTOMS
- Excruciating pain in the toe at the time of injury.
- Walking difficulty.
- Severe pain when attempting to move the injured toe.
- Visible deformity if the dislocated toe has locked in the dislocated position. Bones may spontaneously reposition themselves and leave no deformity, but damage is the same.
- Tenderness over the dislocation.
- Swelling and bruising at the injury site.
- Numbness or paralysis beyond the dislocation from pinching, cutting or pressure on blood vessels or nerves.

CAUSES
- Direct or indirect blow to the foot.

- End result of a severe toe sprain.
- Congenital abnormality, such as a shallow or malformed joint surface.

RISK INCREASES WITH
- Contact or collision sports, especially those that require cleated shoes.
- Previous foot or toe dislocation or sprain.
- Repeated injury to any part of the foot.
- Arthritis of any type (rheumatoid, gout).
- Poor muscle conditioning in the foot.

HOW TO PREVENT—Wear appropriate, well-designed shoes during competition or other athletic activity. Tape the toes to prevent reinjury.

WHAT TO EXPECT

APPROPRIATE HEALTH CARE
- Doctor's treatment. This will include manipulation of the joint to reposition the bones.
- Surgery (sometimes) to restore the joint to its normal position and repair torn ligaments and tendons. Acute or recurring dislocations may require surgical reconstruction or replacement of the joint.
- Self-care during rehabilitation.

DIAGNOSTIC MEASURES
- Your own observation of symptoms.
- Medical history and physical exam by a doctor.
- X-rays of the foot and ankle.

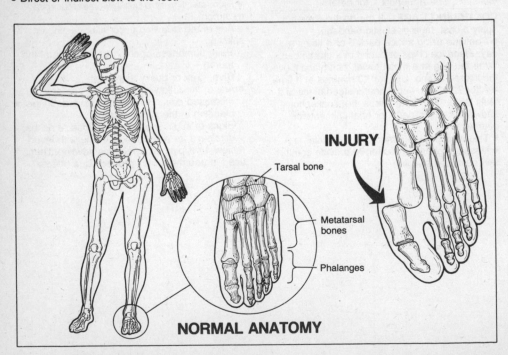

INJURY

Tarsal bone

Metatarsal bones

Phalanges

NORMAL ANATOMY

POSSIBLE COMPLICATIONS
● Pressure or damage to nearby nerves, ligaments, tendons, muscles, blood vessels or connective tissue.
● Excessive internal bleeding in the toe.
● Impaired blood supply to the dislocated area.
● Death of bone cells due to interruption of the blood supply.
● Infection introduced during surgical treatment.
● Continuing recurrent dislocations, often with progressively less severe provocation.
● Prolonged healing if activity is resumed too soon.
● Unstable or arthritic joint following repeated injury.

PROBABLE OUTCOME—After the dislocation has been corrected, the foot may require immobilization with a splint, taping or special shoe for 2 to 3 weeks. Injured ligaments require a minimum of 6 weeks to heal.

 ## HOW TO TREAT

NOTE—Follow your doctor's instructions. These instructions are supplemental.

FIRST AID
● Use instructions for R.I.C.E., the first letters of *rest, ice, compression* and *elevation*. See Appendix 1 for details.
● The doctor will manipulate the dislocated toes to return them to their normal position. Manipulation should be accomplished within 6 hours, if possible. After that time, many tissues lose their elasticity and become difficult to return to a normal functional position.

CONTINUING CARE
● Use an ice pack 3 or 4 times a day. Wrap ice chips or cubes in a plastic bag, and wrap the bag in a moist towel. Place it over the injured area for 20 minutes at a time.
● You may apply heat instead of ice, if it feels better. Use heat lamps, hot soaks, hot showers, heating pads, or heat liniments and ointments.
● Take whirlpool treatments, if available.
● Wrap the injured foot with an elasticized bandage between treatments.
● Massage gently and often to provide comfort and decrease swelling. Stroke from the toes toward the heart.
● Have a metatarsal bar sewed into your shoe by a shoe repairman or brace-maker.

MEDICATION—Your doctor may prescribe:
● Local anesthesia or muscle relaxants to make joint manipulation possible.
● Acetaminophen or aspirin to relieve moderate pain, and narcotic pain relievers for severe pain.
● Stool softeners to prevent constipation due to decreased activity.

ACTIVITY—Resume normal activity when comfortable.

DIET
● Drink only water before manipulation or surgery to correct the dislocation. Solid food in your stomach makes vomiting while under general anesthesia more hazardous.
● During recovery, eat a well-balanced diet that includes extra protein, such as meat, fish, poultry, cheese, milk and eggs. Increase fiber and fluid intake to prevent constipation that may result from decreased activity.

REHABILITATION
● Begin daily rehabilitation exercises when pain subsides.
● Use ice massage for 10 minutes before and after workouts. Fill a large Styrofoam cup with water and freeze. Tear a small amount of foam from the top so ice protrudes. Massage firmly in a circle over the injured area.
● See page 455 for rehabilitation exercises.

 ## CALL YOUR DOCTOR IF

● You have symptoms of a dislocated toe, especially if the toe becomes numb, pale or cold. This is an emergency!
● Any of the following occur after treatment or surgery:
  Swelling above or below the cast.
  Blue or gray skin color, particularly under the toenails.
  Numbness or complete loss of feeling below the dislocation.
  Increased pain, swelling or drainage in the surgical area.
  Signs of infection (headache, muscle aches, dizziness, or a general ill feeling and fever).
● New, unexplained symptoms develop. Drugs used in treatment may produce side effects.
● Toe dislocations that you can "pop" back into normal position occur repeatedly.

TOE EXOSTOSIS

GENERAL INFORMATION

DEFINITION—A painful condition of the tip of the toe (usually the first toe) caused by an exostosis (overgrowth of bone) building up under the nailbed. An exostosis occurs at the site of repeated injury, usually from direct blows. This benign overgrowth of bone can be mistaken for a bone tumor.

BODY PARTS INVOLVED
- Toe (usually the big toe).
- Toenail.
- Soft tissue surrounding the exostosis, including muscles, nerves, lymph vessels, blood vessels and periosteum (covering to bone).

SIGNS & SYMPTOMS
- No symptoms for mild cases.
- Extreme pain at the tip of the toe and under the nail.
- Tenderness over the toe.
- Extreme sensitivity in the toe to pressure or minor injury.
- Change in the contour of the bone, ranging from a slight lump to the appearance of a large calcified spur (1cm or more in length) in the toe. The toenail may appear distorted.

CAUSES
- Repeated injury to the toes.
- Chronic irritation to an already damaged area.

RISK INCREASES WITH
- Contact sports, particularly those with quick stops and turns in which toes are repeatedly jammed into the toes of the shoes.
- Ballet dancing in toe shoes.
- History of bone or joint disease, such as osteomyelitis, osteomalacia or osteoporosis.
- Vitamin or mineral deficiency.
- If surgery or anesthesia is needed, surgical risk increases with smoking, use of mind-altering drugs, muscle relaxants, tranquilizers, sleep inducers, insulin, sedatives, beta-adrenergic blockers or corticosteroids.

HOW TO PREVENT
- Allow adequate recovery time for a toe injury before resuming sports participation.
- Wear adequate protective equipment, especially good shoes and toe padding if necessary, for participation in sports.
- Learn proper moves and techniques for your sport to minimize the risk of injury.

WHAT TO EXPECT

APPROPRIATE HEALTH CARE
- Doctor's care.
- Surgery (sometimes) to remove the exostosis.
- Self-care during rehabilitation.
- Physical therapy.

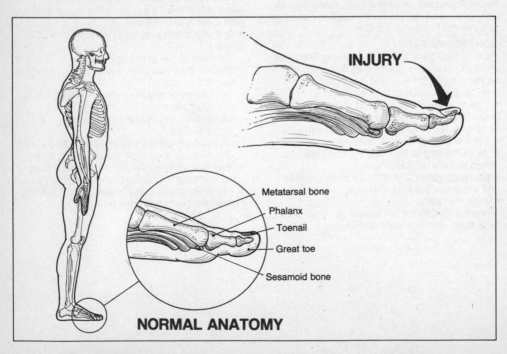

INJURY

Metatarsal bone
Phalanx
Toenail
Great toe
Sesamoid bone

NORMAL ANATOMY

DIAGNOSTIC MEASURES
- Your own observation of signs and symptoms.
- Medical history and physical exam by a doctor.
- X-rays of the toes.

POSSIBLE COMPLICATIONS
- Overlooking a mild exostosis that produces no symptoms, despite signs of diminished performance. Athletes and coaches frequently assume that decreased performance results from loss of competitive drive or emotional causes rather than from the physical disability that actually exists.
- Prolonged healing time if activity is resumed too soon.
- Proneness to repeated injury.
- Unstable or arthritic toe joints following repeated injury.
- Pressure on or injury to nearby nerves, ligaments, tendons, blood vessels or connective tissue.
- Impaired blood supply to the injured toe.

PROBABLE OUTCOME—Toe exostosis usually causes no disability if it is treated properly. Treatment usually involves resting the injured foot and toe for 2 to 4 weeks, heat treatments, corticosteroid injections and protection against additional injury. In a few cases, surgery is necessary to remove the toenail, nailbed, exostosis and the tip of the toe.

 HOW TO TREAT

NOTE—Follow your doctor's instructions. These instructions are supplemental.

FIRST AID—None. This condition develops gradually.

CONTINUING CARE
- Rest the injured area. Use splints or crutches if needed.
- Apply heat frequently. Use heat lamps, hot soaks, hot showers, heating pads, or heat liniments and ointments.
- Take whirlpool treatments, if available.
- Use proper shoes and extra toe padding, if possible, during competition and workouts to avoid recurrence of the injury.

MEDICATION
- Medicine usually is not necessary for this disorder. For minor pain, you may use non-prescription drugs such as aspirin.
- If surgery is necessary, your doctor may prescribe:
  Non-steroidal anti-inflammatory drugs to help control swelling.
  Stronger pain relievers.
  Antibiotics to fight infection.

ACTIVITY—Decrease activity for 2 to 4 weeks. If surgery is necessary, resume normal activity gradually.

DIET—During recovery, eat a well-balanced diet that includes extra protein, such as meat, fish, poultry, cheese, milk and eggs. Increase fiber and fluid intake to prevent constipation that may result from decreased activity. Your doctor may suggest vitamin and mineral supplements to promote healing.

REHABILITATION
- Begin daily rehabilitation exercises when movement is comfortable.
- Use ice massage for 10 minutes before and after exercise. Fill a large Styrofoam cup with water and freeze. Tear a small amount of foam from the top so ice protrudes. Massage gently over the injured area. Do this for 15 minutes at a time, 3 or 4 times a day, and before workouts or competition.
- See page 455 for rehabilitation exercises.

 CALL YOUR DOCTOR IF

- You have symptoms of toe exostosis.
- Any of the following occur after surgery:
  Increased pain, swelling, redness, drainage, or bleeding in the surgical area.
  Signs of infection (headache, muscle ache, dizziness, or a general ill feeling and fever).
  New, unexplained symptoms. Drugs used in treatment may cause side effects.

TOE FRACTURE

GENERAL INFORMATION

DEFINITION—A complete or incomplete break in one or more bones of the toes.

BODY PARTS INVOLVED
- Any of the bones of the toes.
- Joints between the toes, and joints between the foot and toe bones.
- Soft tissue around the fracture site, including nerves, tendons, ligaments and blood vessels.

SIGNS & SYMPTOMS
- Severe pain at the fracture site.
- Swelling of soft tissue around the fracture.
- Visible deformity if the fracture is complete and the bone fragments separate enough to distort normal toe and foot contours.
- Tenderness to the touch.
- Numbness or coldness in the toe if the blood supply is impaired.

CAUSES
- Direct blow to the toe, as when kicking or being stepped on.
- Indirect stress to the toe. Indirect stress may be caused by twisting.

RISK INCREASES WITH
- Sports that require shoes with cleats.
- History of bone or joint disease, especially osteoporosis.
- Obesity.
- Poor nutrition, especially calcium deficiency.

HOW TO PREVENT—Wear appropriate footgear for running and participation in contact sports.

WHAT TO EXPECT

APPROPRIATE HEALTH CARE
- Doctor's treatment to manipulate and set the broken bones.
- Self-care during rehabilitation.
- Whirlpool, ultrasound or massage (to displace excess fluid from the injured joint spaces).

DIAGNOSTIC MEASURES
- Your own observation of symptoms.
- Medical history and physical exam by a doctor.
- X-rays of the toe and foot.

POSSIBLE COMPLICATIONS
- Pressure on or injury to nearby nerves, ligaments, tendons, muscles, blood vessels or connective tissues.
- Delayed union or non-union of the fracture.
- Impaired blood supply to the fracture site.
- Infection in open fractures (skin broken over fracture site), or at the incision if surgical setting was necessary.
- Shortening of the injured bones.
- Unstable or arthritic toe joint following repeated injury.
- Prolonged healing time if activity is resumed too soon.

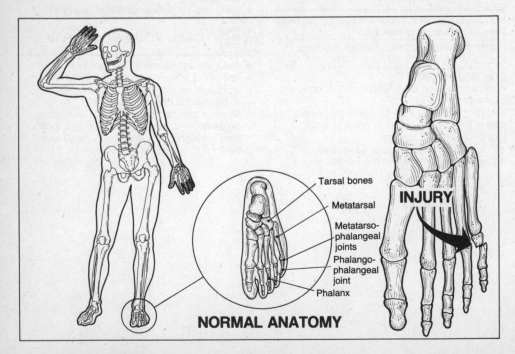

Tarsal bones
Metatarsal
Metatarso-phalangeal joints
Phalango-phalangeal joint
Phalanx

INJURY

NORMAL ANATOMY

• Proneness to repeated toe injury.

PROBABLE OUTCOME—It is impossible to predict exactly how long it will take for any fracture to heal. Variable factors include age, sex, and previous state of health and conditioning. The average healing time for this fracture is 6 to 8 weeks, but you may begin weight-bearing right away. Healing is considered complete when there is no motion at the fracture site and when X-rays show complete bone union.

 HOW TO TREAT

NOTE—Follow your doctor's instructions. These instructions are supplemental.

FIRST AID
• Cut away the shoe and sock, if possible, but don't move the injured toe to do so.
• Follow instructions for R.I.C.E., the first letters of *rest, ice, compression and elevation.* See Appendix 1 for details.
• The doctor will realign the broken bones with surgery or, if possible, without. This manipulation should be done as soon as possible after injury. Six or more hours after the fracture, bleeding and displacement of body fluids may lead to shock. Also, many tissues lose their elasticity and become difficult to return to a normal position.

CONTINUING CARE
• Immobilization will be necessary. Place felt between the fractured toe and a good toe, then fix the two toes together with adhesive strips. Cut the top of the shoe out and have a shoe repairman apply a bar on the sole of the shoe (metatarsal bar). Then bear weight on the foot as pain allows.
• Use frequent ice massage. Fill a large Styrofoam cup with water and freeze. Tear a small amount of foam from the top so ice protrudes. Massage firmly over the injured area in a circle about the size of a baseball. Do this for 15 minutes at a time, 3 or 4 times a day, and before workouts or competition.
• After 48 hours, localized heat promotes healing by increasing blood circulation in the injured area. Use hot baths, showers, compresses, heat lamps, heating pads, heat ointments and liniments, or whirlpools.

MEDICATION—Your doctor may prescribe:
• General anesthesia, local anesthesia, or muscle relaxants to make bone manipulation and fixation possible.
• Narcotic or synthetic narcotic pain relievers for severe pain.
• Stool softeners to prevent constipation due to inactivity.
• Acetaminophen (available without prescription) for mild pain after initial treatment.

ACTIVITY
• Elevate the foot whenever possible.
• Actively exercise all muscle groups in the foot that are not immobilized. These muscle contractions promote fracture alignment and hasten healing.
• Begin reconditioning the injured foot after clearance from your doctor.
• Resume normal activities gradually after treatment. Don't drive until healing is complete.

DIET—During recovery, eat a well-balanced diet that includes extra protein, such as meat, fish, poultry, cheese, milk and eggs.

REHABILITATION—Begin daily rehabilitation exercises when supportive wrapping is no longer needed. Use ice massage for 10 minutes prior to exercise. See page 455 for rehabilitation exercises.

 CALL YOUR DOCTOR IF

• You have signs or symptoms of a toe fracture.
• Any of the following occurs after treatment or surgery:
  Blue or gray skin color, especially under the toenail.
  Numbness or complete loss of feeling in the toe.
  Increased pain, swelling or drainage in the surgical area.
  Signs of infection (headache, muscle aches, dizziness, or a general ill feeling and fever).
  Swelling above the taped area.
  Nausea or vomiting.

TOOTH INJURY & LOSS
(Tooth Avulsion)

 GENERAL INFORMATION

DEFINITION—Damage to a tooth severe enough to separate it completely from the gum and bone without fracture. Children whose front teeth have short, slender roots are most likely to lose teeth through injury.

BODY PARTS INVOLVED
● Teeth.
● Bones that hold teeth.
● Gums and soft tissue surrounding the tooth, including nerves, blood vessels and covering to bone (periosteum).

SIGNS & SYMPTOMS
● Missing tooth.
● Pain and bleeding from the tooth site.
● Swelling of gums soon after injury.

CAUSES—Direct blow to the tooth and gum.

RISK INCREASES WITH
● Contact sports, especially football and boxing.
● Poor nutrition, especially calcium deficiency.
● Poor dental hygiene or gum disease.

HOW TO PREVENT—Wear a helmet, strong face guard and mouthpiece whenever possible during contact sports.

 WHAT TO EXPECT

APPROPRIATE HEALTH CARE
● Dentist's or oral surgeon's evaluation and replantation of an avulsed tooth.
● Blood studies after surgery to evaluate blood loss and infection.

DIAGNOSTIC MEASURES
● Your own observation of symptoms and signs.
● Medical history and physical exam by your dentist or oral surgeon.
● X-rays of the mouth and jaw to detect additional injuries.

POSSIBLE COMPLICATIONS
● Permanent tooth loss if the replantation fails.
● Excessive bleeding.
● Infection.

PROBABLE OUTCOME—Allow about 4 weeks for recovery from surgery if complications don't occur. After it heals, the tooth often appears normal. If it darkens, a plastic dental veneer can be applied to make it cosmetically acceptable.

 HOW TO TREAT

NOTE—Follow your doctor's instructions. These instructions are supplemental.

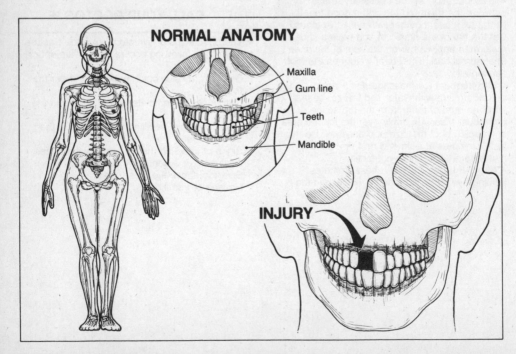

NORMAL ANATOMY

Maxilla

Gum line

Teeth

Mandible

INJURY

FIRST AID
- Find and wash the missing tooth or teeth.
- Replace the tooth in its socket as soon as possible.
- If you cannot replace the tooth in its socket, wash it and keep it wet in a wet cloth until you reach a dentist or doctor. Put a moist cloth in the empty socket and have the patient bite on it.
- Go to the dentist or emergency room immediately. *Hurry!* The longer the tooth stays out of the mouth, the less the chance of saving it.

CONTINUING CARE
The dentist or oral surgeon will:
- Cleanse the socket.
- Remove the nerve from the tooth and fill the root canal with a plasticlike material before the tooth is replaced.
- Replace the tooth in its socket.
- Anchor the tooth to neighboring teeth with wire or plastic. The tooth must be held in place for 6 to 8 weeks.

Home care after replantation:
- Don't rinse your mouth, spit, smoke, or suck on straws for 24 hours after tooth replantation.
- After 24 hours, brush your other teeth often with a soft toothbrush. A clean mouth heals faster. Don't brush the injured tooth until you have clearance from your denist.
- Beginning 24 hours after surgery, rinse your mouth every 1 or 2 hours with a solution of 1/2 teaspoon salt in 8 oz. of lukewarm water.

- Don't bite down on the affected tooth until healing is complete.

MEDICATION
- You may use non-prescription drugs such as acetaminophen for minor pain.
- Your doctor may prescribe:
  Pain relievers. Don't take prescription pain medication longer than 4 to 7 days. Use only as much as you need.
  Antibiotics to fight infection.
  Mouthwashes.

ACTIVITY—Avoid vigorous physical exercise for 4 to 6 weeks following surgery. Wear a face mask after resuming sports activity.

DIET—Adequate food and fluid intake following surgery will promote more rapid healing. If you can't avoid putting pressure on the tooth by eating your normal diet, follow a liquid high-protein diet for 2 or 3 days. Avoid all alcoholic beverages during healing.

REHABILITATION—None.

 CALL YOUR DENTIST IF

- You have a tooth knocked out.
- Any of the following occur after surgery:
  Increased mouth pain, swelling, redness, drainage or bleeding.
  Signs of infection (headache, muscle aches, dizziness, or a general ill feeling and fever).
  New, unexplained symptoms. Drugs used in treatment may produce side effects.

WRIST CONTUSION

GENERAL INFORMATION

DEFINITION—Bruising of skin and underlying tissue of the wrist caused by a direct blow. Contusions cause bleeding from ruptured small capillaries that allow blood to infiltrate muscles, tendons or other soft tissue.

BODY PARTS INVOLVED—Wrist tissues, including blood vessels, muscles, tendons, nerves, covering to bone (periosteum) and connective tissue.

SIGNS & SYMPTOMS
● Wrist swelling—either superficial or deep.
● Wrist pain and tenderness.
● Feeling of firmness when pressure is exerted on the injury site.
● Discoloration under the skin, beginning with redness and progressing to the characteristic "black and blue" bruise.
● Restricted wrist motion proportional to the extent of injury.

CAUSES—Direct blow to the wrist, usually from a blunt object.

RISK INCREASES WITH
● Violent contact sports, especially with inadequate protection of the wrist.
● Medical history of any bleeding disorder such as hemophilia.

● Poor nutrition, including vitamin deficiency.
● Use of anticoagulants or aspirin.

HOW TO PREVENT—Wear appropriate protective gear and equipment, such as wrapped elastic bandages, tape wraps or leather gauntlet gloves, during competition or other athletic activity if there is risk of a wrist contusion.

WHAT TO EXPECT

APPROPRIATE HEALTH CARE
● Doctor's care unless the contusion is quite small.
● Self-care for minor contusions, and following serious contusions during the rehabilitation phase.
● Physical therapy following serious contusions.

DIAGNOSTIC MEASURES
● Your own observation of symptoms.
● Medical history and physical exam by a doctor for all except minor injuries.
● X-rays of the injured area to assess total injury to soft tissue and to rule out the possibility of underlying fracture. The total extent of injury may not be apparent for 48 to 72 hours.

POSSIBLE COMPLICATIONS
● Excessive bleeding leading to disability. Infiltrative-type bleeding can sometimes lead to

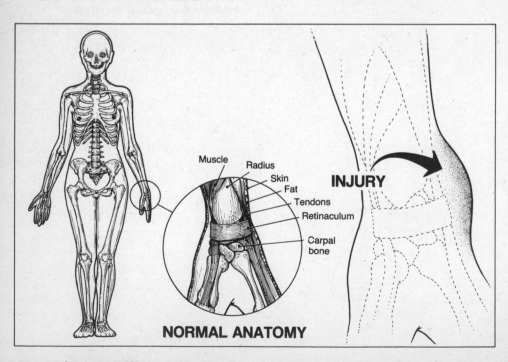

Muscle
Radius
Skin
Fat
Tendons
Retinaculum
Carpal bone

INJURY

NORMAL ANATOMY

calcification and impaired function of injured muscles and tendons.
• Prolonged healing time if usual activities are resumed too soon.
• Infection if skin over the contusion is broken.

PROBABLE OUTCOME—Healing time varies with the extent of injury, but the average healing time for a wrist contusion is 2 days to 2 weeks.

HOW TO TREAT

NOTE—Follow your doctor's instructions. These instructions are supplemental.

FIRST AID—Use instructions for R.I.C.E., the first letters of *rest, ice, compression* and *elevation*. See Appendix 1 for details.

CONTINUING CARE
• Wrap an elasticized bandage over a felt pad on the injured area. Keep the area compressed for about 72 hours.
• Continue ice massage. Fill a large Styrofoam cup with water and freeze. Tear a small amount of foam from the top so ice protrudes. Massage gently over the injured area in a circle about the size of a softball. Do this for 15 minutes at a time, 3 or 4 times a day, and before workouts or competition.
• After 72 hours, apply heat instead of ice if it feels better. Use heat lamps, hot soaks, hot showers, heating pads, heat liniments or ointments, or whirlpool treatments.

• Massage gently and often to provide comfort and decrease swelling. Stroke from the fingers toward the heart.

MEDICATION
• For minor discomfort, you may use:
   Acetaminophen or ibuprofen.
   Topical liniments and ointments.
• Your doctor may prescribe stronger medicine for pain.

ACTIVITY—Begin activities slowly and stop exercise as soon as pain begins. Increase activity as healing progresses.

DIET—Eat a well-balanced diet that includes extra protein, such as meat, fish, poultry, cheese, milk and eggs. Your doctor may prescribe vitamin and mineral supplements to promote healing.

REHABILITATION—Begin daily rehabilitation exercises when supportive wrapping is no longer needed. See page 474 for rehabilitation exercises.

CALL YOUR DOCTOR IF

• Injured wrist doesn't improve in 1 or 2 days.
• Skin is broken and signs of infection (drainage, increasing pain, fever, headache, muscle aches, dizziness or a general ill feeling) occur.

WRIST DISLOCATION, LUNATE

GENERAL INFORMATION

DEFINITION—Injury and displacement of the lunate bone of the wrist (usually) or of other bones in the hand and wrist (less commonly). The dislocated bone no longer touches the adjoining bones in the normal manner.

BODY PARTS INVOLVED
- Joints in the hand adjoining primarily the lunate bone. Other hand bones are affected less frequently.
- Soft tissue surrounding the dislocation, including nerves, tendons, ligaments, muscles and blood vessels.

SIGNS & SYMPTOMS
- Excruciating pain in the wrist at the time of dislocation.
- Loss of hand and wrist function, as well as severe pain when attempting to move them.
- Visible deformity if the dislocated bones have locked in the dislocated position. Bones may spontaneously reposition themselves and leave no deformity, but damage is the same.
- Tenderness over the dislocation.
- Swelling and bruising at the injury site.
- Numbness or paralysis below the dislocation from pressure, pinching or cutting of blood vessels or nerves.

CAUSES
- Direct blow to the wrist—usually a fall on an outstretched hand.

- End result of a severe wrist sprain.
- Congenital abnormality, such as shallow or malformed joint surfaces.

RISK INCREASES WITH
- Any sport where falling or stress on the arm and hand is a possibility.
- Previous wrist dislocation or sprain.
- Repeated wrist injury of any sort.
- Arthritis of any type (rheumatoid, gout).
- Poor muscle conditioning.

HOW TO PREVENT
- Build strength and muscle tone with a long-term conditioning program appropriate for your sport.
- Wear protective devices, such as wrapped elastic bandages, tape wraps or leather gauntlet gloves, to protect vulnerable wrist joints.

WHAT TO EXPECT

APPROPRIATE HEALTH CARE
- Doctor's treatment. This may include manipulating the joint to reposition the bones.
- Surgery (sometimes) to restore the joint to its normal position. Acute or recurring dislocations may require surgical reconstruction or replacement of the joint.
- Self-care during rehabilitation.

DIAGNOSTIC MEASURES
- Your own observation of symptoms.
- Medical history and physical exam by a doctor.

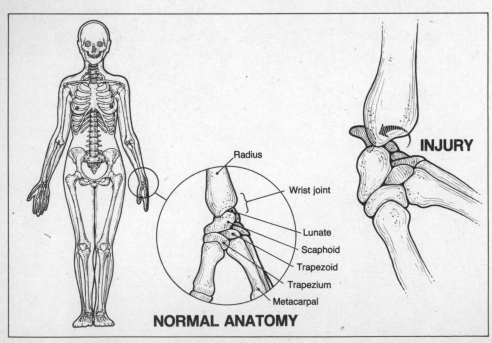

Radius

Wrist joint

Lunate

Scaphoid

Trapezoid

Trapezium

Metacarpal

NORMAL ANATOMY

INJURY

- X-rays of the joint and adjacent bones.

POSSIBLE COMPLICATIONS
- Damage to nearby nerves or major blood vessels, causing numbness, coldness and paleness.
- Excessive internal bleeding at the dislocation site.
- Recurrent dislocations, particularly if the previous dislocation is not healed completely.

PROBABLE OUTCOME—After the dislocation has been corrected, the joint may require immobilization with a cast, splints or sling for 2 to 8 weeks. Complete healing of injured ligaments requires a minimum of 6 weeks.

 HOW TO TREAT

NOTE—Follow your doctor's instructions. These instructions are supplemental.

FIRST AID
- Keep the person warm with blankets to decrease the possibility of shock.
- Cut away clothing if possible, but don't move the injured area to remove clothing.
- Immobilize the wrist joint and the hand with padded splints.
- Follow instructions for R.I.C.E., the first letters of *rest, ice, compression* and *elevation*. See Appendix 1 for details.
- The doctor will manipulate the dislocated bones with surgery or, if possible, without. Manipulation should be done as soon as possible after injury. Six or more hours after the dislocation, internal bleeding and displacement of body fluids may lead to shock. Also, many tissues lose their elasticity and become difficult to return to a normal position.

CONTINUING CARE
If a cast is not necessary:
- Use ice soaks 3 or 4 times a day. Fill a bucket with ice water, and soak the injured area for 20 minutes at a time.
- After 48 hours, apply heat instead of ice if it feels better. Use heat lamps, hot soaks, hot showers, heating pads, or heat liniments and ointments.
- Take whirlpool treatments, if available.
- Wrap the wrist with elasticized bandages between treatments.
- Massage gently and often from the fingers toward the heart to provide comfort and decrease swelling.
If a cast is necessary:
- See Appendix 2 (Care of Casts).
- Actively exercise all muscle groups in the arm and hand that are not immobilized. The resulting muscle contractions promote proper alignment and hasten healing.

MEDICATION—Your doctor may prescribe:
- General anesthesia or muscle relaxants to make joint manipulation possible.
- Acetaminophen or aspirin to relieve moderate pain.
- Narcotic pain relievers for severe pain.
- Antibiotics to fight infection, if surgery is necessary.

ACTIVITY
- Begin reconditioning the wrist after clearance from your doctor.
- If surgery is necessary, resume your normal activities gradually. Don't drive until healing is complete.

DIET
- Drink only water before manipulation or surgery to correct the dislocation. Solid food in your stomach makes vomiting while under general anesthesia more hazardous.
- During recovery, eat a well-balanced diet that includes extra protein, such as meat, fish, poultry, cheese, milk and eggs. Your doctor may suggest vitamin and mineral supplements to promote healing.

REHABILITATION
- Begin daily rehabilitation exercises when supportive wrapping is no longer needed.
- Use ice massage for 10 minutes before and after workouts. Fill a large Styrofoam cup with water and freeze. Tear a small amount of foam from the top so ice protrudes. Massage firmly over the injured area in a circle about the size of a softball.
- See page 474 for rehabilitation exercises.

 CALL YOUR DOCTOR IF

- You have symptoms of a dislocated wrist, especially if the hand becomes numb, pale, or cold. This is an emergency!
- Any of the following occur after treatment or surgery:
  Nausea or vomiting.
  Swelling above or below the cast or splints.
  Blue or gray skin color, particularly under the fingernails.
  Numbness or complete loss of feeling below the dislocation site.
  Increased pain, swelling or drainage in the surgical area.
  Signs of infection (headache, muscle aches, dizziness, or a general ill feeling and fever).
- New, unexplained symptoms develop. Drugs used in treatment may produce side effects.
- Wrist dislocations occur repeatedly that you can "pop" back into normal position.

WRIST DISLOCATION, RADIUS OR ULNA

GENERAL INFORMATION

DEFINITION—An injury to one of the joints in the wrist so that adjoining bones no longer touch each other. *Subluxation* is a minor dislocation. Joint surfaces still touch but not in normal relation to each other.

BODY PARTS INVOLVED
- Lower arm bones (radius and ulna).
- Bones in the hand.
- Ligaments that hold the bones in place.
- Soft tissue surrounding the dislocation site, including periosteum (covering to bone), nerves, tendons, blood vessels and connective tissue.

SIGNS & SYMPTOMS
- Excruciating pain in the wrist at the time of dislocation.
- Loss of hand and wrist function, as well as severe pain when attempting to move them.
- Visible deformity if the dislocated bones have locked in the dislocated position. Bones may spontaneously reposition themselves and leave no deformity, but damage is the same.
- Tenderness over the dislocation.
- Swelling and bruising at the injury site.
- Numbness or paralysis below the dislocation from pressure, pinching or cutting of blood vessels or nerves.

CAUSES
- Direct blow to the wrist—usually a fall on an extended hand.

- End result of a severe wrist sprain.
- Congenital abnormality, such as shallow or malformed joint surfaces.

RISK INCREASES WITH
- Contact sports such as football, basketball, soccer or hockey.
- Previous wrist dislocation or sprain.
- Repeated wrist injury of any sort.
- Arthritis of any type (rheumatoid, gout).
- Poor muscle conditioning.

HOW TO PREVENT
- Build your overall strength and muscle tone with a long-term conditioning program appropriate for your sport.
- Warm up adequately before physical activity.
- After healing, use protective devices such as wrapped elastic bandages or tape wraps, to prevent reinjury during participation in sports.
- Consider avoiding contact sports if treatment does not restore a strong, stable wrist.

WHAT TO EXPECT

APPROPRIATE HEALTH CARE
- Doctor's treatment. This will include manipulation of the joint to reposition the bones.
- Surgery (sometimes) to restore the joint to its normal position and repair torn ligaments and tendons. Acute or recurring dislocations may require surgical reconstruction or replacement of the joint.
- Self-care during rehabilitation.

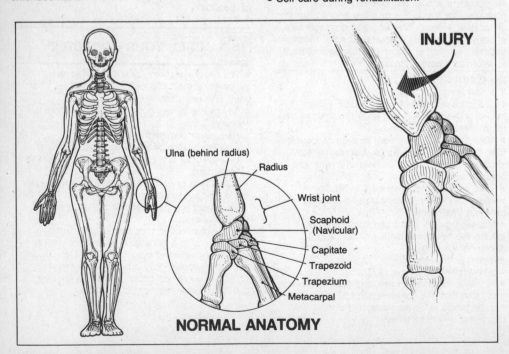

Ulna (behind radius)
Radius
Wrist joint
Scaphoid (Navicular)
Capitate
Trapezoid
Trapezium
Metacarpal

INJURY

NORMAL ANATOMY

DIAGNOSTIC MEASURES
- Your own observation of symptoms.
- Medical history and exam by a doctor.
- X-rays of the wrist, hand and elbow.

POSSIBLE COMPLICATIONS
At the time of injury:
- Shock.
- Pressure or damage to nearby nerves, ligaments, tendons, muscles, blood vessels or connective tissue.

After treatment or surgery:
- Excessive internal bleeding around the wrist.
- Impaired blood supply to the dislocated area.
- Death of bone cells due to the interruption of blood supply.
- Infection introduced during surgical treatment.
- Prolonged healing if activity is resumed too soon.
- Recurrent wrist dislocations.
- Unstable or arthritic wrist following repeated injury.

PROBABLE OUTCOME—After the wrist
dislocation has been corrected, the joint may require immobilization with a cast or splint for 4 to 8 weeks. Complete healing of injured ligaments requires a minimum of 6 weeks.

 HOW TO TREAT

NOTE—Follow your doctor's instructions. These instructions are supplemental.

FIRST AID
- Keep the person warm with blankets to decrease the possibility of shock.
- Cut away clothing if possible, but don't move the injured area to remove clothing.
- Immobilize the wrist joint and arm with padded splints.
- Follow instructions for R.I.C.E., the first letters of *rest, ice, compression* and *elevation*. See Appendix 1 for details.

CONTINUING CARE
If a cast is not necessary:
- Use ice soaks 3 or 4 times a day. Fill a bucket with ice water, and soak the injured area for 20 minutes at a time.
- After 48 hours, apply heat instead of ice if it feels better. Use heat lamps, hot soaks, hot showers, heating pads, or heat liniments and ointments.
- Take whirlpool treatments, if available.
- Massage gently and often to provide comfort and decrease swelling. Stroke from the fingers toward the heart.
- Wrap the injured wrist with an elasticized bandage between treatments.
If a cast or plaster splint is necessary:
- See Appendix 2 (Care of Casts).

- Actively exercise all muscle groups in the arm and hand that are not immobilized. Muscle contractions promote proper alignment and hasten healing.

MEDICATION—Your doctor may prescribe:
- General anesthesia or muscle relaxants to make joint manipulation possible.
- Acetaminophen to relieve moderate pain.
- Narcotic pain relievers for severe pain.
- Antibiotics to fight infection if surgery is necessary.

ACTIVITY
- Begin reconditioning the wrist after clearance from your doctor.
- If surgery is necessary, resume usual activities and reconditioning gradually after surgery. Don't drive until healing is complete.

DIET
- Drink only water before manipulation or surgery to correct the dislocation. Solid food in your stomach makes vomiting while under general anesthesia more hazardous.
- During recovery, eat a well-balanced diet that includes extra protein, such as meat, fish, poultry, cheese, milk and eggs. Increase fiber and fluid intake to prevent constipation that may result from decreased activity.

REHABILITATION
- Begin daily rehabilitation exercises when supportive wrapping is no longer needed.
- Use ice massage for 10 minutes before and after workouts. Fill a large Styrofoam cup with water and freeze. Tear a small amount of foam from the top so ice protrudes. Massage firmly in a circle over the injured area.
- See page 474 for rehabilitation exercises.

 CALL YOUR DOCTOR IF

- You have symptoms of a dislocated wrist, especially if the arm becomes numb, pale, or cold. This is an emergency!
- Any of the following occur after treatment or surgery:
  Nausea or vomiting.
  Swelling above or below the cast or splint.
  Blue or gray skin color, particularly under the fingernails.
  Numbness or complete loss of feeling below the dislocation site.
  Increased pain, swelling or drainage in the surgical area.
  Signs of infection (headache, muscle aches, dizziness, or a general ill feeling and fever).
  Constipation.
- New, unexplained symptoms develop. Drugs used in treatment may produce side effects.
- Wrist dislocations occur repeatedly that you can "pop" back into normal position.

WRIST GANGLION
(Synovial Hernia; Synovial Cyst)

GENERAL INFORMATION

DEFINITION—A small, usually hard nodule lying directly over a tendon or a joint capsule on the back or front of the wrist. Occasionally the nodule may become quite large. Wrist ganglions are quite common.

BODY PARTS INVOLVED
- Back or front of the wrist.
- Tendon sheath (a thin membranous covering to any tendon).
- Any of the joint spaces in the wrist.

SIGNS & SYMPTOMS
- Hard lump over a tendon or joint capsule in the wrist. The nodule "yields" to heavy pressure because it is not solid.
- No pain usually, but overuse of the wrist may cause mild pain and aching.
- Tenderness if the lump is pressed hard.
- Discomfort with extremes of motion (flexing or extending) and with repetition of the exercise that produced the ganglion.

CAUSES
- Mild sprains and chronic sprains of the wrist, causing weakness of the joint capsule.
- A defect in the fibrous sheath of the joint or tendon that permits a segment of underlying synovium (thin membrane that lines the tendon sheath) to herniate through it.

- Irritation accompanying the herniated synovium, causing continued secretion of fluid. The sac gradually fills, enlarges, and becomes hard, forming the ganglion.

RISK INCREASES WITH
- Repeated injury, especially mild sprains. Wrist ganglions frequently occur in bowlers, tennis players, and handball, racquetball and squash players.
- Inadequate warmup prior to practice or competition.
- Poor muscle strength or conditioning.
- If surgery is necessary, surgical risk increases with smoking, poor nutrition, alcoholism, and recent or chronic illness.

HOW TO PREVENT
- Participate in a long-term strengthening and conditioning program appropriate for your sport.
- Warm up before practice or competition.

WHAT TO EXPECT

APPROPRIATE HEALTH CARE
- Doctor's care for diagnosis and possible injections of local anesthetic or corticosteroids.
- Surgery (usually). Surgery will be conducted under local or general anesthesia in an outpatient surgical facility or hospital operating room.

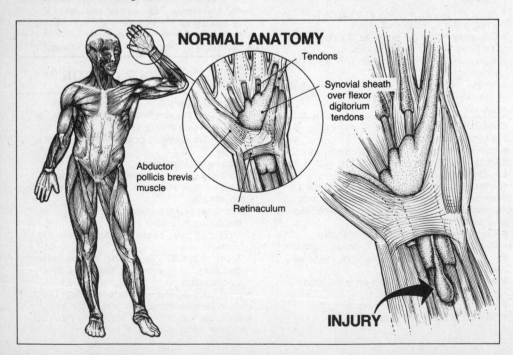

NORMAL ANATOMY

Tendons

Synovial sheath over flexor digitorium tendons

Abductor pollicis brevis muscle

Retinaculum

INJURY

DIAGNOSTIC MEASURES
- Your own observation of signs and symptoms.
- Medical history and physical examination by a doctor.
- X-rays of the area to rule out a bone tumor or unhealed bone fracture.

POSSIBLE COMPLICATIONS
- Calcification of the ganglion (rare).
- After surgery:
  Excessive bleeding.
  Surgical-wound infection.
  Recurrence if surgical removal is incomplete.

PROBABLE OUTCOME—Ganglions sometimes disappear spontaneously, only to recur later. Surgery is usually necessary. After surgery, allow about 3 weeks for recovery if no complications occur.

HOW TO TREAT

NOTE—Follow your doctor's instructions. These instructions are supplemental.

FIRST AID—None. This condition develops gradually.

CONTINUING CARE
Immediately after surgery:
- The affected area is usually immobilized in a splint for 1 to 2 weeks following surgery.
- If the wound bleeds during the first 24 hours after surgery, press a clean tissue or cloth to it for 10 minutes.
- A hard ridge should form along the incision. As it heals, the ridge will recede gradually.
- Use an electric heating pad, a heat lamp, or a warm compress to relieve incisional pain.
- Bathe and shower as usual. You may wash the incision gently with mild unscented soap.
- Between baths, keep the wound dry with a bandage for the first 2 or 3 days after surgery. If a bandage gets wet, change it promptly.
- Apply non-prescription antibiotic ointment to the wound before applying new bandages.
- Wrap the hand with an elasticized bandage until healing is complete.
After the incision has healed:
- Use ice massage. Fill a large Styrofoam cup

with water and freeze. Tear a small amount of foam from the top so ice protrudes. Massage firmly over the injured area in a circle about the size of a baseball. Do this for 15 minutes at a time, 3 or 4 times a day, and before workouts or competition.
- You may apply heat instead of ice if it feels better. Use heat lamps, hot soaks, hot showers, heating pads, or heat liniments and ointments.
- Take whirlpool treatments, if available.

MEDICATION
- Your doctor may prescribe pain relievers. Don't take prescription pain medication longer than 4 to 7 days. Use only as much as you need.
- You may use non-prescription drugs such as acetaminophen for minor pain.

ACTIVITY
- Return to work and normal activity as soon as possible. This reduces postoperative depression and irritability, which are common.
- Avoid vigorous exercise for 3 weeks after surgery.
- Resume driving when healing is complete.

DIET—During recovery, eat a well-balanced diet that includes extra protein, such as meat, fish, poultry, cheese, milk and eggs. Increase fiber and fluid intake to prevent constipation that may result from decreased activity.

REHABILITATION—Begin daily rehabilitation exercises when supportive wrapping is no longer needed. Use ice massage for 10 minutes before and after exercise. See page 474 for rehabilitation exercises.

CALL YOUR DOCTOR IF

- You have signs or symptoms of a wrist ganglion.
- Any of the following occur after surgery:
  Increased pain, swelling, redness, drainage or bleeding in the surgical area.
  Signs of infection (headache, muscle aches, dizziness, or a general ill feeling and fever).
  New, unexplained symptoms. Drugs used in treatment may produce side effects.

WRIST SPRAIN

GENERAL INFORMATION

DEFINITION—Violent overstretching of one or more ligaments in the wrist joint. Sprains involving two or more ligaments cause considerably more disability than single-ligament sprains. When the ligament is overstretched, it becomes tense and gives way at its weakest point, either where it attaches to bone or within the ligament itself. If the ligament pulls loose a fragment of bone, it is called a *sprain-fracture*. There are 3 types of sprains:
● Mild (Grade I)—Tearing of some ligament fibers. There is no loss of function.
● Moderate (Grade II)—Rupture of a portion of the ligament, resulting in some loss of function.
● Severe (Grade III)—Complete rupture of the ligament or complete separation of ligament from bone. There is total loss of function. A severe sprain requires surgical repair.

BODY PARTS INVOLVED
● Ligaments of the wrist.
● Tissue surrounding the sprain, including blood vessels, tendons, bone, periosteum (covering of bone) and muscles.

SIGNS & SYMPTOMS
● Severe pain at the time of injury.
● A feeling of popping or tearing inside the wrist.
● Tenderness at the injury site.
● Swelling in the wrist.
● Bruising that appears soon after injury.

CAUSES—Stress on a ligament that temporarily forces or pries the wrist joint out of its normal location.

RISK INCREASES WITH
● Contact sports such as boxing or wrestling.
● Bowling.
● Skiing.
● Pole-vaulting.
● Previous wrist injury.
● Poor muscle conditioning.
● Inadequate protection from equipment.

HOW TO PREVENT
● Build your strength with a conditioning program appropriate for your sport.
● Warm up before practice or competition.
● To prevent reinjury, tape vulnerable joints before practice or competition.

WHAT TO EXPECT

APPROPRIATE HEALTH CARE
● Doctor's diagnosis.
● Application of a cast, tape or elastic bandage.
● Self-care during rehabilitation.
● Physical therapy (moderate or severe sprain).
● Surgery (severe sprain).

DIAGNOSTIC MEASURES
● Your own observation of symptoms.
● Medical history and exam by a doctor.

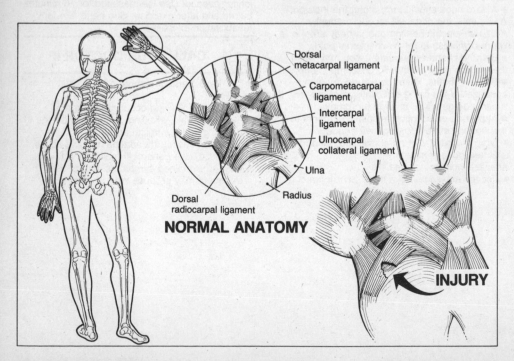

Dorsal metacarpal ligament
Carpometacarpal ligament
Intercarpal ligament
Ulnocarpal collateral ligament
Ulna
Radius
Dorsal radiocarpal ligament

NORMAL ANATOMY

INJURY

- X-rays of the wrist and hand to rule out fractures.

POSSIBLE COMPLICATIONS
- Prolonged healing time if usual activities are resumed too soon.
- Proneness to repeated injury.
- Inflammation at the ligament attachment to bone (periostitis).
- Prolonged disability (sometimes).
- Unstable or arthritic wrist following repeated injury.

PROBABLE OUTCOME—If this is a first-time injury, proper care and sufficient healing time before resuming activity should prevent permanent disability. Ligaments have a poor blood supply, and torn ligaments require as much healing time as fractures. Average healing times are:
- Mild sprains—2 to 6 weeks.
- Moderate sprains—6 to 8 weeks.
- Severe sprains—8 to 10 weeks.

 HOW TO TREAT

NOTE—Follow your doctor's instructions. These instructions are supplemental.

FIRST AID—Use instructions for R.I.C.E., the first letters of *rest, ice, compression* and *elevation.* See Appendix 1 for details.

CONTINUING CARE—If the doctor does not apply a cast, tape or elastic bandage:
- Continue using an ice pack 3 or 4 times a day. Place ice chips or cubes in a plastic bag. Wrap the bag in a moist towel, and place it over the injured area. Use for 20 minutes at a time.
- Wrap the wrist with an elasticized bandage between ice treatments.
- After 72 hours, apply heat instead of ice if it feels better. Use heat lamps, hot soaks, hot showers, heating pads, or heat liniments or ointments.
- Take whirlpool treatments, if available.
- Massage gently and often to provide comfort and decrease swelling.

MEDICATION
- For minor discomfort, you may use:
  Aspirin, acetaminophen or ibuprofen.
  Topical liniments and ointments.
- Your doctor may prescribe:
  Stronger pain relievers.
  Injection of a long-acting local anesthetic to reduce pain.
  Injection of a corticosteroid, such as triamcinolone, to reduce inflammation.

ACTIVITY—Resume your normal activities gradually after clearance from your doctor.

DIET—During recovery, eat a well-balanced diet that includes extra protein, such as meat, fish, poultry, cheese, milk and eggs. Increase fiber and fluid intake to prevent constipation that may result from decreased activity.

REHABILITATION
- Begin daily rehabilitation exercises when the cast or supportive wrapping is no longer necessary.
- Use ice massage for 10 minutes before and after exercise. Fill a large Styrofoam cup with water and freeze. Tear a small amount of foam from the top so ice protrudes. Massage firmly over the injured area in a circle.
- See page 474 for rehabilitation exercises.

 CALL YOUR DOCTOR IF

- You have symptoms of a moderate or severe wrist sprain, or a mild sprain persists longer than 2 weeks.
- Pain, swelling or bruising worsens despite treatment.
- Any of the following occur after casting or splinting:
  Pain, numbness or coldness beyond the wrist.
  Blue, gray or dusky fingernails.
- Any of the following occur after surgery:
  Increased pain, swelling, redness, drainage or bleeding in the surgical area.
  Signs of infection (headache, muscle aches, dizziness, or a general ill feeling with fever).
- New, unexplained symptoms develop. Drugs used in treatment may produce side effects.

WRIST STRAIN

GENERAL INFORMATION

DEFINITION—Injury to the muscles or tendons of the wrist. Muscles, tendons and attached bones comprise units. These units stabilize the wrist and allow its motion. A strain occurs at the weakest part of a unit. Strains are of 3 types:
● Mild (Grade I)—Slightly pulled muscle without tearing of muscle or tendon fibers. There is no loss of strength.
● Moderate (Grade II)—Tearing of fibers in a muscle, tendon or at the attachment to bone. Strength is diminished.
● Severe (Grade III)—Rupture of the muscle-tendon-bone attachment with separation of fibers. Severe strain requires surgical repair. Chronic strains are caused by overuse. Acute strains are caused by direct injury or overstress.

BODY PARTS INVOLVED
● Tendons and muscles of the forearm.
● Bones at the wrist, where the muscles and tendons attach.
● Soft tissue surrounding the strain, including nerves, periosteum (covering to bone), blood vessels and lymph vessels.

SIGNS & SYMPTOMS
● Pain when moving or stretching the wrist.
● Muscle spasm of forearm muscles.
● Redness and swelling over the injury.
● Loss of strength (moderate or severe strain).
● Crepitation ("crackling") feeling and sound when the injured area is pressed with fingers.
● Calcification of the muscle or tendon (visible with X-rays).
● Inflammation of the tendon sheath.

CAUSES
● Prolonged overuse of muscle-tendon units in the forearm.
● Single violent injury or force applied to the forearm.

RISK INCREASES WITH
● Contact sports such as boxing, wrestling or football.
● Gymnastics.
● Weight-lifting.
● Any cardiovascular medical problem that results in decreased circulation.
● Medical history of any bleeding disorder.
● Obesity.
● Poor nutrition.
● Previous wrist injury.
● Poor muscle conditioning.

HOW TO PREVENT
● Participate in a strengthening and conditioning program appropriate for your sport.
● Warm up before practice or competition.
● Tape the wrist area before practice or competition.
● Wear proper protective equipment.

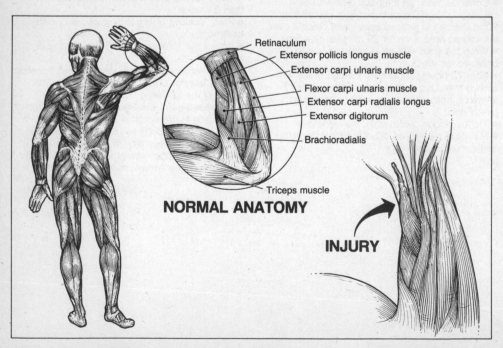

Retinaculum
Extensor pollicis longus muscle
Extensor carpi ulnaris muscle
Flexor carpi ulnaris muscle
Extensor carpi radialis longus
Extensor digitorum
Brachioradialis
Triceps muscle

NORMAL ANATOMY

INJURY

WHAT TO EXPECT

APPROPRIATE HEALTH CARE
- Doctor's diagnosis.
- Application of tape, plaster splints or casts (sometimes).
- Self-care during rehabilitation.
- Physical therapy (moderate or severe strain).
- Surgery (severe strain).

DIAGNOSTIC MEASURES
- Your own observation of symptoms.
- Medical history and exam by a doctor.
- X-rays of the wrist and forearm to rule out fractures.

POSSIBLE COMPLICATIONS
- Prolonged healing time if activity is resumed too soon.
- Proneness to repeated injury.
- Unstable or arthritic wrist joint following repeated injury.
- Inflammation at the attachment to bone (periostitis).
- Prolonged disability (sometimes).

PROBABLE OUTCOME—If this is a first-time injury, proper care and sufficient healing time before resuming activity should prevent permanent disability. Torn ligaments and tendons require as long to heal as fractured bones. Average healing times are:
- Mild strain—2 to 10 days.
- Moderate strain—10 days to 6 weeks.
- Severe strain—6 to 10 weeks.

If this is a repeat injury, complications listed above are more likely to occur.

 HOW TO TREAT

NOTE—Follow your doctor's instructions. These instructions are supplemental.

FIRST AID—Use instructions for R.I.C.E., the first letters of *rest, ice, compression* and *elevation*. See Appendix 1 for details.

CONTINUING CARE—If splints or a cast are used after injury or surgery, leave fingers free and exercise them regularly. If a cast or splints are not used:
- Use ice massage 3 or 4 times a day for 15 minutes at a time. Fill a large Styrofoam cup

with water and freeze. Tear a small amount of foam from the top so ice protrudes. Massage firmly over the injured area in a circle about the size of a softball.
- After the first 24 hours, apply heat instead of ice, if it feels better. Use heat lamps, hot soaks, hot showers, heating pads, or heat liniments and ointments.
- Take whirlpool treatments, if available.
- Wrap the injured wrist and forearm with an elasticized bandage between treatments.
- Massage gently and often to provide comfort and decrease swelling.

MEDICATION
- For minor discomfort, you may use:
  Aspirin, acetaminophen or ibuprofen.
  Topical liniments and ointments.
- Your doctor may prescribe:
  Stronger pain relievers.
  Injection of a long-acting local anesthetic to reduce pain.
  Injections of corticosteroids, such as triamcinolone, to reduce inflammation.

ACTIVITY
- For a moderate or severe strain, use a sling or wrist splint for at least 72 hours—longer with a cast. See Appendix 3 (Care of Casts).
- Resume your normal activities gradually.

DIET—Eat a well-balanced diet that includes extra protein, such as meat, fish, poultry, cheese, milk and eggs. Increase fiber and fluid intake to prevent constipation that may result from decreased activity.

REHABILITATION—Begin daily rehabilitation exercises when supportive wrapping (including cast) is no longer needed. Use ice massage for 10 minutes prior to exercise. See page 474 for rehabilitation exercises.

 CALL YOUR DOCTOR IF

- You have symptoms of a moderate or severe wrist strain, or a mild strain persists longer than 10 days.
- Pain or swelling worsens despite treatment.
- The following occurs with a cast or splints:
  Pain, numbness or coldness below the injury.
  Dusky, blue or gray fingernails.

WRIST TENOSYNOVITIS

GENERAL INFORMATION

DEFINITION—Inflammation of the lining of a tendon sheath in the wrist. The lining secretes a fluid that lubricates the tendon. When the lining becomes inflamed, the tendon cannot glide smoothly in its covering.

BODY PARTS INVOLVED
- Any wrist-tendon lining and covering.
- Soft tissue in the surrounding area, including blood vessels, nerves, ligaments, periosteum (covering to bone) and connective tissue.

SIGNS & SYMPTOMS
- Constant pain or pain with motion of the wrist.
- Limited motion of the wrist and hand.
- Crepitation (a "crackling" sound) when the tendon moves or is touched.
- Redness and tenderness over the inflamed tendon.

CAUSES
- Strain from overuse of the wrist.
- Direct blow or injury to muscles and tendons in the wrist and hand. Tenosynovitis becomes more likely with repeated injury to the wrist or hand.
- Infection introduced through broken skin at the time of injury or through a surgical incision after injury.

RISK INCREASES WITH
- Contact sports.
- "Throwing" sports.

- If surgery is needed, surgical risk increases with smoking, poor nutrition, alcoholism or drug abuse, and recent or chronic illness.

HOW TO PREVENT
- Engage in a vigorous program of physical conditioning before beginning regular sports participation.
- Warm up adequately before practice or competition.
- Wear protective gear appropriate for your sport.
- Learn proper moves and techniques for your sport.

WHAT TO EXPECT

APPROPRIATE HEALTH CARE
- Doctor's examination and diagnosis.
- Surgery (sometimes) to enlarge the tunnel of the tendon covering and restore a smooth gliding motion. The surgical procedure under general anesthesia is performed in an outpatient surgical facility or hospital operating room.

DIAGNOSTIC MEASURES
- Your own observation of symptoms and signs.
- Medical history and physical examination by your doctor.
- X-rays of the wrist, arm and hand to rule out other abnormalities.
- Laboratory studies:
  Blood and urine studies before surgery.
  Tissue examination after surgery.

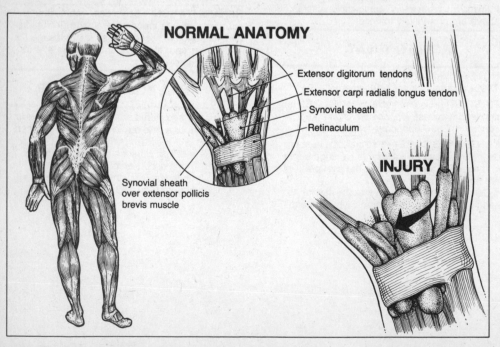

NORMAL ANATOMY

Extensor digitorum tendons
Extensor carpi radialis longus tendon
Synovial sheath
Retinaculum

Synovial sheath over extensor pollicis brevis muscle

INJURY

POSSIBLE COMPLICATIONS
• Prolonged healing time if activity is resumed too soon.
• Proneness to repeated injury.
• Adhesive tenosynovitis: The tendon and its covering become bound together. Loss of motion may be complete or partial. Surgery is necessary to remove the covering or transfer the tendon to a new area.
• Constrictive tenosynovitis: The walls of the covering thicken and narrow, preventing the tendon from sliding through. Surgery is necessary to cut away part of the covering.

PROBABLE OUTCOME—Tenosynovitis is usually curable in about 6 weeks with heat treatments, corticosteroid injections and rest of the inflamed area. Recovery is usually quicker if the inflammation is caused by a direct blow rather than from a strain or sprain.

 ## HOW TO TREAT

NOTE—Follow your doctor's instructions. These instructions are supplemental.

FIRST AID—None. This problem develops slowly.

CONTINUING CARE
• Wrap the hand and wrist with an elasticized bandage until healing is complete.
• Apply heat frequently. Use heat lamps, hot soaks, hot showers, heating pads, or heat liniments and ointments.
• Take whirlpool treatments, if available.

MEDICATION—You may use non-prescription drugs such as acetaminophen for minor pain.

Your doctor may prescribe:
• Stronger pain relievers. Don't take prescription pain medication longer than 4 to 7 days. Use only as much as you need.
• Injection of the tendon covering with a combination of a long-acting local anesthetic and a non-absorbable corticosteroid such as triamcinolone.

ACTIVITY—Resume normal activities gradually.

DIET—During recovery, eat a well-balanced diet that includes extra protein, such as meat, fish, poultry, cheese, milk and eggs. Your doctor may prescribe vitamin and mineral supplements to promote healing.

REHABILITATION
• Begin daily rehabilitation exercises when supportive wrapping is no longer needed.
• Use ice massage for 10 minutes before and after exercise. Fill a large Styrofoam cup with water and freeze. Tear a small amount of foam from the top so ice protrudes. Massage firmly over the injured area in a circle about the size of a softball.
• See page 474 for rehabilitation exercises.

 ## CALL YOUR DOCTOR IF

• You have symptoms of wrist tenosynovitis.
• Any of the following occur after surgery:
Increased pain, swelling, redness, drainage or bleeding in the surgical area.
Signs of infection (headache, muscle aches, dizziness, or a general ill feeling and fever).
New, unexplained symptoms. Drugs used in treatment may produce side effects.

ALTITUDE ILLNESS

GENERAL INFORMATION

DEFINITION—Any of several illnesses associated with higher-than-usual altitudes. Illnesses are of several types, including:
- Acute Mountain Sickness (AMS).
- High Altitude Pulmonary Edema (HAPE).
- High Altitude Cerebral Edema (HACE).
- High Altitude Retinal Hemorrhage (HARH).
- Subacute and Chronic Mountain Sickness (CMS). This illness is a complication that represents failure to recover from AMS over a long period of time.

These illnesses affect most body systems, especially the brain, heart, lungs, gastrointestinal tract, circulatory system and electrolytes.
- Other altitude-related problems include frostbite, blood clots in the legs and lungs, dehydration, swollen feet and ankles.
- Pre-existing illnesses that are aggravated by high altitude include sickle-cell disease or trait, chronic heart disease or chronic lung disease.

SIGNS & SYMPTOMS
- AMS: Headache, nausea, vomiting, shortness of breath, sleep disturbances.
- HAPE: Shortness of breath, cough, weakness, headache, coma.
- HACE: Severe headache, staggering gait, hallucinations, stupor. These indicate swelling of the brain. Death will occur without descent.
- HARH: Visual disturbances, including spots before the eyes. Blood clots and bleeding into the retina occur in 50% of those who go above 17,000 feet.
- CMS: Shortness of breath, fatigue, bloated face and body, congestive heart failure after years of living at high altitude (rare).

CAUSES & RISK FACTORS—Insufficient
oxygen at high altitudes. Following are the altitudes at which each type of illness can occur:
- AMS: 7,000 to 8,000 feet or higher.
- HAPE: 9,000 to 10,000 feet.
- HACE: 10,000 to 12,000 feet.
- HARH: 17,000 feet.
Additional factors that contribute to development of altitude illness include:
- Fatigue or overwork.
- Previous episodes of altitude illness.
- Chronic illness of any sort, particularly cardiovascular and lung diseases.
- Obesity.
- Age over 60.
- Excess alcohol consumption.
- Use of mind-altering drugs, including narcotics and tranquillizers.

HOW TO PREVENT—Don't ascend to heights that cause symptoms. If you must climb,
become acclimatized gradually by a slow ascent.

WHAT TO EXPECT

DIAGNOSTIC MEASURES
- Your own observation of symptoms.
- Medical history and exam by a doctor.
- Laboratory studies such as EKG and chest x-ray.

SURGERY—Not necessary nor appropriate for these disorders.

NORMAL COURSE OF ILLNESS—Usually curable without residual impairment after returning to lower altitudes.

POSSIBLE COMPLICATIONS—Permanent brain, eye, heart and lung damage. Worst cases of HAPE and HACE can lead to death.

HOW TO TREAT

NOTE—Follow your doctor's instructions. These instructions are supplemental.

MEDICAL TREATMENT—See a doctor to determine the extent of damage and possible complications. He may prescribe medication.

HOME TREATMENT—Follow these instructions:
- AMS: Descend to lower altitude if illness lasts 2 or more days.
- HAPE: Oxygen, rest and diuretics help, but rapid descent is usually necessary.
- HACE: Oxygen and corticosteroids help, but rapid descent to lower altitudes is the only certain way to recover.
- HARH: No treatment except to descend.
- CMS: Return to lower altitudes if symptoms persist.

MEDICATION
Your doctor may prescribe:
- For AMS: Diamox (carbonic anhydrase inhibitor).
- For HAPE: Oxygen, furosemide (diuretic), morphine (narcotic pain reliever).
- For HACE: Corticosteroids.

ACTIVITY
- If any altitude illness occurs, decrease activity to a level at which symptoms disappear.
- Resume normal activities gradually upon returning to normal altitude.

DIET—No special diet.

CALL YOUR DOCTOR IF

- You have symptoms of any altitude illness.
- New, unexplained symptoms develop. Drugs used in treatment may produce side effects.

ANEMIA RELATED TO EXERCISE

GENERAL INFORMATION

DEFINITION—A decreased number of circulating red blood cells, or insufficient hemoglobin in the cells, caused from participation in exercise. Anemia is also a symptom of other disorders, and may interfere with athletic performance. For proper treatment, the cause must be found.

SIGNS & SYMPTOMS
Signs of pronounced anemia:
● Decreased performance in maximum-effort activities.
● Tiredness and weakness.
● Paleness, especially in the hands and lining of the lower eyelids.
Less common signs:
● Tongue inflammation.
● Fainting.
● Breathlessness.
● Excessively rapid heartbeat with exercise.
● Appetite loss.

CAUSES & RISK FACTORS
● Participation in exercise such as prolonged walking, running or cross-country skiing. The forces exerted on the red blood cells in the capillaries of the feet may rupture the blood cells and lead to anemia.
● Other heavy physical exercise and exertion.
● Heavy menstrual bleeding.
● Pregnancy.
● Malabsorption of iron from food.
● Profuse sweating.
● Age over 60.
● Recent illness with bleeding, such as an ulcer, diverticulitis, colitis, hemorrhoids or gastrointestinal tumor.

HOW TO PREVENT—Maintain an adequate iron intake by eating a well-balanced diet or taking iron supplements.

WHAT TO EXPECT

DIAGNOSTIC MEASURES
● Your own observation of symptoms.
● Medical history and exam by a doctor.
● Laboratory blood studies every 2 months while involved in vigorous physical activity. Tests should include studies of hematocrit (see Glossary), hemoglobin and red-blood-cell counts.
● X-rays of the gastrointestinal tract.

SURGERY—Necessary only if the underlying cause, such as a tumor, requires surgery.

NORMAL COURSE OF ILLNESS—Usually curable with iron supplements if the underlying cause can be identified and treated. Unless anemia is severe, you may continue training and vigorous physical activity while under treatment with iron supplements for anemia.

POSSIBLE COMPLICATIONS
● Failure to diagnose a bleeding malignancy.
● Without treatment, increasing weakness and eventual congestive heart failure.

HOW TO TREAT

NOTE—Follow your doctor's instructions. These instructions are supplemental.

MEDICAL TREATMENT—See your doctor to identify and treat the underlying cause.

HOME TREATMENT—None except to take iron supplements.

MEDICATION—Your doctor may prescribe iron supplements:
● Take iron on an empty stomach (at least 1/2 hour before meals) for best absorption. If it upsets your stomach, you may take it with a small amount of food (except milk).
● If you take other medications, wait at least 2 hours after taking iron before taking them. Antacids and tetracycline especially interfere with iron absorption.
● Continue iron supplements until 2 to 3 months after blood tests return to normal.
● Too much iron is dangerous. A bottle of iron tablets can poison a child. Keep iron supplements out of the reach of children.

ACTIVITY—No restrictions unless exercise-induced anemia is severe. Then reduce activity level slightly while undergoing treatment and continue at a slower pace until iron levels are back to normal.

DIET
● Limit milk to 1 pint a day. It interferes with iron absorption.
● Eat protein foods and iron-containing foods, including meat, beans and leafy green vegetables.
● Increase dietary fiber to prevent constipation (a common side effect of iron supplements).

CALL YOUR DOCTOR IF

● You have symptoms of anemia.
● Nausea, vomiting, severe diarrhea or constipation occur during treatment.

ASTHMA & EXERCISE-INDUCED BRONCHOSPASM (EIB)

 GENERAL INFORMATION

DEFINITION—A chronic breathing disorder characterized by recurrent attacks of wheezing and shortness of breath. It affects many people who exercise regularly.

SIGNS & SYMPTOMS
- Chest tightness and shortness of breath.
- Wheezing when exhaling.
- Coughing, especially at night, with little sputum.
- Rapid, shallow breathing that is easier with sitting up.
- Breathing difficulty—neck muscles tighten.

Severe late symptoms:
- Bluish skin.
- Exhaustion.
- Grunting respiration.
- Inability to speak.
- Mental changes, including restlessness, confusion or delirium.

CAUSES & RISK FACTORS—Spasm of air passages (bronchi and bronchioles) followed by swelling of the passages and thickening of lung secretions (sputum). This decreases or closes off air to the lungs. These changes are caused by:
- Allergens, such as some medications, pollen, dust, animal dander, molds and some foods.
- Air irritants, such as smoke, smog and odors.
- Exercise, especially exercise in smoggy or cold air. Bronchospasm can occur within minutes while exercising in cool air. Warm, humid air seldom triggers exercise-induced bronchospasm.
- Lung infections such as bronchitis.
- Stress.
- Family history of asthma or allergies.
- Smoking.
- Use of drugs to which you are allergic, such as aspirin.

HOW TO PREVENT
- Avoid known allergens and air pollutants.
- Take prescribed preventive medicines regularly—don't omit them when you feel well.
- Reduce activity level (sometimes).
- Exercise indoors on smoggy or cold days.

 WHAT TO EXPECT

DIAGNOSTIC MEASURES
- Your own observation of symptoms.
- Medical history and exam by a doctor.
- Laboratory blood studies and pulmonary-function test.
- Chest X-rays.

NORMAL COURSE OF ILLNESS—Symptoms

can be controlled with treatment and strict adherence to preventive measures. Children often outgrow asthma. Without treatment, severe attacks can be fatal.

POSSIBLE COMPLICATIONS
- Enlarged chest from repeated asthma attacks over a long period of time.
- Pneumothorax (collapsed lung).
- Repeated lung infections.
- COPD (see Glossary) from recurrent attacks.
- Respiratory failure.

 HOW TO TREAT

NOTE—Follow your doctor's instructions. These instructions are supplemental.

MEDICAL TREATMENT
- Emergency-room care and hospitalization for severe attacks.
- Psychotherapy or counseling, if asthma is stress-related.

HOME TREATMENT
- Eliminate allergens and irritants at home and at work, if possible.
- Keep regular medications with you at all times. Ask your doctor about having emergency drugs available.
- Sit upright during attacks.
- Practice deep breathing and postural drainage (see Glossary) each morning to loosen accumulated lung secretions.

MEDICATION—Your doctor may prescribe:
- Expectorants to loosen sputum.
- Bronchodilators to open air passages.
- Corticosteroid drugs by nebulizer, which have fewer adverse reactions than oral forms.
- Cromolyn sodium by nebulizer. This is a preventive drug.

ACTIVITY
- Stay active, but avoid sudden bursts of exercise. If an attack follows heavy exercise, sit and rest. Sip warm water.
- Continue sports activities if symptoms can be controlled. If not, decrease exercise levels temporarily until symptoms improve.

DIET—No special diet, but avoid foods to which you are sensitive. Drink at least 3 quarts of liquid daily to keep lung secretions thin and loose.

 CALL YOUR DOCTOR IF

- You have frequent symptoms of asthma.
- You have an asthma attack that doesn't respond to treatment. This is an emergency!
- New, unexplained symptoms develop. Drugs used in treatment may produce side effects.

ATHLETE'S FOOT
(Tinea Pedis; Ringworm of the Feet)

 GENERAL INFORMATION

DEFINITION—A common, contagious fungus infection of the skin on the feet between the toes (usually 4th and 5th toes). It is especially common among athletes.

SIGNS & SYMPTOMS
- Moist, soft, gray-white or red scales on feet, especially between toes.
- Dead skin between toes.
- Itching in inflamed areas.
- Damp, musty foot odor.
- Small blisters on the feet (sometimes), caused by a hypersensitivity to the fungus.

CAUSES & RISK FACTORS—Infection by a *trichophyton* fungus or yeast. Contributing factors include:
- Use of locker rooms and public showers.
- Infrequent washing of the feet.
- Infrequent changes of shoes or socks.
- Hot, humid weather.

HOW TO PREVENT
- Observe good locker-room hygiene (see Appendix 4).
- Bathe feet daily. Dry thoroughly, especially between the toes, and dust with talc or antifungal powder.
- Go barefoot when possible.
- Change shoes and socks daily.
- Wear socks made of cotton, wool or other natural, absorbent fibers. Avoid socks made with synthetic fibers.

 WHAT TO EXPECT

DIAGNOSTIC MEASURES
- Your own observation of symptoms.
- Medical history and exam by a doctor.
- Laboratory culture and microscopic examination of scales.

SURGERY—Not necessary nor useful for this illness.

NORMAL COURSE OF ILLNESS—Usually curable in 3 weeks with treatment, but recurrence is common.

POSSIBLE COMPLICATIONS
- Secondary bacterial infection in the affected area.
- "Id" reaction (an allergic autoimmune response to the infection) on hands and face. This is rare.

 HOW TO TREAT

NOTE—Follow your doctor's instructions. These instructions are supplemental.

MEDICAL TREATMENT—See your doctor if infection is severe or persistent.

HOME TREATMENT
- Remove scales and material between the toes daily.
- Keep affected areas cool and dry. Go barefoot or wear sandals during treatment.

MEDICATION
- Use non-prescription antifungal powders, creams or ointments after each bath.
- For severe cases, your doctor may prescribe:
  Oral antifungal medication.
  Corticosteroid drugs if an "id" reaction occurs.

ACTIVITY—No restrictions.

DIET—No special diet.

 CALL YOUR DOCTOR IF

- You have severe symptoms of athlete's foot that persist, despite self-treatment.
- You develop fever or the infection seems to be spreading or complicated by a bacterial infection.

BAROTITIS MEDIA
(Barotrauma)

 GENERAL INFORMATION

DEFINITION—Damage to the middle ear caused by pressure changes. This is very common in scuba divers.

SIGNS AND SYMPTOMS
- Hearing loss (to varying degrees).
- A plugged feeling in the ear.
- Severe pain.
- Dizziness.
- Ringing noise in the ear.

CAUSES & RISK FACTORS—Damage caused by sudden, increased pressure in the surrounding air, such as occurs in the rapid descent of an airplane or while scuba diving. In these activities, air moves from passages in the nose into the middle ear to maintain equal pressure on both sides of the eardrum. If the tube leading from the nose to the ear (eustachian tube) doesn't function properly, pressure in the middle ear is less than outside pressure. The negative pressure in the middle ear sucks the eardrum inward. Blood and mucus may later appear in the middle ear. This damage is more likely if you have a nose or throat infection when scuba diving or traveling by air.

HOW TO PREVENT
- Don't scuba-dive when you have an upper-respiratory infection.
- On feeling ear pain while scuba diving, stop the descent, ascend a few feet and try to equalize pressure. If you cannot equalize the pressure, terminate the dive.
- If flying, take a moderate-size breath, hold the nose and try to force air into the eustachian tube by gently puffing out the cheeks with the mouth closed.

 WHAT TO EXPECT

DIAGNOSTIC MEASURES
- Your own observation of symptoms.
- Medical history and exam by a doctor.

SURGERY—Sometimes necessary to open the eardrum and release fluid trapped in the middle ear. A plastic tube may be inserted through the surgically perforated eardrum to keep it open and equalize pressure. The tube falls out spontaneously in 9 to 12 months.

NORMAL COURSE OF ILLNESS—With treatment, most cases of barotitis media are reversible without permanent damage or hearing loss.

POSSIBLE COMPLICATIONS—Without treatment, fluid may accumulate, become infected and rupture the eardrum. The rupture may affect nerve endings, causing permanent hearing loss.

 HOW TO TREAT

NOTE—Follow your doctor's instructions. These instructions are supplemental.

MEDICAL TREATMENT—See your doctor for prescription of medications and surgery (sometimes).

HOME TREATMENT—If fluid drains from the ear, place a small piece of cotton in the outer-ear canal to absorb it.

MEDICATION
- For minor discomfort, you may use non-prescription decongestants and pain relievers such as acetaminophen.
- Your doctor may prescribe:
  Stronger prescription decongestant nasal sprays or tablets. Use for at least 2 weeks after damage.
  Corticosteroid nasal spray.
  Antibiotics if infection is present.

ACTIVITY—Resume normal activities as soon as symptoms improve. If surgery is necessary to insert tubes in the ears, keep water out of the ears. Consult your doctor about special ear plugs for use during swimming, bathing and shampooing.

DIET—No special diet.

 CALL YOUR DOCTOR IF

- You have symptoms of barotitis media.
- Severe ear pain, severe headache, fever or dizziness occur during treatment.
- New, unexplained symptoms develop. Drugs used in treatment may produce side effects.

BLISTERS

GENERAL INFORMATION

DEFINITION—Collection of fluid in a "bubble" under the outer layer of skin.

SIGNS & SYMPTOMS
- Fluid collection under the superficial skin layer.
- Sensitivity to pressure over the blister.
- Redness and swelling around the blister.

CAUSES & RISK FACTORS—Repeated friction and pressure against the skin, especially during hot, humid weather. Examples of common sites for blisters include the hands of gymnasts, the feet of runners and dancers, the fingers of baseball pitchers, and the buttocks of bicycle riders.

HOW TO PREVENT
- Apply 10% tannic acid to vulnerable areas of skin once or twice daily for 2 to 3 weeks.
- Wear shoes that fit like a glove, but allow enough space for the forefoot and toes. Check for rough seams inside the shoe.
- Don't wear thick socks. Clean, white cotton or cotton-wool socks are less likely to cause blisters than synthetic materials. Avoid tube socks.
- Try wearing no socks, but dusting shoes with talcum powder or rubbing feet and shoes with petroleum jelly.
- Put tape on vulnerable areas prior to exercise.
- Don't run in shoes still wet from previous use.
- Protect hands with gloves appropriate for your sport, if possible.

WHAT TO EXPECT

DIAGNOSTIC MEASURES—Your own observation of symptoms.

SURGERY—Not necessary nor useful for this illness.

NORMAL COURSE OF ILLNESS—Blisters usually heal in 3 to 7 days if they don't become infected.

POSSIBLE COMPLICATIONS—Infection. Fluid becomes pus, pain becomes worse and red streaks develop.

HOW TO TREAT

NOTE—Follow your doctor's instructions. These instructions are supplemental.

MEDICAL TREATMENT—See your doctor if infection develops.

HOME TREATMENT—No treatment is necessary for small, painless blisters (less than 1 inch across). To treat painful blisters or blisters larger than 1 inch:
- Apply ice to the blister for 5 minutes.
- Wash the blistered area with warm soapy water. Pat dry with a clean towel.
- Sterilize a pin or tip of a scissor by dipping in alcohol or by holding it in the flame of a lighted match until it becomes red.
- Puncture the blister in several places around the edge.
- Apply gentle pressure to the top of the blister to squeeze out fluid. Leave the skin in place.
- Repeat all steps above once a day if the blister persists.
- Place moleskin (see Glossary) over a blister pad on top of the blister. Pad blisters on the bottoms of the feet with adhesive felt or foam with a hole cut slightly larger than the blister.

MEDICATION—You may use non-prescription antibiotic medicine, such as Bacitracin or Neosporin, on the skin of the blister.

ACTIVITY—No restrictions unless the blister becomes infected.

DIET—No special diet.

CALL YOUR DOCTOR IF

- Home treatment of blisters hasn't brought relief in 1 to 3 days.
- Signs of infection occur (increased heat, redness, swelling or pus in the blister).

BOIL
(Furuncle)

 ## GENERAL INFORMATION

DEFINITION—A painful, deep, bacterial infection of a hair follicle. The infection—usually from *staphylococcus* bacteria—begins in the hair follicle and penetrates the skin's deeper layers. Boils are common and contagious.

SIGNS & SYMPTOMS
- A domed nodule that is painful, tender, red and has pus at the surface. Boils appear suddenly and ripen in 24 hours. They are usually 1-1/2cm to 3cm in diameter; some are larger.
- Fever.
- Swelling of the closest lymph glands.

CAUSES & RISK FACTORS—Boils are easily transmitted under crowded, unsanitary conditions. Athletic teams who work out with each other daily may have an outbreak of boils among members. Health clubs that do not keep showers clean or put adequate amounts of chemicals in pools or whirlpool hot tubs are particularly likely to harbor germs that cause boils. The following factors make a person more susceptible to boils:
- Poor nutrition.
- Illness that has lowered resistance.
- Diabetes mellitus.
- Use of immunosuppressive drugs.

HOW TO PREVENT—Keep the skin clean. Use only locker rooms, showers, tubs and steam rooms that are maintained according to hygienic regulations.

 ## WHAT TO EXPECT

DIAGNOSTIC MEASURES
- Your own observation of symptoms.
- Medical history and physical exam by a doctor.
- Laboratory culture of the pus to identify the germ.

SURGERY—Incision and drainage of the boil (sometimes).

NORMAL COURSE OF ILLNESS—Without treatment, a boil will heal in 10 to 20 days. With treatment, the boil should heal in less time, symptoms will be less severe, and new boils should not appear. The pus that drains when a boil opens spontaneously may contaminate nearby skin, causing new boils.

POSSIBLE COMPLICATIONS—The infection may enter the bloodstream and spread to other body parts.

 ## HOW TO TREAT

NOTE—Follow your doctor's instructions. These instructions are supplemental.

MEDICAL TREATMENT—Incision and drainage of the boil by a doctor may be necessary.

HOME TREATMENT
- Relieve pain with gentle heat from warm-water compresses, a heating pad, hot-water bottle or heat lamp. Use heat 3 or 4 times daily for 20 minutes.
- Prevent the spread of boils by using clean towels only once or using paper towels and discarding them.

MEDICATION
- Your doctor may prescribe a penicillin drug, such as oxacillin, dicloxacillin or nafcillin, or erythromycin antibiotics to fight infection.
- Don't use non-prescription antibiotic creams or ointments on the boil's surface. They are ineffective.

ACTIVITY—Decrease activity until the boil heals. Avoid sweating which may aggravate the infection.

DIET—No special diet.

 ## CALL YOUR DOCTOR IF

- You have a boil.
- The following occurs during treatment:
  Symptoms don't improve in 3 to 4 days, despite treatment.
  New boils appear.
  Fever rises above 100F (37.8C).
  Other family members develop boils.
  New, unexplained symptoms develop. Drugs used in treatment may produce side effects.

BUNION
(Hallux Valgus)

GENERAL INFORMATION

DEFINITION—Overgrowth of tissue at the base of the great (big) toe. Bunions may be congenital or hereditary. A bunion often impairs athletic performance until it is corrected with medical treatment or surgery.

SIGNS & SYMPTOMS
- An inward-turned great toe that may overlap the second—and sometimes the third—toe.
- Thickened skin over the bony protrusion at the base of the great toe.
- Fluid accumulation under the thickened skin (sometimes).
- Foot pain and stiffness.
- Inflammation and swelling around the bunion.

CAUSES & RISK FACTORS
- Irritation of the bony bump when the big toe is directed toward the little toe.
- Narrow-toed, high-heeled shoes that compress toes together.
- Arthritis.
- Family history of foot disorders.

HOW TO PREVENT
- Wear wide-toed, well-fitting shoes with strong arch supports. Don't wear high heels or shoes without room for toes in their normal position.
- Don't wear socks or stockings that are too tight.
- After treatment, prevent a recurrence by placing a 1/4-inch thickness of foam rubber between the big toe and second toe.

WHAT TO EXPECT

DIAGNOSTIC MEASURES
- Your own observation of symptoms.
- Medical history and exam by a doctor or podiatrist.
- X-rays of the foot.

SURGERY—Often necessary to remove the overgrown tissue and correct the position of the bones.

NORMAL COURSE OF ILLNESS—Usually improves with treatment and preventive measures to guard against recurrence.

POSSIBLE COMPLICATIONS
- Infection of the bunion, especially in persons with diabetes mellitus.
- Inflammation and arthritic changes in other joints caused by walking difficulty, which places abnormal stress on the foot, hip and spine.
- Excessive bleeding or infection if surgery is required.

HOW TO TREAT

NOTE—Follow your doctor's instructions. These instructions are supplemental.

MEDICAL TREATMENT—None necessary for mild cases. Surgery may be required for persistent or severe cases.

HOME TREATMENT
- Before bedtime, separate the great toe from the others with a foam-rubber pad.
- When wearing shoes, place a thick, ring-shaped adhesive pad over the bunion.
- Use arch supports to relieve pressure on the bunion. These are available in shoe-repair shops.

MEDICATION—Usually not necessary for this disorder unless infection develops.

ACTIVITY—No restrictions as long as the bunion is protected from irritation. If surgery is necessary, resume normal activities gradually afterward. Walk on your heels until the surgical site heals. Elevate the foot of the bed to reduce swelling over the incision. Avoid vigorous exercise for 6 weeks following surgery.

DIET—During recovery from surgery, eat a well-balanced diet that includes extra protein, such as meat, fish, poultry, cheese, milk and eggs. Increase fiber and fluid intake to prevent constipation that may result from decreased activity.

CALL YOUR DOCTOR IF

- You have a bunion that is interfering with normal activities.
- Signs of infection (fever, headache, heat, increased tenderness or pain) develop during treatment or after surgery.

CARPAL-TUNNEL SYNDROME

 GENERAL INFORMATION

DEFINITION—A nerve disorder that causes pain, loss of feeling and loss of strength in the hands. It may greatly decrease athletic performance in sports that require strong hand or wrist action, such as tennis, racquetball, squash, golf, skiing, weight-lifting, baseball, football, horseshoes, bowling, archery, rowing, wrestling, boxing, gymnastics, hockey, judo or water-skiing. Carpal-tunnel syndrome is most common in women between ages 29 and 62.

SIGNS & SYMPTOMS
- Tingling or numbness in part of the hand.
- Sharp pains that shoot from the wrist up the arm, especially at night.
- Burning sensations in the fingers.
- Thumb weakness.
- Frequent dropping of objects.
- Poor performance in any sport that requires a strong grip.
- Inability to make a fist.
- Shiny, dry skin on the hand.

CAUSES & RISK FACTORS—Pressure on the median nerve of the wrist caused by swollen, inflamed or scarred tissue. The sources of pressure include:
- Inflammation of the wrist-tendon sheaths, a likely result of any sport that requires gripping or squeezing.
- Fracture of the forearm.
- Sprain or dislocation of the wrist.
- Arthritis.
Contributing factors include:
- Diabetes mellitus.
- Hypothyroidism (underactive thyroid gland).
- Raynaud's disease (a circulatory disorder that affects blood circulation to fingers).
- Menopause.
- Pregnancy.

HOW TO PREVENT—Cannot be prevented at present.

 WHAT TO EXPECT

DIAGNOSTIC MEASURES
- Your own observation of symptoms.
- Medical history and physical exam by a doctor.
- Electromyograms (see Glossary).
- X-rays of the hand and wrist.

SURGERY—Necessary sometimes to free the pinched nerve in the wrist.

NORMAL COURSE OF ILLNESS—Usually curable—sometimes spontaneously, sometimes with surgery.

POSSIBLE COMPLICATIONS—Permanent pain, numbness and a weak thumb or fingers in the affected hand.

 HOW TO TREAT

NOTE—Follow your doctor's instructions. These instructions are supplemental.

MEDICAL TREATMENT—Surgery or medications listed below.

HOME TREATMENT
- Discomfort improves by shaking hands or dangling arms. If you awaken at night with pain in your hand, hang it over the side of the bed; rub or shake it.
- Consult your doctor about wearing a splint on the affected wrist at night.

MEDICATION—Your doctor may prescribe:
- Diuretics to decrease fluid retention that causes swollen tissue.
- Anti-inflammatory drugs to reduce inflammation.
- Corticosteroid injections at the wrist to reduce inflammation.

ACTIVITY—Stay as active as your strength allows. If surgery is necessary, allow 4 weeks for recovery. Resume normal activities gradually during that time. Exercises may be prescribed for the hand.

DIET—Eat a normal, well-balanced diet that is low in sodium. This will help prevent fluid retention that aggravates the condition.

 CALL YOUR DOCTOR IF

You have symptoms of carpal-tunnel syndrome that don't disappear in 2 weeks.

COLD SORE
(Fever Blister; Herpes Simplex)

GENERAL INFORMATION

DEFINITION—A common, contagious viral infection of the lip, gum and mouth areas. It occasionally affects the genitals and rarely affects the cornea (thin transparent layer covering the eye).

SIGNS & SYMPTOMS
● Eruption of very small, painful blisters that are grouped together and surrounded by a red ring. They fill with fluid, then dry up and disappear.
● If the eye is infected:
Eye pain and redness.
Feeling that something is in the eye.
Sensitivity to light and tearing.

CAUSES & RISK FACTORS—Infection from the herpes simplex virus. The virus is transmitted through saliva, stools, urine or eye discharge from the infected eye of someone with active herpes. Most persons are exposed to the virus in childhood. The virus remains in the body indefinitely, becoming active occasionally and causing an outbreak of blisters. The following can trigger flare-ups:
● Injury to the skin from friction with clothing or protective gear.
● Previous eczema.
● Physical or emotional stress.
● Illness or excessive exercise that has lowered resistance.
● Excess sun exposure.
● Use of immunosuppressive drugs.
● Menstrual period.

HOW TO PREVENT
● Avoid physical contact with others who have active lesions.
● Avoid excess direct exposure to sun. Use zinc oxide or a sunscreen on your lips.
● To avoid spreading the virus to others:
Wash your hands often during a flare-up.
Avoid wrestling, judo, boxing and other sports involving physical contact until lesions heal.
Don't use protective equipment, such as a face mask, until lesions heal.

WHAT TO EXPECT

DIAGNOSTIC MEASURES—Your own observation of symptoms.

NORMAL COURSE OF ILLNESS
Spontaneous recovery in a few days to a week, occasionally longer. Recurrence is common. The virus remains in the body for life, but it is usually dormant. Research continues in developing a vaccine.

POSSIBLE COMPLICATION
● Permanent vision impairment, if herpes eye infections are untreated.
● Severe, widespread infection in patients with eczema.
● Meningitis or encephalitis (rare).

HOW TO TREAT

NOTE—Follow your doctor's instructions. These instructions are supplemental.

MEDICAL TREATMENT—Not usually necessary except for a herpes eye infection or if a herpes lesion in any part of the body becomes infected with bacteria.

HOME TREATMENT
● Drink cool liquids or suck frozen juice bars.
● Apply an ice cube for 1 hour during the first 24 hours after a lesion appears. This may make it heal more quickly.
● Don't rub or scratch an infected eye.

MEDICATION
● You may use the following non-prescription medications:
Acetaminophen to relieve minor pain. Don't use aspirin, especially for children and adolescents. Use of aspirin for some viral illnesses has been linked to Reye's syndrome, a form of encephalitis.
Drying medications such as Campho-Phenique, tincture of benzoin or benzoyl peroxide 5-10% for lesions close to the lip.
● Don't treat an infected eye without consulting your doctor. *Don't use corticosteroid ointment or drops in the eye.* Corticosteroids promote growth of the herpes virus in the cornea.
● Your doctor may prescribe:
Antiviral medication at the earliest sign of a flare-up. (Later use is ineffective).
Antibiotics if lesions become infected with bacteria.
Anticancer topical medication for eye infections.

ACTIVITY—Avoid close contact—especially kissing or oral sex—until lesions heal.

DIET—No special diet.

CALL YOUR DOCTOR IF

The following occurs with a cold sore:
● Signs of secondary bacterial infection, such as fever, pus instead of clear fluid in the lesions, headache and muscle aches.
● Eruption of lesions on the genitals similar to those around the mouth.
● Development of new, unexplained symptoms. Drugs in treatment may produce side effects.

COLON, IRRITABLE
(Spastic Colon; Mucous Colitis; Spastic Colitis; Irritable Bowel Syndrome)

 GENERAL INFORMATION

DEFINITION—An irritative and inflammatory disorder involving the large and small intestines. It is not contagious, inherited or cancerous—but it probably is stress-related. Flare-ups may be triggered by approaching competitive events.

SIGNS & SYMPTOMS—The following symptoms usually begin in early adult life. Episodes may last for days, weeks or months:
● Cramplike pain in the middle or to one side of the lower abdomen. Pain is usually relieved with a bowel movement.
● Nausea.
● Bloating and gas.
● Occasional appetite loss that may lead to weight loss.
● Diarrhea or constipation, usually alternating.
● Fatigue.
● Depression.
● Anxiety.
● Concentration difficulty.

CAUSES & RISK FACTORS
● Stress and emotional conflict prior to athletic competition, resulting in anxiety or depression.
● Obsessive worry about everyday problems or about self-image.
● Concern about performance.
● Marital tension.
● Fear of loss of a beloved person or object.
● Death of a loved one.
● Improper diet. Symptoms may be triggered by eating, though no specific food has been identified as responsible.
● Smoking.
● Excess alcohol consumption.
● Use of drugs.
● Fatigue or overwork.
● Poor physical fitness.

HOW TO PREVENT—Reduce stress or try to modify your response to it. An exercise program without competition may protect against flare-ups because it reduces stress.

 WHAT TO EXPECT

DIAGNOSTIC MEASURES
● Your own observation of symptoms.
● Medical history and physical exam by a doctor.
● Laboratory studies, including stool studies, to exclude other disorders such as lactose intolerance, ulcers, parasites, enzyme deficiency and ulcerative colitis.
● X-ray of the colon (barium enema).

SURGERY—Not necessary nor useful for this illness.

NORMAL COURSE OF ILLNESS—Curable if the underlying causes can be eliminated or modified. If not, symptoms can be controlled with treatment.

POSSIBLE COMPLICATIONS
● Decreased athletic performance.
● Poor nutrition caused by malabsorption.
● Psychological fixation on bowel function, leading to neurosis.
● Increased risk of colon cancer.

 HOW TO TREAT

NOTE—Follow your doctor's instructions. These instructions are supplemental.

MEDICAL TREATMENT
● Medication.
● Counseling with a trained therapist to define, confront and solve conflicts in day-to-day living.

HOME TREATMENT
● Diet changes.
● Adequate rest.

MEDICATION—Medication can help control symptoms, but it cannot cure this disorder. Your doctor may prescribe:
● Antispasmodics to relieve severe abdominal cramps.
● Tranquilizers to reduce anxiety.

ACTIVITY—No restrictions. Good physical fitness improves bowel function.

DIET
● Increase fiber in the diet to promote good bowel function.
● Don't eat foods that aggravate symptoms.

 CALL YOUR DOCTOR IF

You have symptoms of an irritable colon, and any of the following occur:
● Fever develops.
● Stool is black or tarry-looking.
● You begin vomiting.
● You lose 5 pounds or more for unknown reasons.
● Symptoms don't improve despite treatment.

CONJUNCTIVITIS
(Pink Eye)

 GENERAL INFORMATION

DEFINITION—An inflammation of the eyelid's underside and white part of the eye. It is contagious and easily transmitted, particularly to athletes on the same team who have close daily contact or in crowded or unsanitary athletic facilities.

SIGNS & SYMPTOMS—The following symptoms may affect one or both eyes:
- Clear, green or yellow discharge from the eye.
- After sleeping, crusts on lashes that cause eyelids to stick together.
- Eye pain.
- Swollen eyelids.
- Sensitivity to bright light.
- Redness and gritty feeling in the eye.
- Intense itching (allergic conjunctivitis only).

CAUSES & RISK FACTORS
- Viral infection. Conjunctivitis may accompany colds or diseases such as measles.
- Bacterial infection.
- Chemical irritation or wind, dust, smoke and other types of air pollution.
- Allergies caused by cosmetics, pollen or other allergens.
- A partially closed tear duct.
- Intense light, such as from sunlamps, snow or water reflection, or electric arcs in welding.

HOW TO PREVENT
- Wash hands frequently with soap and warm water to avoid spreading germs to the eye area.
- Don't use anyone else's towel.
- Avoid exposure to eye irritants.

 WHAT TO EXPECT

DIAGNOSTIC MEASURES
- Your own observation of symptoms.
- Medical history and physical exam by a doctor.
- Laboratory culture of the eye discharge.

SURGERY—Not necessary nor appropriate for this illness.

NORMAL COURSE OF ILLNESS
- Bacterial or viral conjunctivitis is curable in 1 to 2 weeks with treatment.
- Allergic conjunctivitis can be cured if the allergen is removed. It is likely to recur.

POSSIBLE COMPLICATIONS—If untreated, pink eye may spread and damage the cornea permanently, impairing vision.

 HOW TO TREAT

NOTE—Follow your doctor's instructions. These instructions are supplemental.

MEDICAL TREATMENT—Doctor's examination and medication.

HOME TREATMENT
- Wash hands often with antiseptic soap, and use paper towels to dry. Don't touch eyes.
- Gently wipe the discharge from the eye using disposable tissues. Infections are frequently spread by contaminated fingers, towels, handkerchiefs or wash cloths that have touched the infected eye.
- Use warm-water compresses to reduce discomfort.
- Don't use eye makeup.

MEDICATION—Your doctor may prescribe antibiotic eye drops, sulfa eye drops, steroid eye drops or antibiotic ointment to fight infection. Use 3 times daily. If the infection does not improve in 2 or 3 days, it may be caused by an insensitive bacteria, virus or allergy. At this point, an ophthalmologist may need to culture the conjunctivae or make special studies to determine the cause of the conjunctivitis. Most ophthalmologists believe corticosteroid eye drops should not be used until a diagnosis is definite. If the infection is caused by herpes simplex virus, steroids may spread it from the conjunctiva to the cornea, damaging the eye.

ACTIVITY—Resume vigorous physical activities when symptoms improve.

DIET—No special diet.

 CALL YOUR DOCTOR IF

- You have symptoms of conjunctivitis.
- The infection does not improve in 48 hours despite treatment.
- Fever occurs.
- Eye pain increases.
- Vision is affected.

CORN OR CALLUS

 GENERAL INFORMATION

DEFINITION
- A corn is a painful thickening (bump) of the outer skin layer, usually over bony areas such as toe joints.
- A callus is a painless (usually) thickening of skin caused by repeated pressure or irritation. Corns and calluses form to protect a skin area from injury caused by repeated irritation (rubbing or squeezing). Pressure causes cells in the irritated area to grow at a faster rate, leading to overgrowth. They are a frequent problem for all athletes.

SIGNS & SYMPTOMS
- Corn: A small, painful, raised bump on the side or over the joint of a toe. Corns are usually 3mm to 10mm in diameter and have a hard center.
- Callus: A rough, thickened area of skin that appears after repeated pressure or irritation.

CAUSES & RISK FACTORS—Repeated injury
to the skin, particularly on the feet. These occur frequently in athletes due to excessive perspiration, increased heat, friction of clothing and protective gear, or poorly fitting shoes. Athletic activities that cause pressure on the hands or knees include throwing sports, gripping sports and wrestling.

HOW TO PREVENT
- Don't wear shoes that fit poorly.
- Avoid activities that create constant pressure on specific skin areas.
- When possible, wear protective gear such as gloves or knee pads.
- Use corn and callus pads on the feet to reduce pressure on irritated areas.
- Stretch the shoe at the spot where it covers the corn or callus.
- Treat new shoes with leather-softening compounds such as mink oil.

 WHAT TO EXPECT

DIAGNOSTIC MEASURES
- Your own observation of symptoms.
- Medical history and physical exam by a medical doctor or a podiatrist.

SURGERY—Avoid surgery. It does not remove the cause. Postsurgical scarring is painful and may complicate healing.

NORMAL COURSE OF ILLNESS—Usually curable if the underlying cause can be removed. Allow 3 weeks for recovery. Recurrence is likely—even with treatment—if the cause is not removed.

POSSIBLE COMPLICATIONS
- Back, hip, knee or ankle pain caused by a change in one's gait due to severe discomfort.
- Mistaken diagnosis—sometimes a wart, splinter or ulcer can look like a callus.

 HOW TO TREAT

NOTE—Follow your doctor's instructions. These instructions are supplemental.

MEDICAL TREATMENT—Not usually necessary. For resistant cases, your doctor may inject cortisone medication into the corn or callus to reduce inflammation.

HOME TREATMENT
- Rub the thickened area with a pumice stone, sandstone, callus file or sandpaper to remove it. Don't cut it with a razor. Soak the area in warm water to soften it before rubbing.
- After removing the top skin layer, cleanse the treated area with soap and water and apply a non-medicated corn or callus pad. Stretch the hole in the pad to fit over the corn or callus and overlap at least 1/8 inch on all sides. Then wrap the treated area with adhesive tape.
- Remove the source of pressure, if possible. Discard ill-fitting shoes.
- Use corn and callus pads to reduce pressure on irritated areas.
- Ask the shoe repairman to sew a metatarsal bar onto your shoe to use while a corn is healing.

MEDICATION
- After peeling the upper layers of the corn or callus once or twice a day, apply ointment, petroleum jelly or massage oil.
- Your doctor may prescribe cortisone injections.

ACTIVITY—Resume your normal activities as soon as symptoms improve.

DIET—No special diet.

 CALL YOUR DOCTOR IF

- You have a corn or callus that persists, despite self-treatment.
- Any signs of infection, such as redness, swelling, pain, heat or tenderness, develop around a corn or callus.

CORNEAL ULCER

GENERAL INFORMATION

DEFINITION—An open sore in the thin transparent layers that cover the eye. It is particularly likely to occur in sports activities in areas with lots of wind, sand or gravel.

SIGNS & SYMPTOMS
- Eye pain.
- Sensitivity to bright light.
- Eyelid spasm.
- Tearing.
- Blurred vision.
- Redness in the white of the eye.

CAUSES & RISK FACTORS
- Injury to the cornea or the imbedding in the cornea of a foreign body, such as a small piece of steel, sand or glass. A bacterial infection—usually *pneumococcal, streptococcal* or *staphylococcal*—may follow the injury.
- Use of contact lenses, especially extended-wear lenses.
- Complications of the virus, herpes simplex, that produces cold sores on the mouth and can affect the eye.
- Infections of the eyelids and conjunctiva.
- Defective closure of the lid.
- Smoking or other environmental eye irritants.
- All the above infections are contagious from person to person or from one part of the body to another—especially finger-to-eye contact after touching cold sores on the mouth.

HOW TO PREVENT
- Wash hands frequently.
- Avoid injury. Use appropriate equipment such as protective goggles, helmets and face masks to prevent injury to the head, face and eyes.
- Don't touch your eyes if you have cold sores.

WHAT TO EXPECT

DIAGNOSTIC MEASURES
- Your own observation of symptoms.
- Medical history and physical exam by a doctor (ophthalmologist).
- Laboratory studies to identify the bacterium, virus or fungus responsible for the infection and ulcer.

SURGERY—Not necessary nor useful for this disorder, unless a corneal transplant becomes necessary (rare).

NORMAL COURSE OF ILLNESS—A corneal ulcer is a serious eye problem. It is usually curable in 2 to 3 weeks if treated by an ophthalmologist. If scars from previous corneal ulcers impair vision significantly, a corneal transplant (grafting a new cornea onto the eye) may make vision nearly normal.

POSSIBLE COMPLICATIONS—Neglected corneal ulcers may penetrate the cornea, allowing infection to enter the eyeball. This can cause permanent vision loss.

HOW TO TREAT

NOTE—Follow your doctor's instructions. These instructions are supplemental.

MEDICAL TREATMENT—None is usually necessary after diagnosis and prescription of medications.

HOME TREATMENT—Apply cool-water compresses to the eye as often as they feel good.

MEDICATION
- Your doctor may prescribe antibiotic eye drops, ointments or oral antibiotics for bacterial infections. Your doctor will administer medication for viral and fungus infections.
- For minor pain, you may use non-prescription drugs such as acetaminophen.

ACTIVITY—After treatment, resume normal activity as soon as possible.

DIET—No special diet.

CALL YOUR DOCTOR IF

- You have symptoms of a corneal ulcer.
- The following occurs during treatment:
  Fever over 101F (38.3C).
  Pain that is not relieved by acetaminophen.
  Changed vision.
- New, unexplained symptoms develop. Drugs used in treatment may produce side effects.

COUGH

GENERAL INFORMATION

DEFINITION—This is a symptom, not a disease. A cough protects the lungs by raising sputum and irritating substances, but it can prove distracting to the athlete during exercise or sleep. A cough can decrease or prevent athletic participation. Coughs are of two types:
● Non-productive cough (no sputum raised).
● Productive cough (sputum raised with or without blood). Sputum may be clear, mucoid, purulent (looks like pus), bloody or streaked with blood.

SIGNS & SYMPTOMS—Cough *is* the symptom.

CAUSES & RISK FACTORS
For non-productive coughs (no sputum raised):
  Cigarette smoke and other pollutants.
  Postnasal drip.
  Asthma.
  Viral infection.
  Foreign body in the lung.
For productive coughs (sputum raised with or without blood):
  Bacterial lung infection (sometimes viral).
  Chronic bronchitis.
  Bronchiectasis.
  Tuberculosis.
  Fungus infections (such as valley fever and histoplasmosis).
  Lung abscess.
  Lung cancer.

HOW TO PREVENT
● Treat the underlying disease.
● Don't smoke.
● Avoid people with colds or flu if you can. Wash your hands frequently during epidemics of upper-respiratory illness.

WHAT TO EXPECT

DIAGNOSTIC MEASURES
● Your own observation of symptoms.
● Medical history and exam by a doctor.
● Laboratory studies (see Glossary for all):
  Culture of sputum.
  Bronchoscopy.
  Laryngoscopy.
● X-rays of chest and sinuses.

SURGERY—Sometimes necessary if cough is caused by lung abscess or tumor.

NORMAL COURSE OF ILLNESS
● The majority of coughs are related to influenza or the common cold, and they clear spontaneously in 7 to 21 days.
● Outcome of more serious or underlying disease will depend entirely on which disorder is responsible and its extensiveness.

POSSIBLE COMPLICATIONS
● A fainting spell a few seconds after a coughing spell.
● Vomiting.
● Urinary incontinence (particularly in women over 40 who have borne children).

HOW TO TREAT

NOTE—Follow your doctor's instructions. These instructions are supplemental.

MEDICAL TREATMENT—Necessary only if underlying cause does not respond to home treatment, or if signs of infection are present.

HOME TREATMENT—Use a cool-mist humidifier close to your bed when sleeping. Wash the humidifier often to prevent contamination with germs.

MEDICATION—To relieve symptoms, you may use non-prescription drugs, such as throat lozenges or cough remedies containing dextromethorphan. Avoid cough remedies with codeine if you are planning to continue to exercise and compete.

ACTIVITY—Bed rest is not necessary, but avoid vigorous activity. Rest often.

DIET—Drink extra fluids, including water, fruit juice, tea and carbonated drinks. Avoid milk because it thickens lung secretions in some persons.

CALL YOUR DOCTOR IF

The following occurs during the illness:
● Coughing episodes that last longer than intervals between coughing.
● Cough that produces thick, yellow-green or gray sputum.
● Cough that lasts longer than 10 days.
● Difficult or labored breathing between coughing bouts.
● Fever that lasts several days or rises to 101F (38.3C).
● Shaking chills.
● Chest pain or shortness of breath.
● Earache or headache.
● Skin rash.
● Pain in the teeth or over the sinuses.
● Unusual lethargy or unusual irritability.
● Delirium.
● Enlarged, tender glands in the neck.
● Dusky blue or gray lips, skin or nails.

DEHYDRATION

GENERAL INFORMATION

DEFINITION—Loss of water and essential body salts due to excessive sweating during exercise, particularly in hot, humid weather.

SIGNS & SYMPTOMS
- Dry mouth.
- Decreased or absent urination.
- Sunken eyes.
- Wrinkled skin.
- Confusion.
- Low blood pressure.
- Coma.

CAUSES & RISK FACTORS
- Heavy sweating.
- Persistent vomiting or diarrhea from any cause.
- Use of drugs that deplete fluids and electrolytes, such as diuretics ("water pills").
- Overexposure to sun or heat.
- Age over 60.
- Recent illness with high fever.
- Chronic kidney disease.

HOW TO PREVENT
- Drink water frequently in small quantities during exercise that causes excessive sweating.
- If you are vomiting or have diarrhea, take small amounts of liquid with non-prescription electrolyte supplements—or drinks such as Gatorade—every 30 to 60 minutes.
- If you use diuretics, weigh daily. Report to your doctor a weight loss of more than 3 pounds in 1 day or 5 pounds in 1 week.
- Weigh in before and after practice sessions. Skip workouts if a weight loss of 2% or more has not been regained.

WHAT TO EXPECT

DIAGNOSTIC MEASURES
- Your own observation of symptoms.
- Medical history and physical exam by a doctor.
- Laboratory blood studies, including blood counts and electrolyte measurement (see Glossary).

SURGERY—Not necessary nor useful for this disorder.

NORMAL COURSE OF ILLNESS—Curable with control of the underlying cause and replacement of necessary fluids.

POSSIBLE COMPLICATIONS—Blood pressure drop, shock and death from prolonged, severe dehydration.

HOW TO TREAT

NOTE—Follow your doctor's instructions. These instructions are supplemental.

MEDICAL TREATMENT—Hospitalization for intravenous fluids (severe or prolonged illness only).

HOME TREATMENT
- Weigh at the same time each day on an accurate home scale and record the weight so you can be aware of fluid loss.
- If you have vomiting or diarrhea, keep a record of the number of episodes so you can estimate your fluid loss.
- For minor dehydration, take frequent small amounts of clear liquids. Large amounts may trigger vomiting.

MEDICATION—Your doctor may prescribe intravenous fluids to replace lost water.

ACTIVITY—Rest in bed until you recover. You may read or watch TV.

DIET—Depends on the underlying disorder. Salty foods decrease the effect of dehydration.

CALL YOUR DOCTOR IF

You have symptoms of dehydration.

DERMATITIS, CONTACT

GENERAL INFORMATION

DEFINITION—Skin inflammation caused by contact with an irritating substance, such as artificial turf, poorly fitting gear, excessive sweat or repeated application of adhesive tape. Contact dermatitis is not contagious.

SIGNS & SYMPTOMS
- Itching (sometimes).
- Slight redness.
- Cracks and fissures in the skin.
- Bright red, weeping areas (severe cases).

CAUSES & RISK FACTORS
- Contact with irritants, such as adhesive tape, acids or solvents. The irritant removes the fatty layer of skin. This causes dehydration and shrinking of surface cells.
- Hot weather and increased sweating.
- Constant exposure to hot water, soap and detergents, or any irritant that changes the moisture content of skin.
- Burns from hot water or sunburn.

HOW TO PREVENT
- Avoid contact with any irritant which has caused dermatitis in the past.
- Protect skin from sunburn and other burns.

WHAT TO EXPECT

DIAGNOSTIC MEASURES
- Your own observation of symptoms.
- Medical history and physical exam by a doctor.

SURGERY—Not necessary nor useful for this disorder.

NORMAL COURSE OF ILLNESS—Symptoms can be controlled with treatment and avoidance of the irritant. Recurrence is common, so intermittent treatment may be necessary for years.

POSSIBLE COMPLICATIONS—Pain and disfigurement of hands from constant lesions.

HOW TO TREAT

NOTE—Follow your doctor's instructions. These instructions are supplemental.

MEDICAL TREATMENT—Usually not necessary unless infection develops.

HOME TREATMENT
- Avoid the chemical or material causing the skin eruption.
- Use bath oil instead of soap for bathing.
- Pat skin dry rather than rubbing it.
- Reduce water temperature to lukewarm for bathing or other uses.
- Use only cream, lotion or ointment prescribed for the condition. Other commercial products may aggravate the condition. Apply ointment or cream to hands 6 or 7 times a day. For other body parts, lubricate twice a day, especially after bathing.

MEDICATION—Your doctor may prescribe topical creams, ointments or lotions. These may include corticosteroid preparations to reduce inflammation or lubricants to preserve moisture.

ACTIVITY—Resume your normal activities gradually as irritation subsides.

DIET—No special diet.

CALL YOUR DOCTOR IF

- You develop fever.
- Signs of infection (swelling, tenderness, redness, warmth) develop at the site of irritation.
- Treatment does not relieve symptoms in 1 week.

DERMATITIS, SEBORRHEIC

GENERAL INFORMATION

DEFINITION—A skin condition characterized by greasy or dry, white scales on the skin of the scalp (dandruff), eyebrows, forehead, face, folds around the nose, behind ears, in the external ear canal, or on skin of the trunk, especially over the breastbone or in skin folds. It is not contagious. It is especially of concern to athletes because extra heat and sweat can aggravate skin irritation and trigger the production of more scales.

SIGNS & SYMPTOMS—Flaking, white scales over reddish patches on the skin and scalp. Scales anchor to hair shafts. They may itch, but they are usually painless unless complicated by infection.

CAUSES & RISK FACTORS
- Sweating.
- Stress.
- Hot, humid weather or cold, dry weather.
- Infrequent shampoos.
- Oily skin.
- Other disorders, such as acne rosacea, acne or psoriasis.
- Obesity.
- Parkinson's disease.
- Use of drying lotions that contain alcohol.

HOW TO PREVENT—Cannot be prevented. To minimize severity or frequency of flare-ups:
- Shampoo frequently.
- Dry skin folds thoroughly after bathing.
- Wear loose, ventilating clothing.

WHAT TO EXPECT

DIAGNOSTIC MEASURES
- Your own observation of symptoms.
- Medical history and physical exam by a doctor.

SURGERY—Not necessary nor useful for this disorder.

NORMAL COURSE OF ILLNESS—This is a chronic condition, but it is often characterized by long periods of inactivity. During active phases, symptoms can be controlled with treatment.

POSSIBLE COMPLICATIONS
- Embarrassment and social discomfort.
- Secondary bacterial infection in affected areas.

HOW TO TREAT

NOTE—Follow your doctor's instructions. These instructions are supplemental.

MEDICAL TREATMENT—Home treatment is sufficient unless infection develops.

HOME TREATMENT
- Shampoo vigorously and as often as once a day. The shampoo you use is not as important as the way you scrub your scalp. Loosen scales with your fingernails while shampooing, and scrub at least 5 minutes.
- Lubricate skin before drying off after baths and showers.

MEDICATION
- For minor dandruff, you may use non-prescription dandruff shampoos and lubricating skin lotion.
- For severe problems, your doctor may prescribe:
  Shampoos that contain coal tar or scalp creams that contain cortisone. To apply medication to the scalp, part the hair a few strands at a time, and rub the ointment or lotion vigorously into the scalp.
  Topical corticosteroids for other affected parts.

ACTIVITY—No restrictions. Outdoor activities in summer may help.

DIET—No special diet. Avoid foods that seem to worsen your condition.

CALL YOUR DOCTOR IF

- You have symptoms of seborrheic dermatitis that don't respond to self-care.
- Patches of seborrheic dermatitis ooze, form crusts or drain pus. These signs may indicate infection.

DROWNING, NEAR-

GENERAL INFORMATION

DEFINITION—The immediate aftereffects of prolonged submersion under water. This may occur with or without aspirating water into the lungs. Approximately 10% to 15% of all drownings or near-drownings occur without aspiration. There have been a few reports of survival following submersion up to 40 minutes when the water was very cold. Submersion in warm or hot water results in more rapid death. Drowning accounts for approximately 10,000 deaths in North America each year.

SIGNS & SYMPTOMS
- Confusion or unconsciousness.
- Little or no breathing or heartbeat.
- Bluish-white paleness.

CAUSES & RISK FACTORS—Submersion under water, resulting in either of the following:
- Spasm of the larynx (the tube from the throat to the lungs). After rescue, this spasm prevents oxygen from reaching the lungs unless air is forced through the spasm by a respirator or CPR procedures.
- Water in the lungs, causing life-threatening changes in the circulating blood.

HOW TO PREVENT
- Learn cardiopulmonary resuscitation (CPR).
- Encourage all family members—including infants—to learn to swim. Never leave a child, even one who can swim, alone near the water.
- Never swim alone.
- Don't drink alcohol and swim.

WHAT TO EXPECT

DIAGNOSTIC MEASURES
- Your own observation of symptoms.
- Medical history and physical exam by a doctor.
- Laboratory blood tests.

SURGERY—Not necessary nor useful for this disorder.

NORMAL COURSE OF ILLNESS—Depends on the length of time under water. With early rescue and treatment, full recovery is possible. Special body mechanisms may permit full recovery from near-drowning in icy water.

POSSIBLE COMPLICATIONS
- Pulmonary edema (body fluid in the lungs) followed by acute respiratory failure.
- Permanent brain damage.
- Lung infection.
- Heart irregularities, including cardiac arrest and death.

HOW TO TREAT

NOTE—Follow your doctor's instructions. These instructions are supplemental.

FIRST AID
- If the victim is unconscious and not breathing, yell for help. Don't leave the victim.
- Begin mouth-to-mouth breathing immediately.
- If there is no heartbeat, give external cardiac massage.
- Have someone call 0 (operator) or 911 (emergency) for an ambulance or medical help.
- Don't stop CPR until help arrives.
- The near-drowning victim should be taken to the nearest hospital for intensive care—even if the victim has regained consciousness. Complications or death due to heart-rhythm disturbances may occur 24 to 48 hours after the accident.
- Remain with a recovering patient to provide support and reassurance. Near-drowning is a traumatic experience.

MEDICAL TREATMENT
- Immediate cardiopulmonary resuscitation (CPR).
- Hospitalization (sometimes) to lower body temperature, to induce coma with medicines and to monitor spinal-fluid pressure.
- Hospitalization for observation for delayed, serious reactions.

HOME TREATMENT—None appropriate.

MEDICATION—Your doctor may prescribe:
- Oxygen.
- Cortisone drugs to prevent or treat lung inflammation.
- Antibiotics to prevent lung infection.
- Bronchodilators to enable oxygen to enter the lungs.

ACTIVITY—Complete bed rest is necessary until activity is permitted by the doctor.

DIET—Intravenous nutrients, if the victim is unconscious upon hospitalization. After recovery, no special diet is necessary.

CALL YOUR DOCTOR IF

- Someone appears to have drowned. Call for emergency help immediately!
- Signs of infection (fever, cough, muscle aches and fatigue) appear after apparent recovery.

EAR INFECTION, OUTER- (Swimmer's Ear; Otitis Externa)

GENERAL INFORMATION

DEFINITION—Inflammation or infection of the ear canal that extends from the eardrum to the exterior of the ear. This is a particularly common problem in athletes when the ear canal remains moist due to perspiration running into the ear. It is also very likely to be a problem in swimmers, divers and water-polo players.

SIGNS & SYMPTOMS
- Ear pain that worsens when the earlobe is pulled.
- Slight fever (sometimes).
- Discharge of thick white matter or pus from the ear.
- Temporary loss of hearing on the affected side.

CAUSES & RISK FACTORS
- Bacterial or fungal infection of the delicate skin lining of the ear canal.
- Excess moisture from any cause.
- Swimming in dirty, polluted water.
- Frequent swimming in hot or warm chlorinated pools. Chlorinated water dries out the ear canal, allowing bacteria or fungi to enter the skin.
- Irritation from swabs, metal objects, such as bobby pins, or ear plugs, especially if they are left in a long time.
- Previous external-ear infections.
- Skin allergies.
- Diabetes mellitus or other disorders that predispose one to infection.

HOW TO PREVENT
- Don't clean your ears with any object or chemical. A small amount of ear wax helps protect against infection.
- Don't use ear plugs, alcohol in the ears, lamb's wool or anything else to keep ears dry. These are not only useless—they may trap moisture or cause irritation.

WHAT TO EXPECT

DIAGNOSTIC MEASURES
- Your own observation of symptoms.
- Medical history and physical exam by a doctor.

SURGERY—Not necessary nor useful for this illness.

NORMAL COURSE OF ILLNESS—Usually curable with treatment in 7 to 10 days.

POSSIBLE COMPLICATIONS
- Severe pain.
- Chronic inflammation that is difficult to cure.
- A boil in the ear canal caused by secondary bacterial infection.
- Cellulitis (deep-tissue infection).

HOW TO TREAT

NOTE—Follow your doctor's instructions. These instructions are supplemental.

MEDICAL TREATMENT
- Your doctor will probably cleanse the ear canal and insert a cotton wick. The wick allows medication to reach all infected parts.
- Severe cases may require treatment by an ear, nose and throat specialist.

HOME TREATMENT
- If your doctor has inserted a wick, moisten the wick with medication every hour for the first 24 hours. Continue to use drops according to your doctor's instructions after the wick is removed. Clean the tip of the dropper with alcohol after each use. Don't let other persons use the medicine.
- After you have had otitis externa, keep the prescription ear drops on hand. If the ear canals get wet for any reason, such as swimming, showering or shampooing, put drops in both ears at bedtime.

MEDICATION
- You may use non-prescription drugs, such as acetaminophen or aspirin, for minor pain.
- Your doctor may prescribe:
  Ear drops that contain antibiotics and cortisone drugs to control inflammation and fight infection.
  Oral antibiotics for severe secondary bacterial infection.
  Codeine or narcotics for a short time to relieve severe pain.

ACTIVITY—Resume your normal activities as soon as symptoms improve. Avoid getting water in the ears for 3 weeks after all symptoms disappear. Any moisture—even from showering or washing hair—can trigger a recurrence.

DIET—No special diet.

CALL YOUR DOCTOR IF

- You have symptoms of otitis externa.
- Pain persists despite treatment.
- You feel your ears need cleaning.

EPILEPSY

GENERAL INFORMATION

DEFINITION—A disorder of brain function characterized by sudden seizures, brief attacks of inappropriate behavior, change in consciousness or bizarre movements. Seizures—also called "fits" or convulsions—are a symptom, not a disease. Seizures have never been proven to be triggered by athletic activity, but those who have seizures may have to modify athletic participation.

SIGNS & SYMPTOMS—There are several forms of epilepsy (listed below), each with its own characteristics:
- *Petit mal epilepsy* mostly affects children. The person stops activity and stares blankly around for a minute or so—unaware of what is happening.
- *Grand mal epilepsy* affects all ages. The person loses consciousness, stiffens, then twitches and jerks uncontrollably. He or she may lose bladder control. The seizure lasts several minutes, and is often followed by deep sleep or mental confusion. Prior to the seizure, the person may have warning signals: a tense feeling; visual disturbances; smelling a bad odor; or hearing strange noises.
- *Focal epilepsy,* in which a small part of the body begins twitching uncontrollably. The twitching spreads until it may involve the whole body. The person does not lose consciousness.
- *Temporal-lobe epilepsy,* in which the person suddenly behaves out of character or inappropriately, such as becoming suddenly violent or angry; laughing for no reason; or making agitated or bizarre body movements, including odd chewing movements.

CAUSES & RISK FACTORS—Seizures result from abnormal, excessive signals produced by the brain's nerve cells. It is caused by any of more than 50 brain disorders, but the organic cause can be determined in only 25% of cases. Common causes include:
- Brain damage at birth.
- Drug or alcohol abuse.
- Severe head injury.
- Brain infection.
- Brain tumor or expanding lesion that compresses the brain (occasionally).
- Family history of seizure disorders.
- Exposure to toxic fumes.
- Low blood sugar.

HOW TO PREVENT—No specific preventive measures.

WHAT TO EXPECT

DIAGNOSTIC MEASURES
- Medical history and exam by a doctor.
- Laboratory blood studies.
- EEG, PET and MRI (see Glossary for all).
- X-rays of the head.
- CAT scan (see Glossary).

SURGERY—If a tumor, scar or abscess is causing epilepsy, surgery with microsurgical techniques may cure or improve it.

NORMAL COURSE OF ILLNESS—Epilepsy is incurable, except in cases where it is caused by treatable brain damage, tumors or infection. However, anticonvulsant drugs can prevent most seizures and allow a near-normal life. Continuing physical activity is recommended.

POSSIBLE COMPLICATIONS—Continuing seizures despite treatment and mental deterioration (rare).

HOW TO TREAT

NOTE—Follow your doctor's instructions. These instructions are supplemental.

MEDICAL TREATMENT—After diagnosis and possible surgery (rare), psychotherapy or counseling may help the patient and family learn to understand and live with the disorder.

HOME TREATMENT
- Request and carry a Medic-Alert bracelet or pendant that shows you have epilepsy.
- Avoid any circumstance that has triggered a seizure previously.
- See Convulsions, page 326, for additional instructions.

MEDICATION—Your doctor will prescribe one or more anticonvulsant drugs. Your response to treatment will be monitored by checking blood and urine frequently. Medication changes or adjustments are often necessary. Learn as much as you can about your medications.

ACTIVITY—No restrictions (if seizures are under control), but scuba diving and mountain climbing should be avoided by people with epilepsy. Most states allow persons with epilepsy to drive a vehicle after being seizure-free for 1 year.

DIET—No special diet. Don't drink alcohol or take mind-altering drugs. They may decrease the effectiveness of your medication and provoke seizures.

CALL YOUR DOCTOR IF

- You have a seizure seemingly related to exercise.
- New, unexplained symptoms develop during treatment for epilepsy. Drugs used in treatment may produce side effects.

EYE, FOREIGN BODY IN

 GENERAL INFORMATION

DEFINITION—Imbedding of a small speck of lime, stone, sand, paint or other foreign material in the eye. This is particularly likely to occur in athletes who cycle, box, wrestle, or play football, soccer or any other field event.

SIGNS & SYMPTOMS
- Severe pain, irritation and redness in the eye.
- Foreign body visible with the naked eye (usually). Sometimes the foreign body is small, trapped under the eyelid and invisible except with medical examination.

CAUSES & RISK FACTORS
- Windy weather.
- Sports activity in which the eye may come into contact with any foreign material.

HOW TO PREVENT—Wear protective eye coverings if possible.

 WHAT TO EXPECT

DIAGNOSTIC MEASURES
- Your own observation of symptoms.
- Medical history and physical exam by a doctor. This may include staining the eye with a harmless dye (flourescein) to outline the object and examine the eye through a magnifying lens.

SURGERY—Necessary only for deeply imbedded particles.

NORMAL COURSE OF ILLNESS—Most objects can be removed simply under local anesthesia in a doctor's office or emergency room.

POSSIBLE COMPLICATIONS
- Infection, especially if the foreign body is not removed completely.
- Severe, permanent vision damage caused by penetration of deeper eye layers.

 HOW TO TREAT

NOTE—Follow your doctor's instructions. These instructions are supplemental.

MEDICAL TREATMENT—Doctor's or emergency-room care to remove the particle (sometimes).

HOME TREATMENT
- Ask someone else to drive you to the doctor's office. Don't try to drive.
- Don't rub the eye.
- Keep both eyes closed, if possible, until you are examined.
- To protect your eye from bright light, wear an eye patch or dark glasses for 24 hours after treatment.
- Use moist compresses to relieve discomfort after removal. Prepare by folding a clean cloth in several layers. Dip in warm water, wring out slightly and apply to the eye. Dip the compress often to keep it moist. Apply the compress for 1 hour, rest 1 hour and repeat.

MEDICATION—Your doctor may prescribe:
- Antibiotic eyedrops or ointment to prevent infection or to dilate the pupil.
- Pain relievers.
- Local anesthetic eyedrops.

ACTIVITY—Resume your normal activities gradually after removal of the foreign body and the patch, if one is applied.

DIET—No special diet.

 CALL YOUR DOCTOR IF

- You have a foreign body in the eye.
- The following occurs after removal:
  Pain increases or does not disappear in 2 days.
  You develop a fever.
  Your vision changes.

EYE, SUBCONJUNCTIVAL HEMORRHAGE

GENERAL INFORMATION

DEFINITION—Sudden appearance of blood in the white area of the eye (conjunctiva). Although the bleeding may appear frightening, it is not painful or serious.

SIGNS & SYMPTOMS—A small, painless collection of bright red blood over the white of the eye. Swelling may occur in the affected area of the conjunctiva. The condition doesn't interfere with vision.

CAUSES & RISK FACTORS
● Sometimes caused by injury to the eye, but usually is spontaneous bleeding with no known cause. It may follow coughing, sneezing or vomiting. Risk increases with:
● Use of mind-altering drugs.
● Use of anticoagulant drugs.

HOW TO PREVENT—Use appropriate equipment to protect the head and face from injury.

WHAT TO EXPECT

DIAGNOSTIC MEASURE
● Your own observation of symptoms.
● Medical history and physical exam by a doctor (sometimes).

SURGERY—Not necessary nor useful for this disorder.

NORMAL COURSE OF ILLNESS—The blood should be absorbed in 2 or 3 weeks. The blood changes color gradually to brown or green before disappearing.

POSSIBLE COMPLICATIONS—None expected.

HOW TO TREAT

NOTE—Follow your doctor's instructions. These instructions are supplemental.

MEDICAL TREATMENT—Consult a doctor if there has been injury to the eye or a change in vision.

HOME TREATMENT
● Use cold compresses for several days to prevent additional bleeding. Fold a clean cloth in several layers, dip it in cold water and wring it out a little. Apply it to the eye for 10 minutes every hour.
● Use warm compresses when signs of bleeding have stopped for 2 days. This will hasten blood absorption. Apply to the eye for 10 to 30 minutes 3 times a day.

MEDICATION—Medicine is usually not necessary for this disorder.

ACTIVITY—No restrictions.

DIET—No special diet.

CALL YOUR DOCTOR IF

You have symptoms of subconjunctival hemorrhage, especially if you have eye pain or your vision changes.

FAINTING
(Syncope)

GENERAL INFORMATION

DEFINITION—Sudden, temporary loss of consciousness. This is most likely to occur in an athlete involved in prolonged physical exertion in warm weather. It usually occurs *after* exercising.

SIGNS & SYMPTOMS
- Skin that is pale, cold and sweaty.
- Sudden lightheadedness.
- Blurred vision (sometimes).
- Nausea (sometimes).
- General weakness, then unconsciousness.
- Rapid heartbeat (100 to 120 beats per minute) and rapid breathing. If heartbeat or breathing is not present, this may be cardiac arrest rather than fainting.

CAUSES & RISK FACTORS—A sudden decrease in blood pressure, which temporarily deprives the brain of blood. The drop in blood pressure may result from:
- Pooled blood in the extremities caused by a long run.
- Prolonged straining, such as from lifting heavy weights, coughing forcefully or attempting bowel movements when constipated.
- Sudden emotional stress.
- Standing after squatting (orthostatic hypotension). This is quite likely in weight-lifting when also holding breath ("weight-lifter's blackout.")
- Hot, humid weather.
- Low blood sugar.
- Heartbeat abnormalities—too fast, too slow or irregular.
- Heart diseases that limit the amount of blood the heart pumps.
- Heart attack (rare).
- Anemia (rare).
- Use of certain drugs, such as heart medications that slow the heartbeat. These include digitalis, beta-adrenergic blockers and other antihypertensive drugs.

HOW TO PREVENT
- Avoid any of the causes or risk factors listed above if possible.
- Avoid sudden changes in physical activity.
- If fainting episodes are caused by medication, consult your doctor about changing drugs.

WHAT TO EXPECT

DIAGNOSTIC MEASURES
- Observation of symptoms by those nearby.
- Medical history and physical exam by a doctor.

SURGERY—Not necessary nor useful for this disorder.

NORMAL COURSE OF ILLNESS—Simple fainting disappears in 1 to 3 minutes. It may seem longer to bystanders.

POSSIBLE COMPLICATIONS
- Injury while fainting.
- Mistaking cardiac arrest for fainting.

HOW TO TREAT

NOTE—Follow your doctor's instructions. These instructions are supplemental.

FIRST AID—If someone faints, check for breathing and a neck pulse. If neither is present, this represents a cardiac arrest. Treat as an emergency:
- Dial 0 (operator) or 911 (emergency) for an ambulance or medical help. Then give first aid immediately.
- Begin cardiac massage and mouth-to-mouth breathing (CPR). Don't stop until help arrives. If someone faints, is breathing and has a pulse, leave the person on the ground and elevate both legs. This helps return blood to the heart.

MEDICAL TREATMENT—Doctor's treatment, if fainting is caused by an underlying disorder (see Causes).

HOME TREATMENT
- If you feel faint, sit down immediately and bend over, or lie down.
- If you are subject to frequent fainting spells, avoid activities in which fainting may endanger your life, such as climbing to high places, driving vehicles or operating dangerous machinery.

MEDICATION—Medication usually is not necessary for fainting. Medication may be necessary for underlying disorders.

ACTIVITY—Resume your normal activities as soon as you regain consciousness.

DIET—No special diet unless fainting episodes are caused by low blood sugar. If so, eat 5 or 6 small meals a day. The meals should be high in protein, high in complex carbohydrates and low in simple carbohydrates (sugar).

CALL YOUR DOCTOR IF

- An unconscious person has no pulse and is not breathing. Give CPR first.
- Someone faints and is breathing, but does not regain consciousness in 2 minutes.

FROSTBITE
(Cold injury)

 GENERAL INFORMATION

DEFINITION—Temporary or permanent tissue damage from exposure to subfreezing temperature. Ice crystals form in the skin and blood vessels, leading to tissue injury or tissue death, depending on the temperature and length of exposure.

SIGNS & SYMPTOMS
During exposure:
● Gradual numbness, hardness and paleness in the affected area.
After rewarming the skin:
● Pain and tingling or burning (sometimes severe) in the affected area, with color change from white to red, then purple.
● Blisters (severe cases).
● Shivering.

CAUSES & RISK FACTORS—The following factors make frostbite more likely:
● Constriction of blood vessels in the extremities by too-tight clothing.
● Wet skin.
● Blood-vessel disease such as Raynaud's phenomenon (a circulatory-system disorder affecting fingers and toes).
● Smoking.
● Excess alcohol consumption.
● Windy weather, which increases chilling.
● Any chronic disease.

HOW TO PREVENT
● Anticipate sudden temperature changes. Carry a jacket, gloves, socks, hat, knit face mask and scarf.
● Don't drink alcohol or smoke prior to anticipated exposure.

 WHAT TO EXPECT

DIAGNOSTIC MEASURES
● Your own observation of symptoms.
● Medical history and physical exam by a doctor.
● X-rays of damaged areas.

SURGERY—Sometimes necessary to remove permanently damaged (gangrenous) tissue.

NORMAL COURSE OF ILLNESS—For mild cases, full recovery is possible with treatment. Severe cases usually require amputation of the affected part.

POSSIBLE COMPLICATIONS
● Temporarily slurred speech and memory loss after rewarming the skin.

● Death or severe infection, requiring amputation of affected tissue. This is most likely in fingers, toes, nose or ears following severe exposure.
● Cardiac arrest, if frostbite is accompanied by total body hypothermia.

 HOW TO TREAT

NOTE—Follow your doctor's instructions. These instructions are supplemental.

MEDICAL TREATMENT
● Doctor's care for all but the mildest cases.
● Hospitalization (sometimes).

FIRST AID—The following instructions apply to emergency care until medical care is available:
● Upon reaching shelter, remove clothing from the frostbitten parts.
● Never massage damaged tissue.
● Immerse the affected parts in warm water (about l00F or 37.8C). Use a thermometer, if available. Higher temperature may cause further injury.
● Drink warm fluids with a high sugar content, if available.
● Don't smoke.
● After rewarming, cover the affected areas with soft cloth bandages.
● Don't use affected limbs until you have medical attention. If feet are involved, don't walk.

HOME TREATMENT—Appropriate for mildest cases only.

MEDICATION
● Your doctor may prescribe:
  Analgesics, including narcotics, to relieve severe pain. Don't use strong pain killers longer than 4 to 7 days.
  Antibiotics to fight infection.
● You may use non-prescription drugs, such as acetaminophen, for minor pain.

ACTIVITY—Resume normal activities after treatment.

DIET—No special diet.

 CALL YOUR DOCTOR IF

● You have symptoms of frostbite or observe them in someone else.
● The following occurs during treatment:
  Increased pain, swelling, redness or drainage at the site of injury.
  Fever, muscle aches, dizziness or a general ill feeling.
  New, unexplained symptoms. Drugs used in treatment may produce side effects.

HEAD INJURY

 GENERAL INFORMATION

DEFINITION—Injury to the head, with or without unconsciousness or other visible signs.

SIGNS & SYMPTOMS—Depends on the extent of injury. The presence or absence of swelling at the injury site is not related to the seriousness of injury. Signs and symptoms include any or all of the following:
- Drowsiness or confusion.
- Vomiting and nausea.
- Blurred vision.
- Pupils of different size.
- Loss of consciousness—either temporarily or for long periods.
- Amnesia or memory lapses.
- Irritability.
- Headache.
- Bleeding of the scalp if the skin is broken.

CAUSES & RISK FACTORS—In sports, head injury is most common in contact or collision sports, especially football, ice hockey, boxing and wrestling. It is more likely in persons with seizure disorders.

HOW TO PREVENT—Wear protective headgear for contact sports and cycling.

 WHAT TO EXPECT

DIAGNOSTIC MEASURES
- Your own observation of symptoms.
- Medical history and physical exam by a doctor.
- Laboratory studies of blood and cerebrospinal fluid.
- X-rays of the skull and neck.
- CAT scan (see Glossary) of the head.

SURGERY—May be life-saving if diagnostic measures detect a severe injury.

NORMAL COURSE OF ILLNESS—Usually heals without complications with early recognition of danger signs and prompt medical treatment. Complications can be life-threatening or cause permanent disability.

POSSIBLE COMPLICATIONS
- Bleeding under the skull (subdural hemorrhage and hematoma).
- Bleeding into the brain.

 HOW TO TREAT

NOTE—Follow your doctor's instructions. These instructions are supplemental.

MEDICAL TREATMENT
- Careful examination by a doctor to determine the extent of injury.
- Hospitalization for observation if signs and symptoms are severe.

HOME TREATMENT—After a doctor's examination, the injured person may be sent home—but a responsible person must stay with the person and watch for serious symptoms. The first 24 hours after injury are critical, although serious aftereffects can appear later. If you are watching the patient, awaken him or her every hour for 24 hours. Report to the doctor immediately if you can't awaken or arouse the injured person. Report also any of the following:
- Vomiting.
- Inability to move arms and legs equally well on both sides.
- Temperature above 100F (37.8C).
- Stiff neck.
- Pupils of unequal size or shape.
- Convulsions.
- Noticeable restlessness.
- Severe headache that persists longer than 4 hours after injury.
- Confusion.

MEDICATION—Don't give any medicine—including non-prescription acetaminophen or aspirin—until the diagnosis is certain.

ACTIVITY—The patient should rest in bed until the doctor determines the danger of complications is over. Normal activity may then be resumed as symptoms improve.

DIET—Full liquid diet until the danger passes.

 CALL YOUR DOCTOR IF

You have symptoms of a head injury or observe signs of a head injury in someone else.

HEAT ILLNESS
(Heatstroke; Heat Exhaustion; Heat Cramps)

 GENERAL INFORMATION

DEFINITION—Illness caused by prolonged exposure to hot temperatures, high humidity, slow air movement and increased physical activity. Long runs are responsible for most heat illness in athletes. *Heatstroke* represents failure of the body's heat-regulating mechanisms, leading to a heat buildup in the body. *Heat exhaustion* represents a loss of body fluids.

SIGNS & SYMPTOMS
Heatstroke:
● Sudden dizziness, weakness, faintness and headache.
● Skin that is hot and dry.
● No sweating.
● High body temperature—frequently 102F (38.9C) or higher.
● Rapid heartbeat.
● Muscle cramps.
Heat exhaustion:
● Skin that is cool and moist.
● Pale or gray skin color.
● Slow pulse.
● Confusion.
● Muscle cramps.
● Low or normal body temperature.
● Dark yellow or orange urine.

CAUSES & RISK FACTORS
● Excessive sweating.
● Failure to drink enough fluid.
● Recent illness involving fluid loss from vomiting or diarrhea.
● Hot, humid weather.
● Working or exercise in a hot environment.

HOW TO PREVENT
● Wear light, loose-fitting clothing in hot weather.
● Drink extra iced water throughout practice or competition, if you sweat heavily.
● Be adequately trained and fit before a long race.
● Splash water on the body during a race or heavy exercise.
● Don't take salt tablets.
● Pay attention to early symptoms of heat illness. Reduce exercise until symptoms disappear.

 WHAT TO EXPECT

DIAGNOSTIC MEASURES
● Your own observation of symptoms.
● Medical history and physical exam by a doctor.

● Laboratory studies of blood and urine to measure electrolyte levels.

SURGERY—Not necessary nor useful for this disorder.

NORMAL COURSE OF ILLNESS—Prompt treatment usually brings full recovery in 1 to 2 days.

POSSIBLE COMPLICATIONS
● Shock.
● Brain damage caused by prolonged, high body temperature (106F or 41.1C).

 HOW TO TREAT

NOTE—Follow your doctor's instructions. These instructions are supplemental.

MEDICAL TREATMENT
● For heatstroke: Hospitalization to lower body temperature and provide intravenous replacement fluids.
● For heat exhaustion: Call your doctor for advice.

FIRST AID
● If someone with symptoms is very hot and not sweating:
　Cool the person rapidly. Use a cold-water bath or wrap in wet sheets. Arrange for transportation to the nearest hospital. This is an emergency!
● If someone is faint but sweating:
　Give the person cold or ice liquids (water, soft drinks or fruit juice). Don't give salt pills. Arrange for transportation to the hospital, except in mild cases. Call your doctor for advice.

HOME TREATMENT—Not appropriate except for mildest cases of heat exhaustion.

MEDICATION—Medicine usually is not necessary for this disorder.

ACTIVITY—Activity may be resumed slowly when symptoms disappear.

DIET—Drink extra fluids and eat foods high in potassium (orange juice, bananas) or take potassium supplements.

 CALL YOUR DOCTOR IF

You have symptoms of heatstroke or heat exhaustion, or observe them in someone else. Call immediately! These conditions may be serious or fatal.

HEEL PAIN
(Heel Spur; Calcaneal Bursitis or Neuritis)

 GENERAL INFORMATION

DEFINITION—Heel pain or discomfort of the following types:
- Contusion or bone bruise—Inflammation of the tissue that covers bone (periosteum).
- Heel spur—A hard bony shelf as wide as the width of the heelbone caused by repeated pulling away of periosteum from the heelbone (calcaneus). The repeated stress or injury causes inflammation and calcification of tendons and ligaments in the foot.
- Plantar fasciitis—Inflammation of the fibrous band that originates at the bottom of the calcaneus. This hurts worse when running faster or when weight is on the ball of the foot.
- Heel bursitis—Formation in the heel area of an irritated or inflamed protective sac of fluid due to irritation caused by a heel spur.

SIGNS & SYMPTOMS
- Deep discomfort under the heel while walking, running or at rest.
- Redness.
- Tenderness.
- Increased heat.

CAUSES & RISK FACTORS
- Running, jogging or fast walking.
- Previous serious foot, ankle or heel injury.
- Repeated heel injury from any cause.
- Prolonged standing.
- Obesity.

HOW TO PREVENT
- Avoid activities that cause constant foot strain.
- Wear athletic shoes with good shock absorption in the heel, good flexibility and good support to control side-to-side motion.
- Don't wear everyday shoes with more than 1-1/2-inch heels.

 WHAT TO EXPECT

DIAGNOSTIC MEASURES
- Your own observation of symptoms.
- Medical history and exam by a doctor.
- X-rays of the heel.

SURGERY—Occasionally necessary to remove a heel spur, if home treatment does not cure it.

NORMAL COURSE OF ILLNESS—Usually curable with conservative treatment (see How to Treat).

POSSIBLE COMPLICATIONS—Inflammation and arthritic changes in the heel that place abnormal stress on previously pain-free joints, such as those in the knee, hip and spine.

 HOW TO TREAT

NOTE—Follow your doctor's instructions. These instructions are supplemental.

MEDICAL TREATMENT—Usually not necessary.

HOME TREATMENT
- Use ice massage. Fill a large styrofoam cup with water and freeze. Tear a small amount of foam from the top so ice protrudes. Massage firmly over the heel in a circle. Do this for 15 minutes at a time, 3 or 4 times a day.
- Elevate the foot above the level of the heart to reduce swelling and prevent accumulation of fluid. Use pillows for propping, or elevate the foot of the bed.
- Use doughnutlike or horseshoelike padding in shoes, such as cushion pads, homemade felt inlays, sponge-rubber heel pads or shaped pieces of indoor/outdoor carpeting. Put in both shoes, even if only one heel hurts. Otherwise, normal mechanics of standing and moving will be altered and may cause pain in other areas.
- Try a plastic or rubber heel cup (available at sporting-goods stores and drug stores).
- Don't walk on toes while treating heel pain.
- Do this stretch exercise:
  Sit on the floor with legs straight.
  Grasp the toes with your hands.
  Pull toes slowly toward you for 30 seconds.
  Repeat several times for 5 to 10 minutes.
- When returning to athletics or exercise, use ice massage for 10 minutes before warmup and after exercise.

MEDICATION—To relieve minor pain, you may use non-prescription drugs, such as ibuprofen, acetaminophen or aspirin.

ACTIVITY—Stay off your feet as much as possible, especially at beginning of treatment.

DIET—No special diet, unless you are overweight. If so, lose weight to reduce stress on the foot.

 CALL YOUR DOCTOR IF

- You have persistent heel pain, despite treatment.
- Any of the following occur after surgery:
  Pain, swelling, redness, drainage or bleeding increases in surgical area.
  You develop signs of infection (headache, muscle aches, dizziness, or a general ill feeling and fever).
  New, unexplained symptoms develop. Drugs used in treatment may produce side effects.

HEADACHE, MIGRAINE RELATED TO EXERTION (Effort Migraine)

GENERAL INFORMATION

DEFINITION—An intense, incapacitating headache, accompanied by other symptoms, that occurs after all-out physical effort in various sports, such as running, football, basketball, boxing, wrestling or soccer. Migraines related to exertion are most common in persons with a family history of migraines.

SIGNS & SYMPTOMS—The nature of attacks varies between persons and from time to time in the same person. Symptoms of a classic migraine attack appear in the following sequence:
● Inability to see clearly, followed by seeing bright spots and zigzag patterns. Visual disturbances may last several minutes or several hours, but they disappear once the headache begins.
● Dull, boring pain in the temple that spreads to the entire side of the head. Pain becomes intense and throbbing. Sometimes the pain may affect both temples simultaneously.
● Nausea and vomiting.
In other types of migraine attack, the above symptoms (vision disturbances, headache or vomiting) may be absent, or other symptoms may be present. Some persons become pale, with bloodshot eyes and a runny nose or eyes.

CAUSES & RISK FACTORS—Constriction, then dilation and inflammation of blood vessels that go to the scalp and brain. Vision disturbances occur when blood vessels narrow. Headache begins when they widen again. Attacks may be triggered by:
● All-out physical activity, particularly in competitive sports.
● Tension and stress.
● Use of oral contraceptives.
● Use of many prescription and non-prescription drugs.
● Excess alcohol consumption.
● Consumption of certain foods.
● Fatigue.
● Smoking.

HOW TO PREVENT
● Taking one aspirin a day *may* prevent migraine attacks in some adults. You may try it if you have no reasons to avoid aspirin.
● Use of the drug propranolol prevents attacks in some persons, but may decrease successful athletic performance. It can cause unpleasant side effects, including depression and impotence.

WHAT TO EXPECT

DIAGNOSTIC MEASURES
● Your own observation of symptoms.
● Medical history and exam by a doctor.
● Laboratory blood studies.
● CAT scan (see Glossary) of the head.

SURGERY—Not necessary nor useful for this disorder.

NORMAL COURSE OF ILLNESS—Symptoms can usually be controlled with medication, but medication may significantly diminish athletic performance.

POSSIBLE COMPLICATIONS—None expected.

HOW TO TREAT

NOTE—Follow your doctor's instructions. These instructions are supplemental.

MEDICAL TREATMENT—Doctor's examination and medication for persistent migraines.

HOME TREATMENT—At the first sign of a migraine attack:
● Apply a cold cloth or ice pack to your head, or splash your face with cold water.
● Take pain relievers, such as aspirin or acetaminophen.
● Lie down in a quiet, dark room for several hours. Relax if possible. Listen to music, sleep or meditate—but don't read.

MEDICATION—Your doctor may prescribe:
● Antihistamines to expand blood vessels.
● Antiemetics to decrease nausea and vomiting.
● Vasoconstrictors to narrow blood vessels.
● Pain relievers.
● Beta-adrenergic blockers to prevent attacks, if headaches are so frequent or severe that you can't function normally. This medication may have undesirable side effects and it does not help everyone.

ACTIVITY—Rest during attacks. Otherwise, exercise regularly to achieve maximum fitness.

DIET—Because some attacks are triggered by foods, such as cheese or chocolate, keep a record of what you ate before each attack. Avoid foods that seem to trigger migraine attacks. Otherwise, no special diet is necessary.

CALL YOUR DOCTOR IF

● You have a migraine attack that persists longer than 24 hours, despite treatment.
● Recurrent migraine attacks interfere with normal life.

HEADACHE, TENSION OR VASCULAR

GENERAL INFORMATION

DEFINITION—Simple tension or vascular headaches are of 3 types:
- Pain from muscle strain in the scalp, neck and face.
- Pain from constricted blood vessels in the head that cause pressure on blood-vessel walls.
- Pain from dilated blood vessels in the brain.

Tension headaches frequently occur in athletes anticipating an important athletic event. Until the headache subsides, it can greatly impair athletic performance.

SIGNS & SYMPTOMS—Any of the following:
- Moderate pain in the front or back of the head, accompanied by tight muscles in the neck or scalp.
- Constant pain over the temples, accompanied by the feeling that a vise is over the back of the head.
- Throbbing pain all over the head.

CAUSES & RISK FACTORS
- Severe overexertion.
- Tension, producing strain on muscles of the neck, scalp, face and jaw.
- Sleep disturbances.
- Excessive eating, drinking or smoking.
- Anxiety or depression.
- Sun glare.
- Use of drugs or alcohol.
- Low blood sugar.
- Hormone changes during the menstrual cycle.
- Allergic reactions.
- Stress, either mental or physical.
- Environments that are noisy, stuffy, hot, poorly lit, or have irritating odors.
- Exposure to or consumption of nitrites, sulfites, monosodium glutamate or other food additives.

HOW TO PREVENT
- Get enough sleep—an average of 8 hours for men and 7 hours for women.
- Don't skip meals, especially breakfast.
- Don't overeat.
- Exercise regularly to reduce tension and improve circulation. But don't exercise to the point of headache.
- Don't smoke cigarettes, and avoid smoky environments.
- Don't use mood-altering, mind-altering, stimulant or sedative drugs.
- Avoid foods that contain nitrites or other additives to which you are sensitive.

WHAT TO EXPECT

DIAGNOSTIC MEASURES
- Your own observation of symptoms.
- Medical history and exam by a doctor.
- Laboratory studies, such as a CAT scan (see Glossary) for unrelenting pain.

NORMAL COURSE OF ILLNESS—Most tension or vascular headaches can be relieved with simple treatment (see How to Treat).

POSSIBLE COMPLICATIONS—None expected for a simple headache.

HOW TO TREAT

NOTE—Follow your doctor's instructions. These instructions are supplemental.

MEDICAL TREATMENT
- Doctor's treatment, if headache persists or worsens despite self-care.
- Biofeedback training, behavior-modification training or counseling.

HOME TREATMENT
- If possible, stop what you are doing and try to relax.
- Massage shoulders, neck, jaw and scalp.
- Take a hot bath or shower, and allow water to massage tense muscles.
- Lie down. Place a warm or cold cloth, whichever feels better, over the aching area.

MEDICATION—You may take acetaminophen or aspirin to relieve pain.

ACTIVITY—Rest in a quiet room until headache subsides.

DIET
- Most persons feel better if they don't eat until the headache subsides unless the headache is from low blood sugar.
- Don't drink alcohol.
- Avoid food additives to which you are sensitive.

CALL YOUR DOCTOR IF

You have a headache accompanied by any of the following:
- Fever of 101F (38.3C) or higher.
- Recent head injury.
- Drowsiness.
- Nausea and vomiting.
- Pain in one eye.
- Blurred vision.
- High blood pressure.
- Pain and tenderness around the eyes and cheekbones that worsens when you lean forward. This may indicate a sinus infection.
- Vision disturbances and vomiting prior to the headache.
- Persistent headache pain for longer than 24 hours without other symptoms.
- You suspect a prescription, non-prescription or illegal drug of abuse caused the headache.

HEMATURIA

 GENERAL INFORMATION

DEFINITION—Blood in the urine. This may or may not be visible with the naked eye. It is a common occurrence in people who exercise strenuously. Hematuria following vigorous physical exercise does not necessarily represent any disease of the kidney or other parts of the urinary tract.

SIGNS & SYMPTOMS
- Bloody urine with many red blood cells present (gross hematuria).
- "Smoky" colored urine. Red blood cells are visible in large quantities when urine is examined under the microscope (microscopic hematuria). Clear urine may also contain some red blood cells that are visible under the microscope.

Additional symptoms in athletes that indicate the need for laboratory studies of the kidneys:
- Discomfort, frequency or urgency in urinating (may represent infection).
- Colicky pain in either flank (area on the side of the abdomen under the last rib).
- Hematuria lasting longer than 48 hours after exercise.
- Decreased urine output for 12 hours after prolonged, strenuous exercise.

CAUSES & RISK FACTORS
- Prolonged exercise, such as a running a marathon, with no underlying disease (benign hematuria).
- Kidney disease.
- Kidney, ureter, bladder or urethral injury.
- Stone in the ureter, kidney or bladder.
- Infection.
- Tumor of the urinary tract.

HOW TO PREVENT
- Obtain treatment for any illness of the kidney or urinary tract.
- Don't get dehydrated. Drink lots of water—a minimum of 8 glasses per day—and much more during hot weather and prolonged exercise.
- Include urine studies in your routine checkups every 2 to 3 months during periods of vigorous activity.

 WHAT TO EXPECT

DIAGNOSTIC MEASURES
- Your own observation of symptoms.
- Medical history and physical exam by a doctor.
- Laboratory studies such as: urinalysis; urine culture; blood studies; intravenous pyelogram (special kidney X-rays); cystoscopy; angiography; or sonogram (see Glossary for these).

SURGERY—Necessary only if the underlying disorder requires surgery.

NORMAL COURSE OF ILLNESS—If there is no underlying disease of the urinary tract, benign hematuria usually clears spontaneously within 24 to 48 hours.

POSSIBLE COMPLICATIONS—Anemia due to blood loss.

 HOW TO TREAT

NOTE—Follow your doctor's instructions. These instructions are supplemental.

MEDICAL TREATMENT—Doctor's treatment for diagnosis and treatment if an underlying urinary-tract disorder is present.

HOME TREATMENT—Drink extra water, particularly during hot weather and prolonged, strenuous exercise.

MEDICATION—Medicine usually is not necessary unless blood in the urine is caused by illness. If so, your doctor may prescribe antibiotics for infection or medicine appropriate for other forms of kidney disease.

ACTIVITY—No restrictions.

DIET—No special diet.

 CALL YOUR DOCTOR IF

You have signs or symptoms of hematuria.

HEMOPHILIA

GENERAL INFORMATION

DEFINITION—An inherited deficiency of a blood-clotting factor that results in serious and sometimes dangerous bleeding, particularly following injuries. Hemophilia affects 1 in 10,000 males (no females) and appears early in childhood.

SIGNS & SYMPTOMS
● Painful, swollen joints or swelling in the leg or arm (especially the knee or elbow) when bleeding occurs.
● Frequent bruises following even minor injury. Major injuries can be life-threatening.
● Excessive bleeding from minor cuts.
● Spontaneous nosebleeds.
● Blood in the urine.

CAUSES & RISK FACTORS—A deficiency of a coagulation factor passed to male children through the genes of a female carrier. All active athletic activities are risky for children with hemophilia, particularly violent contact sports such as football, soccer, boxing or wrestling.

HOW TO PREVENT—Cannot be prevented at present. If your family has a history of hemophilia, obtain genetic counseling before having children.

WHAT TO EXPECT

DIAGNOSTIC MEASURES
● Your own observation of symptoms and signs.
● Medical history and physical exam by a doctor. General physicians, internists and pediatricians will wish a consultation with a hematologist (medical doctor specializing in diseases of the blood and immune system).
● Complicated and extensive laboratory blood studies.

SURGERY—None useful for hemophilia. Special precautions before and after unavoidable surgery for injuries will be explained in detail by your hematologist and surgeon.

NORMAL COURSE OF ILLNESS—This condition is currently considered incurable, but not fatal. If bleeding can be controlled, patients can reasonably expect a nearly normal life span. Scientific research into causes and treatment continues, so there is always hope for increasingly effective treatment and cure.

POSSIBLE COMPLICATIONS
● Dangerous bleeding episodes requiring emergency treatment.
● Permanent joint disability caused by persistent bleeding into the joints.
● Hepatitis from blood transfusions with contaminated blood. Until recently, those with hemophilia had an increased risk of contracting AIDS, but new techniques allow screening of donated blood. These tests assure an uncontaminated supply.

HOW TO TREAT

NOTE—Follow your doctor's instructions. These instructions are supplemental.

MEDICAL TREATMENT—A hematologist will direct treatment of any bleeding episode when it occurs. You may require hospitalization or care in an outpatient facility for transfusions of plasma and various blood factors.

HOME TREATMENT
● If bleeding occurs spontaneously or following an injury, apply direct pressure by hand or elastic bandage. Apply ice packs or towels wrung out in ice water to the injured or bleeding part of the body. Rest the injured part with a splint or sling. Elevate the arm or leg above the level of the heart. Call your doctor immediately.
● Wear a bracelet or pendant that identifies you as a person who has hemophilia.

MEDICATION
● Your doctor may prescribe:
  Medication to reduce joint pain.
  Transfusion of plasma or clotting factors.
● Don't take aspirin. It may increase the possibility of bleeding.
● Don't take any medicine without first consulting your doctor.

ACTIVITY—Avoid activities that can lead to injury, such as contact sports. Instead, work toward physical fitness by vigorous walking, swimming, jogging, cycling, or other activities that are not likely to cause injury or lead to overuse of a joint.

DIET—No special diet.

CALL YOUR DOCTOR IF

● You have symptoms of hemophilia.
● The following occurs after diagnosis:
  Injury from any cause with swelling. This may indicate bleeding under the skin.
  Bleeding that isn't quickly controlled.
  Tenderness or pain in any joint.

HEPATITIS, ACUTE VIRAL

 GENERAL INFORMATION

DEFINITION—Inflammation of the liver caused by a virus. Hepatitis can be a devastating illness for an athlete and may prevent sports participation for a long period of time. It is easily transmitted among teammates who share locker facilities.

SIGNS & SYMPTOMS
Early stages:
● Flulike symptoms, such as fever, fatigue, nausea, vomiting, diarrhea and loss of appetite.
Several days later:
● Jaundice (yellow eyes and skin) caused by a buildup of excess bile in the blood.
● Dark urine from bile in the urine.
● Light, "clay-colored" or whitish stools.

CAUSES & RISK FACTORS—Caused by any of 3 different but related viruses that may infect the liver:
● Type A: Usually enters the body through water or food, especially raw shellfish, that has been contaminated by sewage.
● Type B: Usually enters the body through blood transfusions contaminated with the virus or from injections with non-sterile needles.
● Type Non-A, Non-B: Usually enters the body by contaminated blood transfusions.
Additional risk factors include:
● Travel to areas with poor sanitation.
● Oral-anal sexual practices.
● Use of intravenous drugs such as heroin.
● Blood transfusions.
● Employment in a hospital.
● Close personal contact in locker rooms.
● Poor nutrition.
● Previous illness that has lowered resistance.
● Alcoholism.

HOW TO PREVENT
● If you are exposed to someone with hepatitis, consult your doctor about receiving gamma-globulin injections to prevent or decrease the risk.
● If you are in a high-risk group, such as hospital workers or male homosexuals, consult your doctor about receiving a vaccine for Type-B hepatitis. Vaccines are not available for other forms.

 WHAT TO EXPECT

DIAGNOSTIC MEASURES
● Your own observation of symptoms.
● Medical history and exam by a doctor.
● Laboratory blood tests to identify infection (Type A and Type B) and study liver function.
● Urine and stool examinations.

NORMAL COURSE OF ILLNESS—Jaundice and other symptoms peak and then gradually disappear over 3 to 16 weeks. Most people in good general health recover fully in 1 to 4 months. A small percentage (1% to 2%) infected with hepatitis virus B may proceed to chronic hepatitis. Recovery from other forms of viral hepatitis usually provides permanent immunity against it. You may expect not to be able to participate fully in athletics or vigorous physical activity for up to 1 year.

POSSIBLE COMPLICATIONS—Liver failure in severe cases. If vigorous activities are resumed too soon, permanent liver damage is likely.

 HOW TO TREAT

NOTE—Follow your doctor's instructions. These instructions are supplemental.

MEDICAL TREATMENT—Hospitalization (severe cases).

HOME TREATMENT
● Most persons with hepatitis can be cared for at home without undue risk. Bed rest, time and good nutrition are essential for a complete recovery. Strict isolation is not necessary, but the ill person should have separate eating and drinking utensils, or use disposable ones.
● If you are caring for someone with hepatitis, wash your hands carefully and often. If you have hepatitis, wash your hands often—especially after bowel movements.

MEDICATION—Your doctor may prescribe corticosteroid drugs for severe cases to reduce liver inflammation.

ACTIVITY
● Bed rest is necessary until jaundice disappears and appetite returns.
● Don't resume your normal activities until:
  You have clearance from your doctor.
  Results of laboratory liver-function studies are normal.
  Normal, hearty appetite returns. You should begin to regain weight lost during illness.

DIET—Despite poor appetite, small well-balanced meals help promote recovery. Drink at least 8 glasses of water daily. Avoid alcohol.

 CALL YOUR DOCTOR IF

● You have symptoms of hepatitis, or have been exposed to someone who has it.
● The following occurs during treatment:
  Increasing loss of appetite.
  Excessive drowsiness or mental confusion.
  Vomiting, diarrhea or abdominal pain.
  Deepening jaundice.
  Skin rash or itching.

HERNIA

 GENERAL INFORMATION

DEFINITION—Protrusion of an internal organ through a weakness or abnormal opening in the muscle around it. The most common types that affect athletes include: inguinal hernia (more common in males); incisional hernia; femoral hernia (more common in females); umbilical hernia (more common in children). Athletic performance will be impaired until the hernia is repaired.

SIGNS & SYMPTOMS—One of the following:
● A lump in the groin or umbilical area that usually returns to its normal position with gentle pressure or by lying down.
● A protrusion at the site of previous surgery.
● Scrotal swelling, with or without pain.
● Fullness or swelling in lips of the vagina.
All types of hernias can cause mild discomfort or pain at the site of the lump, particularly with exercise or competitive sports.

CAUSES & RISK FACTORS—Weakness in connective tissue or a muscle wall. This may be present at birth or acquired later in life. In athletes, hernias are usually associated with straining. Weight-lifters are especially susceptible. In the general population, premature infants, obese persons and pregnant women are most vulnerable to hernias.

HOW TO PREVENT—A weak area may not herniate until it ruptures with heavy lifting or straining. Don't strain when having bowel movements. Don't use weight-lifting equipment until the hernia has been repaired surgically. If you must lift something, lift properly. Bend your knees, lift the object and rise using your leg muscles. Keep the object close to your body. Don't bend from the waist and lift. Prevent complications by having surgery to repair the hernia.

 WHAT TO EXPECT

DIAGNOSTIC MEASURES
● Your own observation of symptoms.

● Medical history and physical exam by a doctor.
● Laboratory blood studies.
● X-rays of the abdomen.

SURGERY—Necessary to repair the opening caused by weakened muscle or connective tissue.

NORMAL COURSE OF ILLNESS—Umbilical hernias usually heal spontaneously by age 4 and rarely require surgery. Other hernias can be repaired with surgery.

POSSIBLE COMPLICATIONS—If the hernia becomes strangulated (loses its blood supply), it may cause severe illness (intestinal obstruction, fever, severe pain and shock).

 HOW TO TREAT

NOTE—Follow your doctor's instructions. These instructions are supplemental.

MEDICAL TREATMENT—Necessary for diagnosis and surgery.

HOME TREATMENT
● Whenever you lie down prior to surgery, push your hernia gently into place if it protrudes visibly.
● Don't wear a hernia truss. It injures or weakens tissues, making surgery difficult or impossible.
● Don't strain to have bowel movements.

MEDICATION—For minor discomfort, you may use non-prescription drugs such as acetaminophen.

ACTIVITY—Avoid heavy lifting—either before or after surgery.

DIET—Eat a high-fiber diet and increase fluid intake to prevent constipation and straining with bowel movements.

 CALL YOUR DOCTOR IF

You have symptoms of a hernia. If you have fever or severe pain, call immediately!

HIDRADENITIS SUPPURATIVA

GENERAL INFORMATION

DEFINITION—A skin disorder characterized by nodules in the armpit. Athletes are more likely to develop the disorder because of excessive sweating and moisture.

SIGNS & SYMPTOMS—Nodules with the following characteristics:
- Nodules are firm, tender and domed.
- Nodules are 1cm to 3cm in diameter.
- Larger nodules soften in the center and become painful. When pressed, they feel like an overfilled inner tube.
- Nodules open and drain pus spontaneously.
- Individual nodules (with or without drainage) heal slowly over 10 to 30 days.
- Nodules leave scars.
- Severity of the disorder varies from a few lesions per year to a constant succession of lesions that form as old ones heal. Lesions frequently recur at the same site.

CAUSES & RISK FACTORS
- Hormonal influences that activate the apocrine glands under the arms. Secretions in these glands enlarge the gland. The outlets become blocked, probably by heat, sweat or incomplete gland development. The secretions that are dammed in the glands force sweat and bacteria into surrounding tissue, which becomes infected.
- Repeated injury to the skin of athletes due to excessive heat, perspiration and friction of clothing and protective gear.
- Obesity.
- Exposure to environmental heat and moisture.
- Genetic factors. This disorder is most common in black females.

HOW TO PREVENT—No specific preventive measures.

WHAT TO EXPECT

DIAGNOSTIC MEASURES
- Your own observation of symptoms.
- Medical history and physical exam by a doctor.
- Laboratory culture of the discharge from the draining abscess.

SURGERY—Often necessary to open and drain abscesses. Surgery is necessary to remove involved skin in desperate cases only.

NORMAL COURSE OF ILLNESS—This disorder may last many years—from puberty through the following 10 to 20 years. Symptoms can be controlled with treatment.

POSSIBLE COMPLICATIONS—Scarring.

HOW TO TREAT

NOTE—Follow your doctor's instructions. These instructions are supplemental.

MEDICAL TREATMENT—None is usually necessary after diagnosis and prescription of medications. Surgery is helpful in some cases.

HOME TREATMENT
- Don't use commercial underarm deodorants or antiperspirants.
- Wear cotton shirts or shirts without sleeves to prevent accumulation of sweat in the armpits during exercise.
- Avoid constrictive clothing.
- Lose weight if you're overweight.
- Apply warm-water compresses to soothe pain or inflammation. Cool-water soaks feel better for itching.

MEDICATION—Your doctor may:
- Inject corticosteroid drugs directly into the lesions.
- Prescribe antibiotics to fight infection.
- Prescribe hormones to help subdue inflammation.
- Provide instructions for acceptable deodorant protection.
- Prescribe pain medication. For minor discomfort, you may use non-prescription drugs such as acetaminophen.

ACTIVITY—Restrict your activity in extremely hot weather. Swimming is an excellent substitute exercise, especially swimming in a warm ocean.

DIET—No special diet unless you need to lose weight.

CALL YOUR DOCTOR IF

- You have symptoms of hidradenitis suppurativa.
- Lesions don't improve after 5 days of treatment.
- Your temperature rises to 101F (38.3C).
- Lesions appear that become soft and seem to have pus, but don't drain spontaneously.
- New, unexplained symptoms develop. Drugs used in treatment may produce side effects.

HYPERVENTILATION SYNDROME
(Panic Attack)

 GENERAL INFORMATION

DEFINITION—Breathing so fast that carbon dioxide levels in the blood are decreased, temporarily upsetting normal blood chemistry. This may occur in athletes during or following vigorous physical activity.

SIGNS & SYMPTOMS
- Feeling of severe air hunger.
- Rapid breathing.
- Numbness and tingling around the mouth, hands and feet.
- Weakness or faintness.
- Muscle spasm or contractions in the hands and feet.
- Dry mouth.
- Palpitations.
- Fatigue.
- Frequent sighing.
- Fainting (occasionally).

CAUSES & RISK FACTORS—A change in the normal ratio of acid to other elements in the blood caused by breathing out too much carbon dioxide. Hyperventilation can accompany fever, disease of the heart and lungs, or severe injury. If disease or injury is not present, hyperventilation is caused by anxiety. The following factors make it more likely to occur:
- Stress such as that associated with competition.
- Feelings of guilt.
- Fatigue or overwork.
- Illness such as those listed above.
- Smoking.
- Excess alcohol consumption.

HOW TO PREVENT—Avoid anxiety-producing situations.

 WHAT TO EXPECT

DIAGNOSTIC MEASURES
- Your own observation of symptoms.
- Medical history and physical exam by a doctor.

SURGERY—Not necessary nor useful for this disorder.

NORMAL COURSE OF ILLNESS—Symptoms can be controlled with the instructions below. If hyperventilation is caused by a disease, it will stop when the disease is cured. Recurrent attacks caused by anxiety should stop if underlying stress can be eliminated.

POSSIBLE COMPLICATIONS
- Seizures.
- Fainting.

 HOW TO TREAT

NOTE—Follow your doctor's instructions. These instructions are supplemental.

MEDICAL TREATMENT
- Doctor's treatment, if the cause is organic or symptoms are prolonged.
- Psychotherapy, biofeedback training or counseling, if hyperventilation occurs often and is caused by anxiety.

HOME TREATMENT—During an attack, the following instructions will increase carbon dioxide in the blood and relieve symptoms:
- Cover your mouth and nose completely with a paper bag.
- Breathe slowly into the bag and rebreathe the air. The air in the bag contains additional carbon dioxide.
- Breathe slowly in and out of the bag at least 10 times.
- Put the bag aside and breathe normally a few minutes.
- Repeat the process until the symptoms diminish or disappear.
- If symptoms return, repeat the process as often as needed.

MEDICATION—Medicine usually is not necessary for this disorder.

ACTIVITY—After treatment, resume normal activity as soon as possible.

DIET—No special diet.

 CALL YOUR DOCTOR IF

- You have symptoms of hyperventilation that don't diminish with self-treatment.
- The following occurs during an attack: fainting, seizure or sudden fever.
- You have repeated attacks of hyperventilation and want a referral to a counselor.

IMPETIGO
(Pyoderma)

 ## GENERAL INFORMATION

DEFINITION—An infectious, contagious, common bacterial skin infection that affects the superficial layers of the skin. This is more common in athletes and those who participate in vigorous physical activity that causes excessive sweating.

SIGNS & SYMPTOMS
• A red rash with many small blisters. Some blisters contain pus, and yellow crusts form when they break. The blisters don't hurt, but they may itch.
• Slight fever (sometimes).

CAUSES & RISK FACTORS—*Staphylococci* or *streptococci* bacteria growing in the upper skin layers. The following conditions make a person more susceptible to impetigo infections:
• Increased perspiration from physical exertion.
• Crowded or unsanitary conditions, such as locker rooms, or sharing of towels.
• Constant friction with clothing and athletic equipment.
• Fair complexion.
• Skin that is sensitive to sun and irritants, such as soap and makeup.
• Warm, moist weather.
• Poor hygiene.
• Recent illness that has lowered resistance.

HOW TO PREVENT
• Bathe daily with soap and water.
• Keep fingernails short. Don't scratch impetigo blisters.
• If there is an outbreak in the team or family, urge all members to use antibacterial soap.
• Use separate towels for each person, or substitute paper towels temporarily.

 ## WHAT TO EXPECT

DIAGNOSTIC MEASURES
• Your own observation of symptoms.
• Medical history and physical exam by a doctor.
• Laboratory skin culture to identify the germ causing the infection.

SURGERY—Not necessary nor useful for this illness.

NORMAL COURSE OF ILLNESS—Curable in 10 days with treatment, usually leaving no scars.

POSSIBLE COMPLICATIONS
• Penetration of the infection to deeper skin layers (ecthyma or cellulitis). This may cause scarring. Treatment is the same as for impetigo.
• Acute glomerulonephritis (kidney disease) if impetigo has been caused by a streptococcal infection that has not been adequately treated.

 ## HOW TO TREAT

NOTE—Follow your doctor's instructions. These instructions are supplemental.

MEDICAL TREATMENT—None usually necessary after diagnosis and prescription of medication.

HOME TREATMENT
• Follow the suggestions listed under How to Prevent.
• Scrub lesions with gauze and antiseptic soap. Break any pustules. Remove all crusts, and expose and cleanse all lesions. If crusts are difficult to remove, soak them in warm soapy water and scrub gently.
• Cover impetigo sores with gauze and tape to keep hands away from them.
• Treat new lesions the same way, even if you are not sure they are impetigo.
• Separate and boil bed linen, towels, clothes and other items that have touched sores.
• Men should shave around sores on the face, not over them. Use an aerosol shaving cream and change razor blades each day. Don't use a shaving brush—it may harbor germs.

MEDICATION—Your doctor may prescribe:
• Oral antibiotics, such as dicloxacillin or erythromycin. To avoid complications, take antibiotics for 10 days even if symptoms disappear.
• Antibiotic ointments for very small areas of infection. Rub antibiotic ointment into the lesions for 60 seconds at least 4 times a day. If your doctor has not prescribed an ointment, you may use a non-prescription ointment containing neomycin and bacitracin.

ACTIVITY—No restrictions.

DIET—No special diet.

 ## CALL YOUR DOCTOR IF

• You have symptoms of impetigo.
• Fever of 101F (38.3C) or higher orally develops.
• The sores continue to spread or don't begin to heal in 3 days, despite treatment.

INSECT BITES & STINGS

GENERAL INFORMATION

DEFINITION—Skin eruptions and other symptoms caused by insect bites or stings from mosquitoes, fleas, chiggers, bedbugs, ants, spiders, bees and other insects. The victim often doesn't remember being bitten or stung.

SIGNS & SYMPTOMS—Red lumps in the skin. The lumps usually appear within minutes after the bite or sting, but some don't appear for 6 to 12 hours. Skin reactions fall into 2 categories:
• A toxic reaction with pain and sometimes fever, such as from bee stings.
• A toxic reaction with itching due to the body's release of histamine at the bite site, such as from mosquitoes.

CAUSES & RISK FACTORS—Bites or stings are most likely in areas with heavy insect infestations, and during outdoor activity in the warm weather of spring and summer.

HOW TO PREVENT
• Recent evidence indicates that vitamins in the B-vitamin group may be a deterrent to mosquito and other insect bites. Try 50mg thiamine orally once a day (unless your doctor advises otherwise) if you expect insects where you exercise or compete.
• Apply an insect repellent with diethyltoluamide (DEET) before exposure.
• Treat animals for fleas and exterminate the house or kennel.

WHAT TO EXPECT

DIAGNOSTIC MEASURES
• Your own observation of symptoms.
• Medical history and physical exam by a doctor.

SURGERY—Not necessary nor useful for this problem.

NORMAL COURSE OF ILLNESS—Most troublesome symptoms disappear in 2 to 3 days, but scratching may prolong symptoms for several weeks or introduce a bacterial infection. Treatment helps, but it doesn't cure quickly.

POSSIBLE COMPLICATIONS
• Secondary bacterial infection at the site of the bite. This may cause swollen lymph glands in the neck, armpit, groin or elbow.

• Anaphylaxis (severe allergic response in hypersensitive persons).

HOW TO TREAT

NOTE—Follow your doctor's instructions. These instructions are supplemental.

MEDICAL TREATMENT—If you have had anaphylaxis (severe allergic reaction) following an insect bite, ask your doctor for an anaphylaxis kit to treat any future recurrences.

HOME TREATMENT
• If anaphylaxis occurs, give CPR if the victim is not breathing and has no heartbeat. Ask someone to get emergency medical help.
• For less severe cases, apply compresses to the bite or sting to relieve itching and hasten healing. Warm-water compresses are usually more soothing for pain or inflammation. Cool-water compresses feel better for itching.

MEDICATION
• For minor discomfort, you may use:
  Non-prescription oral antihistamines to decrease itching.
  Non-prescription topical corticosteroid preparations to reduce inflammation and decrease itching. Use according to label directions. For face and groin, use only low-potency steroid products without fluorine.
• For serious symptoms, your doctor may prescribe:
  Stronger topical or oral corticosteroids if the reaction is severe.
  Epinephrine or corticosteroids (orally or by injection) to prevent or diminish anaphylaxis symptoms.

ACTIVITY—No restrictions.

DIET—No special diet.

CALL YOUR DOCTOR IF

• You have symptoms of anaphylaxis. This is an emergency!
• Self-care does not relieve symptoms, or symptoms don't improve after 2 to 3 days of medical treatment.
• A bitten area becomes red, swollen, warm and tender, indicating infection.
• Temperature rises to 101F (38.3C).

ISCHEMIA DURING EXERCISE

 GENERAL INFORMATION

DEFINITION—Decreased blood flow to the brain, spinal cord and other parts of the body during exercise. In younger people, this is a warning sign that risk factors may exist for stroke. Symptoms may cease, but underlying problems will not. In older persons, ischemia is often a sign of impending stroke.

SIGNS & SYMPTOMS
- Dizziness or falling.
- Leg pain brought on by exercise and relieved by rest.
- Impaired gait or legs "giving out."
- Nystagmus (irregular, involuntary movement of the eyes).
- Vomiting.
- Speech impairment.
- Partial, temporary or permanent paralysis of arm, leg and neck muscles on one or both sides.
- Diminished vision.
- Breathing difficulty.

CAUSES & RISK FACTORS
- Excessive exercise, such as prolonged walking or running, that tires the heart and decreases the amount of blood it can pump.
- Excessive rotation or bending of the neck backward or forward, constricting blood vessels in the neck. This may occur occasionally in gymnastics, calisthenics, wrestling, football and yoga.
Underlying conditions that make ischemia during exercise more likely:
- Hardening of the arteries.
- Cervical spondylosis (degenerative changes in bones of the neck, causing pressure on nerves, blood vessels and muscles).
- Congenital anatomic abnormalities in blood vessels to the brain (aneurysms, for example).
- High blood pressure.
- Diabetes mellitus.
- Obesity.
- Family history of strokes.

HOW TO PREVENT
- Try to avoid specific exercises or activities that bring on ischemia.
- Follow measures to prevent hardening of the arteries:
  Don't smoke.
  Reduce stress to a manageable level.
  Follow a low-fat, low-salt, high-fiber diet.
  Maintain your ideal weight.
- If you have diabetes or high blood pressure, adhere rigidly to your treatment program to keep it under control.
- If you are over 40, ask your doctor about taking 1 aspirin tablet daily to decrease the likelihood of platelet-clumping (see Glossary).

 WHAT TO EXPECT

DIAGNOSTIC MEASURES
- X-rays of the head and spine.
- CAT scan (see Glossary) of the brain and spinal cord.

SURGERY—May be necessary to clear out or bypass blocked or narrowed arteries.

NORMAL COURSE OF ILLNESS—In some cases, symptoms of ischemia disappear within 1 or 2 days without residual effects. In most cases, an underlying disorder is causing the ischemia, and it must be treated. Ischemia symptoms may improve, but they may not disappear entirely.

POSSIBLE COMPLICATIONS—Severe stroke and death.

 HOW TO TREAT

NOTE—Follow your doctor's instructions. These instructions are supplemental.

MEDICAL TREATMENT
- Consult your doctor after the first incident of ischemia, *even if symptoms disappear.* Diagnosis of the underlying cause is essential.
- Hospitalization and surgery may be necessary to correct serious underlying disorders.
- If ischemia leaves residual disability, physical therapy will be helpful until recovery is complete.

HOME TREATMENT—No self-treatment. Seek emergency professional care for any signs of ischemia.

MEDICATION—Your doctor may prescribe anticoagulants such as warfarin, aspirin or others.

ACTIVITY
- Rest in bed until symptoms improve.
- Resume your normal activities gradually, but consult your doctor before resuming the activity that brought on the ischemia.
- If you have lost a great deal of muscle control, physical therapy will help you to use affected limbs to regain basic skills, such as eating, dressing and toilet functions.

DIET—Follow a low-fat, low-salt, high-fiber, low-cholesterol diet. This will help minimize the chance of stroke.

 CALL YOUR DOCTOR IF

You have symptoms of ischemia during or following exercise.

JOCK ITCH
(Tinea Cruris)

GENERAL INFORMATION

DEFINITION—Infection of the skin in the groin with one of several fungus germs. These fungi thrive in the groin where darkness, warmth and moisture stimulate their growth. Jock itch is more likely to occur in men than women. It is contagious from person to person.

SIGNS & SYMPTOMS
● Scaling patches on the skin of the groin, thighs and buttocks. Patches have well-defined edges. Occasionally small, pus-filled blisters appear.
● Itching of involved areas.
● Pain (if the skin becomes secondarily infected with bacteria).

CAUSES & RISK FACTORS
● Athlete's foot, a fungus infection of the feet that can spread to the groin area.
● Contact with infected surfaces, such as towels or benches.
● Hot, humid weather.
● Excessive sweating.
● Obesity, which fosters sweating.
● Friction of skin against skin from constant movement.

HOW TO PREVENT
● Dry thoroughly after bathing.
● Don't sit around in a wet bathing suit.
● Wear absorbent, loose, cotton underwear.
● Wear clean, dry athletic supporters and underwear for each workout.
● Use non-prescription tolnafate (Tinactin) after bathing if you have had jock itch. This powder discourages recurrence.

WHAT TO EXPECT

DIAGNOSTIC MEASURES
● Your own observation of symptoms.
● Medical history and physical exam by a doctor.
● Laboratory studies, including microscopic examination of scraped-off scales suspended in potassium hydroxide liquid.

SURGERY—Not necessary nor useful for this disorder.

NORMAL COURSE OF ILLNESS—Symptoms can be controlled in 2 to 3 weeks with treatment. Recurrences are common.

POSSIBLE COMPLICATIONS
● Contact or allergic dermatitis accompanying jock itch that requires additional treatment, usually with steroid topical applications.
● Slow healing.
● Secondary bacterial infection in the affected area.
● Rash from an "id reaction" (allergic immunological response to the disorder) on the hands and face (rare).

HOW TO TREAT

NOTE—Follow your doctor's instructions. These instructions are supplemental.

MEDICAL TREATMENT—None is usually necessary after diagnosis and prescription of medications by a doctor.

HOME TREATMENT
● Bathe with clear water only. Don't use soaps until the skin clears completely. Soap irritates infected skin.
● Wear loose cotton underwear.
● Change to dry clothes immediately after swimming.
● If you have an athlete's foot infection also, treat both areas with equal care.

MEDICATION—Your doctor may prescribe:
● Topical treatment with antifungal medicines such as clotrimazole, haloprigin or miconazole.
● Oral antifungal medication, such as griseofulvin, if topical medication doesn't bring relief in 7 to 10 days.

ACTIVITY—No restriction.

DIET—No special diet.

CALL YOUR DOCTOR IF

● You have symptoms of jock itch that don't clear spontaneously in 5 days.
● New, unexplained symptoms develop. Drugs used in treatment may produce side effects.

KERATOSIS, ACTINIC

 ## GENERAL INFORMATION

DEFINITION—A small area of sun-damaged skin that is precancerous. This can be a problem for athletes who spend a lot of time in the sun.

SIGNS & SYMPTOMS—Brownish or reddish scaly patches on exposed areas of skin. The patches are painless.

CAUSES & RISK FACTORS—Keratoses occur after prolonged exposure to the sun's radiation. The following factors contribute to their formation:
● Outdoor athletic activities and sports.
● Outdoor occupations such as farming.
● Light complexion.
● Repeated skin injury from excessive perspiration and heat, or friction with clothing and protective gear.

HOW TO PREVENT—Protect yourself against direct sun exposure. When outdoors, wear a hat and protective clothing. Use sunscreen lotions and creams, and reapply them often during prolonged exposure.

 ## WHAT TO EXPECT

DIAGNOSTIC MEASURES
● Your own observation of symptoms.
● Medical history and physical exam by a doctor.

SURGERY—Not necessary nor useful for this disorder, but if skin cancer develops, surgery may be necessary.

NORMAL COURSE OF ILLNESS—An individual keratosis will disappear with treatment, but new lesions are likely to recur. If neglected, actinic keratosis can lead to skin cancer.

POSSIBLE COMPLICATIONS
● Skin damage.
● Skin cancer (including malignant melanoma, basal-cell carcinoma and squamous-cell carcinoma).

 ## HOW TO TREAT

NOTE—Follow your doctor's instructions. These instructions are supplemental.

MEDICAL TREATMENT—All patches require treatment to prevent skin cancer. Your doctor may use:
● Liquid nitrogen to freeze the affected tissue.
● Applications of various medications to the affected area.

HOME TREATMENT
● Minimize direct sun exposure.
● See your doctor for checkups every 6 months to ensure early detection and treatment of skin cancers.

MEDICATION—Your doctor may use:
● Applications of fluorouracil to the affected area. This causes uncomfortable inflammation, but it is very effective.
● Application of vitamin A ointment (still experimental).

ACTIVITY—No restrictions.

DIET—No special diet.

 ## CALL YOUR DOCTOR IF

You have signs of an actinic keratosis. Even though this causes no symptoms, it is precancerous.

LABYRINTHITIS
(Inner-Ear Disorder)

 GENERAL INFORMATION

DEFINITION—Inflammation of the inner ear. Because dizziness is the main symptom of labyrinthitis, this problem can impair performance in any sport until it clears.

SIGNS & SYMPTOMS
- Extreme dizziness with head movement—especially in people over 40 who may have hardening of the arteries in the neck (atherosclerosis). Exercises that exaggerate head, neck and trunk movements can cause kinking or narrowing of these arteries. The dizziness begins gradually and peaks in 48 hours.
- Involuntary eye movement.
- Nausea and vomiting.
- Loss of balance, especially falling toward the affected side.
- Temporary hearing loss.

CAUSES & RISK FACTORS
- Virus infection (usually) in the inner ear.
- Other recent viral illness, especially respiratory infection.
- Bacterial infection in the inner ear.
- Spread of a chronic middle-ear infection.
- Head injury.
- Heavy exercise in hot weather, causing dehydration or electrolyte imbalance from excessive sweating.
- Stress, fatigue or overwork.
- Use of medication or toxic drugs, including aspirin.
- Allergy or family history of allergies.
- Cholesteatoma (an accumulation of debris covered by skin in the outer-ear canal).
- Exaggerated head, neck or trunk movements in people with hardening of the arteries (atherosclerosis).
- Transient ischemic attacks due to hardening of the arteries (atherosclerosis).
- Heart-rhythm irregularity.
- Bleeding or tumor inside the brain.
- Anemia.
- Smoking.
- Excess alcohol consumption.

HOW TO PREVENT
- Obtain prompt medical treatment for ear infections.
- Don't take medication that has produced dizziness without consulting your doctor.
- Follow all preventive measures for hardening of the arteries recommended by the American Heart Association:
  Low-fat, low-salt, high-fiber diet.
  Stress reduction.
  Regular exercise.
  No smoking.

 WHAT TO EXPECT

DIAGNOSTIC MEASURES
- Your own observation of symptoms.
- Medical history and exam by a doctor.
- Audiometry (see Glossary).
- Skull X-rays.
- CAT scan (see Glossary).

SURGERY—Sometimes necessary to open arteries in the neck, if labyrinthitis is caused by decreased blood flow from atherosclerosis.

NORMAL COURSE OF ILLNESS—Recovery —either spontaneous or with treatment—in 1 to 6 weeks.

POSSIBLE COMPLICATIONS
- Permanent hearing loss on the affected side.
- Frequent dizziness, if due to atherosclerosis.

 HOW TO TREAT

NOTE—Follow your doctor's instructions. These instructions are supplemental.

MEDICAL TREATMENT—See your doctor for diagnosis and possible prescription of medications. Hearing tests may be required.

HOME TREATMENT—No specific instructions except those listed under other headings.

MEDICATION—Your doctor may prescribe:
- Antinausea medications.
- Tranquilizers such as diazepam to reduce dizziness.
- Diuretics to decrease fluid accumulation in the inner ear.
- Antibiotics to fight bacterial infection.

ACTIVITY—Keep the head as still as possible. Rest in bed until dizziness subsides. Then resume your normal activities gradually. Avoid heavy exercise, competition or hazardous activities, such as driving, climbing or working around dangerous machinery, until 1 week after symptoms disappear.

DIET—No special diet, but decrease salt and fluid intake until you resume your usual activity.

 CALL YOUR DOCTOR IF

- You get dizzy for more than 1 or 2 minutes.
- The following occurs during treatment:
  Decreased hearing in either ear.
  Persistent vomiting.
  Convulsions.
  Fainting.
  Fever of 101F (38.3C) or higher.
  New, unexplained symptoms. Drugs used in treatment may produce side effects.

LICE
(Pediculosis; Head Lice; Body Lice; "Crabs")

GENERAL INFORMATION

DEFINITION—Skin inflammation caused by tiny parasites (lice) that live on the hairy areas of the body, especially the genital area, scalp, eyelashes, eyebrows, and skin in close contact with clothing. The tiny (3mm to 4mm) parasites bite through skin to obtain nourishment (blood). The bites cause itching and inflammation. Some lice live in clothing near skin. Eggs (nits) adhere to hairs.

SIGNS & SYMPTOMS
- Itching and scratching, sometimes intense and usually in hair-covered areas.
- Eggs (nits) on hair shafts.
- Scalp inflammation and matted hair.
- Enlarged lymph glands at the back of the scalp or in the groin (sometimes).
- Red bite marks and hives.
- Eye inflammation if eyelashes are infected.

CAUSES & RISK FACTORS
- Crowded or unsanitary living conditions or locker rooms.
- Sexual intercourse (genital or oral) with an infected person.

HOW TO PREVENT
- Bathe and shampoo often.
- Avoid wearing the same clothing more than a day or two.
- Change bed linens often.
- Don't share combs, brushes, towels, helmets or hats with others.

WHAT TO EXPECT

DIAGNOSTIC MEASURES
- Your own observation of symptoms. You may see nits (like tiny footballs) on the side of hairs.
- Medical history and physical exam by a doctor.

SURGERY—Not necessary nor useful for this disorder.

NORMAL COURSE OF ILLNESS—Usually curable with medicated creams, lotions and shampoos. Allow 5 days after treatment for symptoms to disappear. Lice often recur.

POSSIBLE COMPLICATIONS
- Infection at the site of deep scratching may cause diseases such as typhus (rare).
- Worst complication is spread to others.

HOW TO TREAT

NOTE—Follow your doctor's instructions. These instructions are supplemental.

MEDICAL TREATMENT—Home care is usually sufficient. Lice on eyebrows and eyelashes must be removed by a doctor.

HOME TREATMENT—The following measures apply to all members of the household, and to any sexual partners of household members:
- Use medicated shampoo, cream or lotion prescribed by your doctor.
- Machine-wash all clothing and linen in hot water. Dry in the dryer's hot-air cycle. Iron the clothing and linen, if possible. Washing removes the lice, and ironing destroys nits.
- If you don't have a washing machine, iron the clothes and linen, or seal for 10 days in a plastic bag to kill lice and nits.
- Dry-clean non-washable items or seal in a plastic bag for 10 days.
- Boil articles such as combs, curlers, hairbrushes and barrettes.
- Hair does not have to be shaved.

MEDICATION—Your doctor may prescribe antilice (pediculocide) cream, lotion or shampoo. Apply creams or lotions to infected body parts according to instructions. To use the shampoo:
- Wet the hair. Apply 1 tablespoon of shampoo. Lather for 4 minutes, working the lather well into the scalp.
- If shampoo gets in eyes, wash out immediately with water.
- Rinse hair thoroughly and towel dry. Don't use this towel again without laundering and boiling.
- Comb the hair with a fine comb dipped in hot vinegar to remove the lice. The comb must run through the hair repeatedly from the scalp outward until the hair is completely free of nits.
- A single application of shampoo is effective in more than 90% of cases. Don't use more frequently than recommended, because the shampoo may cause skin irritation or be absorbed into the body.
- If the lice infect eyelashes or eyebrows, they must be removed carefully by your doctor. The prescribed medications should not go into the eye or on the eyelashes. You may apply petroleum jelly to the eyelashes for 7 or 8 days after removal.

ACTIVITY—No restrictions.

DIET—No special diet.

CALL YOUR DOCTOR IF

- You, your sexual partner, or anyone in your household has symptoms of lice.
- Symptoms recur after treatment.

MONONUCLEOSIS, INFECTIOUS
(Mono; "Kissing Disease")

 GENERAL INFORMATION

DEFINITION—An infectious viral disease that affects the respiratory system, liver and lymphatic system. Mononucleosis causes spleen enlargement, making athletic activity dangerous.

SIGNS & SYMPTOMS
- Fever.
- Sore throat (sometimes severe).
- Appetite loss.
- Fatigue.
- Swollen lymph glands, usually in the neck, underarms or groin.
- Enlarged spleen or liver.
- Jaundice with yellow skin and eyes (sometimes).
- Headache.
- General aching.

CAUSES & RISK FACTORS—A contagious virus (Epstein-Barr virus) that is transmitted from person to person by close contact, such as kissing, shared food or coughing. The following factors increase the risk of getting mononucleosis:
- Stress.
- Illness that has lowered resistance.
- Fatigue or overwork. The high incidence among college students, athletes and military recruits may result from inadequate rest and crowded living conditions.

HOW TO PREVENT
- Avoid contact with persons having infectious mononucleosis.
- Vaccine (possibly). This is still in the experimental stages.

 WHAT TO EXPECT

DIAGNOSTIC MEASURES
- Your own observation of symptoms.
- Medical history and exam by a doctor.
- Laboratory blood tests.

SURGERY—Not necessary nor useful for this illness, unless a ruptured spleen must be removed (rare).

NORMAL COURSE OF ILLNESS
Spontaneous recovery in 10 days to 6 months. Most previously healthy athletes usually have about 3 weeks of disability. Fatigue frequently persists for 3 to 6 weeks after other symptoms disappear.

POSSIBLE COMPLICATIONS
- Meningitis or encephalitis (rare).
- Misdiagnosis as a streptococcal sore throat.
- Ruptured spleen, requiring emergency surgery.
- Destruction or rupture of red blood cells, requiring critical emergency treatment.

 HOW TO TREAT

NOTE—Follow your doctor's instructions. These instructions are supplemental.

MEDICAL TREATMENT—Not usually necessary after diagnosis.

HOME TREATMENT
- To relieve the sore throat, gargle frequently with double-strength tea or warm salt water (1 teaspoon of salt to 8 oz. of water).
- Don't strain hard for bowel movements. This may cause bleeding in or rupture of an enlarged spleen.

MEDICATION
- For minor discomfort, you may use non-prescription drugs such as acetaminophen. Don't take aspirin because of its possible association with Reye's syndrome.
- If symptoms are severe, your doctor may prescribe a short course of corticosteroid drugs.

ACTIVITY
- Rest in bed, especially when you have fever. Resume activity gradually. Rest when you are fatigued.
- Return to full activity when cleared by your doctor. This will usually be when fever has disappeared, when you have regained any lost weight due to illness, and when your sleep pattern has returned to normal.
- If the spleen remains enlarged after other symptoms resolve, return to exercise only after a doctor's clearance. Don't return to contact or collision sports until the spleen is normal size.

DIET—No special diet. Eat as heartily as possible. You may not feel like eating while you are ill. Maintain an adequate fluid intake. Drink at least 8 glasses of water or juice a day—more during periods of high fever.

 CALL YOUR DOCTOR IF

- You have symptoms of infectious mononucleosis.
- Any of the following occur during treatment:
  Fever over 102F (38.9C).
  Constipation, which may cause straining.
  Severe pain in the upper left abdomen that lasts for 5 minutes or more.
  Swallowing or breathing difficulty from severe throat inflammation.

MUSCLE CRAMPS

GENERAL INFORMATION

DEFINITION—Painful involuntary contractions of muscles in swimmers and others caused by abnormalities of the nervous system or exercise-related changes in muscle-cell chemistry.

SIGNS & SYMPTOMS—Painful, involuntary contraction of muscles, usually in the legs. Swimming more than other sports causes leg cramps in athletes during exercise.

CAUSES & RISK FACTORS
● Vigorous physical activity.
● Inadequate warm-up before engaging in strenuous physical activity.
● Calcium deficiency.
● Nerve disorders, such as pressure on nerve roots near the spinal cord, or abnormalities of nerve fibers after they leave the spinal cord.
● Enzyme deficiency (temporary).
● Diabetes, alcoholism, chronic kidney disease, a variety of medications, hardening of the arteries, Buerger's disease (see Glossary), all of which can cause damage to peripheral nerves and thereby cause muscle cramps.
● In swimmers, the cause of leg cramps is frequently unknown, and their presence does not suggest an underlying disorder.

HOW TO PREVENT
● Undertake a slow, thorough conditioning program prior to beginning vigorous physical activity, including swimming.
● Consult your doctor if you take any medicine and develop cramps. Discontinuing or modifying the dosage may prevent recurrent cramps.
● If you have an enzyme deficiency, there is no treatment except to reduce sports activities below the level that produces cramps.
● Don't smoke. Avoid polluted air while exercising. Both may decrease oxygen flow to muscles. Oxygen is needed in the muscles to avoid cramps.

WHAT TO EXPECT

DIAGNOSTIC MEASURES
● Your own observation of symptoms and signs.
● Medical history and exam by a doctor.
● Blood studies (sometimes) to measure enzyme levels.

SURGERY—None useful nor necessary for this disorder.

NORMAL COURSE OF ILLNESS—Can be controlled by treating any underlying medical disorder, using medication (carbamazepine) and undertaking a better conditioning program.

COMPLICATIONS
● Permanent muscle contractures (rare).
● Permanently weakened muscle groups (rare).
● Fear of recurrence, resulting in unwarranted abandonment of the exercise program.

HOW TO TREAT

NOTE—Follow your doctor's instructions. These instructions are supplemental.

MEDICAL TREATMENT—Physical therapy including warm soaks, applications of ice or heat, whirlpool, or gentle massage may help with residual pain and soreness in cramped muscles.

HOME TREATMENT
● Stretch and rub the cramping muscles.
● Voluntarily contract the muscles that directly oppose those that are cramping. For example, if cramps affect the calf of the leg, force the front of the foot upward toward the knee and hold it until the cramp is diminished.

MEDICATION—Your doctor may prescribe the following medications:
● Carbamazepine for muscle cramps due to nerve damage.
● Aspirin or acetaminophen for pain following a muscle cramp.

ACTIVITY—Decrease or discontinue vigorous physical activity until muscle cramp relaxes.

DIET
● If you have frequent muscle cramps from any cause, eat foods high in potassium, such as dried apricots, whole-grain cereal (hot or cold), dried lentils, dried peaches, bananas, peanuts, citrus fruits or fresh vegetables.
● Following a diet high in complex carbohydrates makes good nutritional sense to all those hoping to maintain or reach a good level of health and fitness. However, do not eat such a meal within 3 to 5 hours before competition, and eat only lightly directly afterwards.
● Make sure you have sufficient calcium in your diet through the use of dairy products or calcium supplements.

CALL YOUR DOCTOR IF

● You have persistent or recurrent muscle cramps despite following the suggestions on this page.
● You develop new symptoms after starting any prescribed medicine. All effective medicines have potentially undesirable side effects. These can frequently be controlled by modifying the dosage.

MUSCLE WEAKNESS

 ## GENERAL INFORMATION

DEFINITION—Profound muscle weakness following hard or unaccustomed exercise.

SIGNS & SYMPTOMS
- Unaccustomed exercise.
- Symptoms that appear following a period of rest after the exercise, an hour or 2 later or the next day. Frequently a high-carbohydrate meal is eaten after competition or vigorous physical exercise, followed by a night's sleep. The muscle weakness then appears the next day.
- Weakness that begins in the legs and progresses to the arms or other muscles in the body. Disabling fatigue accompanies the muscle weakness.

CAUSES & RISK FACTORS—Decreased
potassium levels in the circulating blood and muscle cells. The decreased potassium levels can be brought about by any of the following:
- An underlying inherited disorder called *periodic paralysis* (see Glossary) that interferes with muscle cellular metabolism.
- Excessive exercise in hot weather with loss of water, sodium and potassium, leading to dehydration.
- Diuretic medications that cause sodium loss and excessive potassium loss through the kidneys. The sodium loss is desirable; the potassium loss is a significant undesirable side effect that may lead to major body disturbances. Customary doses of diuretics may require reduction during hot weather.

HOW TO PREVENT
- Prevent potassium loss, increase fluid intake and adjust exercise programs and medication dosages during hot weather.
- Avoid the combination of diuretic medications, alcohol and heavy exercise during exceptionally hot weather. This combination can be lethal, causing strokes and life-threatening episodes of irregular heart rhythms.
- Increase potassium-rich foods in your diet.
- Take potassium supplements (with a doctor's prescription) prior to vigorous exercise if you have had an exercise-induced muscle weakness in the past.
- Modify activity level to one below that which triggers attacks.

 ## WHAT TO EXPECT

DIAGNOSTIC MEASURES
- Your own observation of symptoms and signs.
- Medical history and exam by a doctor.
- Blood studies (sometimes) to measure potassium levels.
- Electromyography (see Glossary).

SURGERY—None useful nor necessary for this disorder.

NORMAL COURSE OF ILLNESS—Curable and preventable without long-lasting complications by modifying the exercise program, taking potassium supplements, and avoiding dehydration.

COMPLICATIONS
- Permanently weakened muscle groups (rare).
- Fear of recurrence, resulting in unwarranted abandonment of the exercise program.

 ## HOW TO TREAT

NOTE—Follow your doctor's instructions. These instructions are supplemental.

MEDICAL TREATMENT—Must be individualized according to the underlying disorder.

HOME TREATMENT
- Replace lost potassium with supplements or increase high-potassium foods in the diet.
- Replace fluid loss with water instead of soft drinks.
- After vigorous exercise, avoid a high-carbohydrate meal.

MEDICATION—Your doctor may prescribe potassium supplements for muscle weakness.

ACTIVITY—If exercise-induced muscle weakness is a recurrent problem, it may be necessary to cut back on your activity level permanently.

DIET
- If you have a potassium deficiency, eat foods high in potassium, such as dried apricots, whole-grain cereal (hot or cold), dried lentils, dried peaches, bananas, peanuts, citrus fruits or fresh vegetables.
- Following a diet high in complex carbohydrates makes good nutritional sense to all those hoping to maintain or reach a good level of health and fitness. However, do not eat such a meal within 3 to 5 hours before competition, and eat only lightly directly afterwards.

 ## CALL YOUR DOCTOR IF

- You have persistent or recurrent muscle weakness following exercise.
- You develop new symptoms after starting any prescribed medicine. All effective medicines have potentially undesirable side effects. These can frequently be controlled by modifying the dosage.

NASAL OBSTRUCTION

 GENERAL INFORMATION

DEFINITION—Nasal passageways that are blocked by an anatomic abnormality or disease. Nasal obstruction can force mouth-breathing and decrease athletic endurance and performance.

SIGNS & SYMPTOMS
- Obstruction of air through the nose.
- Crooked nose (with deviated septum, sometimes).
- Impaired sense of smell.
- Nasal discharge.
- Facial pain (sometimes).
- Headaches (sometimes).
- Frequent sneezing.
- Wheezing (sometimes) with allergic rhinitis.

CAUSES & RISK FACTORS
- Deviated nasal septum.
- Previous nose injury.
- Nasal polyps.
- Hay fever (allergic rhinitis), especially during spring and fall when the pollen count is highest.
- Nasal infections (common cold and other infections).
- Sinusitis or chronic nasal infection.
- Smoking.

HOW TO PREVENT—Most forms of obstruction cannot be prevented. To minimize obstruction caused by allergic reactions:
- Obtain medical treatment for underlying allergies with desensitization procedures.
- Install an air-purification unit in your home's heating and air-conditioning system.

 WHAT TO EXPECT

DIAGNOSTIC MEASURES
- Your own observation of symptoms.
- Medical history and exam by a doctor.
- X-rays of the face.
- Allergy skin tests.

SURGERY—Often necessary to correct a deviated nasal septum or to remove nasal polyps.

NORMAL COURSE OF ILLNESS
- Nasal polyps and deviated septum are usually curable with surgery.
- Other causes of obstruction usually can be controlled with treatment.

POSSIBLE COMPLICATIONS
- Hampered athletic performance.
- Recurrent nosebleeds.
- Sleeping difficulty and chronic fatigue.
- Sinus infections.
- Middle-ear infections.
- Repeated nasal infections.

 HOW TO TREAT

NOTE—Follow your doctor's instructions. These instructions are supplemental.

MEDICAL TREATMENT
- Doctor's care for desensitization procedures for allergic disorders.
- Surgery for deviated septum and polyps.

HOME TREATMENT—For allergic rhinitis and nasal polyps, eliminate as many allergens in your environment as possible. Prepare your bedroom as follows:
- Empty the room of furniture, rugs or carpet, and drapes or curtains.
- Clean the walls, woodwork and floors with a damp mop. Wax the floor.
- Take the mattress and box springs outside and vacuum or clean them. Cover the box springs, mattress and pillows with plastic covers.
- Use only rugs that can be washed weekly.
- Use bedclothes that can be washed often, such as cotton sheets, washable mattress pads and synthetic fiber blankets. Don't use chenille bedspreads, quilts or comforters.
- Use wood or plastic chairs—not stuffed chairs. Use plastic curtains, if possible. Dust them daily.
- Keep windows and doors closed.
- Don't handle objects that are very dusty, such as books, stored clothing or stuffed toys.
- Remove all pets (except fish) from the house.

MEDICATION
- To reduce the body's allergic response, your doctor may prescribe: antihistamines; decongestants; corticosteroid eye drops or nasal spray; corticosteroid tablets (severe cases only); or cromolyn nasal spray. These medications relieve symptoms, but they don't cure hay fever.
- Densensitization injections may be helpful for known allergens.
- If surgery is necessary, your doctor may prescribe pain relievers and antibiotics to prevent or treat post-surgical infection.

ACTIVITY—No restrictions except those imposed by the obstruction.

DIET—No special diet.

 CALL YOUR DOCTOR IF

- You have severe symptoms of nasal obstruction that are interfering with your normal activities, including sports performance.
- You have allergies and develop signs of infection, such as fever, headache, muscle aches, or thick, discolored nasal discharge.
- New, unexplained symptoms develop. Drugs used in treatment may produce side effects.

NOSEBLEED
(Epistaxis)

GENERAL INFORMATION

DEFINITION—Bleeding from the nose. This is common in athletes who participate in contact or collision sports, especially football, boxing, wrestling or hockey.

SIGNS & SYMPTOMS
- Blood oozing or gushing from the nostril. If the nosebleed is close to the nostril, the blood is bright red. If the nosebleed is deeper in the nose, the blood may be bright or dark.
- Lightheadedness from blood loss.
- Rapid heartbeat, shortness of breath and pallor (with significant blood loss only.)

CAUSES & RISK FACTORS
- Injury to the nose.
- Nasal or sinus infection.
- Nasal polyps or a foreign body in the nose.
- Use of certain drugs, such as anticoagulants, aspirin, or prolonged use of nose drops.
- Exposure to irritating chemicals.
- High altitude or dry climate.
- Dry nasal membranes from any cause.
- Atherosclerosis (hardening of the arteries).
- High blood pressure.
- Bleeding tendencies associated with aplastic anemia, leukemia, hemophilia, thrombocytopenia or liver disease.
- Hodgkin's disease.
- Scarlet fever.
- Scurvy.
- Rheumatic fever.

HOW TO PREVENT
- Avoid injury if possible. Use appropriate equipment to protect the face and head.
- Obtain medical treatment for any known underlying cause.
- Humidify the air if you live in a dry climate or at high altitude.

WHAT TO EXPECT

DIAGNOSTIC MEASURES
- Your own observation of symptoms.
- Medical history and exam by a doctor.
- Laboratory blood studies.

SURGERY—May be necessary in cases of severe bleeding to tie off the artery feeding the bleeding area.

NORMAL COURSE OF ILLNESS—Symptoms can be controlled with treatment. Severe bleeding requires hospitalization and usually is caused by an underlying disorder, such as liver disease, blood disease or hypertension. In these cases, the disorder must also be treated.

POSSIBLE COMPLICATIONS
- Bleeding severe enough to require transfusion.
- Nasal and sinus infections.

HOW TO TREAT

NOTE—Follow your doctor's instructions. These instructions are supplemental.

MEDICAL TREATMENT
- Doctor's or emergency-room treatment if there is a nose fracture or other injury, or if home treatment is unsuccessful. Gauze packing may be inserted to absorb blood, stop dripping and exert pressure on the ruptured blood vessels. Continued bleeding may require cauterization (see Glossary) and packing.
- Surgery (for severe bleeding only).

HOME TREATMENT—If there has been no serious injury to the nose:
- Sit up with your head bent forward.
- Clamp your nose closed with your fingers for 5 uninterrupted minutes. During this time, breathe through your mouth.
- If bleeding stops and recurs, repeat—but pinch your nose firmly on both sides for 8 to 10 minutes. Holding your nose tightly closed allows the blood to clot and seal the damaged blood vessels.
- You may apply cold compresses at the same time.
- Don't blow your nose for 12 hours after bleeding stops because you may dislodge the blood clot.
- Don't swallow blood. It may upset your stomach, or make you "gag" or vomit, causing you to inhale blood.
- Don't talk excessively, laugh or sing. These may cause gagging.

MEDICATION—Your doctor may prescribe drugs to treat any underlying serious disorder.

ACTIVITY—Resume your normal activities when bleeding has stopped for 24 hours.

DIET—No special diet.

CALL YOUR DOCTOR IF

- You have a nosebleed that won't stop with home treatment described above.
- After the nosebleed, you become nauseated or vomit.
- After the nose has been packed, your temperature rises to 101F (38.3C) or higher.
- Renewed bleeding or signs of infection (fever and a general ill feeling) begin after surgery.

OSGOOD-SCHLATTER DISEASE
(Osteochondrosis)

 GENERAL INFORMATION

DEFINITION—"Growing pain" at the knee, a temporary condition affecting adolescents who exercise vigorously. The powerful quadriceps muscles of the thigh attach to the lower leg bone (tibia) at a growth zone, a relatively vulnerable area of bone. Pain, tenderness and swelling occur at this point with repeated stress. Sometimes both knees are affected.

SIGNS & SYMPTOMS
● Pain following an extended period of vigorous exercise in an adolescent. In more severe cases, pain occurs during less vigorous activity, especially straightening the leg against force, as in stair-climbing, jumping, doing deep knee bends or weight-lifting.
● A slightly swollen, warm and tender bump below the knee.

CAUSES & RISK FACTORS
● Repeated, overzealous conditioning routines, such as running, jumping or jogging.
● Overweight.

HOW TO PREVENT
● Help an overweight child or adolescent lose weight.
● Encourage your child to exercise moderately, avoiding extremes.

 WHAT TO EXPECT

DIAGNOSTIC MEASURES
● Your own observation of symptoms.
● Medical history and physical exam by a doctor.
● X-ray of the knee.

SURGERY—Necessary only in severe cases in which a bone fragment forms and remains painful after growth has ceased.

NORMAL COURSE OF ILLNESS
● Mild cases can be "lived with" successfully with some reduction of activity level.
● Moderate to severe cases may require significantly reduced activity and immobilization for 4 to 8 months.
● No permanent defects are expected.

POSSIBLE COMPLICATIONS
● Bone infection.
● Development of bone fragment (ossicle) below the affected knee.
● Recurrence of the condition in adulthood.

 HOW TO TREAT

NOTE—Follow your doctor's instructions. These instructions are supplemental.

MEDICAL TREATMENT—Not necessary for mild cases. For moderate or severe cases, the knee may be immobilized with a cast for approximately 2 months.

HOME TREATMENT
● Use heat to relieve pain. Warm compresses, heating pads, warm whirlpool baths and heat lamps are effective.
● Wear a knee pad below the knee during exercise.
● Apply ice to the affected area immediately before and after exercise (if your doctor has cleared you for increased activity).
● Avoid kneeling.

MEDICATION
● For minor discomfort, you may use non-prescription drugs such as aspirin or ibuprofen.
● Your doctor may prescribe corticosteroid injections if other treatment fails. Injections may weaken tendons. Avoid them if possible to allow the condition more time to heal with rest and simpler treatment.

ACTIVITY—If pain is incapacitating, resting the affected leg is the most important treatment. This is done with:
● Crutches.
● A leg cast or splint.
● An elastic knee brace that prevents the knee from bending fully.
● During treatment, don't participate in sports that cause pain. Consider switching to a sport that does not cause the same stresses on the knee. The condition is usually temporary, and normal activity can be resumed when inflammation subsides. Mild to moderate activity up to point of pain can sometimes be pursued during treatment phase. Check with your doctor.

DIET—No special diet. Lose weight back to normal if you are overweight.

 CALL YOUR DOCTOR IF

● You have symptoms of Osgood-Schlatter disease.
● The following occurs during treatment:
  Symptoms don't improve in 4 weeks, despite treatment.
  Pain increases.
  Temperature rises to 101F (38.3C)

OSTEOPOROSIS

 GENERAL INFORMATION

DEFINITION—Loss of normal bone density, mass and strength, leading to increased porousness and vulnerability to fracture. This is rare in men. It is most likely to develop in women after menopause, particularly women who lead sedentary lives and have insufficient calcium intake. Conversely, osteoporosis at an early age is also likely in women who exercise so strenuously (such as marathon runners) that menstrual periods cease and estrogen production declines.

SIGNS & SYMPTOMS
Early stages:
● Backache.
● No symptoms (often).
Later stages:
● Fractures, especially of the hip or arm, occurring after minor injury.
● Deformed spinal column with humps, leading to loss of height.

CAUSES & RISK FACTORS—Loss of bony structure and strength. Factors include:
● Prolonged lack of adequate calcium and protein in the diet.
● Long-term, excessive exercise in women.
● Low estrogen levels after menopause.
● Decreased activity with increased age.
● Smoking (possibly).
● Use of corticosteroid drugs.
● Prolonged disease, including alcoholism.
● Vitamin deficiency (especially of vitamin D).
● Hyperthyroidism.
● Cancer that spreads to bone.
● Surgery to remove the ovaries.
● Radiation treatment for ovarian cancer.
● Chronic or recurrent urinary-tract or other pelvic infections.
● Family history of osteoporosis.
● Body type. Thin women with a small frame are more susceptible.
● Genetic factors. Caucasian or Oriental women are most at risk.

HOW TO PREVENT
● Moderate exercise helps prevent or reverse osteoporosis by making bones thicker and stronger. Begin an exercise program before menopause and continue for life. Get clearance from your doctor before beginning.
● Ensure an adequate calcium intake—approximately 1500mg a day—with milk and milk products or calcium supplements.
● Protect yourself against falls, especially in the home.
● Consult your doctor about taking estrogen, calcium and fluoride after menopause begins or the ovaries have been removed—even if you have no signs of osteoporosis.

 WHAT TO EXPECT

DIAGNOSTIC MEASURES
● Your own observation of symptoms.
● Medical history and exam by a doctor.
● X-rays of bones and blood studies.

NORMAL COURSE OF ILLNESS—Diet, calcium and fluoride supplements, vitamin D, exercise and estrogen can halt progress of the disease. Fractures heal slowly with treatment.

POSSIBLE COMPLICATIONS—Bone fracture after a fall. The hip and spine are most vulnerable. Fractured hips require surgery. Sometimes a bone will break or collapse without injury or a fall.

 HOW TO TREAT

NOTE—Follow your doctor's instructions. These instructions are supplemental.

MEDICAL TREATMENT—If estrogen is prescribed, visit your doctor for regular pelvic exams, breast exams and Pap smears. Examine your breasts for lumps once a month. Report vaginal bleeding or discharge.

HOME TREATMENT
● If you already have osteoporosis, avoid all circumstances that may lead to injury. Stay off icy streets and wet or waxed floors.
● Use heat or ice in any form to ease pain.
● Sleep on a firm mattress.
● Use a back brace, if prescribed by your doctor.
● Use correct posture when lifting.

ACTIVITY—Stay active, but avoid the risk of falls. Exercise—especially weight-bearing exercise, such as walking or running—helps maintain bone strength.

MEDICATION
● You may use non-prescription drugs such as acetaminophen to relieve minor pain.
● Your doctor may prescribe:
   Calcium and vitamin D.
   Fluoride.
   Estrogen-replacement therapy.

DIET—Eat a normal, well-balanced diet high in protein, calcium and vitamin D.

 CALL YOUR DOCTOR IF

● You have symptoms of osteoporosis.
● Pain develops, especially after injury.
● New, unexplained symptoms develop, such as vaginal bleeding. Drugs used in treatment may produce side effects.

PITYRIASIS VERSICOLOR
(Tinea Versicolor)

 GENERAL INFORMATION

DEFINITION—A yeast infection of the skin that changes the color of skin it affects. It usually affects skin of the chest, back, shoulders, upper arms, trunk or groin.

SIGNS & SYMPTOMS—Lesions with the following characteristics:
- Lesions on exposed skin are white; on covered areas, they are brown or brownish red.
- Lesions are flat with clearly defined borders. They don't scale unless scraped.
- Lesions begin at 3mm to 4mm in diameter and spread. They often join together to form large patches.

CAUSES & RISK FACTORS
- Infection with the developing stage of a yeast, *pityrosborum orbiculare*. The infection is contagious, but how it spreads is unknown.
- Environmental exposure to heat and high humidity make infection more likely.
- Repeated injury to the skin of athletes increases the likelihood due to excessive perspiration, increased heat, friction of clothing and protective gear.

HOW TO PREVENT—No known prevention. Avoid risk factors when possible.

 WHAT TO EXPECT

DIAGNOSTIC MEASURES
- Your own observation of symptoms.
- Medical history and physical exam by a doctor.
- Laboratory culture of scrapings for positive diagnosis.

SURGERY—Not necessary nor helpful for this disease

NORMAL COURSE OF ILLNESS— Untreated pityriasis versicolor persists indefinitely but seems to come and go unpredictably. It frequently recurs, even with treatment. Following treatment, the white patches will remain for months after the yeast infection has been cured. These white patches become more prominent when the surrounding skin becomes tanned from exposure to the sun.

POSSIBLE COMPLICATIONS—Unlimited recurrence without treatment.

 HOW TO TREAT

NOTE—Follow your doctor's instructions. These instructions are supplemental.

MEDICAL TREATMENT—None necessary after diagnosis and prescription of special medications.

HOME TREATMENT
- Apply prescribed medicine with cotton balls to affected parts once a day for 3 weeks. Rinse off in 30 minutes if you wish.
- Expose affected skin to air as much as possible.
- Repeat treatment prior to tanning season each year.

MEDICATION—Your doctor may prescribe:
- Selenium sulfide shampoo to use in one of two ways:
  One 6- to 12-hour application and reapplication in 1 week.
  One daily application of 15 to 30 minutes for 10 to 14 days.
- An alternate antifungal medication, such as sodium thiosulfate or imidazole. This is applied to the involved area twice daily for 10 days.

ACTIVITY—No restrictions.

DIET—No special diet.

 CALL YOUR DOCTOR IF

- You have symptoms of pityriasis versicolor.
- Infection doesn't improve despite treatment.

PLANTAR NEUROMA
(Morton's Toe)

 GENERAL INFORMATION

DEFINITION—A small benign tumor in the nerve that serves the 2nd, 3rd and 4th toes. It may affect one or both feet.

SIGNS & SYMPTOMS
Early stages:
● Excruciating pain in the front part of the foot, particularly when running or bearing weight while jumping, turning or dancing.
Later stages:
● Localized pain in the sides of the 3rd and 4th toes (usually). Pain occurs suddenly when least expected. Removing the shoe and massaging the painful area brings dramatic relief almost immediately. Pain is less when barefooted.
● Tenderness at the base of the 3rd and 4th toes.
● Feelings of electric shock or numbness running out into one or both toes.

CAUSES & RISK FACTORS
● Relaxation of the ligaments of the foot causing thickening of the plantar nerve.
● Ill-fitting shoes (possibly), particularly shoes used for athletic activity.
● Repeated foot injuries.
● Obesity and poor nutrition.
● Recent or chronic illness.
● If surgery is used for treatment, surgical risk increases with: smoking; use of drugs such as antihypertensives, muscle relaxants, tranquilizers, sleep inducers, insulin, sedatives, beta-adrenergic blockers or cortisone; use of mind-altering drugs, including narcotics, psychedelics, hallucinogens, marijuana, sedatives, hypnotics or cocaine.

HOW TO PREVENT—Unknown.

 WHAT TO EXPECT

DIAGNOSTIC MEASURES
● Before surgery: Blood and urine studies; X-rays of the foot.
● After surgery: Laboratory examination of removed tissue.

SURGERY—Necessary to remove the neuroma if conservative treatment fails.

NORMAL COURSE OF ILLNESS—Treatment with a metatarsal bar in the shoe usually relieves pain, although the tumor will remain until removed surgically. If surgery is necessary, allow about 3 weeks for recovery.

POSSIBLE COMPLICATIONS—Continuous pain and partial disability if the tumor is untreated. Complications following surgery include excessive bleeding and surgical-wound infection.

 HOW TO TREAT

NOTE—Follow your doctor's instructions. These instructions are supplemental.

MEDICAL TREATMENT—Your doctor may prescribe a trial treatment with a metatarsal bar in the shoe. If this fails, surgery will be necessary.

HOME TREATMENT—After surgery, the foot will be snugly wrapped in a bandage. Keep the bandage dry and the foot elevated as much as possible during recovery. After removal of bandages, apply heat with soaks, tub baths or heat lamps. When healed, massage with ice for 10 minutes before and after vigorous physical activity.

MEDICATION—After surgery, your doctor may prescribe:
● Pain relievers. Don't take prescription pain medication longer than 4 to 7 days. Use only as much as you need.
● Antibiotics to fight infection.
● Non-prescription drugs, such as acetaminophen, for minor pain.

ACTIVITY—No restrictions except those imposed by foot pain. After surgery, avoid vigorous exercise for 6 weeks. Gradually return to light activity after clearance from your doctor once the bandage is removed.

DIET—No special diet.

 CALL YOUR DOCTOR IF

● You have signs and symptoms of plantar neuroma.
● Any of the following occur after surgery:
Pain, swelling, redness, drainage or bleeding increases in the surgical area.
You develop signs of infection (headache, muscle aches, dizziness or a general ill feeling and fever).
New, unexplained symptoms develop. Drugs used in treatment may produce side effects.

PNEUMONIA, BACTERIAL

 ## GENERAL INFORMATION

DEFINITION—Infection and inflammation of the lungs with bacterial germs. Respiratory disorders of this type are the most common non-injury disorder seen in athletes.This is not usually contagious. Pneumonia is especially likely during cold or harsh weather, or with exhaustive exercise prior to developing sufficient cardiovascular-respiratory conditioning.

SIGNS & SYMPTOMS
- High fever (over 102F or 38.9C) and chills.
- Shortness of breath.
- Cough with sputum that may contain blood or blood streaks.
- Rapid breathing.
- Chest pain that worsens with inhalations or exercise.
- Abdominal pain.
- Fatigue.
- Bluish lips and nails in advanced, untreated pneumonia (rare).

CAUSES & RISK FACTORS—Infection with
bacteria, such as *pneumococci, hemophilus, streptococci* or *staphylococci,* especially in those athletes who smoke or have recently had an illness that lowered resistance.

HOW TO PREVENT
- Obtain prompt medical treatment for respiratory infections (except for uncomplicated common colds).
- Arrange for pneumococcal and influenza immunizations if you are in a high-risk group. Persons at risk include those with heart disease, cancer, tuberculosis, congestive heart failure, diabetes, alcoholism, chronic lung disease or who have had recent surgery.

 ## WHAT TO EXPECT

DIAGNOSTIC MEASURES
- Your own observation of symptoms.
- Medical history and exam by a doctor.
- Laboratory studies, including sputum culture, blood culture and blood count.
- X-rays of the lungs.

NORMAL COURSE OF ILLNESS— Usually
curable in 1 to 2 weeks with treatment, but may take longer for older persons.

POSSIBLE COMPLICATIONS
- Pleurisy.
- Lung abscess.
- Pleural effusion (fluid between the membranes that cover the lung).
- Spread of infection to the brain or meninges (meningitis).
- Prolonged healing or relapse due to resuming activity too soon.

 ## HOW TO TREAT

NOTE—Follow your doctor's instructions. These instructions are supplemental.

MEDICAL TREATMENT—Hospitalization is sometimes necessary for severe cases. Otherwise bacterial pneumonia may be treated at home following doctor's instructions.

HOME TREATMENT
- Use a cool-mist humidifier to increase air moisture. This helps thin lung secretions so they can be coughed out more easily. Putting medicine in the humidifier probably will not help. Wash the humidifier with warm water and detergent at least once a day to prevent growth of harmful germs.
- Don't suppress the cough with medicine if the cough produces discolored or clear sputum or mucus. It is useful in ridding the body of lung secretions.
- Suppress the cough with medicine if it is dry, non-productive and painful. Consult your doctor about a cough suppressant.
- Use a heating pad or hot compresses to relieve chest pain.

MEDICATION
- Your doctor may prescribe:
  Antibiotics to fight infection.
  Cough suppressants.
- You may use non-prescription drugs such as acetaminophen to relieve minor discomfort.

ACTIVITY—Rest in bed until fever declines and pain and shortness of breath disappear. You may read or watch TV. After treatment, resume normal activity and exercise at reduced levels until your strength returns.

DIET—No special diet. Increase fluid intake. Drink at least 1 glass of water or other beverage every hour. Extra fluid helps thin lung secretions.

 ## CALL YOUR DOCTOR IF

- You have symptoms of pneumonia.
- The following occurs during treatment:
  Fever higher than 102F (38.9C).
  Pain not relieved by heat or prescribed medication.
  Increased shortness of breath.
  Dark or bluish fingernails, skin or toenails.
  Blood in the sputum.
  Nausea, vomiting or diarrhea.
  New, unexplained symptoms. Drugs used in treatment may produce side effects.

PNEUMONIA, VIRAL

GENERAL INFORMATION

DEFINITION—Lung infection caused by a virus. It is unlikely that others will develop pneumonia from exposure to a person with viral pneumonia. Respiratory infections of all sorts constitute the most common non-injury disorder seen among those who exercise. This is especially true with team sports, with exposure to cold or harsh weather, or with exhaustive exercise before developing sufficient cardiovascular-pulmonary conditioning.

SIGNS & SYMPTOMS
- Fever and chills.
- Nasal stuffiness.
- Muscle aches and fatigue.
- Cough, with or without sputum.
- Rapid, labored (sometimes) breathing.
- Chest pain.
- Sore throat.
- Loss of appetite.
- Enlarged lymph glands in the neck.
- Bluish nails in advanced, untreated viral pneumonia (rare).

CAUSES & RISK FACTORS—Viral pneumonia is caused by a virus infection, including influenza, chickenpox (especially in adults), common cold viruses, and measles or other systemic virus infections. These viruses are most likely to cause pneumonia in those who:
- Are over age 60.
- Have asthma.
- Have cystic fibrosis.
- Have inhaled a foreign body into the lung.
- Smoke.
- Live in crowded or unsanitary conditions, or use an unsanitary locker room.

HOW TO PREVENT
- Avoid anyone with a viral illness.
- Avoid overexertion, and condition your entire body, including the cardiovascular-pulmonary system, before engaging in strenuous sports.

WHAT TO EXPECT

DIAGNOSTIC MEASURES
- Your own observation of symptoms.
- Medical history and physical exam by a doctor.
- Laboratory blood studies.
- X-rays of the chest.

SURGERY—Not necessary nor useful for this disease.

NORMAL COURSE OF ILLNESS— Usually curable in 4 weeks if no complications occur.

POSSIBLE COMPLICATIONS
- Secondary bacterial infection of the lungs.
- Post-infectious depression.

HOW TO TREAT

NOTE—Follow your doctor's instructions. These instructions are supplemental.

MEDICAL TREATMENT—None usually necessary, except for hospitalization in rare cases.

HOME TREATMENT
- Use a cool-mist humidifier to increase air moisture. This helps thin lung secretions so they can be coughed out more easily. Keep the humidifier clean.
- Use a heating pad on the chest to relieve chest pain.

MEDICATION
- If the cough produces sputum, it is ridding the lungs of secretions and should not be suppressed with medicine. If the cough is dry, non-productive and painful, you may suppress it with non-prescription cough medicine that contains dextromethorphan.
- For minor nasal congestion, pain and fever, you may use non-prescription drugs such as acetaminophen or decongestant nose drops, nasal sprays or tablets.
- Your doctor may prescribe antibiotics to fight secondary bacterial infections or stronger cough suppressants.

ACTIVITY—Bed rest is necessary until fever, pain and shortness of breath have been gone at least 48 hours. Then normal activity may be resumed slowly. Many people are fatigued and weak for up to 6 weeks after recovery, so don't expect a quick return to normal strength or normal exercise tolerance.

DIET—No special diet, but do everything possible to maintain a normal intake of nutritious foods and drinks. Drink at least 1 full glass of fluid each hour. This helps thin lung secretions.

CALL YOUR DOCTOR IF

- You have symptoms of pneumonia.
- The following occurs during treatment:
  Temperature spike over 102F (38.9C).
  Intolerable pain, despite medication and heat treatment.
  Increasing shortness of breath.
  Increasing blueness of nails and skin.
  Blood in the sputum.
  Nausea, vomiting or diarrhea.

PNEUMOTHORAX

GENERAL INFORMATION

DEFINITION—Collapse of part or all of a lung caused by pressure from free air in the chest between the two layers of the pleura (thin membranes that cover the lung). Peak incidence is in males between ages 20 to 40.

SIGNS & SYMPTOMS—The following symptoms vary according to the degree of lung collapse and extent of underlying lung disease. Symptoms may be less acute if the pneumothorax develops slowly:
- Sharp chest pain. Pain may extend to a shoulder or across the chest or abdomen.
- Shortness of breath and rapid breathing.
- Dry, hacking cough (occasionally).
- Bluish nails.
- Coughing bloody sputum (sometimes).
- Rapid pulse.
- In worst cases (tension pneumothorax), fainting and shock.

CAUSES & RISK FACTORS
Spontaneous pneumothorax:
- Physical exertion in a healthy individual, with no obvious preceding injury, infection or disease. Activities most likely to produce pneumothorax include:
   Ascent while scuba diving.
   Diving or high-altitude flying.
   Activities that require stretching the chest and rib cage, such as track and field events, throwing sports and bowling.
- Rupture of small air sacs in the lung. Asthma, emphysema, chronic bronchitis, lung abscess, empyema, or other lung disease may cause the rupture of air sacs.
Pneumothorax due to trauma:
- Penetrating wound to the chest, which permits outside air to rush into the pleural space and causes the lung to collapse.
- Complication of removing fluid from the lung (thoracentesis).

HOW TO PREVENT
- Learn and use proper techniques for activities at risk listed above (especially ascending in scuba diving).
- Obtain medical treatment for lung disorders such as asthma or emphysema.
- Don't smoke.

WHAT TO EXPECT

DIAGNOSTIC MEASURES
- Your own observation of symptoms.
- Medical history and physical exam by a doctor.
- X-rays of the chest to confirm the diagnosis.

SURGERY—Sometimes necessary to remove free air that has leaked out of the lungs into the chest.

NORMAL COURSE OF ILLNESS—A small pneumothorax is inconsequential and heals itself. However, if the collapse is extensive and it occurs in middle-aged or older adults whose lungs are damaged by asthma, chronic bronchitis or emphysema, it can lead to respiratory failure and critical illness. Treatment depends on the size of the pneumothorax and the condition of the lungs.

POSSIBLE COMPLICATIONS
- Respiratory failure.
- Lung infection.
- Recurrence of pneumothorax. If it is going to recur, 20% to 40% of cases usually do so within 2 years of initial pneumothorax.

HOW TO TREAT

NOTE—Follow your doctor's instructions. These instructions are supplemental.

MEDICAL TREATMENT—Hospitalization and treatment with special equipment following minor surgery may be necessary.

HOME TREATMENT
- Don't exercise during healing, but resume normal activities—including the one that triggered the pneumothorax—after clearance from your doctor.
- Don't smoke.
- Try not to cough.
- Avoid loud talking, laughing or singing.
- You may be more comfortable if you rest in a sitting or semi-reclining position.

MEDICATION—Medication usually is not necessary. However, you may use non-prescription drugs such as acetaminophen for minor pain. For severe pain, your doctor may prescribe stronger pain relievers.

ACTIVITY—Stay as active as your strength allows. Rest often. Resume your normal activities as soon as possible. Allow about 2 to 3 weeks for lung to re-expand. Allow 6 weeks before returning to maximal exercise.

DIET—No special diet.

CALL YOUR DOCTOR IF

- You have symptoms of pneumothorax.
- The following occurs during treatment:
   Temperature rises to 101F (38.3C).
   Chest pain or shortness of breath increases.
   Painful, debilitating coughing or sputum production begins.

POTASSIUM IMBALANCE

GENERAL INFORMATION

DEFINITION—Above-normal levels (hyperkalemia) or below-normal levels (hypokalemia) of potassium in the blood, body fluids and body cells.

SIGNS & SYMPTOMS
Hypokalemia:
- Muscle cramps, particularly following or accompanying exercise.
- Weakness and paralysis.
- Low blood pressure.
- Life-threatening rapid, irregular heartbeat. This is more severe than with hyperkalemia.

Hyperkalemia:
- Weakness and paralysis.
- Dangerously rapid, irregular heartbeat or slow heartbeat (sometimes).
- Nausea and diarrhea.

CAUSES & RISK FACTORS
Hypokalemia:
- The use of diuretic drugs for any purpose. Taking diuretics is a frequent—but unwise and unethical—practice among athletes who must meet a certain weight limit before competing (jockeys, boxers, wrestlers).
- Prolonged loss of body fluids from vomiting or diarrhea.
- Chronic kidney disease with kidney failure. At certain stages, this may cause the body to lose potassium.
- Uncontrolled diabetes mellitus.
- Adrenal disease.
- Use of drugs, including diuretics, potassium supplements and digitalis. Low potassium levels—especially in persons who take digitalis—often lead to serious heartbeat disturbances.

Hyperkalemia:
- Chronic kidney disease with kidney failure. Failing kidneys eliminate potassium too slowly, causing an excess in the body.
- Use of oral potassium supplements without monitoring of potassium levels.
- Burns or crushing injuries. These may cause potassium to be released from body tissues into body fluids.

HOW TO PREVENT
- If you have a disorder or take drugs that affect potassium levels (see Causes & Risk Factors), learn as much as you can about your condition, your drugs and how you can prevent a potassium imbalance.
- If you take digitalis and diuretics, have frequent blood studies to monitor potassium levels.
- For prolonged vomiting or diarrhea, reduce athletic activities and seek medical care.

OTHER—A medium to high blood level of potassium (in the normal range) may help protect against coronary-artery disease.

WHAT TO EXPECT

DIAGNOSTIC MEASURES
- Your own observation of symptoms, especially muscle weakness and heart-rhythm changes.
- Medical history and exam by a doctor.
- Laboratory blood and urine studies of potassium, sodium and other electrolytes.
- EKG (see Glossary).

NORMAL COURSE OF ILLNESS—Usually can be corrected with intravenous fluids and treatment of the underlying disorder.

POSSIBLE COMPLICATIONS—Cardiac arrest and death.

HOW TO TREAT

NOTE—Follow your doctor's instructions. These instructions are supplemental.

MEDICAL TREATMENT
- Monitoring of blood potassium levels, treatment of underlying disorders and prescription of medications by a doctor.
- Hospitalization (severe cases).

HOME TREATMENT—If you take diuretics and digitalis, your friends and family members should learn cardiopulmonary resuscitation (CPR). Learn to count your own pulse at the wrist or neck, and report significant variations to your doctor.

MEDICATION—Your doctor may prescribe:
- Oral potassium supplements to raise low levels.
- Diuretics to increase urination and decrease high potassium levels.
- Intravenous fluids to correct a serious imbalance.
- Medications appropriate for the underlying disease.

ACTIVITY—Resume your normal activities after clearance from your doctor when symptoms improve.

DIET—Depends on the condition. Mild hypokalemia can be corrected by increasing consumption of potassium-containing foods, such as apricots, cantaloupes, bananas and citrus. There is no special diet for hyperkalemia.

CALL YOUR DOCTOR IF

You have symptoms of a potassium imbalance or are having problems with a disorder that affects potassium levels.

PULMONARY EMBOLISM

GENERAL INFORMATION

DEFINITION—A blood clot or fat cells that block one of the arteries carrying blood to the lungs. The blood clot usually begins in an inflamed deep vein of the leg or pelvis (phlebitis). A fat embolus usually begins at a fracture site. This blockage decreases breathing ability and sometimes destroys lung tissue.

SIGNS & SYMPTOMS
- Sudden shortness of breath.
- Faintness or fainting.
- Pain in the chest.
- Cough (sometimes with bloody sputum).
- Rapid heartbeat.
- Low fever.

These symptoms are often preceded by swelling and pain in the leg or thigh.

CAUSES & RISK FACTORS—Clots are most likely to form in association with any of the following:
- Injury to the pelvis, thigh or leg, especially dislocations, contusions and fractures.
- Use of oral contraceptives, especially in women over age 35.
- Any injury, illness or surgery that requires prolonged bed rest. This can lead to pooling of blood in veins.
- Sitting in one position for a prolonged period.
- Heart-rhythm disturbance.
- Hemolytic anemia.
- Polycythemia (see Glossary).
- Smoking.
- Pregnancy.

HOW TO PREVENT
- Observe safety regulations and wear protective equipment for contact sports to prevent injury whenever possible.
- Don't smoke, especially if you are a woman 35 or older who takes birth-control pills.
- Avoid prolonged bed rest during illnesses. Wear elastic support stockings during recuperation from surgery or illness. Start moving lower limbs and walking as soon as possible.
- When traveling, stand and walk every 2 hours.

WHAT TO EXPECT

DIAGNOSTIC MEASURES
- Medical history and exam by a doctor.
- Laboratory blood studies to regulate anticoagulant medication dose.
- X-rays of the chest.
- CAT scan (see Glossary) and radioactive studies to establish presence and extent of a clot in the lung.

SURGERY—(Rare) To tie off the big vein

leading to the heart and lungs (vena cava) or for insertion of a filter to trap recurrent clots.

NORMAL COURSE OF ILLNESS—Usually curable in 10 to 14 days with treatment.

POSSIBLE COMPLICATIONS
- Rapid death from a large clot that obstructs more than 50% of the blood to the lungs.
- Massive bleeding in the lungs caused by smaller clots.
- Congestive heart failure and chronic lung disease after repeated episodes of embolism.

HOW TO TREAT

NOTE—Follow your doctor's instructions. These instructions are supplemental.

MEDICAL TREATMENT—Hospitalization for anticoagulation, oxygen and possible surgery.

HOME TREATMENT
- Wear elastic stockings or leg wraps with elastic bandages.
- Don't sit with your legs or ankles crossed.
- Elevate your feet higher than your hips when sitting for long periods.
- Elevate the foot of your bed.

MEDICATION—Your doctor probably will prescribe anticoagulant drugs to dissolve and prevent clots. The anticoagulant level must be monitored to keep it in a safe range.

ACTIVITY
- Rest in bed until all symptoms and signs of clots and embolism disappear. While in bed, move your legs often to stimulate circulation.
- Resume light exercise only after clearance from your doctor—usually within 2 weeks. Don't participate in active exercise or training until the deep vein clot has disappeared and anticoagulants can be safely discontinued.
- It will probably be 3 or 4 additional weeks before your doctor clears you for exercise or reconditioning. Having a pulmonary embolus *does not* prevent you from participating in athletics in the future.

DIET—No special diet.

CALL YOUR DOCTOR IF

- You have symptoms of pulmonary embolism or phlebitis (vein inflammation). This is an emergency!
- The following occurs during treatment:
  Chest pain, coughing up blood or shortness of breath.
  Increased swelling and pain in the leg.
- You take anticoagulants and develop any signs of internal bleeding, such as vomiting blood, blood in stool or severe abdominal or back pain.

RINGWORM
(Tinea Infection)

 ## GENERAL INFORMATION

DEFINITION—Fungus (tinea) infection of the skin or scalp. This is transmitted by person-to-person contact or by contact with infected surfaces, such as towels, shoes or shower stalls. *Tinea corporis* affects the non-hairy skin of the body. *Tinea capitis* affects the scalp.

SIGNS & SYMPTOMS—Red, itchy, circular, flat, scaling lesions with well-defined borders. They cause patchy hair loss on the scalp.

CAUSES & RISK FACTORS—Infection with *tinea corporis* or *tinea capitis* fungus. Infection is most likely when combined with the following:
- Diabetes mellitus.
- Exposure to darkness, moisture and warmth.
- Crowded or unsanitary locker-room or living conditions.
- Repeated abrasion of the skin or scalp from friction with clothing and protective gear. An athlete is especially vulnerable during hot weather when exercising while wearing an athletic uniform or head covering such as a swimming cap, football helmet or baseball cap.

HOW TO PREVENT—The fungi are so prevalent that total prevention is impossible. To minimize risk:
- Avoid continuous exposure to overheated humid environments.
- Don't touch pets that have skin problems.

 ## WHAT TO EXPECT

DIAGNOSTIC MEASURES
- Your own observation of symptoms.
- Medical history and physical exam by a doctor.
- Microscopic exam of skin scrapings suspended in potassium hydroxide solution.
- Laboratory culture of skin scrapings.

SURGERY—Not necessary nor useful for this disease.

NORMAL COURSE OF ILLNESS—Usually curable in 6 weeks with treatment, but recurrence is common. Ringworm becomes chronic in 20% of cases.

POSSIBLE COMPLICATIONS—Secondary bacterial infection of ringworm lesions.

 ## HOW TO TREAT

NOTE—Follow your doctor's instructions. These instructions are supplemental.

MEDICAL TREATMENT—None necessary after diagnosis.

HOME TREATMENT
- Observe rules of locker-room hygiene (see Appendix 4).
- Don't use towels used by others.
- Boil or chemically sterilize all clothing, towels or bed linens that have touched the lesions.
- Keep the skin dry. Moist, dark areas favor fungus growth.
- Wear cotton underwear. Change more than once a day. Avoid tight clothes.
- If the area is red, swollen and weeping, use salt-water compresses (1 teaspoon salt to 1 pint water). Apply 4 times a day for 2 to 3 days before starting the local antifungal medication.
- Shampoo the hair every day.
- Have the hair cut short, but don't shave the scalp. Place large sheets of paper under and around the hair and chair to catch all the clippings. Place a cloth drape around the shoulders, chest and back. Don't wear street clothes for a haircut. Wear something that can be sterilized, such as pajamas, a housecoat or smock. Repeat this procedure every 2 weeks for 6 months.

MEDICATION—Your doctor may prescribe oral or topical antifungal drugs, such as imidazole creams and lotions applied twice a day for 1 month.

ACTIVITY—No restrictions.

DIET—No special diet.

 ## CALL YOUR DOCTOR IF

- You have symptoms of ringworm.
- Ringworm lesions become redder, painful and ooze pus.
- Symptoms don't improve in 3 or 4 weeks, despite treatment.
- New, unexplained symptoms develop. Drugs used in treatment may produce side effects.

RUNNER'S KNEE
(Chondromalacia Patellae)

 GENERAL INFORMATION

DEFINITION—Aching pain behind the kneecap. Pain begins and progresses slowly. It appears in healthy, athletically active young people between 12 and 35 years old, and is twice as common in women as in men. This is the most common knee problem for runners.

SIGNS & SYMPTOMS
- Soreness and aching pain around or under the kneecap, especially on the inner side. Symptoms worsen after walking or running up ramps or hills, squatting, or jumping up and running.
- "Giving way" at the knee (sometimes).
- "Water on the knee" (sometimes).

CAUSES & RISK FACTORS
- Muscle imbalance or compression at the knee that pulls the kneecap sideways out of normal alignment.
- Direct blow to the kneecap.
- Injury resulting from extreme flexing of the knee, as in squatting and kneeling.
- Congenital abnormal development in the knee.
- Overstress of the knee as can occur in any running sport, such as jogging, sprinting, football, basketball or soccer.

HOW TO PREVENT
- Strengthen and condition upper leg and hip muscles for maximum strength, flexibility and endurance before you start competition or vigorous physical activity.
- Avoid deep squats or activities that compress the kneecap.
- Don't use knee wraps for weight-lifting. Wraps increase knee compression.

 WHAT TO EXPECT

DIAGNOSTIC MEASURES
- Your own observation of symptoms.
- Medical history and exam by a doctor.
- X-rays of the knee to rule out fracture. Special views can reveal misalignment or tilting of the patella.

SURGERY—Sometimes necessary as a last resort. In surgery, cartilage is shaved using an arthroscope (see Glossary). Open-knee surgery may be necessary to realign the kneecap.

NORMAL COURSE OF ILLNESS—With successful treatment, 80% should be able to return to vigorous physical activity. In the remaining 20%, the condition will return if vigorous activity is resumed.

POSSIBLE COMPLICATIONS—Non-healing with conservative measures, leading to a need for surgery (a last resort).

 HOW TO TREAT

NOTE—Follow your doctor's instructions. These instructions are supplemental.

MEDICAL TREATMENT
- Often none is necessary after diagnosis and prescription of medications and special shoes (sometimes).
- Rehabilitation of the quadriceps muscles and hamstrings is sometimes necessary following surgery.

HOME TREATMENT
- Rest is essential. Trying to "work through" or "run through" pain worsens the condition.
- Don't kneel or climb stairs unless you must.
- Apply ice bags for 10 minutes 3 or 4 times a day for 3 to 4 days.
- After ice treatments end, apply heat frequently. Use heat lamps, hot soaks, hot showers, heating pads, or heat liniments and ointments.
- Your doctor may prescribe orthotic shoe devices, knee straps or braces.

MEDICATION—Your doctor may prescribe aspirin, ibuprofen or other non-steroidal anti-inflammatory medicine.

ACTIVITY—When pain has subsided, start on quadriceps drills for rehabilitation (see page 471). Resume athletic training when the injured leg reaches 75% of the strength of the other leg.

DIET—Eat a well-balanced diet that includes extra protein, such as meat, fish, poultry, cheese, milk and eggs. Increase fiber and fluid intake to prevent constipation that may result from decreased activity.

 CALL YOUR DOCTOR IF

You have symptoms of runner's knee that don't improve after resting for 2 or 3 days.

SCABIES

 GENERAL INFORMATION

DEFINITION—A disease of the skin caused by a parasitic mite (the "itch" mite) with a characteristic pattern of distribution involving skin of the finger webs and folds under the arms, breasts, elbows, genitals and buttocks. Scabies is contagious from person to person (by shared clothing or bed linen) and from one site to another in the same person. Outbreaks are likely among teammates using crowded locker facilities.

SIGNS & SYMPTOMS
● Small, itchy blisters in several parts of the body. The blisters break easily when scratched.
● Broken blisters leave scratch marks and thickened skin, crisscrossed by grooves and scaling.

CAUSES & RISK FACTORS—Infestation by a mite that burrows into deep skin layers, where the female mite deposits eggs. Eggs mature into adult mites in 3 weeks. Mites are 0.1mm in diameter and can only be seen under a microscope. Scratching collects mites and eggs under the fingernails, so they spread to other parts of the body. Spreading increases with crowded or unsanitary living conditions.

HOW TO PREVENT
● Avoid contact with persons or linen and clothing that you suspect may be infected with scabies.
● Maintain personal cleanliness: Bathe daily, or at least 2 or 3 times a week.
● Wash hands before eating.
● Launder clothes often.
● Observe the rules of locker-room hygiene (see Appendix 4).

 WHAT TO EXPECT

DIAGNOSTIC MEASURES
● Your own observation of symptoms.
● Medical history and physical exam by a doctor. The diagnosis is confirmed by discovering the mite, lifting it with a needle or sharp scalpel point from its burrow, and identifying it under a microscope.

SURGERY—Not necessary nor useful with this disease.

NORMAL COURSE OF ILLNESS— Itching usually disappears quickly, and evidence of the disease is gone in 1 to 2 weeks with treatment. If skin irritation persists longer than this, oral antihistamines or topical steroids may be necessary to break the itch-scratch cycle. When untreated, scabies can last for years.

POSSIBLE COMPLICATIONS—Secondary bacterial infection of mite-infested areas of inflammation.

 HOW TO TREAT

NOTE—Follow your doctor's instructions. These instructions are supplemental.

MEDICAL TREATMENT—None necessary after diagnosis.

HOME TREATMENT
● Bathe thoroughly before applying the prescribed medicine.
● Apply medicine from the neck down, and cover the entire body.
● Wait 15 minutes before dressing.
● Carefully wash all clothes and toys used prior to or during treatment. You don't need to clean furniture or floors with special care.
● Leave medicine on the skin for 2 hours before bathing.
● You may need to repeat in 1 week. Ask your doctor.
● If many members of a team are infested, it will be most effective to treat the entire team, including those without symptoms, at one time. Lockers should also be disinfected.

MEDICATION—Your doctor may prescribe a pediculocide such as gamma benzene hexachloride or crotamiton cream. Infants and pregnant women may need a pediculocide that is less toxic, such as a 6% solution of sulfur.

ACTIVITY—No restrictions.

DIET—No special diet.

 CALL YOUR DOCTOR IF

● You have symptoms of scabies.
● After treatment, the lesions show signs of infection (redness, pus, swelling or pain).
● New, unexplained symptoms develop. Drugs used in treatment may produce side effects.

SHIN SPLINTS

GENERAL INFORMATION

DEFINITION—A catchall phrase for pain in the lower leg brought on by exercise or athletic activity. The discomfort is due to inflammation of one or several body tissues. Pain worsens with exercise using the legs. The muscles (causing myositis), tendons (causing tendinitis) or the bone covering (causing periostitis) may be involved.

SIGNS & SYMPTOMS
• Anterior shin splints: Pain in front of the lower leg. Pain radiates down the front and outer side of the leg.
• Posterior shin splints: Pain along the back and inner side of the lower leg and ankle.

CAUSES & RISK FACTORS—Inflammation of muscles, tendons and covering to bone (periosteum), usually due to an imbalance of the calf muscles (which pull the forefoot down) and the shin muscles (which pull the forefoot up). Shin splints are most common with marathon running, walking, or jogging, particularly on rough terrain.

HOW TO PREVENT
• Avoid hard and uneven surfaces—use soft surfaces such as dirt or grass for jogging, running and walking.
• Warm up adequately before exercise or competition. Keep shins warm during exercise.
• Wear well-fitting shoes with good arch support during physical activities.

WHAT TO EXPECT

DIAGNOSTIC MEASURES
• Your own observation of symptoms.
• Medical history and physical by a doctor.
• X-rays of the lower leg, knee and ankle.

NORMAL COURSE OF ILLNESS— Complete cure requires rest and slow rehabilitation. Total time may range from 2 weeks to 2 months. Tough competition should be delayed until you can exercise regularly for 4 to 6 weeks without pain.

POSSIBLE COMPLICATIONS
• Mistaken diagnosis. Similar symptoms can be caused by stress fractures or increased pressure caused by constricted tissue covering muscles or nerves.
• Prolonged healing time if activity is resumed too soon.
• Proneness to recurrence.
• Inflammation and arthritic changes in nearby joints (such as ankle, knee, hip, back) caused by a changed gait and posture due to lower-leg pain.

HOW TO TREAT

NOTE—Follow your doctor's instructions. These instructions are supplemental.

MEDICAL TREATMENT—Physical therapy is sometimes necessary.

HOME TREATMENT
• Stop your exercise until you can resume without pain. If you have pain with walking, don't try to run.
• Use ice massage. Fill a large Styrofoam cup with water and freeze. Tear a small amount of foam from the top so ice protrudes. Massage firmly over the painful area in a circle about the size of a softball. Do this for 15 minutes at a time, 3 or 4 times a day, and before workouts or competition.
• Apply heat instead of ice, if it feels better. Use heat lamps, hot soaks, hot showers, heating pads, or heat liniments or ointments.
• Take whirlpool treatments, if available.
• Massage gently and often to provide comfort and decrease swelling. Apply lubricating oil to skin over the painful area during massage.
• For anterior shin splints, raise the heel of the shoe with 1/8 inch of adhesive felt.
• For posterior shin splints, wear an extra pair of socks and run with the body erect, not leaning forward. Try not to land directly on the toes.

MEDICATION
• For minor discomfort, you may use non-prescription drugs such as aspirin or ibuprofen.
• Your doctor may prescribe other non-steroidal anti-inflammatory medicines.

ACTIVITY—After treatment, when ready to resume your normal athletic activity:
• Cut back on your training schedule in proportion to the time it took for pain to stop.
• Ice the legs 6 to 10 minutes before warmup and after running.
• Wear long socks to keep legs warm.
• Run only every other day during first few weeks after treatment.
• For anterior shin splints, shave the legs and use criss-cross adhesive taping over the front half of the lower leg, with or without the elbow brace.

DIET—Eat a well-balanced diet that includes extra protein, such as meat, fish, poultry, cheese, milk and eggs. Increase fiber and fluid intake to prevent constipation that may result from decreased activity.

CALL YOUR DOCTOR IF

You have symptoms of shin splints that persist despite treatment.

SKIN CANCER, BASAL-CELL

GENERAL INFORMATION

DEFINITION—Skin cancer affecting the skin's basal layer (the 5th layer). Basal-cell skin cancer invades areas under skin, but it does not spread to distant areas. Skin of the face, ears, backs of hands, shoulders and arms is most frequently affected.

SIGNS & SYMPTOMS—A small skin lesion that does not heal in 3 weeks with the following characteristics:
● The lesion appears flat and "pearly." Its edges are translucent and rounded or rolled. The edges may have small, curvy, new blood vessels. The ulcer in the center is dimpled. Lesion size varies from 4mm to 6mm, but it may grow larger if untreated.
● The lesion occurs on skin that is exposed to the sun and shows evidence of sun damage.
● The lesion grows slowly. It does not hurt or itch.

CAUSES & RISK FACTORS—Skin damage from sun that occurs many years prior to the cancer's appearance. Persons most at risk include:
● Athletes who exercise, train and play outdoors.
● Persons over age 60.
● Persons with a fair skin complexion.

HOW TO PREVENT—Limit exposure to sun. Protect skin from sun exposure with a head covering, clothing or sunscreen.

WHAT TO EXPECT

DIAGNOSTIC MEASURES
● Your own observation of symptoms.
● Medical history and physical exam by a doctor.
● Pathological exam of tissue after removal to confirm diagnosis.

SURGERY—Usually necessary. See "Medical Treatment" below.

NORMAL COURSE OF ILLNESS— Curable in 2 to 4 weeks if cancer is removed. This does not become life-threatening unless it is ignored completely.

POSSIBLE COMPLICATIONS—Without treatment, cancers may enlarge, ulcerate and disfigure. Less than 1% spread to other sites, but they should be removed to prevent local damage.

HOW TO TREAT

NOTE—Follow your doctor's instructions. These instructions are supplemental.

MEDICAL TREATMENT—Removal of cancer by one of the following methods. The treatment method is chosen in a doctor-patient conference:
Surgery in the doctor's office or an outpatient surgical unit of the hospital.
Electrosurgery (see Glossary).
Cryosurgery (see Glossary).
Radiation treatment.

HOME TREATMENT—After surgery:
● Apply rubbing alcohol to the scab twice a day.
● Apply an adhesive bandage to the scab during the day. Leave it uncovered at night.
● Remove the bandage to wash the wound. Dry gently and completely after bathing and swimming. Reapply the bandage until healed.

MEDICATION—After surgery:
● For minor pain, you may use non-prescription drugs, such as acetaminophen or aspirin.
● If the scab cracks or oozes, apply a non-prescription antibiotic ointment several times a day.
● Your doctor may prescribe an antibiotic ointment to prevent wound infection.

ACTIVITY—No restrictions.

DIET—No special diet.

CALL YOUR DOCTOR IF

● You have symptoms of basal-cell skin cancer.
● The wound bleeds after surgery, and the bleeding cannot be stopped by applying pressure for 10 minutes.
● The wound shows signs of infection, such as pain, redness, swelling or increased tenderness.

SKIN CANCER, MALIGNANT MELANOMA

 GENERAL INFORMATION

DEFINITION—A skin cancer that spreads to other areas of the body, primarily the lymph nodes, liver, lungs and central nervous system. Most melanomas begin in a mole or other pre-existing skin lesion. Excessive exposure to sun is a major factor in causing malignant melanoma. It usually affects the skin of the head, neck, legs or back, but rarely occurs in the eye, mouth, vagina or anus. Melanomas are more likely to occur in adults, but some affect children. The incidence of melanomas has increased since 1970.

SIGNS & SYMPTOMS—A flat or slightly raised skin lesion that can be black, brown, blue, red, white or a mixture of all colors. Its borders are often irregular and may bleed.

CAUSES & RISK FACTORS—Uncontrolled growth of cells that give skin its brownish color (melanocytes). When the cells grow down into deep skin layers, they invade blood vessels and lymph vessels and are spread to other body areas. The following factors increase the likelihood of developing a melanoma:
- Moles on the skin.
- Excessive sun exposure.
- Pregnancy.
- Genetic factors. This is most common in light-complexioned, blonde people, and is rare in black people.
- Radiation treatment or excessive exposure to ultraviolet light, as with sun lamps.

HOW TO PREVENT—If you are in a high-risk group:
- Protect yourself from excessive sun exposure. Wear broad-rimmed hats and protective clothing. Use maximum protection sun-block preparations on exposed skin.
- Examine your skin, including genitals and soles of the feet, regularly for changes in pigmented areas. Ask a family member to examine your back. See your doctor about any skin area (especially brown or black) that becomes multicolored, develops irregular edges or surfaces, bleeds or changes in any way.

 WHAT TO EXPECT

DIAGNOSTIC MEASURES
- Your own observation of symptoms.
- Medical history and physical exam by a doctor.
- Biopsy (see Glossary) of suspicious lesions. The melanoma's depth must be established to determine appropriate treatment.

SURGERY—Necessary to remove suspicious skin lesions or to remove nearby lymph glands if the tumor has spread.

NORMAL COURSE OF ILLNESS—Varies greatly. Early melanomas that have not grown downward are curable with surgical removal. Once the tumor has spread to distant organs, this condition is currently considered incurable. However, symptoms can be relieved or controlled. Scientific research into causes and treatment continues, so there is hope for increasingly effective treatment and cure.

POSSIBLE COMPLICATIONS—Fatal spread to lungs, liver, brain or other internal organs.

 HOW TO TREAT

NOTE—Follow your doctor's instructions. These instructions are supplemental.

MEDICAL TREATMENT
- Surgery.
- Hospitalization for radiation treatment and chemotherapy, if the tumor has spread.

HOME TREATMENT—No specific instructions except those listed under other headings.

MEDICATION—Your doctor may prescribe anticancer drugs.

ACTIVITY—No restrictions.

DIET—No special diet.

 CALL YOUR DOCTOR IF

- You have a skin lesion with any characteristics of a malignant melanoma.
- During treatment, changes occur in another skin area.
- New, unexplained symptoms develop. Drugs used in treatment may produce side effects.

SKIN CANCER, SQUAMOUS-CELL

 GENERAL INFORMATION

DEFINITION—A malignant growth of the epithelial layer (external surface) of the skin, especially in areas exposed to the sun, such as the face, ears, hands or arms.

SIGNS & SYMPTOMS—A small, disfiguring, scaling, raised bump on the skin with a crusting ulcer in the center. The bump doesn't hurt or itch.

CAUSES & RISK FACTORS—Risk increases with any of the following:
- Excessive exposure to sunlight.
- Overexposure to X-rays.
- Light complexion.
- Recent illness with chronic skin ulcers from any cause.
- Repeated injury to the skin of athletes due to excessive perspiration, increased heat, friction of clothing and protective gear.
- Age over 60.

HOW TO PREVENT—Wear sunscreen or a hat and protective clothing to protect skin from sun damage.

 WHAT TO EXPECT

DIAGNOSTIC MEASURES
- Your own observation of symptoms.
- Medical history and physical exam by a doctor.
- Biopsy (see Glossary).

SURGERY—Sometimes necessary to remove the growth.

NORMAL COURSE OF ILLNESS—This type of skin cancer responds well to treatment. It is usually curable in 2 weeks with treatment.

POSSIBLE COMPLICATIONS
- Cancer must be treated again in 10% of cases.
- Cancer will spread to other tissue if untreated.

 HOW TO TREAT

NOTE—Follow your doctor's instructions. These instructions are supplemental.

MEDICAL TREATMENT—Removal of the growth may be with any of the following methods:
- Surgical removal.
- Scraping and removal by electrocautery (see Glossary) or laser beam.
- Radiation therapy.

HOME TREATMENT—After removal of the tumor, keep the area clean, dry and protected from clothing until healed. Your doctor will provide additional instructions, depending on the treatment used.

MEDICATION
- For minor discomfort, you may use non-prescription drugs such as acetaminophen.
- Your doctor may prescribe topical antibiotic ointment or cream to prevent infection after surgery.

ACTIVITY—After treatment, resume normal activity as soon as possible.

DIET—No special diet.

 CALL YOUR DOCTOR IF

- You have symptoms of squamous-cell skin cancer.
- The following occurs after treatment:
  Redness, swelling, bleeding or tenderness occurs at the treatment site.
  Pain cannot be controlled by non-prescription pain relievers.
  The sore has not healed 3 weeks after treatment.

SNAKEBITE

GENERAL INFORMATION

DEFINITION—Bite from a venomous snake, including rattlesnake, copperhead, water moccasin or coral snake. Bites on the extremities are most common, but bites on the head and trunk are most dangerous. They are likely to happen to runners, joggers, walkers, hikers, backpackers, fishers, boaters and campers, or anyone playing or working where snakes live.

SIGNS & SYMPTOMS—If the bite is from a coral snake, it will have multiple fang marks and small cuts. Coral-snake symptoms may not appear for 3 to 4 hours. If the bite is from another snake, it will have deep single or double-fang marks. Symptoms from other snakes begin quickly. Symptoms of any venomous snakebite include:
- Severe pain and swelling around the bite.
- Skin discoloration that resembles bruising around the bite.
- Bleeding spots under the skin all over the body.
- Numbness and tingling around the mouth and in the hands and feet.
- Excessive sweating.
- Fever.
- Low blood pressure and life-threatening shock.
- Breathing difficulty.
- Blurred vision.
- Headache.
- Seizures.
- Coma.

CAUSES & RISK FACTORS—Bites from venomous snakes are most likely to occur during outdoor activities in warm months in areas where venomous snakes are abundant.

HOW TO PREVENT—Wear protective shoes, boots and clothing for hiking, camping, fishing and hunting. Prevent complications by carrying a snakebite kit and instructions when you enter high-risk areas.

WHAT TO EXPECT

DIAGNOSTIC MEASURES
- Your own observation of symptoms.
- Medical history and physical exam by a doctor.
- Laboratory blood studies.

SURGERY—Occasionally necessary to remove injured or gangrenous tissue 2 to 3 days after the bite.

NORMAL COURSE OF ILLNESS—Usually curable with rapid medical care. Severe bites involving a large amount of venom may be fatal—even with treatment. After one snakebite, succeeding snakebites may produce a more severe reaction.

POSSIBLE COMPLICATIONS
- Gangrene, requiring amputation of the affected part.
- DIC (disseminated intravascular coagulation). This is a serious disruption of blood-clotting mechanisms, resulting in hemorrhaging or internal bleeding.
- Severe immunological response if the victim has had a previous venomous snakebite.

HOW TO TREAT

NOTE—Follow your doctor's instructions. These instructions are supplemental.

MEDICAL TREATMENT—Treatment as soon as possible at an emergency facility.

HOME TREATMENT
- Don't panic! Venom will spread more quickly through the body if the victim runs or becomes excited.
- Before giving first aid, identify the snake.
- Don't pack the affected part in ice.
- If the bite is from a coral snake, elevate and immobilize the bitten part and go to the nearest emergency facility.
- If it is from another venomous snake:
  Put a light tourniquet (constricting band of any sort) 3 or 4 inches above the bite, toward the body. Don't use a tourniquet if 30 minutes or more have passed since the bite.
  Wash the bite with soap and water.
  Immobilize the bitten area.
  Go immediately to the nearest emergency facility.

MEDICATION—Your doctor may prescribe:
- Antivenin to neutralize snake poison.
- Tetanus booster injection.
- Antibiotics to prevent infection.
- Pain relievers. (Narcotics cannot be used for coral-snake bites. They may cause shock.)

ACTIVITY—Resume normal activities as soon as symptoms improve.

DIET—No special diet.

CALL YOUR DOCTOR IF

- You or someone you are with receives a snakebite that could be venomous.
- New, unexplained symptoms develop. Drugs used in treatment may produce side effects.

SODIUM IMBALANCE

 GENERAL INFORMATION

DEFINITION—Above-normal level (hypernatremia) or below-normal level (hyponatremia) of sodium in the blood.

SIGNS & SYMPTOMS—Any of the following:
- Muscle cramps (usually in the legs), particularly following or accompanying exercise.
- Confusion.
- Restlessness and anxiety.
- Weakness.
- Changes in pulse rate and blood pressure.
- Tissue swelling (edema).
- Stupor or coma.

Sodium imbalance may be part of a disease with other symptoms that predominate, such as fever, vomiting, diarrhea or excessive sweating.

CAUSES & RISK FACTORS
Hyponatremia:
- Use of diuretics. Diuretics are used for serious medical problems such as hypertension and disorders of the kidney, liver and heart. They are sometimes used unwisely and unethically by athletes who need to meet a certain weight limit (boxers, wrestlers, jockeys). Diuretics, coupled with excessive sweating, heat and exercise, can cause severe sodium imbalance.
- Poor kidney function.
- Prolonged loss of body fluids from vomiting or diarrhea.
- Infections with high fever.
Hypernatremia:
- Inability to drink water, as with stroke or gastrointestinal diseases.
- Use of cortisone drugs or anabolic steroids.
- Excessive intake of salty food or liquid, as in near-drowning in salt water.
- Diabetes mellitus.
- Congestive heart failure.
- Kidney diseases. Healthy kidneys can usually control sodium levels.

HOW TO PREVENT—If you take diuretics for any reason and exercise strenuously, make sure you drink extra water. Eat a generous diet. Do not drink salt mixtures such as Gatorade or take salt tablets. They may compound any developing problem.

 WHAT TO EXPECT

DIAGNOSTIC MEASURES
- Your own observation of symptoms.
- Medical history and physical exam by a doctor.
- Laboratory blood and urine studies of sodium and other electrolytes.

SURGERY—Not necessary nor useful for this disorder.

NORMAL COURSE OF ILLNESS—Usually can be corrected with intravenous fluids and treatment of the underlying disorder.

POSSIBLE COMPLICATIONS—Shock and death from severe fluid and sodium imbalance following vigorous exercise in hot weather.

 HOW TO TREAT

NOTE—Follow your doctor's instructions. These instructions are supplemental.

MEDICAL TREATMENT—Hospitalization (sometimes).

HOME TREATMENT—If you have a disorder or take drugs that affect sodium balance, learn as much as possible about your drugs, your condition and how to prevent a sodium imbalance.

MEDICATION—Your doctor may prescribe:
- Intravenous sodium if sodium levels are low.
- Medications to correct underlying disorders.

ACTIVITY—Resume your normal activities after recovery.

DIET
- No special diet for low sodium levels. Low-salt diets contain enough sodium to prevent hyponatremia. However, sodium levels are not influenced by diet alone.
- If you take diuretics, don't drink alcohol. Diuretics combined with alcohol use and excessive sweating can cause life-threatening shock.

 CALL YOUR DOCTOR IF

- You have symptoms of a sodium imbalance.
- You are having problems with a disorder that affects sodium levels.

STRESS INCONTINENCE

 GENERAL INFORMATION

DEFINITION—An involuntary loss of urine in women that accompanies any action that suddenly increases pressure in the abdomen. This is most common when jumping, running or straining (as with lifting weights).

SIGNS & SYMPTOMS—Unintentional loss of urine with exercise, lifting, sneezing, singing, coughing, laughing, crying or straining to have a bowel movement.

CAUSES & RISK FACTORS—Shortening of the urethra and loss of the normal muscular support for the bladder and floor of the pelvis. These changes occur during pregnancy and after childbirth, particularly repeated childbirth. They may also occur as a natural consequence of aging. They are made worse by obesity.

HOW TO PREVENT
- Empty your bladder before exercise.
- Eat a normal, well-balanced diet and exercise regularly to build and maintain muscle strength.
- Learn and practice Kegel exercises (see Home Treatment) after childbirth, before symptoms of stress incontinence begin. If you have passed menopause, practice Kegel exercises even if you have not given birth.

 WHAT TO EXPECT

DIAGNOSTIC MEASURES
- Your own observation of symptoms.
- Medical history and physical exam by a doctor.
- Urinalysis to determine if a urinary-tract infection is causing the symptoms.

SURGERY—Sometimes necessary to tighten relaxed or damaged muscles that support the bladder. This surgical procedure is called *anterior colporrhaphy*. It may be performed alone or in conjunction with other gynecological surgery, especially vaginal hysterectomy.

NORMAL COURSE OF ILLNESS—If the stress incontinence is not severe enough to require surgery, exercise can improve the muscle function. If it is severe, it can be cured with surgery.

POSSIBLE COMPLICATIONS
- Complete loss of urinary control. This requires surgery.
- Recurrent or chronic urinary-tract infections.

 HOW TO TREAT

NOTE—Follow your doctor's instructions. These instructions are supplemental.

MEDICAL TREATMENT—Not usually necessary nor useful unless complications develop, especially urinary-tract infection or total loss of control.

HOME TREATMENT—Learn to recognize, control and develop the muscles of the pelvic floor. These are the ones you use to interrupt urination in midstream. The following exercises (Kegel exercises) strengthen these muscles so you can control or relax them completely:
- To identify which muscles are involved, alternately start and stop urination when using the toilet. Another method is to place a finger just inside the opening of your vagina and squeeze the finger with your vaginal muscles.
- Practice tightening and releasing these muscles while sitting, standing, walking, driving, watching TV or listening to music.
- Tighten the muscles a small amount at a time "like an elevator going up to the 10th floor." Then release very slowly, "one floor at a time."
- Tighten the muscles from front to back, including the anus, as in the previous exercise.
- Practice exercises every morning, afternoon and evening. Start with 5 times each, and gradually work up to 20 or 30 each time.

MEDICATION—Medicine usually is not necessary for this disorder, but your doctor may prescribe:
- Antibiotics if you have a complicating urinary-tract infection.
- A pessary (support device) made of plastic, rubber or other material to fit inside the vagina to support the uterus and lower muscular layer of the bladder.

ACTIVITY—No restrictions.

DIET—Follow a weight-loss diet if you are obese.

 CALL YOUR DOCTOR IF

- You have symptoms of stress incontinence.
- Any sign of infection develops, such as fever, pain on urination, frequent urination or a general ill feeling.
- Symptoms don't improve after 3 months of Kegel exercises, or symptoms become intolerable and you wish to consider surgery.

SUN POISONING

GENERAL INFORMATION

DEFINITION—Reaction to overexposure to the sun. This is likely to be a problem in any hot-season sport such as swimming, surfing, sailing, tennis or water skiing.

SIGNS & SYMPTOMS
- Red skin rash, sometimes with small blisters, in areas exposed to sunlight.
- Fever.
- Fatigue or dizziness.

CAUSES & RISK FACTORS—Exposure to sun during hot seasons when ultraviolet light is strongest. It is triggered by exposure to the sun, usually in conjunction with sunburn. Risks increase with any of the following:
- Use of medications that cause photosensitivity (increased sensitivity to ultraviolet light). The most common drugs include tetracycline antibiotics, thiazide diuretics, sulfa drugs and oral contraceptives. Some cosmetics, including lipstick, perfume and soaps, can also cause a photosensitive reaction.
- Underlying infection.
- Previous episodes of sun poisoning.
- Metabolic disorders, such as diabetes mellitus or thyroid disease.
- Use of immunosuppressive drugs.

HOW TO PREVENT—Stay out of the sun when possible if you have a history of sun poisoning. Change vigorous workouts to a cooler part of the day.

WHAT TO EXPECT

DIAGNOSTIC MEASURES
- Your own observation of symptoms.
- Medical history and physical exam by a doctor.

SURGERY—Not necessary nor useful for this disorder.

NORMAL COURSE OF ILLNESS—Symptoms can be controlled with treatment if you stay out of the sun. Allow up to 1 week for recovery.

POSSIBLE COMPLICATIONS—Recurrence of the rash and other symptoms when exposed to the sun—even for short periods—especially in spring and summer.

HOW TO TREAT

NOTE—Follow your doctor's instructions. These instructions are supplemental.

MEDICAL TREATMENT—None usually needed after diagnosis and prescription of medications.

HOME TREATMENT
- Stay out of the sun during the hours of strongest ultraviolet light (10 a.m. to 2 p.m.).
- If you must go out in the sun for your athletic workouts, wear protective clothing and the most protective sunscreen preparation available. Beware of heat exhaustion and dehydration.

MEDICATION—You may take aspirin or acetaminophen to relieve mild pain or itching. Your doctor may prescribe:
- Beta-carotene to reduce discomfort.
- Chloroquine prior to sun exposure to prevent a recurrence of symptoms.
- Corticosteroids for severe cases.

ACTIVITY—No restrictions, except to avoid prolonged sun exposure.

DIET—No special diet. Drink extra fluids to prevent dehydration.

CALL YOUR DOCTOR IF

- You have symptoms of sun poisoning.
- New, unexplained symptoms develop. Drugs used in treatment may produce side effects.

SUNBURN

GENERAL INFORMATION

DEFINITION—Skin inflammation and damage that follows overexposure to the sun, sun lamps or occupational light sources.
- First-degree burn consists of mild redness.
- Second-degree burn has redness and blisters.
- Third-degree burn includes redness, blisters and skin ulceration.

Sunburn is common in athletes because of frequent exposure to sunlight for long periods.

SIGNS & SYMPTOMS
- Red, swollen, painful, blistered and sometimes ulcerated skin.
- Chills and fever.
- Nausea and vomiting (severe burns).
- Delirium (severe, extensive burns) accompanied by fever and dehydration.
- Tanning or peeling of the skin after recovery, depending on severity of the burn.

CAUSES & RISK FACTORS—Excess
exposure to ultraviolet (UV) light. The following factors make a person more susceptible to sunburn:
- Genetic factors, especially fair skin, blue eyes, and red or blonde hair.
- Use of drugs, including sulfa, tetracyclines, amoxicillin or oral contraceptives.

HOW TO PREVENT
- Avoid sun exposure from 12 noon to 3 p.m.
- Use a sun-block preparation for outdoor activity. Products with a sun-protective value of 10 or more protect almost totally. Reapply after swimming or after prolonged exposure. Baby oil, mineral oil or cocoa butter offer no protection from the sun.
- For maximum protection, use a physical-barrier agent such as zinc-oxide ointment. Reapply after swimming and at frequent intervals during exposure. Barrier agents are especially helpful on skin areas that are most susceptible to burns, such as the nose, ears, backs of the legs and back of the neck.
- If you rarely burn, you may use a sunscreen product that permits tanning and provides minimal protection.
- Wear clothes that have muted colors such as tan to protect skin from sun. Avoid brilliant colors and whites, which reflect the sun into your face.
- If you insist on tanning, limit your sun exposure on the 1st day to 5 or 10 minutes on each side. Add 5 minutes per side each day.
- Some reports suggest that aspirin taken before sun exposure will prevent or reduce the harmful effects of sunlight—including burns.

WHAT TO EXPECT

DIAGNOSTIC MEASURES
- Your own observation of symptoms.
- Medical history and exam by a doctor.

NORMAL COURSE OF ILLNESS—Recovery in 3 days to 3 weeks, depending on the severity of the sunburn.

POSSIBLE COMPLICATIONS
- Skin changes leading to skin cancer, including life-threatening malignant melanoma.
- Keratoses, premalignant skin lesions.
- Premature wrinkling and loss of skin elasticity.
- Temporary delirium in worst cases.
- Triggering of a variety of sun-damage-related disorders, such as erythema multiforme, vitiligo, heatstroke, porphyria, lupus erythematosus or sun poisoning.

HOW TO TREAT

NOTE—Follow your doctor's instructions. These instructions are supplemental.

MEDICAL TREATMENT—A doctor's care will be necessary for severe burns and for complications of sunburn.

HOME TREATMENT
- To reduce heat and pain, dip gauze or towels in cool water and lay these on the burn.
- After skin swelling subsides, apply cold cream or baby lotion.
- For badly blistered skin, apply a light coating of petroleum jelly. This prevents anything from sticking to the blisters.

MEDICATION
- Use non-prescription drugs, such as aspirin or acetaminophen, to relieve pain and reduce fever. Non-prescription burn remedies that contain benzocaine or lidocaine may be useful, but they produce allergic reactions in some.
- Your doctor may prescribe pain relievers or cortisone drugs to use briefly.

ACTIVITY—Rest in any comfortable position until fever and discomfort diminish. Keep bed sheets off burned skin by making an upside-down "cradle" or tent of cardboard or other material.

DIET—No special diet. Increase fluid intake.

CALL YOUR DOCTOR IF

The following occurs after sunburn:
- Oral temperature spikes to 101F (38.3C).
- Vomiting or diarrhea occurs.
- Delirium begins.
- Pain and fever persist longer than 48 hours.

THORACIC-OUTLET-OBSTRUCTION SYNDROME (Cervical-Rib Syndrome; Serratus Anticus Syndrome)

GENERAL INFORMATION

DEFINITION—Pain and weakness from compression of nerves in the neck. These nerves affect the shoulders, arms and hands.

SIGNS & SYMPTOMS—One or more of the following:
- Pain, numbness and tingling in the neck, shoulders, arms and hands.
- Weakness in the arms and fingers.
- Absent pulse in the wrist when raising the arm and turning the head toward the opposite shoulder, if symptoms are caused by a cervical rib.

CAUSES & RISK FACTORS—The nerves and blood vessels that supply the shoulder, arms and hands start in the neck and pass as a bundle near the cervical ribs and collarbone. Pressure on this nerve and blood-vessel bundle creates symptoms. Pressure may be caused by:
- An extra rib in the lower neck (cervical rib).
- Overdevelopment of neck muscles, as may be required with some contact sports or may result from overzealous weight-lifting programs.
- Prolonged period with the arm or neck in an abnormal position, as can occur during surgery, during unconsciousness for any reason, or while sleeping with a too-firm object under the neck.
- Injury from overextending the arm or shoulder.
- Tumor that has spread to the head and neck area from another part of the body.
- Muscle weakness and drooping in the shoulder.

HOW TO PREVENT
- Avoid shoulder and neck injury whenever possible. Wear seat belts and use padded headrests in cars. Use shoulder pads or other protective equipment appropriate for your sport.
- Don't use mind-altering drugs or drink excessive amounts of alcohol, which can lead to unconsciousness.
- Change sleeping positions. Try sleeping on one side or sleep without a firm pillow.
- If symptoms are caused from overdeveloped muscles in the neck, reduce neck-muscle-building exercises.

WHAT TO EXPECT

DIAGNOSTIC MEASURES
- Your own observation of symptoms.
- Medical history and exam by a doctor.

- X-rays of the neck and shoulder area to look for an extra cervical rib or tumor.

SURGERY—Sometimes necessary if a cervical rib is causing pressure on nerves and blood vessels.

NORMAL COURSE OF ILLNESS
- If caused by overdevelopment of neck muscles, the disorder is usually curable with physical therapy and decreased neck-muscle exercises.
- If caused by injury while unconscious or asleep, the disorder is usually curable with retrained sleeping habits and physical therapy.
- If caused by a cervical rib, the disorder is usually curable with surgery.
- If caused by a tumor, treatment may be unsuccessful.

POSSIBLE COMPLICATIONS
- Permanent numbness or loss of arm or hand strength if thoracic-outlet-obstruction syndrome is not treated.
- Post-surgical complications (rare).

HOW TO TREAT

NOTE—Follow your doctor's instructions. These instructions are supplemental.

MEDICAL TREATMENT
- Doctor's treatment.
- Surgery to relieve pressure on the nerves and blood vessels if a cervical rib is the underlying cause.
- Physical therapy.

HOME TREATMENT—Use heat to relieve pain. Use a heating pad, heat lamp, hot showers or warm compresses.

MEDICATION—You may use non-prescription drugs, such as acetaminophen or aspirin, to relieve pain. Medication cannot correct the underlying condition.

ACTIVITY—Your doctor may prescribe physical therapy and exercises less likely to cause neck-muscle overdevelopment.

DIET—No special diet.

CALL YOUR DOCTOR IF

- You have symptoms of thoracic-outlet-obstruction syndrome.
- Symptoms don't improve in 2 weeks, despite treatment.

TOENAIL, INGROWN

 GENERAL INFORMATION

DEFINITION—A condition in which the sharp edge of a nail grows into the flesh of a toe, usually the great (big) toe. Until treated, this problem may markedly hamper maximum athletic performance.

SIGNS & SYMPTOMS—Pain, tenderness, redness, swelling and heat in the toe where the sharp nail edge pierces the surrounding fold of tissue. Once tissue surrounding the nail becomes inflamed, infection usually develops in the injured area.

CAUSES & RISK FACTORS—An ingrown toenail is likely to accompany one of the following conditions:
- The nail formation is more curved than normal.
- The toenail is clipped back too far, allowing tissue to grow up over it.
- Shoes fit poorly, forcing the toe of the shoe against the nail and surrounding tissue.
- The person participates in activities that require sudden stops ("toe jamming").

HOW TO PREVENT
- Wear roomy, well-fitting shoes and socks.
- Cut toenails carefully. Persons with diabetes mellitus or peripheral vascular disease should be especially careful in trimming toenails. Foot injury is dangerous with these disorders because of impaired blood circulation to the feet.
- Keep feet and toenails scrupulously clean.
- Cut toenails the way they are shaped—not straight across.
- Avoid excessive shoe pressure.

 WHAT TO EXPECT

DIAGNOSTIC MEASURES
- Your own observation of symptoms.
- Medical history and physical exam by a doctor.

SURGERY—Often necessary to remove the nail.

NORMAL COURSE OF ILLNESS—Curable with treatment. Oral antibiotics usually relieve symptoms of infection within 1 week. If an ingrown toenail occurs repeatedly despite preventive measures, then part or all of the toenail may be removed surgically and the nailbed scraped so the problem will not recur. The nail should grow back, but it might not look the same.

POSSIBLE COMPLICATIONS
- Chronic infection that cannot be cured without surgery.
- Inflammation and arthritic changes in other parts of the body (such as ankle, knee, hip or back) due to the abnormal stress placed on them when normal standing and walking are not possible because of pain.

 HOW TO TREAT

NOTE—Follow your doctor's instructions. These instructions are supplemental.

MEDICAL TREATMENT—Necessary for diagnosis and surgery.

HOME TREATMENT—The following home treatment is appropriate either before or after surgery:
- Soak the toe for 20 minutes, twice a day, in a gallon of warm water with either 2 tablespoons of epsom salts or 2 tablespoons of a mild detergent.
- Lift the nail corners gently and wedge a small piece of cotton under the ingrown nail edges.
- Between soaks, apply Merthiolate and an antiseptic cream such as Neosporin or Bacitracin. Then apply an adhesive bandage strip to protect from injury.

MEDICATION—Your doctor may prescribe antibiotics to fight infection.

ACTIVITY—Resume your normal activities as soon as symptoms improve. You may need to wear a shoe with the toe cut out until the toe heals.

DIET—Eat a well-balanced diet that includes extra protein, such as meat, fish, poultry, cheese, milk and eggs. Increase fiber and fluid intake to prevent constipation that may result from decreased activity.

 CALL YOUR DOCTOR IF

- You have symptoms of an ingrown toenail.
- The following occurs during treatment or after surgery:
  Fever.
  Increased pain.
  Signs of infection (pain, redness, tenderness, swelling or heat) in the toe.

VAGINITIS

GENERAL INFORMATION

DEFINITION—Irritation, infection or inflammation of the vagina. These are slightly more common in women athletes than in the female population at large.

SIGNS & SYMPTOMS
- Vaginal discharge, with or without an unpleasant odor.
- Swollen, red, tender vaginal lips (labia) and surrounding skin.
- Burning on urination, if urine touches inflamed tissue.
- Change in vaginal color from pale-pink to red.
- Genital itching and pain.
- Discomfort during sexual intercourse.

CAUSES & RISK FACTORS
For irritation:
Friction of clothing, especially tight clothing, that rubs against the skin or mucous membranes in the vaginal area. This occurs often in sports such as cycling, gymnastics or horseback riding.
For infection:
When the vagina's hormone and pH balance is disturbed, germs multiply and cause infection. Germs may be yeast, fungi, parasites or bacteria. Factors that may disturb the vagina's balance include:
- Pregnancy.
- Diabetes mellitus.
- Use of oral contraceptives.
- High intake of simple carbohydrates.
- Non-ventilating clothing or underwear made from man-made fibers, which increases darkness, moisture and warmth in the vaginal area.
- Hot weather.
- Immunosuppression from drugs or disease, including antibiotic treatment.

HOW TO PREVENT
- Take showers rather than tub baths.
- Shower and dry off carefully after any vigorous physical activity.
- Wear cotton panties or pantyhose with a cotton crotch. Avoid panties made from non-ventilating materials.
- Don't sit around in wet clothing—especially a wet bathing suit.
- Avoid frequent douches.
- When you take antibiotics, ask your doctor about eating yogurt, sour cream or buttermilk containing active cultures, or taking acidophilus tablets.
- After urination or bowel movements, cleanse by wiping or washing from front to back (vagina to anus), never back to front.
- Lose weight if you are obese.
- If you have diabetes, adhere strictly to your treatment program.

WHAT TO EXPECT

DIAGNOSTIC MEASURES
- Medical history and physical exam (including pelvic exam) by a doctor.
- Laboratory studies, such as a Pap smear, and culture and microscopic exam of the vaginal discharge.

NORMAL COURSE OF ILLNESS
- Vaginal irritation usually disappears once the irritant is removed.
- Vaginal infection is usually curable with 2 weeks of medication. Recurrence is common.

POSSIBLE COMPLICATIONS—Spread of infection from vagina or skin surrounding the genitals to other female organs (cervix, uterus, fallopian tubes, ovaries).

HOW TO TREAT

NOTE—Follow your doctor's instructions. These instructions are supplemental.

MEDICAL TREATMENT—You may need to visit your doctor for application of special medication to the vagina.

HOME TREATMENT
- Follow the first 5 instructions under How to Prevent.
- Don't douche unless your doctor recommends it.
- If urination burns, urinate through a tubular device, such as a toilet-paper roll or plastic cup with the end cut out, or urinate while bathing.

MEDICATION—Your doctor may prescribe:
- Antibiotics, hormones or topical cortisone cream or ointment.
- Antifungal drugs, either in oral form (rare) or in vaginal creams or suppositories (usually). Keep creams or suppositories in the refrigerator.

ACTIVITY
- For irritation, modify athletic activity if causes and risk factors have been eliminated and intolerable irritation persists.
- For infection, avoid overexertion, heat and excessive sweating during treatment. Delay sexual relations until symptoms cease.

DIET—Increase consumption of yogurt, acidophilus milk, buttermilk or sour cream.

CALL YOUR DOCTOR IF

- You have symptoms of vaginitis.
- Symptoms worsen or persist longer than 1 week despite treatment.
- Unusual vaginal bleeding or swelling develops.

WARTS
(Verruca Vulgaris)

GENERAL INFORMATION

DEFINITION—Benign tumors caused by a virus in the outer skin layer. Warts are not cancerous. They are contagious from person to person and from one area to another on the same person. They appear most often on the fingers, hands and arms. They are common in athletes who share locker facilities and have close personal contact with each other.

SIGNS & SYMPTOMS—A small, raised bump on the skin with the following characteristics:
● Warts begin very small (1mm to 3mm) and grow larger.
● Warts have a rough surface and clearly defined borders.
● They are usually the same color as the skin, but sometimes darker.
● Warts often appear in clusters around a "mother wart."
● If you cut into the wart surface, it contains small black dots or bleeding points.
● Warts are painless and don't itch.

CAUSES & RISK FACTORS—Invasion of the outer skin layer (epidermis) by the papilloma virus. The virus stimulates some cells to grow more rapidly than normal. Warts are very common. By adulthood, 90% of all people have antibodies to the virus, indicating a history of at least one wart infection.

HOW TO PREVENT—To keep from spreading warts, don't scratch them. Warts spread readily to small cuts and scratches.

WHAT TO EXPECT

DIAGNOSTIC MEASURES
● Your own observation of symptoms.
● Medical history and physical exam by a doctor.

SURGERY—Normal surgery with hospitalization and anesthetics is not necessary. Electrosurgery or cryotherapy is sometimes used (see Medical Treatment below).

NORMAL COURSE OF ILLNESS—20% of warts disappear spontaneously in 1 month. Without treatment, the remainder may persist for many months up to 2 or 3 years.

POSSIBLE COMPLICATIONS
● Spread to other body parts.
● Secondary infection of a wart.

HOW TO TREAT

NOTE—Follow your doctor's instructions. These instructions are supplemental.

MEDICAL TREATMENT
● Cryotherapy (freezing cells to destroy them). This is an office procedure that doesn't require anesthesia or cause bleeding. Freezing stings or hurts slightly during application, and pain may increase a bit after thawing. 3 to 5 weekly treatments may be necessary to destroy the wart.
● Electrosurgery (using heat to destroy cells). This treatment can usually be completed in one office visit, but healing takes longer, and secondary bacterial infections and scarring are more common.

HOME TREATMENT
● If you have electrosurgery, keep the treatment site clean with soap and water. Cover with an adhesive bandage, if you wish.
● If you have cryotherapy, a blister (sometimes with blood) will develop at the treatment site. The roof of the blister will come off without further treatment in 10 to 14 days. You should have little or no scarring. Wash and use make-up or cosmetics as usual. If clothing irritates the blister, cover with a small adhesive bandage.

MEDICATION—Your doctor may prescribe chemicals, such as mild salicylic acid, Retin-A Gel or Cream, 1% fluorouracil, or Duofilm (a one-time overnight treatment using a mixture of collodion and lactic acid) to destroy warts.

ACTIVITY—No restrictions.

DIET—No special diet.

CALL YOUR DOCTOR IF

● You have warts and you want them removed.
● After removal by cryosurgery or electrocautery, signs of infection (fever, swelling, redness, pain or pus) appear at the treatment site.
● Warts don't disappear completely after treatment.
● Other warts appear after treatment.

WARTS, PLANTAR

GENERAL INFORMATION

DEFINITION—Warts on the soles of the feet. Plantar warts seem to grow inward ("into the skin"). They are sometimes mistaken for calluses or corns, but the little dark spots in plantar warts help distinguish them from other skin problems.

SIGNS & SYMPTOMS
- Pinhead-sized bump that grows to 2mm or 3mm. Shaving off the top reveals small black dots, pinpoint bleeding and an underlying translucent core.
- Pain on walking. The wart compresses underlying tender tissue.
- Plantar warts may occur singly or in adjacent clusters.

CAUSES & RISK FACTORS—Infection with the human *papilloma* virus, which passes from person to person by direct contact. The virus invades the skin, making infected cells reproduce faster than normal cells. Plantar warts are contagious and are most common in association with the following:
- Repeated injury to the skin due to puncture wounds, excessive perspiration, increased heat, friction of foot covering and protective gear.
- Fall and spring seasons.
- Persons who have other warts.

HOW TO PREVENT
- Don't touch warts on other people.
- Don't wear another person's shoes.
- Wear footwear in public locker rooms or showers.

WHAT TO EXPECT

DIAGNOSTIC MEASURES
- Your own observation of symptoms.
- Medical history and physical exam by a doctor.

SURGERY—Frequently performed in a doctor's office to remove painful, non-healing plantar warts. Hospitalization is not usually necessary.

NORMAL COURSE OF ILLNESS—Usually curable in 6 to 12 weeks with treatment, but some cases are slow to heal or are resistant to treatment. Recurrence is common.

POSSIBLE COMPLICATIONS—Inflammation and arthritic changes in other parts of the body due to abnormal gait and posture caused by painful plantar warts.

HOW TO TREAT

NOTE—Follow your doctor's instructions. These instructions are supplemental.

MEDICAL TREATMENT—Your doctor will probably pare away the overlying callused skin, and apply chemical cauterants, such as trichloracetic acid, 20% salicylic acid or 20% formalin. Sometimes plantar warts are removed with lasers.

HOME TREATMENT
- Insert pads or cushions in your shoes to make walking more comfortable.
- Soak feet in 1/2 gallon of warm water with 2 tablespoons of mild detergent.
- Apply the sticky side of medicated plaster directly onto the wart. Push down, keep it dry and in place for 2 days.
- After 2 days, remove bandage and plaster. If skin tears as you remove the tape, loosen the tape with nail polish remover on a cotton-tip applicator between the skin and the tape. (Wart will look whitish). Wash 2 times daily for 2 days with soap and water and scrub with a brush or toothbrush. Expose the wart to air.
- Scrape gray wart tissue with the point of a sterilized nail file after a bath or shower.
- Repeat entire process for 2 weeks. If warts become sore, skip treatment for 2 or 3 days.
- Wear a pad cut from adhesive foam. Cut a hole for the wart and attach the pad to prevent pressure directly on the wart.
- If the wart is close to the base of the toes, have a shoe repairman sew a metatarsal bar on the bottom of the shoe.

MEDICATION
- For minor discomfort, you may use non-prescription drugs such as acetaminophen.
- Your doctor may prescribe chemically treated plaster for you to apply. Follow instructions carefully.

ACTIVITY—No restrictions. Because walking aggravates the wart, find the most comfortable way to walk without putting weight on the wart.

DIET—No special diet.

CALL YOUR DOCTOR IF

- You have a plantar wart.
- The treated area becomes infected, with redness, heat, increased pain and tenderness.

REHABILITATION & CONDITIONING

Rehabilitation restores full flexibility, strength, endurance and motion to an injured athlete. Conditioning develops these in a new athlete. Rehabilitation and conditioning of a particular body part should be accompanied by exercise of the rest of the body, especially the cardiovascular-pulmonary system. If injured, begin to exercise the uninjured parts as soon and as actively as your injury allows.

The frequency, duration, length of exercises and weights recommended in this section are averages and should not replace the instructions of your doctor or trainer. You must not begin rehabilitation exercises following any serious injury, such as fracture, dislocation, or 2nd- or 3rd-degree sprain, until you have clearance from your doctor. Beginning too soon may cause permanent damage or retard full recovery.

ANKLE EXERCISES

SET 1: TOE RAISES
Do this when ankle stiffness and pain decreases enough to allow exercise without increased pain.

Position: Stand on the floor, feet comfortably apart.
Weight Used: None.
Action: Rise up onto the balls of the feet as far as possible. Immediately lower yourself to the beginning position.
Repetitions: 20 to 25 times, 3 or 4 times a day.

SET 2: ADVANCED TOE RAISES
Begin these exercises when ankle is no longer stiff.

EXERCISE 1
Position: Stand on the edge of a step or other elevated structure so that your heels stretch below the level of your toes.
Weight Used: None.
Action: Rise up onto the balls of the feet as far as possible. Immediately lower yourself to the starting position.
Repetitions: 20 to 25 times, 3 or 4 times a day.

EXERCISE 2
Begin when able to perform Exercise 1 successfully.

Position: Stand on the edge of an elevated structure on one foot only, with the heel lower than the toes.
Weight Used: None.
Action: Rise up onto the ball of the foot as far as possible. Immediately lower yourself to the starting position.
Repetitions: 20 to 25 times, 3 or 4 times a day.

EXERCISE 3
Begin when able to perform Exercise 1 successfully.

Position: Stand on the edge of an elevated structure on one foot only, with the heel lower than the toes.
Weight Used: Hold a weighted object (5 to 10 pounds) in either hand.
Action: Rise on the ball of the foot and lower yourself as in Exercise 1.
Repetitions: 20 to 25 times, 3 or 4 times a day.

ANKLE EXERCISES (continued)

SET 3: HEEL WALKING

EXERCISE 1
Begin at the same time as Set 2.

Position: Stand on the heels, keeping toes as high off the ground as possible. Use a firm, smooth surface. Wear shoes with good solid heels.
Weight Used: None.
Action: Walk, continuing to keep toes as high as possible. Take short, choppy steps. Walk this way as long as possible, up to 2 minutes or about 100 feet.
Repetitions: 3 or 4 times a day.

EXERCISE 2
Begin when Exercise 1 is completed successfully.

Position: As in Exercise 1, stand on the heels, keeping toes as high off the ground as possible. Use a firm, smooth surface. Wear shoes with good solid heels.
Weight Used: 5 to 10 pounds.
Action: Same as Exercise 1. You may also do this exercise "walking" up a hill or incline, with or without weights (see Figure 1).
Repetitions: 3 or 4 times a day.

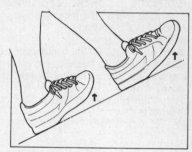

FIGURE 1

SET 4: ISOMETRIC ANKLE "WRESTLING"

EXERCISE 1
Begin as soon as pain has decreased enough to permit light exercise. This may be as soon as 1 day after injury.

Position: Sit comfortably, and place one ankle over the other.
Weight Used: None.
Action: Press outward with both ankles so that your feet are firmly pressing against each other. Hold for 10 seconds. Relax. Hold for 10 seconds.
Repetitions: 5 times for each ankle, 3 or 4 times a day.

EXERCISE 2
Begin when ankle is less stiff and painful than in Exercise 1.

Position: As in Exercise 1, sit comfortably and place one ankle over the other.
Weight Used: None.
Action: Begin as in Exercise 1. When ankles are pressed firmly, rotate the front of feet away from each other and back to the starting position (see Figure 2). Make each rotation last 10 full seconds.
Repetitions: 5 times for each ankle, 3 or 4 times a day.

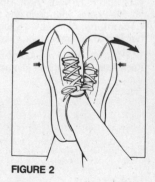

FIGURE 2

Continued on next page.

ANKLE EXERCISES (continued)

SET 5: BALANCE EXERCISES
Begin these at the same time as Set 4, Exercise 2.

EXERCISE 1
Position: Stand on a level surface.
Weight Used: None.
Action: Raise one foot off the floor and balance on the other foot for a count of 10. Change feet and repeat.
Repetitions: 2 or 3 on each foot, 3 or 4 times a day.

EXERCISE 2: CONTROLLED TIPPING
Position: Stand on a flat board resting on a croquet ball cut in half.
Weight Used: None.
Action: Balance on the board using both feet (see Figure 3). As board tips to either side, regain your balance control. Maintain for a count of 10.
Repetitions: Continue for 5 to 10 minutes, 3 or 4 times a day.

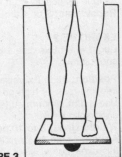

FIGURE 3

LOWER-BACK EXERCISES

These exercises are beneficial for inflammatory conditions or for rehabilitation following back injury. Inflammatory conditions include bursitis, tendinitis, gout, osteoarthritis, myositis and fibrositis.

SET 1: ABDOMINAL CURL
These exercises should permanently replace regular sit-ups in your training. Begin as soon as pain has decreased enough to permit light exercise.

Position: Lie flat on floor or mat, with knees bent and arms folded on the chest.
Weight Used: None.
Action: Roll your body up as if you were rolling a carpet. Start by pulling the neck forward so that your chin in on your chest. Roll your shoulders forward (see Figure 4). Then pull your head toward your legs until your head and shoulders are at a 45-degree angle from the floor.
Repetitions: Athletes—25 to 40 times, 3 or 4 times a day. Others—at least 10 times, gradually building to 25 times, 3 or 4 times a day.

WARNING: Avoid regular sit-ups. They can aggravate back injuries and inflammatory conditions. If necessary, show these instructions to your coach or trainer.

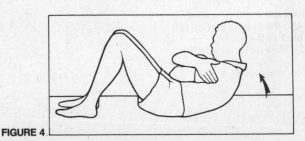

FIGURE 4

LOWER-BACK EXERCISES (continued)

SET 2: KNEES-TO-CHEST STRETCHING
These exercises should permanently replace double-leg raises in your training.

Position: Lie flat on a mat or floor, with knees bent and arms folded on the chest.
Weight Used: None.
Action: Pull the knees as close to your chest as possible while forcing your head toward your stomach (see Figure 5). Hold for 10 to 30 seconds. Return to starting position. Hold for 10 seconds.
Repetitions: Repeat until you feel a relaxing stretch to the back. Do 3 or 4 times a day.

WARNING: Avoid double-leg raises. They can aggravate back problems severely.

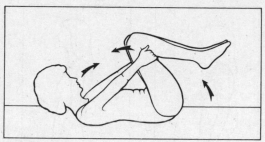

FIGURE 5

SET 3: BACK STRETCH ON CHAIR
If you feel pain when you try this exercise, go back to Set 2. Don't do this exercise until you have less pain.

Position: Sit on the edge of a chair that is supported against the wall (see Figure 6).
Weight Used: None.
Action: Drop your head and shoulders between your knees while trying to touch your elbows to the floor (see Figure 7). Relax and stay in this position 10 to 30 seconds. Return to starting position.
Repetitions: 10 times, 3 or 4 times a day.

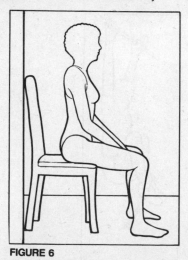

FIGURE 6

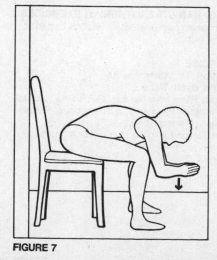

FIGURE 7

Continued on next page.

LOWER-BACK EXERCISES (continued)

SET 4: POSTURE:

Position: Proper posture can be explained in terms of the relationship between the knees and the spine. When a person stands or walks continually with the knees held very straight (even locked-out), as in Figure 8, his spine will exhibit an excess curve. This will cause pain and weakness in the small of the back. If the individual maintains a slight bend at the knees (10 to 15 degrees), as in Figure 9, then back alignment is normal and stresses are reduced.
Weight Used: None.
Action: Assume posture shown in Figure 9.
Repetitions: Practice maintaining proper posture at all times.

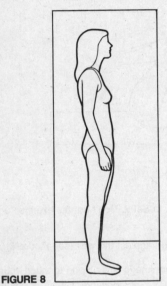

FIGURE 8

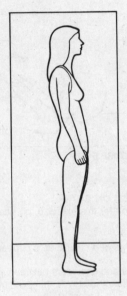

FIGURE 9

SET 5: BAR STRENGTHENING EXERCISES
Begin when pain decreases enough to permit light exercise.

EXERCISE 1
Position: Grip overhead bar.
Weight Used: None.
Action: Hang from the bar. Pull knees to chest (see Figure 10). Hold 5 to 10 seconds. Return slowly to starting position.
Repetitions: Up to 10 times, 3 or 4 times a day.

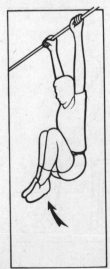

FIGURE 10

LOWER-BACK EXERCISES (continued)

EXERCISE 2
Position: Grip overhead bar.
Weight Used: None.
Action: Hang from the bar. Do "frog kick" (see Figure 11).
Repetitions: Up to 10 times, 3 or 4 times a day.

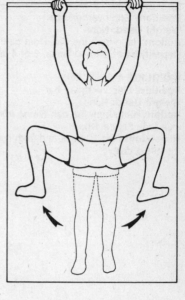

FIGURE 11

UPPER-BACK EXERCISES

These exercises are beneficial for inflammatory conditions or for rehabilitation following back injury. Inflammatory conditions include bursitis, tendinitis, gout, osteoarthritis, myositis and fibrositis. Sets 1 and 2 are very beneficial in stretching and strengthening for injuries caused by throwing.

SET 1: OVERHEAD BAR EXERCISES
Begin as soon as pain has decreased enough to permit light exercise.

EXERCISE 1
Position: Grip overhead bar (see Figure 12).
Weight Used: None.
Action: Hang until grip fails.
Repetitions: Once every hour while awake.

EXERCISE 2
Position: Grip overhead bar.
Weight Used: None.
Action: Hang from the bar. Pull knees to chest (see Figure 10). Hold 5 to 10 seconds. Return slowly to starting position.
Repetitions: Up to 10 times, 3 or 4 times a day.

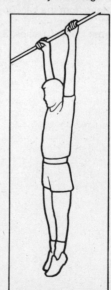

FIGURE 12

Continued on next page.

UPPER-BACK EXERCISES (continued)

EXERCISE 3
Position: Grip overhead bar.
Weight Used: None.
Action: Hang from the bar. Do a partial (not full) pullup. Return to starting position.
Repetitions: Up to 10 times, 3 or 4 times a day.

EXERCISE 4
Position: Grip overhead bar.
Weight Used: None.
Action: Hang from the bar. Swing from side to side (see Figure 13).
Repetitions: Do 10 back-and-forth cycles, 3 or 4 times a day.

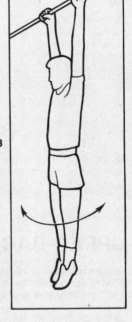

FIGURE 13

EXERCISE 5
Position: Grip overhead bar.
Weight Used: None.
Action: Hang from the bar. Do "frog kick" (see Figure 14).
Repetitions: Up to 10 times, 3 or 4 times a day.

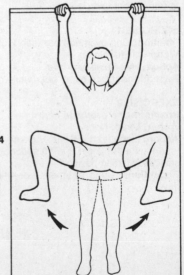

FIGURE 14

UPPER-BACK EXERCISES (continued)

SET 2: PUSH-UP EXERCISE
Begin at same time as Set 1.

Position: Assume a "push-up" position, with feet on the floor and hands on parallel bars or chair seats placed 24 inches apart. (Chairs must be sturdy!) See Figure 15.
Weight Used: None.
Action: Lower body into stretched, fully lowered position. Remain in this position 15 seconds. Then push up into the starting position.
Repetitions: 5 to 10 times, 3 or 4 times a day.

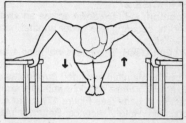

FIGURE 15

SET 3
Begin when you can do Sets 1 and 2 without difficulty or pain. Do exercises in Sets 1 and 2 with weights strapped to the waist for added resistance.

SET 4: UPPER-BACK EXTENSION
Begin as soon as pain has decreased enough to permit light exercise.

EXERCISE 1
Position: Lie face down across an exercise bench. Fold hands behind neck and point elbows outward (see Figure 16). You may need to secure your legs under another bench.
Weight Used: None.
Action: Lift the upper body to a full-extended ("up") position. Hold 2 seconds. Return to starting position. Hold 2 seconds.
Repetitions: 10 times, 3 or 4 times a day.

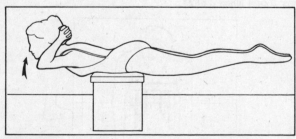

FIGURE 16

Continued on next page.

UPPER-BACK EXERCISES (continued)

EXERCISE 2
Position: Lie face down across an exercise bench, securing legs under another bench if necessary.
Weight Used: Dumbbells weighing 1 to 2.5 pounds.
Action: Maintain extended position as in Exercise 1 while raising dumbbells away from center of body (see Figure 17) as far as possible. Hold 2 seconds. Return to starting position. Hold 4 seconds.
Repetitions: 10 times, 3 or 4 times a day.

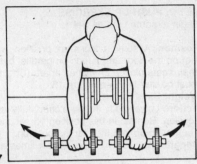

FIGURE 17

EXERCISE 3
Position: Lie face down across an exercise bench, securing legs under another bench if necessary.
Weight Used: Dumbbells weighing 2.5 to 5 pounds.
Action: Maintain extended position as in Exercise 1 while raising dumbbells forward as far as possible (see Figure 18). Hold 2 seconds. Return to starting position. Hold 4 seconds.
Repetitions: 10 times, 3 or 4 times a day.

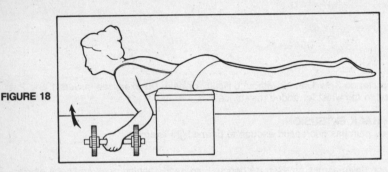

FIGURE 18

EXERCISE 4
Position: Lie face down across an exercise bench, securing legs under another bench if necessary.
Weight Used: Barbell with 2.5 to 5 pounds on each end.
Action: Maintain extended position as in Exercise 1 while pulling barbell to chest (see Figure 19). Hold 2 seconds. Return to starting position. Hold 4 seconds.
Repetitions: 10 times, 3 or 4 times a day.

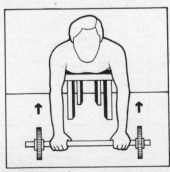

FIGURE 19

ELBOW EXERCISES

EXERCISE 1

Begin as soon as pain has decreased enough to permit light exercise.

Position: Hold a dumbbell or weighted bag at your side so that your thumb points straight forward (see Figure 20).
Weight Used: Begin with 2.5 to 5 pounds. Increase when strength allows.
Action: Bend elbow slowly to 90 degrees *and no farther* (see Figure 21). Allow no upper-arm movement. Hold for 2 to 3 seconds. Lower slowly to original position. Hold for 2 to 3 seconds.
Repetitions: Up to 15 tlmes, 3 or 4 times a day.

EXERCISE 2

Begin when 15 repetitions of Exercise 1 can be performed in perfect form with no pain.

Position: As in Exercise 1, hold a dumbbell or weighted bag at your side so that your thumb points straight forward.
Weight Used: Increase weekly as comfort allows. Stop at any weight that causes pain.
Action: Same as in Exercise 1.
Repetitions: Attempt to do 12 repetitions, 3 or 4 times a day. Increase weekly up to 20 repetitions as comfort allows. Stop at any number of repetitions or frequency of exercise that causes pain.
Then add weight and attempt to do 12. Again increase number as comfort allows. Add more weight and return to 12 as before. Stop at any number or weight that causes pain.

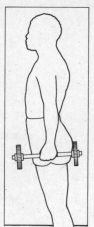
FIGURE 20

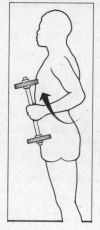
FIGURE 21

FOOT EXERCISES

Begin these exercises as soon as pain has decreased enough to permit light exercise.

SET 1: TOE EXERCISE

EXERCISE 1
Position: Sit, placing foot on a flat, smooth surface.
Weight Used: None.
Action: Lift toes, holding the ball of the foot on the flat surface (see Figure 22). Hold as high as possible for 3 seconds. Lower toes to surface. Hold for 3 seconds.
Repetitions: 10 times, twice a day, increasing to 30 times, twice a day.

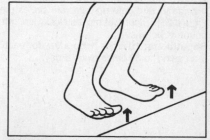
FIGURE 22

Continued on next page.

FOOT EXERCISES (continued)

EXERCISE 2
Position: Sit, placing foot at the edge of a smooth, flat surface, with toes extending beyond the edge.
Weight Used: None.
Action: Bend (flex) toes downward (see Figure 23). Hold down as far as possible for 3 seconds. Return to starting position. Hold for 3 seconds.
Repetitions: 10 times, twice a day, increasing to 30 times, twice a day.

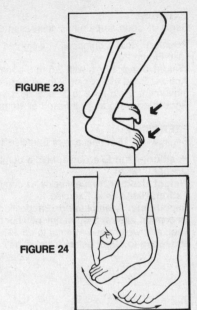

FIGURE 23

EXERCISE 3
Position: Sit comfortably.
Weight Used: None.
Action: Spread toes apart as far as possible, using hand to assist you if necessary (see Figure 24). Hold for 3 seconds. Relax toes. Hold for 3 seconds.
Repetitions: 10 times, twice a day, increasing to 30 times, twice a day.

FIGURE 24

SET 2: FOOT EXERCISES

EXERCISE 1
Position: Sit, placing foot on a flat, smooth surface.
Weight Used: None.
Action: Raise inner edge of foot, with weight on outer edge. Curl toes downward and inward (see Figure 25). Hold as tight as possible for 3 seconds. Relax for 3 seconds.
Repetitions: 10 times twice a day, increasing to 30 times twice a day.

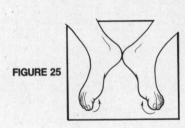

FIGURE 25

EXERCISE 2
Position: Sit comfortably, holding one foot firmly on the floor. Hold other foot in front of it, weight on the heel.
Weight Used: None.
Action: Rotate front of forward foot from outside inward, making complete circles (see Figure 26). Right foot moves clockwise, left foot counterclockwise.
Repetitions: 10 times twice a day for each foot, increasing to 30 times twice a day.

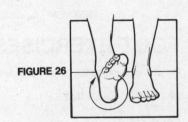

FIGURE 26

HAND EXERCISES

EXERCISE 1
Position: Squeeze a tennis ball or other gripping device with all fingers.
Weight Used: None.
Action: Apply moderate-intensity grip. Hold 2 to 3 seconds. Release.
Repetitions: Up to 15 times, 6 to 8 times a day.

EXERCISE 2
Same as Exercise 1, but squeeze with one finger at a time.

EXERCISE 3
Begin when Exercises 1 and 2 can be performed without hand pain. Same as Exercise 1, but increase frequency and intensity of grip to correspond to increased strength.

HIP & PELVIS EXERCISES

Begin these exercises when normal walking no longer hurts.

SET 1: HAMSTRING STRETCH

Position: Sit on the floor with one leg stretched straight in front of you and the other bent under itself in back of you.
Weight Used: None.
Action: While keeping the knee straight, attempt to bring the chin as close to the knee as possible. If necessary, loop a belt over the foot and pull (see Figure 27). Stretch slowly and steadily until the stretch is complete, usually in 15 seconds (it will be painful). Release slowly. Never jerk or fall into a stretched position. Alternate to the other knee after 4 or 5 stretches.
Repetitions: Alternate one hamstring stretch and one thigh stretch (Set 2, page 458). Repeat 4 or 5 times for each leg, once or twice a day.

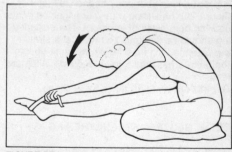

FIGURE 27

HIP & PELVIS EXERCISES (continued)

SET 2: THIGH STRETCH

Position: As in Set 1, sit on the floor with one leg stretched straight in front of you and the other bent under itself in back of you.
Weight Used: None.
Action: While keeping the point of the knee on the floor and the ankle directly under your hips, bend your entire body backward as far as you can. The full range is with the elbows resting on the floor in back of you (see Figure 28).
Repetitions: Alternate one thigh stretch and one hamstring stretch (Set 1, page 457). Repeat 4 to 5 times, once or twice a day.

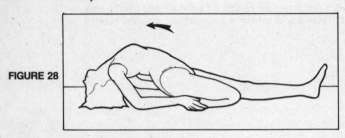

FIGURE 28

SET 3: GROIN STRETCH

Position: Stand with your feet about double-shoulder-width apart. Feet should point forward and remain flat on the floor. Keep them this way throughout the exercise.
Weight Used: None.
Action: Lower your body to one side (see Figure 29), balancing with your fingertips on the floor on both sides of your foot. The extended leg should be straight. You will feel a stretch in the extended leg from inside the knee up into the groin area. Hold 5 to 10 seconds. Alternate legs.
Repetitions: 5 to 10 times for each leg.

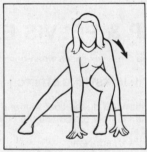

FIGURE 29

SET 4: GLUTEAL STRENGTHENING

Position: Lie face-down on a flat surface.
Weight Used: None.
Action: Lift one leg 3 or 4 inches off the floor (see Figure 30). Keep the knee stiff. Hold for a count of 5. Return to starting position. Repeat with other leg.
Repetitions: 4 or 5 for each leg, 3 or 4 times a day.

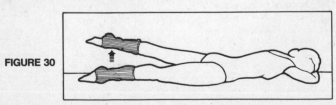

FIGURE 30

HIP & PELVIS EXERCISES (continued)

SET 5: STRENGTHENING BAR EXERCISES
Begin as soon as pain has decreased enough
to permit light exercise.

EXERCISE 1
Position: Grip overhead bar.
Weight Used: None.
Action: Hang from the bar. Pull knees to chest
(see Figure 31). Hold 5 to 10 seconds. Return
slowly to starting position.
Repetitions: Up to 10 times, 3 or 4 times a
day.

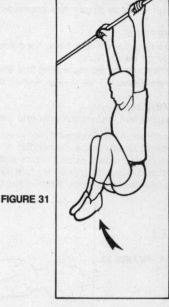

FIGURE 31

EXERCISE 2
Position: Grip overhead bar.
Weight Used: None.
Action: Hang from the bar. Do "frog kick" (see
Figure 32).
Repetitions: Up to 10 times, 3 or 4 times a
day.

WARNING: Avoid overflexing an injured knee.
Never do deep knee bends.

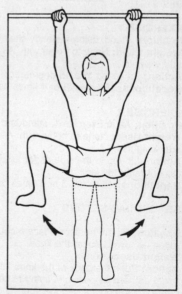

FIGURE 32

KNEE EXERCISES

SET 1
Begin as soon as pain has decreased enough to permit light exercise.

EXERCISE 1
Position: Lie on your back. Keep the injured knee absolutely straight.
Weight Used: None.
Action: Raise the injured leg to a 45-degree angle. Lower it slowly. Do not relax the leg.
Repetitions: 15 times, 3 or 4 times daily.

EXERCISE 2
Begin when you are stronger and Exercise 1 can be performed without additional pain.

Position: As in Exercise 1, lie on your back. Keep the injured knee absolutely straight.
Weight Used: Drape the handles of a gym bag or flight bag over the ankle (see Figure 33). Add weight to it slowly as pain allows and strength increases.
Action: Raise the injured leg to a 45-degree angle. Lower it slowly. Do not relax the leg.
Repetitions: 15 times, 3 or 4 times daily.

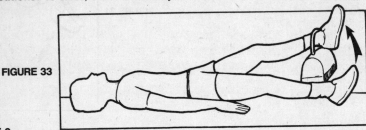

FIGURE 33

SET 2

EXERCISE 1
Position: Stand, using a steady chair or wall as support if necessary.
Weight Used: None to begin with. As your strength increases and pain allows, use a gym bag and add weights.
Action: Raise leg to a 45-degree angle. Lower it slowly. Keep knee straight.
Repetitions: 15 times, 3 or 4 times daily.

EXERCISE 2
Position: As in Exercise 1, stand and use a chair or wall for support.
Weight Used: None to begin with. As your strength increases and pain allows, use a gym bag and add weights.
Action: Lift leg to the side as far as possible, keeping the knee absolutely straight. Lower it slowly. Do not relax the leg.
Repetitions: 15 times, 3 or 4 times daily.

SET 3: QUAD-SETTING

Position: Sit on the floor. Place a couple of rolled-up towels under the knee.
Weight Used: None.
Action: Push the back of the knee into the towel as hard as possible, trying to keep the entire leg in contact with the floor (see Figure 34). Hold 5 seconds. Relax for 5 seconds.
Repetitions: 10 times, 3 or 4 times a day.

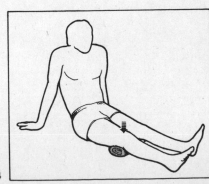

FIGURE 34

KNEE EXERCISES (continued)

SET 4

EXERCISE 1
Position: Sit on a high table with the back of the knee at the edge of the table. You may use towels to pad the back of the knee.
Weight Used: None.
Action: From a fully bent position, straighten the knee as much as possible and hold for 3 seconds. Lower leg and relax for 3 seconds.
Repetitions: 15 times, 3 or 4 times a day.

EXERCISE 2
Begin when strength allows. Continue only as long as pain and swelling do not increase as a result of this exercise.

Position: Sit on a high table as in Exercise 1.
Weight Used: Drape the handles of a gym bag or flight bag over the ankle (see Figure 35). Add weight to it slowly as strength increases and pain allows.
Action: As in Exercise 1, straighten the knee as much as possible and hold for 3 seconds. Lower leg and relax for 3 seconds.
Repetitions: 15 times, 3 or 4 times a day.

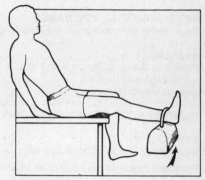

FIGURE 35

SET 5

Position: Stand erect and balance by holding onto a stable piece of furniture or a wall.
Weight Used: None to begin with. Drape the handles of a gym bag or flight bag over the back of the ankle. Add weight to it slowly as strength increases and pain allows.
Action: Bend the leg backward as far as possible (see Figure 36). Hold 5 seconds. Return to starting position. Rest 5 seconds.
Repetitions: 15 times, 3 or 4 times a day.

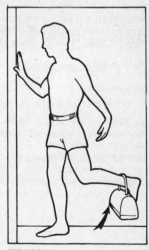

FIGURE 36

LOWER-LEG EXERCISES

SET 1: TOE RAISES
Do this while leg is stiff and painful, after clearance from your doctor.

Position: Stand on the floor, feet comfortably apart.
Weight Used: None.
Action: Rise up onto the balls of the feet as far as possible. Immediately lower yourself to the beginning position.
Repetitions: 20 to 25 times, 3 or 4 times a day.

SET 2: ADVANCED TOE RAISES
Begin these exercises when leg is no longer stiff.

EXERCISE 1
Position: Stand on the edge of a step or other elevated structure so that your heels stretch below the level of your toes.
Weight Used: None.
Action: Rise on the balls of your feet, and immediately lower yourself to the starting position.
Repetitions: 20 to 25 times, 3 or 4 times a day.

EXERCISE 2
Begin when able to perform Exercise 1 successfully.

Position: Stand on the edge of an elevated structure on one foot only, with the heel lower than the toes.
Weight Used: None.
Action: Rise on the ball of your foot, and immediately lower yourself to the starting position.
Repetitions: 20 to 25 times for each foot, 3 or 4 times a day.

EXERCISE 3
Begin when able to perform Exercise 1 successfully.

Position: Stand on the edge of an elevated structure on one foot only, with the heel lower than the toes.
Weight Used: Hold a weighted object (5 to 10 pounds) in either hand.
Action: Rise on the ball of the foot and lower yourself as in Exercise 1.
Repetitions: 20 to 25 times for each foot, 3 or 4 times a day.

SET 3: HEEL WALKING

EXERCISE 1
Begin at the same time as Set 2.

Position: Stand on the heels, keeping toes as high off the ground as possible. Use a firm, smooth surface. Wear shoes with good solid heels.
Weight Used: None.
Action: Walk, continuing to keep toes as high as possible. Take short, choppy steps. Walk this way as long as possible, up to 2 minutes or about 100 feet.
Repetitions: 4 or 5 times a day.

LOWER-LEG EXERCISES (continued)

EXERCISE 2
Begin when Exercise 1 is completed successfully.

Position: As in Exercise 1, stand on the heels, keeping toes as high off the ground as possible. Use a firm, smooth surface. Wear shoes with good solid heels.
Weight Used: 5- to 10-pound ankle weights.
Action: Same as Exercise 1. You may also do this exercise "walking" up a hill or incline, with or without weights (see Figure 37).
Repetitions: 3 to 5 times a day.

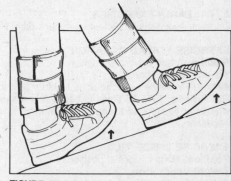

FIGURE 37

SET 4: ISOMETRIC ANKLE "WRESTLING"

EXERCISE 1
Begin as soon as pain has decreased enough to permit light exercise. This may be as soon as 1 day after injury.

Position: Sit comfortably, and place one ankle over the other.
Weight Used: None.
Action: Press outward with both ankles so that your feet are firmly pressing against each other. Hold for 10 seconds. Relax for 10 seconds.
Repetitions: 5 times for each leg, 3 or 4 times a day.

EXERCISE 2
Begin when leg is less stiff and painful than in Exercise 1.

Position: As in Exercise 1, sit comfortably and place one ankle over the other.
Weight Used: None.
Action: Begin as in Exercise 1. When ankles are pressed firmly, rotate the front of feet away from each other and back to the starting position (see Figure 38). Make each rotation last 10 full seconds.
Repetitions: 10 times for each leg, 3 or 4 times a day.

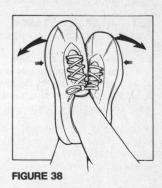

FIGURE 38

NECK EXERCISES

SET 1: EARLY EXERCISES
Do these exercises while you have neck pain. Don't progress to Set 2 while pain is present.

EXERCISE 1: HEAD ROTATION
Position: Head in normal position.
Weight Used: None.
Action: Rotate head to the right. Hold for 5 seconds. Rotate head to the left. Hold for 5 seconds.
Repetitions: 10 to 15 times to begin, 3 or 4 times a day. Gradually increase to 50 repetitions. Stop whenever you feel additional pain. Return to a comfortable level and maintain it as long as necessary.

EXERCISE 2: SIDE TILT
Position: Head in normal position.
Weight Used: None.
Action: Move ear toward right shoulder. Hold for 5 seconds. Move ear toward left shoulder. Hold for 5 seconds.
Repetitions: 3 or 4 times a day, 10 to 15 times to begin. Gradually increase to 50 repetitions. Stop whenever you feel additional pain. Return to a comfortable level and maintain it as long as necessary.

EXERCISE 3: FORWARD THRUST
Position: Head in normal position.
Weight Used: None.
Action: Move chin forward and down, touching it low on the chest. Hold for 5 seconds. Return to normal position for 5 seconds.
Repetitions: 10 to 15 times to begin, 3 or 4 times a day. Gradually increase to 50 repetitions. Stop whenever you feel additional pain. Return to a comfortable level and maintain it as long as necessary.

WARNING: Do not move the head backward past the neutral or "natural" position. This will aggravate most neck problems.

SET 2: NECK RESISTANCE
Start these exercises only when you have no pain or stiffness.

Exercises are done as in Set 1, but resistance to movements is added in one of the following ways:
1) Partner resists movement in all directions with his hands.
2) Injured athlete resists his own movements with his hands or with a towel.
3) Under supervision of a trainer or physical therapist, resistance is applied with a spring-loaded or weight-loaded head strap.

SHOULDER EXERCISES

These exercises are beneficial for inflammatory conditions or for rehabilitation following shoulder injury. Inflammatory conditions include bursitis, tendinitis, gout, osteoarthritis, myositis and fibrositis. Sets 1 and 2 are very beneficial in stretching and strengthening for injuries caused by throwing.

SET 1: OVERHEAD BAR EXERCISES
Begin as soon as pain has decreased enough to permit light exercise.

EXERCISE 1
Position: Grip overhead bar (see Figure 39).
Weight Used: None.
Action: Hang until grip fails.
Repetitions: Once, 3 or 4 times a day.

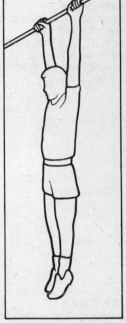

FIGURE 39

EXERCISE 2
Position: Grip overhead bar.
Weight Used: None.
Action: Hang from the bar. Pull knees to chest (see Figure 40). Hold 5 to 10 seconds. Return slowly to starting position.
Repetitions: Up to 10 times, 3 or 4 times a day.

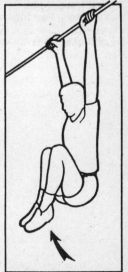

FIGURE 40

Continued on next page.

SHOULDER EXERCISES (continued)

EXERCISE 3
Position: Grip overhead bar.
Weight Used: None.
Action: Hang from the bar. Do a partial (not full) pullup. Return to starting position.
Repetitions: Up to 10 times, 3 or 4 times a day.

EXERCISE 4
Position: Grip overhead bar.
Weight Used: None.
Action: Hang from the bar. Swing from side to side (see Figure 41).
Repetitions: Do 10 back-and-forth cycles, 3 or 4 times a day.

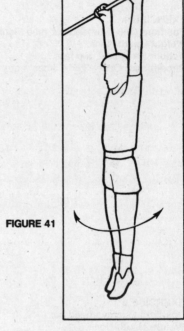

FIGURE 41

EXERCISE 5
Position: Grip overhead bar.
Weight Used: None.
Action: Hang from the bar. Do "frog kick" (see Figure 42).
Repetitions: Up to 10 times, 3 or 4 times a day.

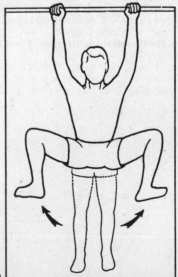

FIGURE 42

SHOULDER EXERCISES (continued)

SET 2: PUSH-UP EXERCISE
Begin at same time as Set 1.

Position: Assume a "push-up" position, with feet on the floor and hands on parallel bars or chair seats placed 24 inches apart. (Chairs must be sturdy!) See Figure 43.
Weight Used: None.
Action: Lower body into stretched, fully lowered position. Remain in this position 15 seconds. Then push up into the starting position.
Repetitions: 5 to 10 times, 3 or 4 times a day.

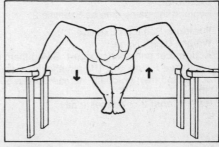

FIGURE 43

SET 3
Begin when when you can do Sets 1 and 2 without difficulty or pain. Do exercises in Sets 1 and 2 with weights strapped to the waist for added resistance.

SET 4: GRAVITY EXERCISES FOR INFLAMMATORY CONDITIONS

EXERCISE 1
Begin as soon as pain has decreased enough to permit light exercise.

Position: Bend far forward holding the shoulders and trunk still.
Weight Used: None.
Action: Hold position for 30 seconds.
Repetitions: 3 or 4 times a day.

EXERCISE 2
Begin when you can do Exercise 1 without pain.

Position: Bend far forward holding the shoulders and trunk still.
Weight Used: None.
Action: Let arms hang loosely. Swing them like a pendulum *back* and *forth* across the front of the body 50 times.
Repetitions: 3 or 4 times a day.

EXERCISE 3
Begin at the same time as Exercise 2.

Position: Same as Exercise 1.
Weight Used: None.
Action: Let arms hang loosely. Swing them like a pendulum *backward* and *forward* 50 times.
Repetitions: 3 or 4 times a day.

Continued on next page.

SHOULDER EXERCISES (continued)

EXERCISE 4
Begin at the same time as Exercise 2.

Position: Same as Exercise 1.
Weight Used: None.
Action: Let arms hang loosely. Swing them in a circle (see Figure 44). The arc should be small at first and then gradually increase. Make 50 circles.
Repetitions: 3 or 4 times a day.

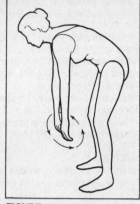

FIGURE 44

SET 5: ANTI-GRAVITY EXERCISES FOR INFLAMMATORY CONDITIONS
Begin when gravity exercises in Set 4 can be performed without pain.

EXERCISE 1
Position: Stand approximately one shoulder width from the wall. Your arm should be in a normal position at your side.
Weight Used: None.
Action: Raise and lower your arm by "climbing" your fingers up and down the wall (see Figure 45).
Repetitions: 10 up-and-down cycles, 3 or 4 times a day.

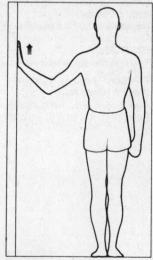

FIGURE 45

SHOULDER EXERCISES (continued)

EXERCISE 2

Position: Face the wall, standing approximately 2 feet from it. Your arm should be in normal position at your side.
Weight Used: None.
Action: Raise and lower your arm by "climbing" your fingers up and down the wall (see Figure 46).
Repetitions: 10 up-and-down cycles, 3 or 4 times a day.

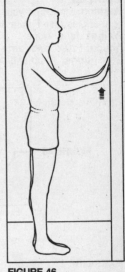

FIGURE 46

SET 6: EXTERNAL ROTATION EXERCISES

EXERCISE 1

Position: Stand with your back, upper arms and elbows against the wall. Bend your arms at a 90-degree angle.
Weight Used: None.
Action: Move your lower arms in arcs between the wall and the front of the body (see Figure 47).
Repetitions: 10 forward-and-back cycles, 3 or 4 times a day.

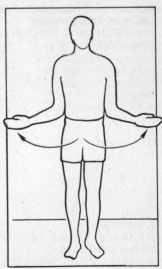

FIGURE 47

Continued on next page.

SHOULDER EXERCISES (continued)

EXERCISE 2
Position: Lie flat on your back, upper arms against your sides, lower arms and hands on floor at right angles (see Figure 48).
Weight Used: None.
Action: Raise lower arms and hands to vertical position. Return to starting position.
Repetitions: 10 up-and-down cycles, 3 or 4 times a day.

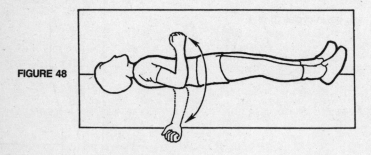

FIGURE 48

EXERCISE 3
Position: Lie flat on your back with hands under your head, elbows pointing up.
Weight Used: None.
Action: Lower elbows to floor (see Figure 49). Return to starting position.
Repetitions: 10 up-and-down cycles, 3 or 4 times a day.

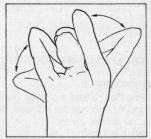

FIGURE 49

EXERCISE 4
Position: As shown in Figure 50.
Weight Used: None.
Action: As shown. Perform at a comfortable speed.
Repetitions: 5 minutes, 3 or 4 times a day.

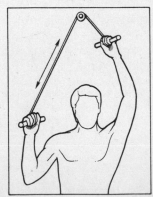

FIGURE 50

THIGH EXERCISES

SET 1
Begin as soon after injury as possible, before and after knee surgery, or during healing of a fractured femur.

EXERCISE 1: QUADRICEPS DRILL
Position: Any comfortable position.
Weight Used: None.
Action: Forcibly contract the quadriceps muscle of the thigh. Hold 10 seconds. Relax it slowly to a count of 10.
Repetitions: 15 to 20 times, once per hour while awake.

EXERCISE 2
Begin after Exercise 1 can be performed without increasing pain at the injury site.

Position: Lie comfortably.
Weight Used: None.
Action: Raise the leg as far as possible and hold for 10 seconds. Lower the leg to the starting position as you count to 10.
Repetitions: 15 to 20 times, once per hour while awake.

EXERCISE 3
Begin when you are able to raise the extended leg against the force of gravity with no difficulty.

Position: Lie comfortably.
Weight Used: Elastic resistive apparatus (see Figure 51). This can be made from surgical tubing or a bicycle innertube.
Action: Raise the leg as far as possible against resistance and hold for 10 seconds. Lower the leg to the starting position as you count to 10.
Repetitions: 10 to 30 times, 3 or 4 times a day.

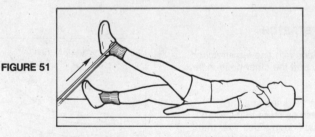

FIGURE 51

SET 2
Begin when you can do the following without increased pain.

EXERCISE 1: BICYCLING
Position: Sit on an exercise bicycle.
Weight Used: None.
Action: Normal bicycling movement.
Repetitions: 5 to 15 minutes, 3 or 4 times a day.

Continued on next page.

THIGH EXERCISES (continued)

EXERCISE 2: STAIR-CLIMBING
Begin when you can do all preceding thigh exercises without difficulty.

Position: Stand in front of a footstool or at the bottom of stairs.
Weight Used: None.
Action: Step up and step down, stepping up with the injured side and down with the uninjured side.
Repetitions: 10 to 30 times, 3 or 4 times a day.

EXERCISE 3
Position: See Figure 52.
Weight Used: Begin with the weight at which you can barely extend the leg. After 1 week, increase the weight to whatever the leg can elevate to full extension. Continue to add weight each week in this way.
Action: Slowly move the leg up and down fully without pausing.
Repetitions: 7 to 10 sets of 10 repetitions each. Rest between each set. Do once or twice a day.

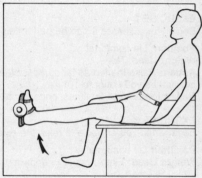

FIGURE 52

SET 3: HAMSTRING STRETCH

Position: Sit on the floor with one leg stretched straight in front of you and the other bent under itself in back of you.
Weight Used: None.
Action: While keeping the knee straight, attempt to bring the chin as close to the knee as possible. If necessary, loop a belt over the foot and pull (see Figure 53). Stretch slowly and steadily until the stretch is complete, usually in 15 seconds (it will be painful). Release slowly. Never jerk or fall into a stretched position. Alternate to the other knee after 4 or 5 stretches.
Repetitions: Alternate one hamstring stretch and one thigh stretch (Set 4, opposite page). Repeat 4 or 5 times for each leg, once or twice a day.

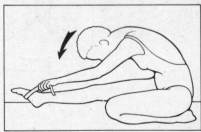

FIGURE 53

THIGH EXERCISES (continued)

SET 4: THIGH STRETCH

Position: As in Set 3, sit on the floor with one leg stretched straight in front of you and the other bent under itself in back of you.
Weight Used: None.
Action: While keeping the point of the knee on the floor and the ankle directly under your hips, bend your entire body backward as far as you can. The full range is with the elbows resting on the floor in back of you (see Figure 54).
Repetitions: Alternate one thigh stretch and one hamstring stretch (Set 3, opposite page). Repeat 4 to 5 times for each leg, once or twice a day.

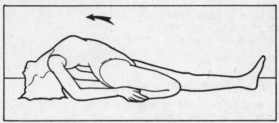

FIGURE 54

SET 5: GROIN STRETCH

Position: Stand with your feet about double shoulder-width apart. Feet should point forward and remain flat on the floor. Keep them this way throughout the exercise.
Weight Used: None.
Action: Lower your body to one side, balancing with your fingertips on the floor on both sides of your foot. The extended leg should be straight. You will feel a stretch in the extended leg from inside the knee up into the groin area. Hold 5 to 10 seconds. Alternate legs.
Repetitions: 5 to 10 times for each leg, once or twice a day.

WARNING: Avoid overflexing an injured knee. Never do deep knee bends.

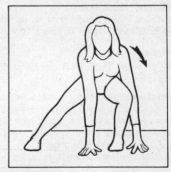

FIGURE 55

WRIST EXERCISES

SET 1: WRIST FLEXION

EXERCISE 1
Begin as soon as pain has decreased enough
to permit light exercise.

Position: Hand palm-up, wrist supported at the
edge of a table or on the knee so that only the
hand is able to move. Grasp the weighted
dumbbell or a weighted bag (see Figure 56).
Weight Used: Begin with 2.5 to 5 pounds.
Increase as strength allows.
Action: Flex the wrist as far as possible. Hold 2
to 3 seconds. Lower fully. Hold 2 to 3 seconds.
Repetitions: Up to 15 times, 3 or 4 times a
day.

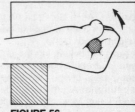
FIGURE 56

EXERCISE 2
Begin when Exercise 1 can be performed with no wrist pain.

Position: Hand palm-up, wrist supported at the edge of a table or on the knee so that only the
hand is able to move. Grasp the weighted dumbbell or a weighted bag, as in Exercise 1.
Weight Used: Increase 5 to 10 pounds weekly as comfort allows. Stop at any weight that triggers
pain, and return to a comfortable weight for as long as necessary.
Action: Flex the wrist as far as possible. Hold 2 to 3 seconds. Lower fully. Hold 2 to 3 seconds.
Repetitions: Up to 15 times, 3 or 4 times a day.

SET 2: WRIST EXTENSION

EXERCISE 1
Begin as soon as pain has decreased enough to permit light exercise.

Position: Hand flat on table, palm-down.
Weight Used: None.
Action: Raise hand up as far as possible, keeping wrist flat on table.
Repetitions: Up to 15 times, 3 or 4 times a day.

EXERCISE 2
Begin when Exercise 1 can be performed with
no wrist pain.

Position: Hand palm-down, wrist supported as
in Set 1, Exercise 1 above. Grasp the weighted
dumbbell or a weighted bag (see Figure 57).
Weight Used: Begin with 2.5 to 5 pounds.
Increase as strength allows.
Action: Lower the wrist as far as possible. Hold
2 to 3 seconds. Raise as far as possible. Hold 2
to 3 seconds.
Repetitions: Up to 15 times, 3 or 4 times a
day.

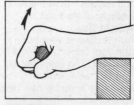
FIGURE 57

WRIST EXERCISES (continued)

SET 3: GRIPPING EXERCISE

EXERCISE 1
Begin as soon as pain has decreased enough to permit light exercise.

Position: Squeeze a tennis ball or other gripping device with all fingers.
Action: Grip with moderate intensity. Hold 2 to 3 seconds. Release.
Weight Used: None.
Repetitions: Up to 15 times, 3 or 4 times a day.

EXERCISE 2
Same as Exercise 1, but squeeze with one finger at a time.

EXERCISE 3
Begin when Exercises 1 and 2 can be performed with no wrist pain.
Position and action are the same as Exercise 1, but increase grip to correspond to increased weight in wrist-flexion and wrist-extension exercises (opposite page).

SET 4: LEVER-BAR ROTATION

EXERCISE 1
Begin as soon as pain has decreased enough to permit light exercise.

Position: Place the wrist at the edge of the table, as in the wrist-flexion exercise (opposite page). Grip the bar at the non-weighted end, with the weight away from the body (see Figure 58).
Weight Used: 5 pounds to begin. Increase as strength allows.
Action: Rotate the hand inward as far as possible. Hold momentarily. Allow the weight to return to the starting position slowly (2 to 3 seconds).
Repetitions: Up to 15 times, 3 or 4 times a day.

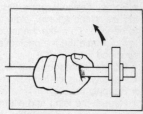

FIGURE 58

EXERCISE 2
Begin when Exercise 1 can be performed with no wrist pain.

Instructions are the same as for Exercise 1, but use additional weight and increase the space along the bar between the grip and the weight.

EXERCISE 3
Begin at same time as Exercise 1.

Position: Place the wrist at the edge of the table, as in Exercise 1. Grip the bar at the non-weighted end, with the weight on the inside (see Figure 59).
Weight Used: 2.5 to 5 pounds.
Action: Rotate the hand outward as far as possible. Hold momentarily. Allow the weight to return to a starting position slowly (2 to 3 seconds).
Repetitions: Up to 15 times, 3 or 4 times a day.

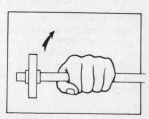

FIGURE 59

APPENDIX 1

R.I.C.E. (Rest, Ice, Compression, Elevation)

R.I.C.E. is an acronym (a word coined from first letters) for the most important elements—*rest, ice, compression* and *elevation*—in first aid of many injuries. This acronym appears repeatedly throughout this book—and in medical literature in general—in reference to athletic injuries. Use the word *R.I.C.E.* to jog your memory when you are faced with such injuries as contusions, sprains, strains, dislocations or uncomplicated fractures.

REST

Stop using the injured part and rest it as soon as you realize an injury has taken place. Continued exercise or other activity could cause further injury, delay healing, increase pain, and stimulate bleeding. Use crutches to avoid bearing weight on injuries of the foot, ankle, knee or leg. Use splints for injuries of the hand, wrist, elbow or arm. After medical treatment, the injured part may require immobilization with splints or a cast to keep the area at rest until it heals.

ICE

Ice helps stop internal bleeding from injured blood vessels and capillaries. Sudden cold causes small blood vessels to contract. This contraction of blood vessels decreases the amount of blood that can collect around the wound. The more blood that collects, the longer the healing time. Ice can be safely applied in several ways using the following instructions:

● For injuries to small areas, such as a finger, toe, foot, or wrist, immerse the injured area in a bucket of ice water. Use ice cubes to keep the water cold as ice dissolves.
● For injuries to larger areas, use ice packs. Avoid placing ice directly on the skin. Before applying the ice, place a towel, cloth, or one or two layers of an elasticized compression bandage on the skin to be iced. To make the ice pack, put ice chips or ice cubes in a plastic bag or wrap them in a thin towel. Place the ice pack over the cloth. The pack may sit directly on the injured part, or it may be wrapped in place.
● Ice the injured area for about 30 minutes (no matter what form of ice treatment you are using).
● Remove the ice to allow the skin to warm for 15 minutes.
● Reapply the ice.
● Repeat the icing and warming cycles for 3 hours, as well as following the instructions below for compression and elevation. If pain and swelling persist after 3 hours, consult your doctor (if you have not already done so). Your doctor may change the icing schedule after the first 3 hours. Regular ice treatment is often discontinued after 24 to 48 hours. At that point, heat is often more comfortable.

COMPRESSION

Compression decreases swelling by slowing bleeding and limiting the accumulation of blood and plasma near the injured site. Without compression, fluid from adjacent normal tissue seeps into the injury area. The more blood and fluid that accumulates around an injury, the slower the healing. Following are instructions for applying compression safely to an injury:

● Use an elasticized bandage (Ace bandage) for compression, if possible. If you do not have one available, any kind of cloth will suffice for a short time. Wrap the injured part firmly, wrapping over the ice also. Begin wrapping below the injury site and extend above the injury site. Be careful not to compress the area so tightly that the blood supply is impaired. Signs of blood-supply deprivation include pain, numbness, cramping, and blue or dusky-colored nails. Remove the compression bandage immediately if any of these symptoms appear. Leave the bandage off until all signs of impaired circulation disappear. Then rewrap the area—less tightly this time.

ELEVATION

Elevating the injured part above the level of the heart is another way to decrease swelling and pain at the injury site. Elevate the iced, compressed area in whatever way is most convenient. Prop an injured leg on solid objects or pillows. Elevate an injured arm by lying down and placing pillows under the arm, or placing them on the chest with the arm folded across. The whole upper part of the body may be elevated gently with pillows, a reclining chair, or by raising the top of the bed on blocks.

APPENDIX 2

Care of Casts

A cast immobilizes a part of the body that has been injured. Casts are used most commonly after bone fractures.

Casts are usually applied by placing a splint along the injured part and wrapping it with gauze saturated with plaster of Paris. Before the injury heals, it may be necessary to change the cast one or more times. The time needed for healing determines how long a cast remains in place. Some casts are needed for only 2 weeks. Others are necessary for several months.

X-rays through a cast reveal whether bone alignment is satisfactory. They are also used in later stages to check for signs of healing.

AFTER YOU LEAVE THE DOCTOR'S OFFICE

- Don't allow pressure on any part of the cast—no matter what type of casting material was used—until it is completely dry. Any depression that develops will create pressure on the skin underneath, making ulcer formation likely. Drying time varies depending on the type of material used, thickness of the cast, temperature and humidity. Drying can require 24 hours or longer.
- Keep the cast dry, especially at first. If the cast accidentally gets wet and a soft area appears, return to the doctor's office, emergency room or outpatient surgical facility for repairs.
- Whenever possible, raise the body part enclosed in the cast. This decreases the chance of tissue swelling inside the cast. Prop a leg in a cast on a pillow when in bed, and on a footstool or chair when sitting. Prop an arm in a cast on a pillow placed on the chest. Elevate the foot of the bed at night for any injury requiring a cast below the abdomen.

SWELLING INSIDE A CAST

No matter how carefully the injured tissues are handled, and no matter how expertly the cast is applied, swelling sometimes occurs inside a cast. Swelling should be reported immediately to the doctor. The following are common symptoms and signs of swelling:

- Severe, persistent pain.
- Change in color of tissues beyond the cast, such as a change to blue or gray under the fingernails or toenails.
- Coldness of the tissues beyond the cast, even though the rest of the body is warm.
- Numbness or complete loss of feeling in the skin beyond the cast.
- Feeling of tightness under the cast after it dries.
- For a leg cast, inability to raise the big toe.

INFECTION INSIDE A CAST

Sometimes the injured area becomes infected during healing. Detecting the infection in early stages may be difficult if the infected area is covered by a cast. Infection should be reported immediately to the doctor. Following are common signs and symptoms of infection:

- Leakage of fluid through the cast.
- Pain or soreness of the skin under the cast.
- Fever accompanied by a general ill feeling.

ITCHING INSIDE A CAST

Itching can be a maddening problem for a person with a cast—especially during hot weather. Even if you can reach the itch, don't scratch the skin inside the cast. Because the skin is in a hot, moist environment, it is very vulnerable to damage. Scratching is more likely to injure the skin than under normal circumstances. If no incision was made, you may sprinkle cornstarch into the cast to relieve itching. If an incision was made, consult your doctor for pain medication. Itching is a form of mild pain.

BATHING WITH A CAST

You may find bathing difficult when wearing a cast. The cast must be kept dry at all times, so do not take showers. If the cast is on a limb, such as your arm or leg, you may take tub baths. Position a chair or other support by the tub so you can prop the injured part out of the water while bathing. If the cast is on the trunk of the body, you should take sponge baths until the cast is removed.

APPENDIX 3

Safe Use of Crutches

Crutches are often a necessary aid to walking when a person has injured a foot, ankle, leg or hip. Proper use of crutches can allow safe, satisfactory mobility. Improper use can cause further accidents.

BEFORE YOU USE CRUTCHES
- Practice using crutches under supervision before trying them out on your own.
- Reread these instructions frequently while getting used to crutches until using the crutches becomes automatic.
- Use a backpack to carry necessary belongings while using crutches. Never try to carry anything in your hands or arms.

FITTING CRUTCHES
You will be fitted for your crutches at the place where you rent or buy them—usually a medical-supply store. The following points are important in ensuring a proper fit:

1. Stand straight.
2. Adjust the length of the crutches so 2 or 3 fingers can fit between the top of the crutch and the armpit (about 2 inches).
3. Adjust the hand grip so your elbow bends about 25 degrees, as shown in Figure 1.
   Warning: Don't bear any weight in the armpits. This can cause permanent damage to the nerves of the arm and hand.

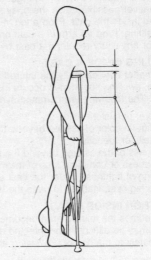

FIGURE 1

MOVING ON CRUTCHES
There are 4 major gaits used by people who need crutches:

Swing-through Gait—Fastest and most difficult.
Swing-to Gait—Slower and easier, and good to use until you become skillful with crutches and can advance to a faster gait.
Shuffle Gait—Slowest of all, and most appropriate for older people.
3-Point Gait—Can be used only when a slight amount of weight can be borne on the weak side.

The last three gaits are described here. When you are ready to progress to a faster gait, such as the swing-through gait, you will need instructions and supervision from your trainer, nurse or doctor. Also described are instructions on ascending and descending stairs and curbs. These are general suggestions that apply to everyone on crutches.

APPENDIX 3 (continued)

SWING-TO GAIT

This is a good gait for beginners.

1. Place both crutches forward simultaneously, 12 inches in front of your feet, 6 to 8 inches wider than your toes on both sides (see Figure 2).
2. Push your hands down against the handles and shift your weight forward.
3. Swing your body to a point directly between the crutches. Let the heel on the healthy side land first.

Note: The Swing-through Gait is the same as the Swing-to Gait except that the body swings through and lands in front of the crutches (see Figure 3).

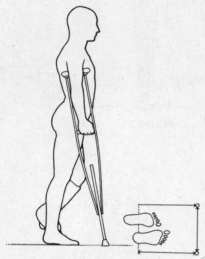

FIGURE 2

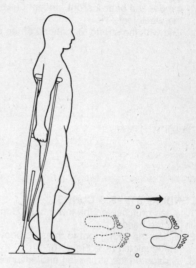

FIGURE 3

SHUFFLE GAIT

This gait should be used when the Swing-to Gait is too difficult:

1. Place both crutches forward simultaneously, 12 inches in front of your feet, 6 to 8 inches wider than your toes on both sides (see Figure 4).
2. Push hands down against the handles as you shift your body weight forward.
3. Slide the strong leg forward a few inches to a point between the crutches.
4. Follow with the weak leg, ending with the legs together.

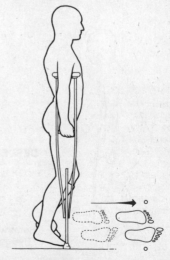

FIGURE 4

APPENDIX 3 (continued)

3-POINT GAIT

Use this gait only when you are able to bear slight, increasing weight on the weak leg (see Figure 5).

1. Place both crutches and the weak foot forward simultaneously, with the weak foot between the crutches. The weight is borne on the strong foot.
2. Push against the handles and shift your weight forward.
3. Swing your body forward with weight on your hands, and bear a slight amount of weight on the weak foot.
4. End with the strong foot ahead of the crutches.

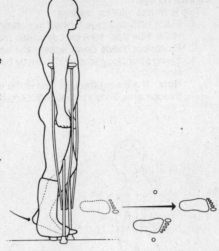

FIGURE 5

ASCENDING STEPS & CURBS

1. Keep crutches on the lower step. Body weight is on the hands.
2. Raise the strong foot to the step above, trailing the weak leg (see Figure 6).
3. Straighten the strong leg and advance the crutches to the next step above.

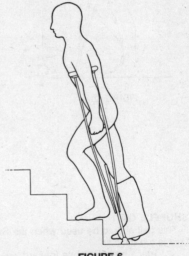

FIGURE 6

DESCENDING STEPS & CURBS

1. Place crutches on the lower step, and extend the weak leg forward. Body weight is on the hands (see Figure 7).
2. Bend the strong leg and slowly lower the body.
3. Quickly move the strong leg to the lower step.

Reminder for ascending and descending steps with crutches: "The good goes up, the bad goes down."

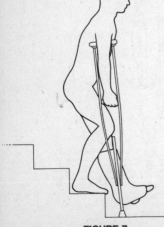

FIGURE 7

APPENDIX 4

Locker-Room Hygiene

Locker rooms, shower rooms and other athletic-club facilities can provide an ideal environment for harmful germs to grow and spread. Many bacteria and fungi thrive in dark, moist environments such as these, and crowded facilities enable germs to spread easily from person to person. Following are some suggestions to help you minimize your risk of illness.

● Shower with soap and warm water as soon as possible after each workout. If you avoid or delay showers, you leave yourself susceptible to *workout-breakout*—a skin condition caused when dry sweat plugs the openings of sweat glands. Moreover, warm showers make you feel better and disperse some of the accumulated lactic acid near muscles that sometimes causes muscle soreness.

● After each shower, use a clean towel that has been laundered with very hot water and detergent in a home or commercial laundry. Never share someone's towel. Unhygienic towels can spread disease such as pink eye, skin eruptions, virus infections or fungus infections.

● Bring your own stool to sit on, if possible. Store your stool in your locker when not in use. Avoid sitting on benches used by others. A damp bench can harbor bacteria, virus, and fungal infections, spreading them easily from one person to another. If you must sit on benches, dry off first and put your clothes on before doing so.

● Wear shoes whenever possible in the locker room. After showering, dry your feet last. Make sure you dry carefully between the toes, and dust your feet with non-prescription antifungal powder to help prevent athlete's foot.

● Avoid touching team members or other persons who share the athletic facilities, especially during outbreaks of colds or the flu. When you can't avoid touching others, wash your hands with soap and warm water before putting fingers or food touched by fingers into your mouth. Colds, flu and other viruses are more likely to be spread by hand-to-mouth contact than by breathing air contaminated with sneezes and coughs.

● Lockers must be well-ventilated to reduce odors and to enable athletic clothing and equipment to dry. Locker rooms should have automatic temperature and ventilation controls. Spray your locker with an antiseptic spray at least once a week.

● Insist that shower rooms and floors of locker rooms be periodically treated with antiseptic solutions.

APPENDIX 5

Nutrition for Athletes

Good nutrition at all times is essential for excellent athletic performance, even if competition is only seasonal. The basic nutritional requirements for athletes and fitness enthusiasts are the same as those for the general population. However, a few minor modifications prior to competition may enhance athletic performance.

Two decades ago, athletes were advised to: eat a high-protein diet; eat little on days of competition; stay away from refreshments and cold drinks during competition; take salt tablets during periods of heavy sweating; consume large doses of vitamins; and eat less than usual for a day following competition. These recommendations have proven more harmful than helpful, and have been discredited in recent years.

PRESENT DIETARY GUIDELINES

Following are the general guidelines advocated currently by nutritionists for a well-balanced diet for athletes and fitness enthusiasts. These guidelines may also be modified eventually as research provides additional information about nutrition and athletic performance, but they represent sound nutritional sense.

Protein—Contrary to what many coaches and athletes believe, the protein requirement for athletes is not significantly greater than it is for others. Most persons need about 1 gram of protein for each kilogram of weight. This amount is easily obtained in a diet in which protein comprises 10 to 15 percent of total calories.

Carbohydrates—The recommended percentage of total daily caloric intake for carbohydrates is 65%. Complex carbohydrates—as opposed to simple carbohydrates (sugar)—should make up the majority of the carbohydrate requirement. Complex carbohydrates are found in potatoes, brown rice, dried beans, fresh fruits and vegetables, and whole-grain breads and cereals. These foods also provide dietary fiber, an important element in regulating bowel function. In addition, complex carbohydrates provide the liver and muscle cells with glucose. This is stored as glycogen and converted back to glucose for use when needed during exercise.

Fat—No more than 20% of the dietary calories should come from fat.

Special Diets—Many good books provide detailed dietary and diet supplement-regimens for athletes. However, beware of advice given by anyone making extraordinary claims for fad foods or for protein, vitamin and mineral supplements. Most of these are not based on sound nutritional research, and are not recommended by nutritionists.

Weight-Loss Diets—Athletes engaged in vigorous physical activity should not skimp on their diets to "lose weight." Vigorous exercise will replace some body fat with muscle at the same time the body weight remains constant. A strenuous exercise program is accompanied by an increased metabolic rate, requiring an increased caloric intake. If you stop exercising for any reason, be sure to reduce your caloric intake. Otherwise, you may gain weight rapidly.

ADDITIONAL RECOMMENDATIONS FOR WOMEN ATHLETES

Some supplements may be necessary for women.

Calcium supplements are recommended for women who exercise so strenuously (as in marathon running) that menstrual periods cease. These women are at a higher risk of developing osteoporosis (softening of the bones) at an early age.

Iron supplements are also recommended for some women. Normally, iron stores are not diminished directly by exercise. However, if iron-deficiency anemia develops from other causes (such as excessive menstruation), an iron supplement is essential to assure normal physical performance in women.

EATING SCHEDULES FOR ATHLETES

Before Competition—A meal should be eaten 3 to 5 hours before competition. This meal should contain: lots of carbohydrates (pasta, fruits, cooked vegetables, gelatin desserts); decreased fat; decreased protein (small amounts of lean meat, fish or poultry are acceptable); decreased foods that cause extra "gas." The food can be digested in the 3 to 5 hours before competition, allowing nutrients to be stored before excitement begins.

After Competition—Glucose stores in the liver and muscles diminish during strenuous exercise. To replenish these, carbohydrate intake should increase for 3 days following competition. Otherwise, training should be reduced during that time.

APPENDIX 5 (continued)

FLUID INTAKE & EXERCISE

Water—Drink cold water during competition. It is absorbed faster and is less likely to cause cramps than warm water. In addition to drinking extra water during competition, drink at least eight 8-ounce glasses of water a day. An occasional soft drink or cup of tea or coffee is not harmful, but these should not make up the majority of your daily fluid intake. Clear, pure water is best to meet your daily fluid requirement.

Fluid and Glucose Replacement—During extended athletic activity, such as jogging or running a marathon, fluid and glucose must be replaced as they are used by the body. The recommended concentration of glucose is 2 to 2.5 grams of glucose (sugar) to each deciliter of water. Don't drink more than 800ml of fluid during any hour of endurance activity. To exceed this will overload the stomach and may impair performance.

APPENDIX 6

Common Injuries Associated with Various Sports

Almost any of the injuries and medical problems described in this book could occur during participation in any sport or vigorous physical activity. The most likely ones associated with popular sports are listed below, sport by sport.

Aerobic Dance: Muscle, ligament or tendon sprain or strain in any area of the shoulder, arms, abdominal wall, pelvis, legs, ankles and feet; "runner's knee"; shin splints; hamstring injury; foot or leg exostosis or stress-fracture.

Archery: Epicondylitis ("tennis elbow"); finger sprain or strain; strain of upper-arm muscles, especially biceps; pneumothorax; puncture wounds (from off-target arrows).

Baseball: Epicondylitis ("tennis elbow" or "pitcher's elbow"); strain of upper-arm muscles; olecranon elbow fracture; radio-humeral elbow-joint sprain; shoulder dislocation; acromio-clavicular strain; shoulder bursitis; shin splints; finger fracture or dislocation; lacerations; contusion; abrasion; puncture wound (from cleats); hematoma under fingernail or toenail.

Basketball: Finger dislocation or fracture; thumb sprain; ankle sprain; groin-muscle sprain; "runner's knee"; shin splints; shoulder dislocation; acromio-clavicular strain; shoulder bursitis; hematoma under toenail; contusion; abrasion; laceration.

Boating (includes Sailing, Canoeing, Kayaking): Cold injury (hypothermia); heat illness; wrist sprain or strain; shoulder tendinitis and bursitis; epicondylitis ("tennis elbow"); knee contusion or abrasion (from kneeling).

Bowling: Epicondylitis ("tennis elbow"); toe contusion; back, shoulder or arm sprain or strain.

Boxing: Facial laceration, especially around the eyes; jaw fracture; head injury, including concussion, epidural hematoma, subdural hematoma, or cauliflower ear; neck sprain or dislocation; internal abdominal injury to spleen, liver or kidney; hematoma under fingernail or toenail; contusions; abrasions.

Cycling: Perineum (area between the scrotum and anus in males, between the vagina and anus in females) contusion or pressure injury, causing numbness in genitals and upper legs; boils on buttocks due to heat and moisture; carpal-tunnel syndrome; "runner's knee"; sprain or strain of pelvic, upper-leg or lower-leg muscles, tendons, and ligaments; ankle sprain; contusions; abrasions; lacerations.

Diving: Hand, thumb, wrist or shoulder sprain or strain; head and neck injuries; back strain; Osgood-Schlatter's disease.

Fencing: Hematoma under toenail; contusions; abrasions; lacerations; puncture wounds; back, shoulder or arm sprain or strain.

Football: Every injury listed in this book. Most common ones include those to head, neck, knee, ankle, and pelvic and leg muscles.

Handball: Finger dislocation or fracture; thumb sprain; ankle sprain; groin-muscle sprain; "runner's knee"; shin splints; shoulder dislocation; acromio-clavicular strain; shoulder bursitis; hematoma under fingernail or toenail; contusions; abrasions; lacerations.

Hiking & Backpacking: Muscle, ligament or tendon strain or sprain in any areas of the shoulder, arms, abdominal wall, pelvis, legs, ankles or feet; "runner's knee"; shin splints; hamstring pull; foot or leg exostosis; stress-fracture; hematoma under toenail; contusion; abrasion; laceration; puncture wound; snakebite.

Hockey: Every injury listed in this book. The most common ones include those to the head, neck, knee, ankle, and pelvic or leg muscles.

Golf: Epicondylitis ("tennis elbow"); shoulder bursitis and tendinitis; upper back sprain; contusions or head injury from flying balls.

Gymnastics: Neck or back strain; radius (bone in forearm) stress-fracture; shoulder, elbow, wrist, knee, ankle or foot sprain or strain; Osgood-Schlatter's disease; shin splints; hematoma under nailbed; contusions; abrasions; lacerations.

Jogging: Muscle, ligament or tendon sprain or strain in any area of the shoulder, arms, abdominal wall, pelvis, legs, ankles and feet; "runner's knee"; shin splints; hamstring injury; foot or leg exostosis or stress-fracture; contusions; abrasions; lacerations; puncture wounds; snakebite.

Mountain-Climbing: Abrasions; contusions; lacerations; shin splints; dislocation, fracture, sprain or strain of any muscle group or joint; snakebite; head injuries; internal chest or abdomen injury; altitude sickness; dehydration; cold injury (hypothermia or frostbite).

APPENDIX 6 (continued)

Racquetball: Eye injury; hematoma under toenail; contusions; abrasions; lacerations; shoulder-area bursitis; sprain or strain of the shoulder, neck, back, arm, wrist, hip, upper leg, knee, lower leg or ankle; shin splints; epicondylitis ("tennis elbow").

Track & Field Events (Sprints, Relays, High Jump, Discus, Long Jump, Hurdles, Javelin Throw, Pole Vault, Shot Put): Muscle, ligament or tendon sprain or strain of all areas of the shoulder, arms, abdominal wall, pelvis, legs, ankles and feet; "runner's knee"; shin splints; hamstring injury; foot or leg exostosis or stress-fracture; hematoma under toenail; contusions; abrasions; lacerations; puncture wounds.

Skating (Ice Skating, Roller Skating): Coccyx (tailbone) fracture or contusion from falling; cold injury (ice skating only); foot stress fracture; "runner's knee"; shin splints; Osgood-Schlatter's disease; sprain or strain in the upper leg, knee, lower leg, ankle or foot; hematoma under toenail; contusions; abrasions; lacerations;.

Skiing (Downhill Skiing, Slalom Skiing, Cross-Country Skiing): Osgood-Schlatter's disease; shin splints; hematoma under toenail; contusions; abrasions; lacerations; sprain or strain of ligaments, muscles or tendons of the back, neck, shoulder, chest, abdominal wall, arm, wrist, pelvis, leg, knee, ankle or foot; knee-cartilage injury; tendinitis and bursitis of the shoulder, knee or hip; epicondylitis ("tennis elbow"); dehydration; altitude sickness; cold injury (hypothermia); sunburn; injury to the retina of the eye from sun glare.

Soccer: Every injury listed in this book. The most common ones are those to the hips, pelvis and lower extremities.

Softball: Epicondylitis ("tennis elbow" or "pitcher's elbow"); strain of upper-arm muscles; olecranon elbow fracture; radio-humeral elbow-joint sprain; shoulder dislocation; acromio-clavicular strain; shoulder bursitis; shin splints; finger fracture or dislocation; lacerations; contusions; abrasions; puncture wound (from cleats); hematoma under fingernail or toenail.

Squash: Eye injury; hematoma under toenail; contusions; abrasions; lacerations; shoulder-area bursitis; sprain or strain of the shoulder, neck, back, arm, wrist, hip, upper leg, knee, lower leg or ankle; shin splints; epicondylitis ("tennis elbow").

Swimming: Eye injury (from pool chemicals); verruca (warts) from poolside damp areas; sprain or strain of the shoulder, lower back, hip or knee areas; cold injury (hypothermia); sunburn.

Scuba Diving: Decompression illness; contact dermatitis (skin rash) if hypersensitive to wet suit material.

Surfing: Head injuries; sprain or strain of the shoulder, lower back, hip or knee; shin splints; cold injury (hypothermia); sunburn; contact dermatitis from wax on surfboard and sensitivity to wet suits; contusions; abrasions; lacerations.

Tennis: Epicondylitis ("tennis elbow"); shoulder-area bursitis; eye injury; shin splints; hematoma under toenail; contusions; abrasions; lacerations; sprain or strain of the shoulder, neck, back, arm, wrist, hip, upper leg, knee, lower leg or ankle.

Trampoline: Sprain or strain of hand, thumb, wrist or shoulder; head and neck injuries; back strain; Osgood-Schlatter's disease.

Volleyball: Finger dislocation or fracture; thumb sprain; ankle sprain; shin splints; groin-muscle sprain; "runner's knee"; shoulder dislocation; acromio-clavicular strain; shoulder bursitis; hematoma under fingernail or toenail; contusions; abrasions; lacerations.

Waterskiing: Head injuries; epicondylitis ("tennis elbow"); contusions; abrasions; lacerations; sprain or strain of the back, neck, shoulder, chest, abdominal wall, arm, wrist, pelvis, leg, knee, ankle or foot; shin splints; knee-cartilage injury; tendinitis and bursitis of the shoulder, knee or hip; cold injury (hypothermia); sunburn; injury to the retina of the eye from sun glare.

Walking: Injuries are unlikely, but possibilities include muscle, ligament or tendon strain or sprain in any areas of the shoulder, arms, abdominal wall, pelvis, legs, ankles or feet; "runner's knee"; hamstring pull; foot or leg exostosis; stress-fracture; contusions; abrasions; lacerations; snakebite.

Water Polo: Eye injury (from pool chemicals); verruca (warts) from poolside damp areas; sprain or strain of the shoulder, lower back, hip or knee; cold injury (hypothermia); sunburn; contusions; abrasions; lacerations.

Weight-Lifting: Strain or sprain of the muscles, tendons or ligaments of the neck, shoulder, arm, wrist, fingers, abdominal wall, hip, pelvis, leg (especially quadriceps), knee, ankle, foot or toes; elbow dislocation; dehydration from fluid loss due to sweating.

Wrestling: Laceration of areas around the eyes; head injury, including concussion, epidural hematoma, subdural hematoma and cauliflower ear; neck sprain or dislocation; internal abdominal injuries to the spleen, liver or kidney; hematoma under fingernail or toenail; contusions; abrasions; shoulder dislocation. Almost any other injury is possible, but because this sport is usually well-supervised, injuries are minimal.

APPENDIX 7

Disqualifying Medical Conditions for Sports Participation

NON-COLLISION, NON-CONTACT SPORTS
(Competitive running or marathons; track and field events; racket sports; competitive swimming; bowling; golf; archery.)

Temporary Disqualifications
- Active infection including:
  Respiratory infection.
  Kidney infection.
  Infectious mononucleosis.
  Hepatitis.
  Acute rheumatic fever.
  Active tuberculosis.
- Joint inflammation resulting from infection or recent injury.

Permanent Disqualifications
- Chronic diseases, including:
  Those that involve serious bleeding tendencies, such as hemophilia.
  Inadequately controlled diabetes.
  Severe chronic obstructive pulmonary disease.
  Valvular heart disease (mitral stenosis, aortic stenosis).
  Previous heart surgery (sometimes).
  High blood pressure with a known cause, such as chronic kidney disease, coarctation (constriction of a small segment) of the aorta, adrenal tumors or congenital arteriosclerosis. This disqualification does not include essential hypertension or high blood pressure from an unknown cause that is under control with medications. Vigorous exercise after adequate training is recommended for persons with this condition.

Exceptions
Persons with mild forms of the preceding conditions may benefit from non-contact, non-collision exercise programs if they have medical supervision and frequent monitoring of their conditions. Consult your doctor for guidance if you have any of the following:

- High blood pressure.
- Asthma.
- Early obstructive pulmonary disease.
- Well-controlled diabetes.
- Convulsive disorders controlled by medication.
- Absence of one kidney.
- Absence of one testicle or undescended testicles.
- Previous heart attack.
- Previous heart surgery.

APPENDIX 7 (continued)

COLLISION AND CONTACT SPORTS
(Football; hockey; rugby; lacrosse; baseball; basketball; soccer; wrestling; boxing.)

Temporary Disqualifications
- Active infection including:
  Respiratory infection.
  Kidney infection.
  Infectious mononucleosis.
  Hepatitis.
  Acute rheumatic fever.
  Active tuberculosis.
- Joint inflammation resulting from infection or recent injury.
- Skin disease in an active phase (boils, impetigo, herpes).

Permanent Disqualifications
- Physical immaturity in comparison with others competing in the same group.
- Chronic diseases, including:
  Those that involve serious bleeding tendencies, such as hemophilia.
  Inadequately controlled diabetes.
  Severe chronic obstructive pulmonary disease.
  Valvular heart disease (mitral stenosis, aortic stenosis).
  Previous heart surgery (sometimes).
  High blood pressure with a known cause, such as chronic kidney disease, coarctation (constriction of a small segment) of the aorta, adrenal tumors or congenital arteriosclerosis. This disqualification does not include essential hypertension or high blood pressure from an unknown cause that is under control with medications. Vigorous exercise after adequate training is recommended for persons with this condition.
- Hernia (no disqualification after successful surgical repair).
- Congenital musculo-skeletal abnormalities that prevent competitive function, such as clubfoot or osteogenesis imperfecta.
- Loss of one eye or blindness in one eye.
- Repeated head injuries or repeated concussions accompanied by unconsciousness.
- Epilepsy or other convulsive disorder not controlled with medication.
- Previous head or brain surgery.
- Absence of one kidney.
- Absence of one testicle.

APPENDIX 8

Stress & Psychosomatic Illness in Athletics

Competitive sports—by their nature—cause stress. Vigorous exercise programs can also cause stress if one takes a program seriously or tries to keep up with friends or others. To a certain degree, stress can have positive effects and push us to greater achievement. But how much stress one can easily handle varies from person to person.

Stress, particularly that due to competitive excitement, fear or anger, causes the body to liberate chemicals that stimulate the adrenal glands. The glands release adrenalin (sometimes called epinephrine). Adrenalin has the following effects on the body:
- Rapid heartbeat.
- Increased blood pressure.
- Tremor.
- Headache.
- Excessive sweating.
- Body hair "standing on end."
- Dry mouth and throat.

Under ordinary circumstances, vigorous exercise "burns off" the breakdown products (catecholamines) of adrenalin. If all the chemicals produced by stress are not burned off, the positive effects of exercise may become negative and self-defeating. Common stress-related disorders are:
- Insomnia.
- Mental and emotional upheavals.
- Skin eruptions, such as eczema and neurodermatitis.
- Digestive-system problems, including peptic ulcers, colitis and irritable colon.
- Endocrine disorders, including overactive thyroid, adrenal-gland or pituitary-gland overactivity or underactivity, changes in menstrual patterns, impotence or premature ejaculation in men, or orgasmic dysfunction in women.
- Lung disorders associated with spasm of the bronchial tubes, such as in asthma.
- Pain syndromes, such as chronic or recurrent disabling headaches or back pain.

Other causes of stress that can occur to anyone, athlete or not, include:
- Regular conflict with others.
- Recent death of a loved one—spouse, child, friend.
- Loss of anything valuable.
- Injury or severe illness.
- Being fired or changing jobs.
- Recent move to a new home.
- Sexual difficulties.
- Business, academic or financial reverses, or taking on a large debt.
- Constant fatigue.

Many doctors believe that stress has a role in almost any disorder. Few doubt that stress can complicate an illness or delay healing from an injury or surgery by preventing normal recovery, prolonging pain and sustaining disability.

SELF-HELP TIPS FOR COPING WITH STRESS

Here are some tips that may help you reduce stress:
- Learn a meditation technique and practice it regularly—daily if possible. There are many methods available. Most of them include "tuning in to" and giving complete attention to a word, sound, sentence or concept that you silently repeat to yourself. Don't try to banish other thoughts that enter your mind during your period of concentration, but don't focus on them enough to stop you from meditating. The purpose of meditation is to empty your mind of all disturbing thoughts for a given period of time to encourage mental relaxation. Mental relaxation, in turn, will help reduce stress.

The Transcendental Meditation Program is a different technique that has been shown through extensive physiological research to be effective in reducing stress. It is taught in most communities in individualized instruction through the International Meditation Society.

APPENDIX 8 (continued)

• Take a short period of time away from any stressful situation you encounter during a day. Practice a muscle-tensing and muscle-relaxing technique. Close your eyes. Take a series of deep breaths. Then start with the muscle groups in your face. Consciously tense them and hold the contraction for a few seconds. Then consciously relax them. Continue through all major muscle groups in the body—neck, shoulders, hands, abdomen, back and legs. When you become skillful, you can use this technique to relax quickly any time you need to and in almost any environment.

• Avoid taking your problems to bed with you. At the end of the day, spend a few minutes reviewing your entire day's experiences, event by event, as if you're replaying a tape. Release all negative emotions you have harbored (anger, feelings of insecurity or anxiety). Relish all good energy or emotion (loving thoughts, praise, feeling good about your work or yourself). Reach a decision about unfinished events, and release mental or muscular tension. Then you're ready for a relaxing and emotionally healing sleep.

PSYCHOSOMATIC ILLNESS

Psychosomatic illness is a term used to describe an illness in which factors other than physical ones dominate. These factors may also play an important part in complications. Such illnesses are real—not imagined, as many people think. We can't separate our body from our mind or our spirit. Most illnesses have some connection with these elements, even if the links between mind, spirit and body are poorly defined at times.

Although medical researchers are beginning to understand the basic mechanisms, we still have much to learn about psychosomatic illness. One group of researchers believes that mental, emotional or spiritual stress can trigger almost any illness in a person genetically predisposed to that illness. Such illnesses include asthma, cancer, digestive disturbances, heart disease—all these and others are more common in certain families. Yet all people in these families do not succumb to the same illnesses.

SUGGESTIONS FOR IMPROVING, PREVENTING OR
COPING WITH PSYCHOSOMATIC ILLNESS

• Define and resolve all personal conflicts, if possible. Confront areas of personal conflict in your spiritual, emotional, occupational, civic or recreational involvements. If you can't resolve these conflicts alone, seek help from family, friends or competent counselors.

• Seek a balanced life of work, intellectual and physical challenges, recreation, intimacy, reflection and rest. Be moderate in all your activities.

• Maintain a positive attitude whenever possible.

• Allow yourself to give and receive love.

• Be a friend. Considerate, respectful and loving attitudes toward yourself and others are powerful allies.

APPENDIX 9

Aging & Exercise

People of all ages benefit from regular exercise. Many persons aged 65 and older exercise regularly and stay as physically fit as their general health allows. These persons grow older with a style and vigor far surpassing that of their sedentary contemporaries. Following are some specific ways in which exercise and fitness are beneficial in aging:

• More people reach age 65 and older who are physically fit than those who are not. Those who remain physically active continue to have more stamina than their inactive counterparts.

• Although exercise probably does not retard the aging process, it reduces the likelihood of untimely death from medical problems that are caused in part by a sedentary lifestyle. These include coronary-artery disease, high blood pressure, stroke, kidney disease, chronic lung disease and depression.

Aerobic exercise is the most effective way to achieve physical and psychological benefits. An exercise is aerobic if it provides:

• Sustained physical activity that uses major muscle groups of the body.

• Regulated intensity, long-duration exercise for 20 minutes or more.

Proper aerobic benefit is based on sufficient exercise to accelerate the heart rate to a prescribed level and keep it there a certain length of time. Three to five aerobic-exercise sessions a week are necessary for maximum benefit. Best forms of aerobic exercise include brisk walking, swimming, bike riding, jogging, rope jumping and rowing. Sports such as bowling, tennis or golf have good recreational effects, but they do not require enough effort to reach sustained aerobic levels.

Persons over 65 receive the same benefits from aerobic exercise as do younger persons—even if they choose the less strenuous forms of exercise. Following is an explanation of the effects of aerobic exercise on the body.

EXERCISE & THE CARDIOVASCULAR SYSTEM

Older persons are most at risk for cardiovascular problems. Exercise benefits the cardiovascular system in the following ways:

• Increased number of circulating red blood cells (thus providing more oxygen and better nourishment to all body cells).

• Increased blood flow during exercise.

• Increased enzymes necessary for changing glucose into usable energy by body cells.

• Increased high-density lipoproteins in the circulating blood. These protect against hardening of the arteries, which is responsible for heart attacks, strokes and chronic kidney failure.

EXERCISE & CIRCULATION TO THE BRAIN AND OTHER BODY PARTS

Exercise in a healthy person produces an increase in an enzyme that helps prevent the deposit of fibrin (a clotting factor in the blood) in blood vessels to the brain and other body parts. Fibrin deposits on the lining of the blood vessels narrow the arteries and decrease blood supply to the cells supplied by the affected blood vessels. Narrowed arteries and decreased blood flow can result in stroke, heart attack and lack of sufficient blood supply to the kidneys and legs, causing kidney failure.

EXERCISE & THE LUNGS

Regular exercise can increase maximum breathing capacity, improving or preventing chronic lung disease.

EXERCISE & THE MUSCULO-SKELETAL SYSTEM

Regular, adequate exercise helps maintain normal size and contour of muscles and bones. The combination of exercise and adequate calcium intake is an important factor in preventing osteoporosis (softening of the bones), a common disorder in women past menopause. (In addition to exercise and calcium, estrogen replacement in women may also be necessary to prevent osteoporosis). Exercise promotes healthy new bone formation in all age groups. This new bone protects against bone fractures that commonly occur in older people of both sexes.

APPENDIX 9 (continued)

EXERCISE & THE MIND

Exercise helps rid the body of ("burn off") undesirable levels of catecholamines (breakdown products of adrenalin, which is released by the body as a reaction to physical or mental stress). The following results have been documented in many studies:

• Regular exercise has a positive influence on one's sense of well-being and self-esteem.

• An exercise program can be very beneficial in relieving depression—it is now commonly prescribed as part of therapy.

BENEFICIAL EFFECTS ON SEXUALITY

• Men who remain physically active maintain a higher level of testosterone than their sedentary contemporaries.

• People who exercise regularly are generally healthier emotionally, have a better self-image and enjoy increased muscular strength. These factors are all important in meaningful sexual relationships.

• People who are fit—no matter what their age—are more sexually attractive to others.

CONCLUSIONS

Regular exercise has proved of great benefit in minimizing the negative effects of aging. If you are an older person who has not remained physically fit, discuss a fitness program with your doctor. Follow his or her suggestions about what you can safely perform.

APPENDIX 10

Chronic Disease & Exercise

Some persons suffer from serious disease that can last many years. Each case must be evaluated on an individual basis, but many of these persons can benefit from regular exercise. It can play a vital role in improving their sense of well-being. In a few instances, it may help retard progress of the disease. Three of the most serious and common forms of chronic disease—heart disease, chronic obstructive pulmonary (lung) disease and diabetes—are discussed in this section.

HEART DISEASE & EXERCISE

The most-common types of heart disease are coronary-artery disease and hardening of the arteries (atherosclerosis or arteriosclerosis). Three important risk factors for developing heart disease are hypertension (high blood pressure), obesity and a sedentary lifestyle. Exercise plays an important role in controlling hypertension and obesity, making it significant in the treatment of heart disease. The known benefits of cardiovascular fitness include:

- An increased blood supply to the heart.
- Decreased oxygen demand.
- Increased blood flow through the coronary arteries.
- Increased efficiency of heart-muscle function.
- Indirect evidence of decreased electrical irritability of the heart, lessening the chance that abnormal or life-threatening heartbeat irregularities will occur.
- Indirect evidence of delayed development of hardening of the arteries.

These benefits are possible for men and women in all age groups, but the most positive evidence of benefit is in men over 40.

After Heart Disease is Diagnosed—Many medical centers throughout the world have developed rehabilitation centers for patients who have had a heart attack. The American College of Sports Medicine has established guidelines and certification programs for exercise leaders trained in cardiac rehabilitation techniques. These centers prescribe exercise after a thorough evaluation, and supervise the exercise carefully with monitors. Cardiac patients following a heart attack can frequently benefit from enrolling in one of these programs in a YMCA, college or university physical education department, or cardiac rehabilitation center. It is unsafe for a recent cardiac patient to try to develop an exercise program at home. A specialized facility, under the supervision of trained professionals, can offer monitoring of your responses to individually designed exercise programs. Repeated studies have shown that such careful programs have brought quicker recovery, earlier return to work, enhanced feeling of well-being, and less likelihood of developing a subsequent heart attack. Ask your physician for a referral.

CHRONIC OBSTRUCTIVE LUNG DISEASE & EXERCISE

C.O.P.D. (chronic obstructive lung disease) is any long-term lung disorder characterized by gradually increasing breathing difficulty. Some underlying diseases that produce C.O.P.D. include chronic bronchitis, bronchiectasis, emphysema, asthma and other disorders associated with spasm of the bronchial tubes. For a full description of each of these diseases, see *Complete Guide to Symptoms, Illness & Surgery,* by H. Winter Griffith, M.D., published by The Body Press.

Exercise Programs—Supervised exercise and activity can enhance breathing function and improve the patient's sense of well-being. However, exercise programs for people with this disorder must be individualized. A physical therapist or doctor can teach the patient how to increase breathing skill and capacity. Breathing retraining begins with exercises using forced expiration against pursed lips, and other techniques to use the diaphragm and accessory muscles of the chest wall. When breathing rehabilitation reaches an acceptable level, a program of walking can increase breathing capacity and general health. See your doctor for detailed instructions.

APPENDIX 10 (continued)

DIABETES & EXERCISE

Diabetes is a disease of metabolism characterized by the body's inability to produce enough insulin to process carbohydrates, fat and protein efficiently. Non-insulin-dependent diabetes can often be controlled with a treatment program that includes diet, exercise, weight loss and oral medication (sometimes). Insulin-dependent diabetes can usually be controlled with regular injections of insulin, in addition to the diet and exercise program. Therefore diabetic patients, whether insulin-dependent or non-insulin-dependent, benefit from exercise—even though the role of exercise in treatment is still not well understood. However, people with diabetes should be medically evaluated and educated before beginning an exercise or athletic program.

Benefits

• Exercise helps control appetite in diabetic persons who need to lose weight. Exercise by itself does not necessarily lead to weight loss, but it does affect the "appetite control center" in the hypothalamus, decreasing appetite. In some persons with non-insulin-dependent diabetes, weight loss alone reduces blood-sugar levels.

• Exercise helps improve glucose (sugar) tolerance in some diabetic persons. This allows a reduction of insulin (for insulin-dependent individuals) or oral medication (for non-insulin-dependent individuals).

• Exercise appears to reduce the likelihood of cardiovascular disease (heart attack, stroke, kidney failure, hypertension). These conditions are more likely to occur in people with diabetes, so exercise becomes an aid in prevention. To sustain the protective effect, exercise must be performed regularly throughout one's lifetime.

Risks

• Prolonged or overly vigorous exercise may increase the effect of insulin or oral antidiabetic medicines, causing them to lower blood sugar too much. This could produce hypoglycemia (low blood sugar) symptoms, including confusion, weakness, sweating, paleness or loss of consciousness. Treatment includes drinking a high-sugar drink, such as orange juice with added sugar, and notifying your doctor as soon as possible.

• Complications of diabetes (diabetic retinopathy, peripheral neuropathy, decreased kidney function) may worsen with overly enthusiastic training or activity, depending on the activity chosen. See recommendations below and consult your doctor for more information.

Recommendations

• Don't start or return to an intensive exercise program until your diabetes is under control. Then consult your doctor about the suitability of the exercise program you have chosen.

• Under medical guidance, learn to balance insulin dosage with exercise and diet. For instance, prior to heavy exercise, you may need to reduce the insulin dose and increase food intake.

• If you use insulin, inject it into a non-exercising part—such as the abdomen—rather than the arm or leg.

• If you have diabetic retinopathy, don't jog, lift weights or attempt any exercise that jars the head or increases pressure in the eye.

• Because diabetes increases the risk of developing cardiovascular problems, all persons with diabetes (particularly those over 40) should have medical clearance before beginning any strenuous exercise program or sports activity.

• Special precautions are necessary for individuals with diabetes who drink alcohol or must take other medications, such as aspirin, beta-adrenergic blockers, and non-steroidal anti-inflammatory medicines. Each of these can cause hypoglycemia during exercise. If you must take these drugs, you must reduce your exercise level to compensate for resulting blood-sugar changes.

APPENDIX 11

Mental Retardation, Sports & Exercise

Athletic activity and recreation are important for everyone, regardless of mental capacity. Sports and athletic activities can make a positive difference in problems experienced by mentally retarded persons. These problems include poor physical fitness, obesity, restlessness, boredom, hyperactivity and social immaturity. Most health professionals and social workers believe that mild to moderately retarded children and adults can and should participate safely in many athletic activities, as long as they are supervised adequately. This section presents guidelines to parents or guardians of mentally retarded children and adults who are considering an exercise program or athletic competition for them.

RECOMMENDATIONS

- Encourage and stress activities that require gross motor (large-muscle) coordination rather than fine motor coordination.
- Stress the right kinds of activities. Mentally retarded children and adults find more satisfaction and success in participating in dual and individual sports rather than team sports. Retarded children may benefit from non-competitive sports with normal children.
- Teach and encourage games, which are more interesting than exercises.The following sports and activities are recommended: tennis, folk-dancing, shooting baskets, running races, playing catch, boating, bicycling and hiking. Less suitable activities that are not recommended include basketball, football or baseball.
- Match competitors evenly so each person has a chance to win sometimes. Have children participate with each other according to developmental age rather than chronological age. Otherwise, some individuals may fail repeatedly, damaging their self-esteem—and turning a positive situation into a negative one.
- Keep records of improvement, and share them with the retarded child.
- Support development of athletic opportunities at the community level. For more information about programs for the mentally retarded, contact either of the following:

The Special Olympics, Inc.
1701 K St., N.W.
Washington, D.C. 20006

Division of Innovation and Development
Department of Education
Donahue Bldg., Rm. 3159
400 Maryland Ave., S.W.
Washington, D.C. 20202

APPENDIX 12

Sexual Activity & Contraception in Athletes

Several medical studies and reports conclude that men and women who are well-conditioned and vigorously engaged in sports and competition have more frequent sexual intercourse—and enjoy it more—than their sedentary counterparts. The energy drain that results from sexual intercourse is negligible among athletes who are physically fit. The amount of energy expended is estimated to be equal to running a 100-yard dash.

CONTRACEPTIVE CONSIDERATIONS

Athletes use the same contraceptive measures as others, but some forms of birth control may require special considerations for athletes. The use of diaphragms, cervical caps or rubber condoms obviously has no effect on sports ability or performance. However, the following forms of contraception for women merit examination:

• Contraceptive creams and jellies sometimes cause vaginal and vulvar irritation that can interfere with athletic performance. These side effects usually disappear readily once the cream or jelly is discontinued. Occasionally, local treatment with topical steroid creams is necessary.

• Oral contraceptive pills cause significant physiological changes. At present, we do not know enough to encourage or discourage their use in women athletes. Some women retain excess fluid while on the pill, and this may decrease performance. On the other hand, the pill increases the body's blood volume. Exercise enhances the body's ability to deal with the body's blood volume because the heart functions more efficiently and circulation is better. Both of these factors can enhance endurance and other aspects of performance. The physiological changes experienced with oral contraceptives vary from woman to woman, so the decision to use the pill should be based on factors other than physical activity.

• Injections of long-acting progesterone are used in some countries, but they are not approved by the FDA for use in the U.S., so we have few studies on this form of contraception. It has been established, however, that progesterone can cause fluid retention and irregular periods. Fluid retention may decrease athletic performance.

• Intrauterine devices (IUDs) have significant negative effects on women athletes and should not be used. Following are some of the reported problems associated with using IUDs:

(1) Higher percentage of pelvic infections in athletes than in sedentary women using IUDs.

(2) Higher degree of unpredictable intervals between menstrual periods in athletes than in sedentary women using IUDs.

(3) Much higher frequency of heavy, prolonged bleeding. Some medical studies have reported that 60% to 75% of IUD users experience excessive flow. This significant increase in bleeding can lead to anemia and decreased oxygen-carrying capacity of the blood, eventually affecting athletic performance.

APPENDIX 13

Pregnancy, Sports & Vigorous Exercise

Fitness and continued recreational activities during pregnancy are important for mother and unborn child. (Increased oxygenation provided by exercise helps nourish the fetus). Continuing exercise and recreation at the pre-pregnancy level (within the limitations described below) are feasible and recommended for the first several months of pregnancy. However, starting a new vigorous fitness program during pregnancy is not wise. Pregnancy affects posture, the respiratory system, the cardiovascular system, total body weight, and the body's ability to dissipate heat.

RECOMMENDATIONS DURING PREGNANCY

● If you are planning to become pregnant, start a fitness program and attain as high a level of physical fitness as possible prior to conception. This maximizes your chances for a healthy pregnancy.

● If you continue to exercise after conception, you should increase your caloric nutritional intake to allow for a 23- to 27-pound weight gain during pregnancy. Carefully follow your doctor's nutritional recommendations regarding vitamins, folic acid, iron and other supplements.

● After conception, continue to exercise at your pre-pregnancy level, but don't increase the frequency or vigor of your program. During the first 3 or 4 months, avoid repeated prolonged exercise. Reduce activity by the 5th month. Toward the end of your pregnancy, your body will let you know you should decrease activity. The signals for this include increased weight, decreased breathing capacity, increased clumsiness and change in the center of gravity. Pay attention to your body's signals—don't push beyond your capacity. By the 7th month and until 4 weeks after delivery, confine exercise to the limited amount prescribed by your doctor.

● Avoid activities in hot weather that increase your body temperature. If you are not sure what your temperature is, take it rectally after an average workout under average conditions. If your body temperature is greater than 101F, take steps to prevent the temperature elevation. Consider these measures:

Select a cooler time of day for exercise.
Wear loose, light clothing.
Increase water intake to prevent dehydration.
Temporarily decrease the vigor or duration of your exercise program.

● Avoid saunas, hot tubs, whirlpools and steam rooms during pregnancy. Any of these may cause harmful increases in body temperature.

● Don't train at high altitudes because oxygen levels are lower.

● Avoid scuba diving while pregnant. Increased pressure can have adverse effects on the fetus.

● Avoid contact or collision sports, which can lead to harmful abdominal injuries. It is probably better to avoid or restrict fast running, cross-country skiing, aerobic-dance exercises (except for special prenatal classes), or speed sports of any sort.

● During later months of pregnancy, avoid downhill skiing. Your center of gravity will have changed and made spills much more likely—even if you are a skilled athlete.

● Stop all exercise and report to your doctor immediately if any of the following occurs:

Abdominal pain.
Bleeding from the vagina.
Rupture of the fetal membranes—signaled by a gush of water from the vagina.
Cessation of fetal movement.

RECOMMENDATIONS FOLLOWING DELIVERY

● Resume your training program and full vigorous exercise and competition as soon as all pain in the genitals and abdomen has disappeared. If you had an episiotomy (an incision that enlarges the vaginal opening), the recovery time will be a little longer. You should be able to gradually resume your regular activities within 3 to 4 weeks after delivery.

● Avoid inserting anything into the vagina (such as tampons or douching chemicals) for 3 to 4 weeks following delivery. Until that time, the dilated cervix that allowed delivery of your baby forms a fertile entry for germs into the reproductive organs, making you susceptible to infection. Use sanitary napkins for continued bleeding. Talk to your doctor about resuming sexual relations. The usual recommendation is to avoid vaginal intercourse for 3 to 6 weeks following delivery, whether or not there has been an episiotomy.

● If you wish to breast-feed your baby, it should cause no major problems that would interfere with your exercise program. Be careful to use adequate breast support and to increase fluid intake during exercise to prevent dehydration.

APPENDIX 14

Drugs in Sports

The use of drugs by amateur and professional athletes has received much publicity in recent years. Many athletes believe that drugs are essential for optimum performance. The issue of whether drugs can enhance physical performance remains controversial and unresolved. However, the physiological effects that drugs have on the body can be documented. This section is devoted to examining the most-common drugs used by athletes. Questions of legality or ethics are best answered by the prevailing view in sports medicine: The use of drugs is generally considered unethical—in some cases illegal—and such use is usually forbidden by organizations that govern competitive athletics.

ANABOLIC STEROID HORMONES

Some athletes take synthetic male hormones (anabolic steroids) in the hope of increasing strength or muscle mass. The most common synthetic male hormones taken by athletes include testosterone, methandrostenolone and nandrolone.

Effects in Women—Muscle mass increases when the hormone is taken for a sufficiently long period of time. However, side effects and adverse reactions include the following:
- Growth of hair on the face and other body parts.
- Enlargement of the clitoris.
- Deepening of the voice.
- Acne.
- Baldness.
- Change in sex drive (usually increased).
- Irregular menstrual periods.
- Depression.

Effects in Men—Strength and body weight sometimes increase. However, many side effects and adverse reactions are possible. These include:
- Decreased levels of FSH (follicle-stimulating hormone) and leutenizing hormone. These in turn cause decreased male-hormone production, decreased sperm production, and testicular atrophy.
- A decrease in high-density lipoprotein, which may increase the likelihood of hardening of the arteries, stroke and kidney disease.
- Increased incidence of liver tumors.
- Increased aggressiveness.
- Acne.
- Depression.
- Change in sex drive (sometimes lessened, sometimes increased).

The consensus among medical experts is that the use of anabolic steroid hormones by both men and women poses greater risk and danger from adverse effects than is justified by any possible benefit. Physicians uniformly advise against using them. Their use is condemned by the Medical Commission of the International Olympic Committee.

AMPHETAMINES

These drugs are central-nervous-system stimulants. Athletes take them believing they will help performance in competition. Studies show that performance is actually diminished, despite the feeling on the part of the athlete that performance is outstanding. The toxic effects of amphetamines are:
- Tremor.
- Confusion.
- Restlessness.
- Loss of appetite.
- Delusions and hallucinations.
- High blood pressure.
- Heartbeat irregularities.

Amphetamines are particularly dangerous if taken with other stimulants such as cocaine, appetite suppressants and caffeine.

APPENDIX 14 (continued)

CAFFEINE

Caffeine is also a central-nervous-system stimulant. When taken in small, infrequent doses, caffeine seems to have few if any long-lasting ill effects. However, new evidence suggests a correlation between consumption of any coffee—including decaffeinated coffee—and an increase in low-density lipoproteins. High levels of these fatty elements in the blood are known to increase the likelihood that atherosclerosis (hardening of the arteries), heart disease, kidney disease and stroke will develop. This effect is noted with the consumption of as little as 2 cups of coffee per day.

The immediate effects of caffeine consumption vary from person to person, depending on individual factors. Most people can tolerate 2 cups a day. However, too much caffeine will produce the following:

- Nervousness, irritability and rapid heartbeat.
- Insomnia.
- Increased urine output.
- Symptoms of low blood sugar (hypoglycemia), including tremor, weakness and increased irritability.

Some people believe caffeine consumption relieves fatigue, but this is an artificial effect. Use of caffeine does not result in increased athletic performance.

COCAINE

This central-nervous-system stimulant has similar effects to those of amphetamines and caffeine—except stronger. Cocaine is illegal and addicting. Its use can lead to delusions, psychosocial problems, tremor, restlessness, and damage to nasal tissues (if "snorted"). An overdose of cocaine can be fatal. Its damaging effects on the central nervous system increase greatly when it is taken with other stimulants such as amphetamines, appetite suppressants or caffeine. Medical experts have documented no benefits from the use of cocaine among athletes.

NICOTINE

This is the addicting factor in tobacco smoke that makes smoking cessation so difficult for many persons. Nicotine causes constriction of peripheral blood vessels. It also causes an increase in heart rate that does not result in increased cardiac output. The result of these two effects is increased fatigue and diminished athletic performance.

PRESCRIPTION & NON-PRESCRIPTION DRUGS

All effective medications have potential side effects for at least some individuals. Do not expect to be able to perform at your accustomed level if you are taking any medication.

Safety precautions for athletes are similar to those for the general population. The most important additional precaution for athletes relates to fluid loss that accompanies heavy sweating. Drugs most likely to become dangerous under these conditions are:

- Digitalis (a heart medicine).
- Diuretics (medicine to treat high blood pressure and heart problems).
- Steroid hormones.

All the above can cause excessive loss of sodium and potassium from the body. The effect of these drugs may be accelerated by fluid loss, as in heavy sweating, diarrhea and vomiting, particularly in hot weather. Excessive sweating from any cause may require a dose modification of digitalis, diuretics or hormones. Let your doctor know if you exercise vigorously. If you take these or any other medication that affects sodium and potassium metabolism in the body, see Sodium Imbalance and Potassium Imbalance in the Sports Medicine section of this book.

APPENDIX 15

Physical Therapy Methods & Techniques

Rehabilitation, when applied to athletic injuries, means to restore to health. Traditionally this has meant exercising muscles to restore strength, endurance, and normal range-of-motion. A broader interpretation includes other methods and techniques that facilitate the healing process.

Physical agents such as heat, cold, massage and electric current can be used in conjunction with exercise programs—and sometimes medications—to hasten rehabilitation. The first three can often be used at home under the supervision of a doctor, physical therapist or trainer. These trained professionals can oversee progress, shifting from one type of exercise to another when advisable. The different methods are explained in greater detail below. Electrical current can only be performed with specialized equipment in a clinical setting, but it is very effective in muscle retraining and restoration of strength.

HEAT

When heat is applied to an injury, it dilates (enlarges) small blood vessels in the area, increasing blood flow. The increased blood supply nourishes the tissues and hastens healing. Heat also reduces pain in an injured area and reduces muscle spasm. But heat increases the chance that small capillaries will leak blood and plasma into soft tissues around the injury. While dilation of the blood vessels and increased blood flow are desirable in healing, capillary leakage is undesirable. It leads to greater fluid accumulation and swelling, which retards the healing process. To be beneficial, heat should not be applied until the capillaries have had a chance to seal and stop leaking. This usually requires 24 to 48 hours following injury—if ice, compression and elevation were used immediately.

Depending on the type of injury, heat can be applied in several ways: hot compresses, hydrocollator packs (see Glossary), heat lamps, heating pads, whirlpool baths or hot tubs, ultrasound, or diathermy (seldom used now—see Glossary).

Your doctor or therapist must prescribe the best program for you and provide supervision and guidance throughout your rehabilitation program. You will need instructions about when to start, how long to apply heat during each treatment, and how long to continue with heat treatments. These factors are determined by many variables, such as type and extent of injury, previous medical history and healing rate.

COLD (CRYOTHERAPY)

During the past several years, cold treatment has been used increasingly in first aid and in rehabilitation of athletic injuries. Localized cold treatments provide these important benefits:

- Reduction and control of swelling (edema).
- Facilitation of active or passive joint motion, allowing a return to exercise sooner than is possible without cryotherapy. Ice is applied before exercise during the healing phase.
- Reduction of pain and muscle spasm.

Because ice can be applied prior to exercise, reducing pain and muscle spasm, muscle and joint movements can start sooner without interfering with the healing process. A thin margin of safety regarding when exercise should start and continue makes clinical supervision necessary during rehabilitation.

Ice can be applied as ice packs, ice compresses or ice massage. Ice massage is particularly helpful for sore muscles or muscles in spasm.

Techniques of ice massage:

- Fill a large Styrofoam cup with water and freeze.
- Tear a small amount of foam from the top so ice protrudes.
- Massage firmly over the injured area in a circle about the size of a softball.
- Do this for 15 minutes at a time, 3 or 4 times a day, and before workouts or competition.

MASSAGE

Gentle massage is useful for treating sore muscles. It consists of gentle or firm stroking of the injured area. Strokes should be directed toward the heart. The appropriate amount of pressure and length of the massage should be determined by the person receiving the massage. Massage that increases pain is too hard. When properly administered, massage can reduce fluid accumulation and swelling around an injury. It will stimulate circulation through the veins and lymphatic vessels. However, *overzealous* massage can aggravate an injury and increase bleeding.

APPENDIX 16

Exercise & Air Pollution

Exercising while breathing polluted air not only decreases performance—it may be hazardous to your health. Polluted air can take either of two forms: it can be polluted by chemicals in the general environment around you, or it can be polluted by tobacco smoke as you inhale it into your lungs.

TOBACCO SMOKE

Tobacco smoke contains up to 4 per cent by volume of carbon monoxide, which greatly reduces the blood's capacity to transport oxygen efficiently to all cells in the body. It may take 24 hours for the blood to return to its normal oxygen-carrying capacity after inhaling the smoke of one cigarette. In addition, smoking tobacco increases airway resistance, preventing the inhaled oxygen from reaching the alveoli (air sacs in the lungs) where oxygen filters into the bloodstream. These effects have a profound effect on athletic performance. An athlete cannot reach peak fitness levels and smoke cigarettes.

ENVIRONMENTAL AIR POLLUTION

Environmental air pollutants can have similar—if not so dramatic—effects on an athlete. However, breathing polluted air may be somewhat inescapable in some urban areas. Environmental pollutants include hydrocarbons, oxidants, carbon monoxide, sulfur oxides, peroxyacetyl nitrates and others. Any or all of these can cause bronchial irritation, excessive mucus production, decreased efficiency of the bronchial cilia (hairlike structures) that move and filter mucus, and decreased resistance to respiratory-tract infections. Exercising in highly polluted areas, such as along expressways, may adversely affect performance and health. When you exercise, try to find the cleanest air possible.

APPENDIX 17

Common Types of Bone Fractures

AVULSION
A small portion of bone, with ligament or tendon attached, is pulled away from the main bone segment.

COMMINUTED
The bone is fractured into three or more segments. This type of fracture usually must be immobilized with surgical screws or pins for healing.

COMPLETE
The fractured bone fragments are completely separated. A clean break usually heals relatively quickly.

COMPOUND (OPEN)
At least one bone fragment penetrates the skin. By opening the injury area to the outside, the risk of complicating infections increases.

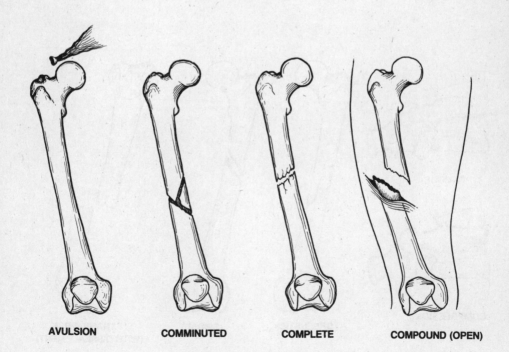

AVULSION   COMMINUTED   COMPLETE   COMPOUND (OPEN)

APPENDIX 17 (continued)

COMPRESSION

Fracture occurs when the mass of bone is compressed, usually by forces in opposite directions. Compression fractures are most common in the spinal vertebrae.

FATIGUE

A complete or incomplete hairline fracture that develops after repeated stress to the bone.

GREENSTICK

This is an incomplete fracture, with bone fragments joined by at least some bone. Greenstick fractures heal more quickly than other fractures.

SPIRAL

Shearing forces cause the fractured segments to separate in a spiral fashion.

STRESS (SEE FATIGUE)

TRANSVERSE (WITH DISPLACEMENT)

The complete fractured bone segments are displaced in relation to each other. These fractures require strength and skill to return bone fragments to a functional position for healing.

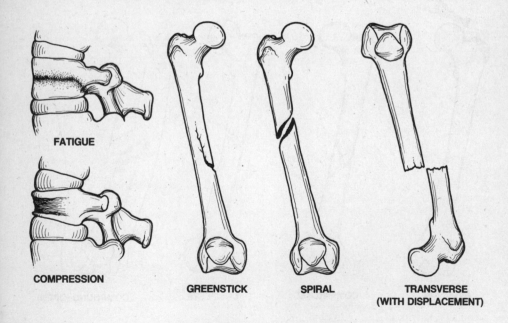

FATIGUE

COMPRESSION

GREENSTICK

SPIRAL

TRANSVERSE
(WITH DISPLACEMENT)

GLOSSARY

A

Abduction—Moving or pushing an arm or leg away from the median line of the body.

Acute—Symptoms that are severe and/or brief in duration.

Adduction—Moving or pulling an arm or leg toward the median line of the body.

Angiography—An X-ray study of blood vessels. The blood vessels to be studied are injected with a chemical that is opaque to X-rays, so abnormalities can be easily detected on the X-ray film.

Angulation—Deviation from a straight line, as in a badly set bone.

Anterior—The front part.

Anterior Cruciate Ligament Injury—A frequent injury to one of the important ligaments in the knee. Sometimes the extent of injury can be diagnosed simply, at other times, arthroscopic surgery is necessary for diagnosis. Most injuries to the anterior cruciate ligament can be repaired surgically with good results. Rehabilitation is as important in recovery as precise surgical repair.

Athlete's Heart—A normal, healthy, efficient heart in a well-conditioned athlete, but larger than the heart of someone of the same age, height and weight who is not well-conditioned. An athlete's heart usually returns to "normal" size when conditioning ceases.

Antihypertensives—Medications used to treat high blood pressure (hypertension).

Arteriography—An X-ray procedure to study arteries. The arteries to be studied are injected with a chemical that is opaque to X-rays, so abnormalities can be easily detected on the X-ray film.

Arthroscopy—A procedure carried out with an arthroscope. An arthroscope is an instrument with a system of lenses and lights that enables a surgeon to view the inside of a joint. It is used most often to study the knee joint. Arthroscopy reveals abnormalities inside the joint. Some surgical procedures can also be accomplished with it. The opening into the joint is minimal and healing is usually more rapid after arthroscopic surgery than after traditional surgery.

Aspirate—A surgical procedure to remove accumulated blood or fluid by suctioning through a needle and syringe.

Atrophy—Wasting away of any part, organ, tissue or cell.

Audiometry—A test of the sense of hearing. Audiometry is usually done in a special soundproof room with sensitive devices that record the intensity of tone heard by the one being tested.

Aura—Unusual or bizarre sensations of sight, hearing, smell or taste that precede a seizure or migraine headache.

Avulsion—Forceful tearing away of any part of a structure.

B

Backboard—An inflexible board made of wood or plastic to keep an injured person's back from bending while being transported to an emergency room or hospital.

Beta-adrenergic Blockers—A class or family of drugs that blocks the effects of adrenalin at selected sites in the sympathetic nervous system. There are many brands available in the United States by prescription. "Beta-blockers" are used to reduce angina attacks, lower blood pressure, stabilize irregular heartbeat, and reduce frequency of migraine headaches. They are very useful and important drugs, but they must be taken under a doctor's supervision.

Biofeedback—A training process of providing visual or auditory evidence of the status of the musculo-skeletal system, cardiovascular system, skin-surface temperature and autonomic nervous system. Biofeedback practitioners work with patients for a number of problems including sessions to learn to reduce stress levels, lower blood pressure, treat headaches, and reduce muscle spasm and pain. The instruments used in biofeedback training are very sensitive galvanometers that record minute changes in body function with great sensitivity.

Biopsy—Removal by surgery or aspiration of a small amount of tissue or fluid for laboratory examination and diagnosis. Biopsy is most often used to differentiate between cancerous and non-cancerous tissue.

GLOSSARY

Blocker's Disease—An overgrowth of bone in the middle third of the arm (approximately where the deltoid muscle attaches to the humerus). It is caused by repeated injury at that site. This overgrowth may be termed an *exostosis* or *myositis ossificans* if the bony part infiltrates a muscle.

Bronchi (Bronchial tubes)—Hollow air passages that branch from the largest segment (the windpipe or trachea) into the lungs. Oxygen-containing air passes into the lungs through the bronchial tubes, and waste gases (mostly carbon dioxide) pass out of the lungs.

Bronchioles—Tiny air passages (too small to be seen except through a microscope) that serve the same purpose as the bronchi.

Bronchoscopy—A surgical procedure using a bronchoscope, an instrument with lenses and lights that is inserted through the throat, vocal cords and into the bronchial tubes. After administering anesthesia, a surgeon passes the bronchoscope into the trachea and the largest branching segments of the bronchi. Foreign bodies that may have been inhaled accidentally can be removed. In addition, fluid may be removed or tissue may be biopsied and examined to detect tumors or infections.

Buerger's Disease (Thromboangiitis Obliterans)—A serious disease of unknown cause that leads to blockage of the small and medium arteries—usually in the legs and feet. Smoking, exposure to cold, or any form of physical or emotional stress are important factors that make Buerger's disease more likely to occur.

C

Calcium Deposit—Abnormal hardening of soft tissue, usually from repeated injury.

Capillaries—The smallest (microscopic) blood vessels in the body. Capillaries form a network throughout the body through which substances can be exchanged between cells and the circulating blood. The exchanged substances include fluid, nourishment, waste material, electrolytes, oxygen and carbon dioxide.

Carbohydrates, Complex—Starches and fiber found in food (mostly whole grains, fresh fruits and vegetables). Carbohydrates are essential for human nutrition, and complex carbohydrates are healthier than simple carbohydrates (sugars).

Carbohydrates, Simple—Sugars found in foods. Many high-carbohydrate foods are refined and depleted of their fiber and starch. Simple sugars are not as nutritious to human bodies as complex carbohydrates. "Junk foods" are frequently very high in simple carbohydrates. They cause a quick rise in blood sugar, followed by a sudden drop in blood sugar.

Carbonic Anhydrase Inhibitors—A class or family of drugs that inhibits the action of carbonic anhydrase, an enzyme. These medicines force the kidney to excrete increased amounts of sodium and water, reducing excess body fluid.

Cardiovascular—Relating to the heart and blood vessels.

Cartilage—Rubbery, fibrous, dense connective tissue—harder than ligaments, softer than bone. Cartilage usually is found between bones and permits smooth movement of joints. It also helps shape flexible parts of the nose and external ear. The most frequent and significant cartilage injury associated with athletics is damage to the crescent-shaped cartilage in the knee (meniscus).

Cast—A stiff dressing or casing made of dressings impregnated with plaster of Paris or other hardening material such as plastic. Casts are used to immobilize various parts of the body in cases of fractures, dislocations, and moderate or severe sprains.

CT Scan (Computerized Axial Tomography)—Previously called CAT scan. A computerized X-ray procedure that provides exceptionally clear images of parts of the body. CT scans aid in the diagnosis of disorders that may not be diagnosed by less sophisticated X-ray studies. They require costly, specialized equipment.

Caudad—Directed toward the tail. Caudad is opposite of *cephalad*.

Cephalad—Directed toward the head; opposite of *caudad*.

Cauterization—A surgical procedure to destroy tissue using a hot instrument, an electric current or a chemical substance.

Cerebrospinal Fluid—Fluid that bathes the brain and the spinal cord.

Chondral—Pertaining to cartilage.

Chronic—The opposite of acute. Chronic means prolonged or slow to heal.

Circulatory System—The system that provides blood to the body. Parts of the system include the heart, arteries, arterioles, capillaries, venules, veins, blood, plasma, and lymphatic vessels and fluid.

Circumduction Exercises—Active or passive circular exercise movements of any part of the body.

Colicky—Intermittent or fluctuating pain. Colicky pain usually refers to abdominal pain caused by spasms of the urinary tract or intestinal tract. Pain corresponds to strong contractions of surrounding involuntary muscles.

Collagen—A protein chemical substance that is the main support of skin, tendon, bone, cartilage and connective tissue.

Congestive Heart Failure—A complication of many serious diseases in which the heart loses its full pumping capacity. Blood backs up into other organs, especially the lungs, producing shortness of breath. Blood also backs up into the liver, causing production of fluid that distends the abdomen or accumulates in the feet, ankles and legs.

Connective Tissue—The body's supporting framework of tissue consisting of strands of collagen, elastic fibers between muscles and around muscle groups and blood vessels, and simple cells.

Contracture—Shortening or distortion of a tissue, usually a muscle. Contractures may be temporary, or permanent if caused by scar tissue.

Contusion—A bruising injury that does not break the skin. The brain can also be contused through the skull, usually leading to temporary unconsciousness.

COPD (Chronic Obstructive Pulmonary Disease)—A disease that results from any of several lung diseases—usually incurable—that lead to increasing breathing difficulty. The chronic diseases that lead to COPD include emphysema, asthma, chronic bronchitis, tuberculosis, fungus infections of the lung and bronchiectasis.

Corticosteroids—Synthetic medications similar in structure and function to natural hormones produced by the core of the adrenal glands. Cortisone, hydrocortisone, dexamethasone and others belong to the family of corticosteroid drugs.

Costochondral—*Costo* means rib. *Chondral* means cartilage. Costochondral is the rib and its attached cartilage.

Cottonmouth—Dry mouth from dehydration or anxiety. People with "cottonmouth" spit whitish sputum that looks like cotton.

Crepitation—The sensation that small balloons or pockets of air beneath the skin are breaking when the skin is pressed with fingers. Crepitation also means the grating feeling produced when two joint surfaces rub against each other.

Cryokinetics—The use of cold for physical therapy.

Cryosurgery—A simple surgical procedure in which tissue is destroyed by below-freezing temperatures. Liquid nitrogen is frequently used as the freezing chemical agent in cryosurgery.

Culture—The growth of microscopic organisms (viruses, bacteria or fungi) or cells in a special environment that supports them so they can be examined.

Cutaneous—Relating to the skin.

Cystoscopy—Examination of the inside of the lower urinary tract using a cystoscope. A cystoscope has a special system of lenses and lights. It is passed from the urethra into the bladder. The cystoscope is used for examination of the bladder and ureters, some surgical procedures on the prostate gland, and biopsies of tissue inside the bladder.

GLOSSARY

D

Delirium—A brief, reversible mental disturbance characterized by delusions, hallucinations, emotional excitement, physical restlessness and incoherence. Delirium can be caused by infections, head injury, decreased blood supply to the brain, medications and psychotic disorders.

Diathermy—Heating deep within body tissues that is done with a special machine. Tissues can be heated without damaging the skin. Diathermy was once popular in physical therapy, but other treatments are now more common.

Displacement—Removal from the normal position or place.

Distal—Distant from a midline or other point of reference. The opposite of distal is proximal.

Diuretics—A class or family of drugs used to force the kidney to excrete more sodium than usual. Increased sodium excretion causes increased water excretion, so urine volume increases. The increased sodium excretion is desirable and therapeutic in disorders causing abnormal fluid retention (edema) due to heart failure, liver failure or kidney failure. Unfortunately, some diuretics increase excretion of potassium, which must be replaced—usually with potassium supplements—to avoid serious adverse effects.

Dorsiflexion—Backward bending, especially of the hand or foot.

E

Ear, Nose & Throat (E.N.T.) Specialist—A physician with special post-graduate training in diagnosing and treating disorders and diseases of the ear, nose and throat.

Ecchymosis—A small area of bleeding under the skin or mucous membrane forming a non-elevated, rounded or irregular blue or purplish patch.

Edema—Accumulation of abnormal quantities of fluid in spaces between the cells of the body. Edema can accumulate in almost any location in the body. Most common sites include the feet and ankles, skin, abdomen, liver and brain.

EEG (Electroencephalogram)—A recording of electrical activity in the brain. An EEG is done with a galvanometer connected to electrodes attached to the skull. The EEG is useful in detecting brain damage and in diagnosing seizure and sleep disorders.

EKG (Electrocardiogram)—A graphic representation of the electrical current generated by the electrical system that controls heart-muscle cells. The EKG is a useful tool in diagnosing the presence and severity of many forms of heart disease. However, the heart may be severely impaired, and still show no typical or characteristic EKG changes, so the EKG is only one of the tools used to detect and monitor heart disorders.

Electrolytes—Chemicals dissolved in the blood and inside body cells. Electrolytes play an essential role in all body functions and must be maintained within narrow limits to preserve health. The major electrolytes include sodium, potassium, chloride, calcium, phosphorous, magnesium and carbon dioxide. They are ingested through food. The kidneys and lungs regulate the rate at which they are excreted. Levels that are too high or too low in body cells can lead to serious illnesses, including heart-rhythm disturbances, fluid accumulation, dehydration and dangerously low blood pressure. In the worst cases, electrolyte disturbances can be life-threatening.

Electromyogram—A recording of the electrical activity of nerve and muscle cells, measured with an extremely sensitive galvanometer. The electromyogram is used to help detect and diagnose a variety of disorders of peripheral nerves and muscles.

Erythema—Redness and warmth of the skin caused by congestion of the capillaries. Erythema may be caused by many factors, including infection, sunburn, inflammation or direct injury.

Erythema multiforme—A disease characterized by a vivid red skin eruption that appears suddenly on the face, neck, forearms, legs, feet and hands. This disorder results from hypersensitivity to some drugs and also sometimes appears spontaneously—probably as a result of a defect in the immune system.

Etiology—The cause of a disease or injury.

Eversion—To turn outward.

F

Fibrosis—The formation of fibrous tissue. Fibrosis is caused by many factors including injury, inflammation and infection.

Fibrositis—An inflammatory condition affecting connective tissue and muscles, joints, ligaments and tendons. Fibrositis has many causes, including repeated injury, infections or overuse of a part. The disease usually resolves itself without treatment, but recurrence is frequent.

Flank—The area of the body that extends from the bottom of the ribs to the upper edge of the hip on either side of the body.

Flatulence—Intestinal gaseousness caused by failure of the intestines to completely process some complex carbohydrates, such as those found in beans, onions and bran. Exercise may increase flatulence because it hastens the passage of food through the intestinal tract, sometimes not allowing enough time for complete digestion.

Fracture—A break in a bone, cartilage, tooth or other rigid body tissue.

Fungus—A microorganism that causes infection of the skin, mucous membranes of the mouth, vagina or rectum, or other organs (particularly the lungs).

"Funny Bone" ("Crazy Bone")—The ulnar nerve in the groove on the inner side of the elbow joint. When injured, it produces a disabling, temporary burning and numbness along the inner side of the forearm and hand.

G

Gastrointestinal (GI) Tract—The digestive tract, beginning with the mouth, continuing through the esophagus, stomach, duodenum, small intestine, large intestine, and ending in the rectum. The GI tract is about 26 feet long.

H

Heartburn—A burning sensation in the chest perceived as arising from the region of the heart. Heartburn is not related to heart disease. It is caused by stomach acid or stomach contents that spill into the lower esophagus, irritating the sensitive lining membrane.

Hemarthrosis—Collection of blood in a joint from broken capillaries or larger blood vessels.

Hematocrit—A blood test to detect anemia and other blood disorders. The test shows what percentage of whole blood is occupied by red blood cells. Normal hematocrit range is 35% to 45%. The remainder of the blood is made up of white blood cells, platelets, serum, plasma and electrolytes. Hematocrit range varies with age and sex.

Hematoma—A dome-shaped collection of blood—usually clotted—under the skin, the scalp or inside the abdomen. The hematoma is formed by bleeding from a broken blood vessel.

Hemoglobin—A chemical component of red blood cells that carries oxygen from air breathed in to all cells in the body. The blood test for hemoglobin is used to detect anemia and other blood disorders. Normal hemoglobin range is 12 to 18 grams per 100 cubic centimeters.

Hernia—Protrusion of an organ or tissue through an abnormal opening.

Hip Pointer—A bruise or contusion of the top part of the ilium, one of the bones of the pelvis.

Hyaluronidase—An enzyme that neutralizes adverse effects of hyaluronic acid, the cement substance of tissues.

Hyper—A prefix meaning above, beyond or excessive. For examples, *hyperextended* means bent beyond normal limits. *Hyperventilation* means excessive breathing.

Hypo—A prefix meaning below or deficient. For examples, *hypogastric* means below the stomach. *Hypoglycemia* means too little sugar in the blood.

I

Id Reaction—A rash associated with, but located remotely from, the main lesions of a disease. The cause is probably an allergic or hypersensitive reaction to the germ causing the original disease. A common example is an itchy rash with blisters that appears on the hands and forearms of people who have athlete's foot.

Iliotibial Band Syndrome—Pain in the knee region (common in runners). Pain is caused by injury to the iliotibial tract—a fibrous band that forms a ligament that helps support and stabilize the knee. Treatment consists of rest, physical therapy, rehabilitation, and occasionally surgery.

Incision—A cut made with a sharp instrument through the skin or other tissue.

Insulin—A hormone manufactured in the pancreas that facilitates the metabolism of glucose (sugar) by the body's cells. A deficiency in the production of insulin results in the disease *diabetes mellitus* (sugar diabetes).

Intravenous—Inside a vein. Medications, electrolyte solutions (such as saline or potassium) and blood transfusions are given intravenously through a needle inserted into a vein.

Inversion—To turn inward.

Ipsilateral—The same side of the body.

J

Joint Capsule—The thin, cartilagenous, fatty, fibrous, membranous structure that envelops a joint. Fluid inside the joint capsule lubricates the area, allowing bones to glide smoothly against each other.

K

Knee, Internal Derangement—Injury to any of the internal structures of the knee joint, including the meniscus (articular cartilage), ligaments, tendons, fat pad under the patella (kneecap), and the uppermost part of the tibia (the major bone in the lower leg).

L

Laryngoscope—An instrument used to inspect and treat the muscular structures in the larynx and vocal cords.

Lateral—Toward the outside or away from a midline.

Lesion—A wound, injury or abnormal skin growth.

Ligament—A band of fibrous tissue that connects bone to bone or cartilage to bone, supporting and strengthening a joint.

Lupus Erythematosus—An inflammatory disease of connective tissues believed to be caused by a defect in the body's immune system, in which the body attacks its own normal tissues.

Luxation—Bones in a joint that are no longer in the correct functional position to each other. Means the same as dislocation. *Subluxation* means a less definable dislocation. With subluxation, there is only partial deformity, and it is usually associated with an injury to attached ligaments.

M

Massage—Therapeutic kneading and stroking of skin and muscles.

Medial—Toward the midline or closest to a midline than any other structure. For example, the breastbone (sternum) is medial to the right rib cage.

Mind-Altering Drugs—Any drug or medication that interferes with normal function of the brain. The group includes: narcotics such as heroin, morphine, Demerol and codeine; major tranquilizers; hallucinogenic agents such as LSD; marijuana; cocaine; amphetamines; and barbiturates and other sedatives.

Moleskin—A heavy, downy cotton-twill material used to wrap around joints for support or to protect the skin under bandages, splints or casts. It is also used to reduce friction over tender skin.

MRI (Magnetic Resonance Imaging)—Special radiological study that allows visualization of scarred or damaged areas of the brain. MRI is useful in diagnosing epilepsy and other disorders of the brain and central nervous system.

Muscle—An organ that produces movement by contractions. There are two major kinds of muscles: voluntary (striated) and involuntary (non-striated). Striated muscles are under voluntary control and include most of the muscles in the body. Involuntary muscle cells form the largest mass of the heart, and surround blood vessels, lymphatic vessels, the urinary tract and the intestinal tract.

N

Necrosis—Death. Tissue death (necrosis) results from deprivation of blood supply.

Neuritis—Any inflammatory condition of a nerve. Neuritis may have many causes, including injury. Treatment is difficult and recurrence frequent.

O

Ophthalmologist—A medical doctor who specializes in medical or surgical disorders of the eye.

Oral Surgeon—A dentist who specializes in tooth extractions and surgery on the gums and other structures in the mouth.

Osteomalacia—A condition characterized by softening of the bones. Symptoms include pain, tenderness, muscle weakness and weight loss. The cause is a deficiency in vitamin D and calcium.

Osteomyelitis—Infection of the bone and bone marrow, frequently associated with open (compound) fractures of bones. The broken skin accompanying such fractures allows bacteria to enter the injured area and infect injured tissue. Bone has relatively poor resistance to infection because of its sparse blood supply.

Overtraining Syndrome—A group of symptoms caused by overwork of muscles and other tissues during vigorous athletic activity. The outstanding symptom is pain in muscles, bones or joints. First symptoms include dull aching of the joints after a hard workout. If training continues at the same level of intensity, pain will occur during and after workouts. The only successful treatment is to decrease the level of activity until symptoms disappear. Training can then resume as long as symptoms don't reappear.

P

Pain—A sensation of discomfort, hurt, stress or agony, resulting from stimulation of specialized nerve endings. Pain means something is wrong, and should not be ignored. The saying of "no pain, no gain" is outmoded.

Periodic Paralysis—A rare disease characterized by a rapidly progressive form of paralysis associated with abnormal serum potassium levels. This is an inherited disease. Attacks may be triggered by vigorous exercise. They are more likely to occur on the day following a workout rather than during the workout.

PET (Positron Emission Tomography)—An expensive, sophisticated radiological procedure that allows visualization of various parts of the body not observable by more traditional X-ray studies.

Plantar Flexion—Bending or pointing the toe toward the floor.

Plantar Fasciitis—A partial or complete tear in the fascia (fibrous connective tissue) of the bottom of the foot. It is characterized by pain just under the heel bone. Causes include: inadequate arch supports; poorly-fitting shoes or shoes with soles that are too stiff; sudden turns or stops; and weak ankles. Rest is the only successful treatment.

Plastic Surgeon—A medical doctor who specializes in surgery concerned with the restoration, reconstruction, correction, or improvement in the shape and appearance of body structures that are defective or misshapen by injury, disease, or growth and development.

Platelets—Blood cells (smaller than red or white blood cells) that assist in the blood-clotting process.

Podiatrist—A doctor who specializes in the diagnosis and treatment of medical and surgical problems of the feet.

Polycythemia—An abnormal increase in the red blood cells of the body. The disease has 3 forms: (1) Polycythemia vera, which involves overproduction of red blood cells, white blood cells and platelets. (2) Secondary polycythemia, a complication of diseases or factors other than blood-cell disorders. (3) Stress polycythemia, which is associated with decreased blood plasma. Stress polycythemia can occur in athletes who become dehydrated during competition or heavy workouts in very hot weather. Secondary polycythemia and stress polycythemia are curable by correcting the underlying cause.

GLOSSARY

Popliteal Space—The space behind the knee joint. The space is bounded by ligaments and contains soft tissue including nerves, fat, membranes and blood vessels.

Porphyria—A serious inherited disease of metabolism characterized by excretion of porphyrins. Attacks can be triggered by pregnancy, excessive exposure to sunlight, and use of barbiturates or birth-control pills.

Posterior—The rear part.

Postural Drainage—A physical therapy procedure for chronic lung disease such as bronchiectasis or lung abscess. The patient is placed so that the involved part of the lung is higher than the trachea and the head. Forced coughing in this position helps clear the lungs and bronchial tubes of harmful accumulated secretions.

Progressive Resistance Exercise (P.R.E.)—Exercise that forces muscles into bearing heavier and heavier loads.

Prognosis—Prediction of the course of an injury or disease, including its end result.

Pronation—Rotation of a body part (usually the hand or foot) backward, inward or downward. Muscles in the forearm can produce pronation of the hand; muscles in the lower leg can produce pronation of the foot.

Proteinuria—Passing protein in the urine. This is sometimes associated with kidney disease, but it may occur normally following many forms of strenuous exercise such as rowing, football, track, long-distance running, swimming and calisthenics. There is no evidence that exercise-induced proteinuria increases the risk for developing chronic kidney disease.

Proximal—Nearest to a point of reference. The opposite of proximal is distal.

Pulmonary—Pertaining to all parts of the lung.

Pyelogram—A special X-ray study of the urinary tract in which dye is injected into a vein, and X-rays are done repeatedly to follow the dye's progress through the urinary tract.

R

Radioactive Technetium Study—Special X-rays following injection of radioactive technetium. These studies can outline various parts of the body that are normally inaccessible to X-ray examination.

Radioactive Uptake Studies—Special X-ray studies showing concentration of injected radioactive materials in various tissues and organs of the body.

Retina—One of the three major segments of the eye. The retina is located in the back of the eyeball, and it has many layers. The layers of the retina contain blood vessels, nerve endings, and the specialized rods and cones that make it possible for us to distinguish shapes and colors.

Rotator Cuff—A structure around the shoulder-joint capsule composed of intermingled muscle and tendon fibers. The rotator cuff provides stability and strength to the shoulder joint.

Rupture—Forcible tearing or disruption of a tissue.

S

Secondary Infection—An infection that follows and sometimes complicates a primary infection. Secondary infections are usually caused by a different germ than the one that caused the first infection. For example, a secondary bacterial skin infection on the feet can occur over a pre-existing fungus infection on the feet.

Sedatives—Drugs to lessen anxiety or excitement. Most effective sedatives are habit-forming.

Soft Tissue—All tissue of the body except bone.

Sonogram—A diagnostic test in which high-frequency sound waves are transmitted into the body. Their reflections or echoes create images of body organs or the outline of a fetus.

Spearing—An aggressive move in which a person butts his or her helmeted head into the chest or midsection of an opponent. This is a hazardous maneuver that may cause neck injury to the aggressor, and severe direct injury to the opponent.

Spineboard—An inflexible board (also called backboard) made of wood or plastic that immobilizes the spine while an injured person is transported to an emergency facility.

Splint—A rigid support made from metal, plaster or plastic and used to immobilize an injured or inflamed part of the body.

Spondylolysis—A congenital defect in which a small area of bone in the spine does not fuse completely. This causes weakness in the spine and makes it subject to more frequent and more serious injury. People with spondylolysis should probably not engage in heavy lifting or in contact sports.

Spondylolisthesis—Spondylolysis with displacement of one of the vertebral bones forward of the one below.

Stitch in Side—Pain, usually in the upper abdomen, accompanying vigorous physical activity. This is probably caused by spasm of the diaphragm, the big muscle that separates the chest from the abdomen and that moves with breathing. Treatment is to stop exercise until the pain disappears.

Subacute—An intermediate stage in the progress of an injury or disease that is between acute and chronic, closer in nature to the acute stage than the chronic.

Subcutaneous—Below the skin.

Supination—Rotating a hand or foot outward on its long axis. The movement is done with the muscles in the forearm or lower leg.

Syncope—Fainting—a mild form of shock with a short period of unconsciousness and usually a rapid recovery.

Synovium—A thin layer of connective tissue with a free smooth surface that lines the capsule of a joint. Synovial fluid lubricates and facilitates movements of the joint.

T

Tenderness—Discomfort produced when any injured area is touched or pressed.

Tendon—A fibrous cord by which a muscle is attached to a bone.

Tinnitus—Ringing in the ears, caused by disorder of the eighth cranial nerve. Disorders can occur from virus infections, occasionally by blood clots to the brain, and commonly by taking medications such as aspirin.

Traction—A form of physical therapy in which a pulling force is exerted on a muscle or joint.

Tranquilizers—A class or family of drugs used to lessen anxiety or nervousness. Most major tranquilizers are habit-forming.

Trauma—A direct wound or injury.

Triad, Unhappy—A classic football injury that results from being hit on the lateral side of the knee with the foot on the ground. The blow causes sprains of the medial collateral ligament and the anterior cruciate ligament, and tears the meniscus (knee cartilage). This injury usually requires surgery to repair.

U

Ultrasound—A form of physical therapy in which deep heat is applied to an injured area using sound waves that are outside the normal range of human hearing. Ultrasound treatments require special equipment and professional supervision.

V

Vesicle—A fluid-containing, blisterlike skin eruption. For example, the lesions of chickenpox are vesicles.

Vitiligo—A loss of pigment in scattered areas of the skin.

W

Whiplash—A non-medical popular term meaning an injury to the neck caused by hyperextension and/or hyperflexion.

Whirlpool—Equipment that provides turbulent water used to treat many athletic injuries.

X

X-rays—Diagnostic procedures to study internal structures not visible to the naked eye.

Y

Yeast—A general term applied to single-budding microscopic fungus cells. Yeast infections can occur on the skin, mucous membranes, and organs of the body such as the lung.

INDEX

INDEX

EMERGENCY FIRST AID

ANAPHYLAXIS (Severe Allergic Reaction)

Symptoms

Itching, rash, hives, runny nose, wheezing, paleness, cold sweats, low blood pressure, coma, cardiac arrest.

Treatment

If Victim is Unconscious, Not Breathing:
1. Yell for help. Don't leave the victim.
2. Begin mouth-to-mouth breathing immediately.
3. If there is no heartbeat, give external cardiac massage.
4. Have someone call 0 (Operator) or 911 (emergency) for an ambulance or medical help.
5. Don't stop cardiopulmonary resuscitation (CPR) until help arrives.

If Victim is Unconscious and Breathing:
1. Dial 0 (Operator) or 911 (emergency) for an ambulance or emergency medical help.
2. If you can't get help immediately, take patient to nearest emergency facility.

BLEEDING

Symptoms

Bright-red blood pumping from an injured artery, or darker blood if a large vein has been injured. Bleeding caused by any serious injury should be treated in an emergency facility.

Treatment

Call for ambulance or take victim to emergency facility. In the meantime, render the following first aid:
1. Cover entire injured area with a cloth, or bare hands if no cloth is available.
2. Apply strong pressure directly on injured area for 10 minutes while awaiting ambulance or while transporting victim to emergency facility.
3. If direct pressure doesn't control brisk bleeding, use a tourniquet. Make a tourniquet from a length of cloth or similar material. Wrap and tie the tourniquet around the extremity above the wound. Place a stick or other rigid object between the cloth and the extremity. Twist the rigid object several times until tight pressure has been applied and bleeding stops. Note how long the tourniquet is in place so emergency medical personnel can take appropriate action.

CONVULSIONS

Symptoms

Unconsciousness; jerking or twitching of the arms, legs or face; loss of bowel or bladder control (sometimes).

Treatment

1. When the victim begins to fall, soften the fall by catching his body, laying it down gently and turning the head to one side.
2. Don't restrain the person. Clear the area of any objects so the victim won't be injured.
3. Don't try to separate the teeth or insert objects to keep the patient from biting his tongue. Doing so can cause injury.
4. Don't throw ice water on the patient.
5. Don't attempt to force water or any fluid until the patient is fully conscious and asks for fluids.
6. Call for medical help and stay with any patient who has a convulsion immediately after the first convulsion. Stay also with any pregnant woman who has a convulsion.

FRACTURES, DISLOCATIONS OR SEVERE SPRAINS

Symptoms

Extreme pain and tenderness in the injured area; change in appearance of injured part, such as swelling, protruding bone or blood under skin. Extremity, such as finger, arm or leg, may be bent out of normal alignment.

Treatment

1. Control any bleeding (see page 525).
2. Immobilize the injured area and keep movement to a minimum. To do so for obvious fractures of the finger, wrist, arm, leg, ankle or foot, improvise a splint from stiff rolled-up paper, scrap wood or metal.
3. Attach the splint firmly to injured extremity with strips of cloth, twine or similar material.
4. Prevent swelling by applying ice and elevating the splinted part, compressing it with a snug elastic bandage whenever possible.
5. If leg, back or neck is severely injured and possibly fractured or dislocated, keep patient warm and immobilized until the ambulance arrives. Don't move the victim.
6. Watch for signs of shock (see page 528).

HEAD, NECK OR BACK INJURY

Symptoms

Head injury: Drowsiness or confusion; vomiting and nausea; blurred vision; pupils of different size; loss of consciousness—either temporarily or for long periods; amnesia or memory lapses; irritability; headache; bleeding of the scalp, if the skin is broken.

Neck or back injury: Pain in the neck or back; paralysis or difficulty in moving.

Treatment

1. Assume that all injuries to the head (including face), neck or back—whether the patient is conscious or unconscious—may also involve damage to the spinal cord.
2. Call 0 (Operator) or 911 (emergency) for an ambulance or medical help.
3. Avoid moving the patient, if at all possible.
4. If the injured person is unconscious and lying face-down so he or she cannot breathe, obtain assistance from several people to carefully support and roll the entire body to one side.
5. Give mouth-to-mouth breathing if the victim is not breathing but has a heartbeat.
6. If there is no heartbeat, give external cardiac massage.
7. Don't stop cardiopulmonary resuscitation (CPR) until help arrives.
8. If an ambulance is not available, take the patient to the nearest emergency center. Make sure that the neck and back are carefully supported and moved as little as possible.

HEART ATTACK

Symptoms

Chest pain that lasts more than 2 minutes and radiates into the jaw or arm; unexplained heavy sweating; weakness; nausea; pale skin; irregular pulse.

Treatment

If Victim is Unconscious, Not Breathing:
1. Yell for help. Don't leave the victim.
2. Begin mouth-to-mouth breathing immediately.
3. If there is no heartbeat, give external cardiac massage.
4. Have someone call 0 (Operator) or 911 (emergency) for an ambulance or medical help.
5. Don't stop cardiopulmonary resuscitation (CPR) until help arrives.

If Victim is Unconscious and Breathing:
1. Dial 0 (Operator) or 911 (emergency) for an ambulance or emergency medical help.
2. If you can't get help immediately, take patient to nearest emergency facility.

SHOCK

Symptoms

Moist, cold, pale skin; fast weak pulse; rapid breathing; disorientation; anxiety with feelings of impending doom; low blood pressure (sometimes so low that it cannot be read); unconsciousness (sometimes).

Treatment

- Keep patient warm with a blanket or other covering.
- Stop any external bleeding by applying pressure.
- Keep the patient lying down with the legs elevated.

If Victim is Unconscious, Not Breathing:

1. Yell for help. Don't leave the victim.
2. Begin mouth-to-mouth breathing immediately.
3. If there is no heartbeat, give external cardiac massage.
4. Have someone call 0 (Operator) or 911 (emergency) for an ambulance or medical help.
5. Don't stop cardiopulmonary resuscitation (CPR) until help arrives.

If Victim is Unconscious and Breathing:

1. Dial 0 (Operator) or 911 (emergency) for an ambulance or emergency medical help.
2. If you can't get help immediately, take patient to nearest emergency facility.

Conversion to Metric Measure

When You Know	Symbol	Multiply By	To Find	Symbol
VOLUME				
teaspoons	tsp.	4.93	milliliters	ml
tablespoons	tbsp.	14.79	milliliters	ml
fluid ounces	fl. oz.	29.57	milliliters	ml
cups	c.	0.24	liters	l
pints	pt.	0.47	liters	l
quarts	qt.	0.95	liters	l
gallons	gal.	3.79	liters	l
LENGTH				
inches	in.	25.4	millimeters	mm
inches	in.	2.54	centimeters	cm
feet	ft.	30.48	centimeters	cm
yards	yd.	0.91	meters	m
TEMPERATURE				
Fahrenheit	F	0.56 (after subtracting 32)	Celsius	C